Pharmacotherapy of Depression

Second Edition

Domenic A. Ciraulo • Richard Irwin Shader
Editors

Pharmacotherapy of Depression

Second Edition

Humana Press

Editors
Domenic A. Ciraulo
Boston University School of Medicine
Boston, MA
USA

Richard Irwin Shader
Tufts University School of Medicine
Boston, MA
USA

ISBN 978-1-60327-434-0 e-ISBN 978-1-60327-435-7
DOI 10.1007/978-1-60327-435-7
Springer New York Dordrecht Heidelberg London

Printed on acid-free paper

Humana Press is part of Springer Science+Business Media (www.springer.com)

Preface

The first edition of the *Pharmacotherapy of Depression* was published in 2004 and the editors wish to express appreciation for the positive reviews of that book. The second edition is similar in organization to the first, but has undergone major revisions of every chapter, the addition of new chapters, and expansion of our expert contributors. We have tried to provide sufficient depth in our reviews of the research literature to support our clinical recommendations without burdening the reader with information that is not of clinical importance for the prescriber.

The first chapter reviews the neurobiology of depression, which lays the groundwork for understanding the mechanisms of action of antidepressants. In the next chapter, we review the general principles guiding the diagnosis and medication treatment of unipolar depression. The clinical pharmacology of antidepressants is reviewed in some detail, supplemented by tables that provide information on dosing, indications, and metabolism. Augmentation strategies are reviewed, including the use of nontraditional agents. The chapters that follow address the use of antidepressants in special populations, such as the elderly and depressed individuals with psychosis, bipolar disorder, substance abuse, and posttraumatic stress disorder. The complex issues involving the diagnosis and treatment of depression during pregnancy are thoroughly reviewed in Chap. 8 and provide a synthesis of the scientific literature in the area, one that is noted for contradictory and controversial findings, and guidelines for prescribing. The following chapter provides an overview of the treatment of depression in the pediatric population, highlighting clinical concerns such as suicide risk. The book concludes with two chapters at the interface of medicine and psychiatry in the treatment of mood disorders: managing depression in primary care settings and depression associated with medical illnesses.

We are indebted to the outstanding clinician scientists who have contributed to this volume. They all are leaders in their fields and represent a broad spectrum of institutions, including current and former NIMH senior scientists, Harvard Medical School, Boston University School of Medicine, Tufts University School of Medicine, and Indiana University School of Medicine. The skill sets of the contributors include bench to bedside talents that have produced a strong scientific foundation that seamlessly transitions into recommendations for clinical practice. The book is based on our courses and lectures on the clinical psychopharmacology of depression that we have developed for practicing physicians, residents in psychiatry, neurology, and medicine, as well as psychologists, medical students, social workers, nurses, mental health counselors, and graduate students. We are grateful for the feedback of our colleagues, trainees, and students, who have been essential in modifications of the content of this edition.

The editors wish to thank Ms. Michele Procida for her ability to motivate us to complete this project. She was able to keep us directed, energized, and enthusiastic at times when progress stalled. She also tolerated late night emails and last minute manuscript changes with grace. We would also like to thank Ann Marie Ciraulo RN for her critical review of the content of the chapters, review of relevant literature, and helpful suggestions for modifications.

We sincerely hope that the reader will find this book a helpful guide to treating depression.

Boston, MA Domenic A. Ciraulo
Boston, MA Richard Irwin Shader

Contents

Biological Theories of Depression and Implications for Current and New Treatments 1
David J. Goldstein, William Z. Potter, Domenic A. Ciraulo, and Richard I. Shader

Clinical Pharmacology and Therapeutics of Antidepressants 33
Domenic A. Ciraulo, Richard I. Shader, and David J. Greenblatt

Antidepressant Treatment of Geriatric Depression 125
Domenic A. Ciraulo, James A. Evans, Wei Qiao Qiu, Richard I. Shader, and Carl Salzman

Treatment of Psychotic Disorders 185
Oliver Freudenreich and Donald C. Goff

Treatment of Bipolar Depression 197
Robert M. Post

Substance Abuse and Depression 239
John A. Renner, Jeffrey Baxter, Joji Suzuki, and Domenic A. Ciraulo

Antidepressant Treatments in PTSD 275
Janet E. Osterman, Brandon Z. Erdos, Mark Oldham, and Ana Ivkovic

Diagnosis and Treatment of Depression During Pregnancy and Lactation 309
Daniel Shaw

Antidepressant Treatment of Pediatric Depression 355
Ricardo M. Vela, Carol A. Glod, Timothy M. Rivinus, and Rebecca Johnson

Managing Depression in Primary Care 375
Larry Culpepper and Peggy Johnson

Treatment of Depression in the Medically Ill 399
Wei Jiang and K. Ranga Rama Krishnan

Index 415

Contributors

Jeffrey Baxter, MD
Department of Family Medicine, University of Massachusetts Medical School, Worcester, MA, USA

Domenic A. Ciraulo, MD
Department of Psychiatry, Boston University School of Medicine, 720 Harrison Avenue, Suite 914, Boston, MA, USA

Larry Culpepper, MD
Department of Family Medicine, Boston University School of Medicine, Boston, MA, USA

Brandon Z. Erdos, MD
Department of Psychiatry, Boston University School of Medicine, Boston, MA, USA

James A. Evans, MD
Department of Psychiatry, Harvard University School of Medicine, Boston, MA, USA

Oliver Freudenreich, MD
Schizophrenia Program, Massachusetts General Hospital, Freedom Trail Clinic, Boston, MA, USA

Carol A. Glod, PhD, APRN
Bouvé College of Health Sciences, Northeastern University, Boston, MA, USA

Donald C. Goff, MD
Schizophrenia Program, Massachusetts General Hospital, Freedom Trail Clinic, Boston, MA, USA

David J. Goldstein, MD, PhD
Department of Toxicology and Pharmacology, Indiana University School of Medicine, and PRN Consulting, Indianapolis IN, USA

David J. Greenblatt, MD
Department of Pharmacology and Experimental Therapeutics,
Tufts University School of Medicine,
Boston, MA, USA

Ana Ivkovic
Department of Psychiatry, Boston University School of Medicine,
Boston, MA, USA

Wei Jiang, MD
Department of Psychiatry and Behavioral Science, Duke University,
Durham NC, USA

Peggy Johnson, MD
Department of Psychiatry, Boston University School of Medicine,
Boston, MA, USA

Rebecca Johnson, MD
Department of Psychiatry, Boston University School of Medicine,
Boston, MA, USA

K. Ranga Rama Krishnan, MD
Department of Psychiatry and Behavioral Sciences,
Duke University, Durham, NC, USA

Mark Oldham
Department of Psychiatry, Boston University School of Medicine,
Boston, MA, USA

Janet E. Osterman, MD
Department of Psychiatry, Boston University School of Medicine,
Boston, MA, USA

Robert M. Post, MD
Bipolar Collabarative Network, Bethesda, MD, USA

William Z. Potter MD, PhD
Vice President, Transitional Neuroscience (retired), Merck Industry,
Philadelphia, PA 19118, USA

Wei Qiao Qiu, MD
Department of Psychiatry and Pharmacology and Experimental Therapeutics,
Boston University School of Medicine,
Boston, MA, USA

John A. Renner MD
Department of Veterans Affairs, Boston University School of Medicine,
Boston, MA, USA

Timothy M. Rivinus, MD
Department of Psychiatry and Human Behavior, Brown University,
Providence, RI, USA

Carl Salzman, MD
Department of Psychiatry, Harvard University School of Medicine,
Boston, MA, USA

Richard I. Shader, MD
Department of Psychiatry and Pharmacology and Experimental Therapeutics,
Tufts University School of Medicine,
Boston, MA, USA

Daniel Shaw, MD
Department of Psychiatry, Boston University School of Medicine,
Boston, MA, USA

Joji Suzuki, MD
Department of Psychiatry, Harvard Medical School, Boston, MA, USA

Ricardo M. Vela, MD
Department of Child and Family Services, Harvard Medical School,
Boston, MA, USA

Biological Theories of Depression and Implications for Current and New Treatments

David J. Goldstein, William Z. Potter, Domenic A. Ciraulo, and Richard I. Shader

Introduction

Unipolar major depressive disorder is a common condition that has both emotional (mood and anxiety) and physical aspects (1). The physical manifestations are common features of depression present in up to 80% of depressed patients (2). These physical symptoms occur in nearly all body systems and are often the presenting features in the nonpsychiatric setting. The most common physical symptoms are sleep disruption, fatigue, pain and discomfort, and appetite disturbance.

Thus, because depression impacts all body systems (3, 4), it is no surprise that investigations attempting to determine the effects of depression on hormones, neurotransmission, brain imaging, sleep architecture, immune function, etc. have tended to identify differences between depressed patients and normal subjects. However, many of these investigations have not been replicated, or show significant overlap between depressed and nondepressed groups, leading to subsequent investigations of subgroups. Such investigations are further complicated by the temporal adaptation that occurs in many biological systems. For example, the hormonal effects of acute stress are different from those of chronic stress. A few studies have attempted to account for such temporal influences.

Genetic studies have shown high heritability for depression, although much stronger for the bipolar than the unipolar form. The heritability of depression has been estimated at 0.33 (5), although slightly greater in individuals exposed to stressful life events or parental maltreatment (6). Most studies have focused on the gene coding for the serotonin transporter, a candidate gene emerging from a focus on serotonin following the introduction of selective serotonin uptake inhibitors (SSRIs). A repeat length polymorphism in the promoter region for the 5-HT transporter gene (SCL6A4) regulates gene expression (7). A series of studies showed that individuals carrying one or two copies of the short (S) allele of the serotonin transporter had high levels of neuroticism, a trait linked to depression vulnerability (8).

W.Z. Potter (✉)
Vice President, Transitional Neuroscience (retired), Merck Industry,
Philadelphia, PA 19118, USA
e-mail: wzpottermd@gmail.com

D.A. Ciraulo and R.I. Shader (eds.), *Pharmacotherapy of Depression*,
DOI 10.1007/978-1-60327-435-7_1, © Springer Science+Business Media, LLC 2011

Other studies found that S-carriers in experimental paradigms showed elevated amygdala activity assessed by functional MRI when they were exposed to threatening stimuli. These findings are consistent with other studies indicating that S-carriers who experienced stressful life events or childhood abuse were prone to depression and suicide (9). This line of research has been important in supporting the concept of genetic–environmental interactions, leading to the development of depression and other psychiatric disorders (7, 10). S-carriers are believed to have impaired transporter function resulting in decreased synaptic reuptake of serotonin – an effect that would at first appear to mimic the effects of SSRI. It has been suggested that the lifelong impairment of the serotonin transporter alters the sensitivity of serotonin receptors, increasing vulnerability to stress, although the exact mechanism has not been established. Interestingly, the presence or absence of the S allele has not been proven to predict response to SSRIs.

Many investigators in the field believe that the core action of antidepressants is to normalize the HPA axis by reversing impaired activity of the glucocorticoid receptor. The candidate gene focus emerging from this theory has been on FKBP5 which decreases binding affinity of the glucocorticoid receptor for cortisol. On the other hand, when FKBP4 replaces FKBP5, the receptor complex has high affinity for cortisol. Three polymorphisms in FKBP5 (rs1360780, rs4713916, and rs3800373) have been associated with response to antidepressants (11). Homozygotes for the rare allele had a more rapid response to antidepressants (10 days earlier) than the other two genotypes. Perhaps most importantly, it was not limited to treatment with any specific antidepressant (12). Other studies have examined other genes regulating neurotransmitter synthesis and function, including the serotonin 2A receptor gene, tyrosine hydroxylase gene (dopamine synthesis), tryptophan hydroxylase 1 (serotonin synthesis), and COMT (dopamine metabolism) although the importance of these genes in the development of depression is not established (13). To date, however, no genetic finding has been widely enough replicated to serve as a basis for identifying a depression subgroup and/or predicting response to one or another class of treatment.

Given that the concordance of depression even in identical twins is considerably less than 100%, it is likely that environmental events such as psychosocial and physiological stress play a substantial role. With unipolar depression, our focus here, a positive family history of depression predisposes individuals to earlier onset, longer time to recovery, greater severity, and more chronicity (14, 15). Thus, there are significant genetic factors, probably including both susceptibility and resistance genes, that modify the risk of developing depression. For example, downregulation of the expression of substance P, upregulation of voltage gated calcium channels, which moderate BDNF signaling in the NAcc, and the release of neuropeptide Y onto amygdala neurons have all been proposed as resilience mechanisms that reduce vulnerability to stress and depression (16). Another study reports that patients with high genetic risk for affective disorders are more vulnerable for developing depression following stressful events than patients who have a low genetic risk (17). There may be a genetic contribution to the association of early childhood maltreatment with elevated rates of depression, anxiety, and other psychiatric disturbance (18). Although early stress can alter the hypothalamic-pituitary axis, cortisol-releasing hormone, monoamines, γ-aminobutyric acid, and glutamate systems, the subsequent caretaking environment or pharmacologic interventions, such as serotonin reuptake inhibitors, benzodiazepine agonists, adrenal steroid inhibitors, tricyclic antidepressants, and electroconvulsant therapy (ECT), can moderate, prevent, or reverse these effects (19–21).

Before leaving the area of genetics of depression, it is important to understand the concept of epigenetics. Another explanation of the low concordance of depression in identical twins has been attributed to epigenetic phenomena. Environmental factors may influence gene function without altering DNA sequence changes. One example of this is increased methylation of the glucocorticoid receptor gene promoter, which has the effect of inhibiting gene expression. Interestingly, this can be reversed by a class of agents called histone deacetylase inhibitors, which have demonstrated antidepressant activity in animal models.

Up until the 1990s, most attempts to evaluate the neurobiology of major depression were based directly or indirectly upon research into the mechanisms of known antidepressant medications. The inherent circularity of exploring a mechanism already shown to be related to antidepressant activity has limited the discovery of novel treatments that have activity at sites other than the one of the previously known mechanism. In the last decade, there have been more attempts to understand manifestations of depression that are not based upon known antidepressant mechanisms and to present rationales for novel therapeutic agents. A major theme emerging from recent studies is that structural and functional changes in the hippocampus and/or prefrontal cortex produced by stress in genetically susceptible individuals are part of the pathophysiology of depression (20, 22–26). Functional neuroimaging studies have shown that MDD is associated with hyperactivity of the amygdala and subgenual anterior cingulate gyrus (ACC), whereas the DLPFC and supragenual ACC are hypoactive in depressed individuals (27–29). Altered functional connectivity between these structures has also been reported in MDD (30). Electrical stimulation of the white tracks surrounding Cg25, which is located in the prefrontal cortex, has resulted in successful treatment of depression (31) as has stimulation of the nucleus accumbens (32). For a detailed review of the brain structural and functional abnormalities in depression, the reader is referred to the review of Drevets et al. (33). For the purposes of this chapter, it is important to recognize that brain imaging findings have supported other studies that have provided a rational strategy for investigating novel antidepressant therapies that go beyond the monoamine theories and suggest roles for corticosteroid receptor antagonists, GABA agonists, NMDA agonists, and other agents that differ from existing therapeutic agents.

Current research does not support a unified theory of the neurobiological basis of depression. Substantial clinical and experimental evidence suggests that there are a number of mechanisms that may lead to major depressive disorders, and it is likely that as these are elucidated through additional research, they will yield therapeutically relevant subtypes. In the review that follows, we will highlight the leading biological theories of unipolar depression and the implications for medication development for mood disorders. The areas of focus are neuroendocrine disturbances, neural degeneration, neurotrophic factors, and neurotransmitter and neuromodulator alterations (see Table 1).

Table 1 Hormones and neurotransmitters that demonstrate alterations in depression and the potential effects on producing symptoms. See text for references

Hormone or neurotransmitter	Change	Symptom
CRF (plasma, cerebrospinal fluid)	Increased	Reduced hunger
		Diminished sex drive
		Heightened arousal
		Reduced delta sleep
		Increased core body temperature during sleep
Norepinephrine (total turnover)	Decreased	Anergia
		Anhedonia
		Anxiety
		Irrational beliefs
		Diminished libido
		Sleep disturbance
		Decreased REM latency
		Increased REM duration
		Decreased pain suppression
Serotonin (function)	Decreased	Depressed mood
		Aggression
		Reduced impulse control
		Diminished libido
		Sleep disturbance
		Decreased time in REM sleep
		Decreased REM latency
		Decreased slow wave sleep
		Appetite disturbance
		Decreased pain suppression
Dopamine (cerebrospinal fluid)	Decreased	Impaired cognition
		Reduced motivation
		Anhedonia
		Decreased motor activity
		Increased appetite
Cortisol (plasma)	Increased	Insomnia
		Hippocampal volume loss
		Treatment resistance
		Loss of concentration and memory
GABA (plasma, cortical postmortem samples)	Decreased	Reduced grooming
		Reduced appetite
Brain-derived neurotrophic factor (BDNF) (postmortem samples)	Decreased	Hippocampal volume loss
c-AMP response element binding protein (CREB) (postmortem samples)	Increased	Hippocampal volume loss
Growth hormone (GH) (plasma)	IncreasedBlunted diurnal rhythm	
	Blunted response to α_2 agonist	
Somatostatin (plasma)	Decreased	
Melatonin (plasma)	Increased	Sleep disturbance

Neuroendocrine Systems

Numerous perturbations of the neuroendocrine system have been described in depressed patients. Most of these findings appear to be related to changes that occur subsequent to, or as part of, a stress response.

Hypothalamic Pituitary Adrenal (HPA) Axis in Depression CRF

The HPA axis is the primary neuroendocrine system mediating the stress response and includes the hormones and structures mediating the production of glucocorticoids. Corticotrophin-releasing hormone (CRH), also known as corticotrophin-releasing factor (CRF), is produced in the paraventricular nucleus of the hypothalamus. It acts on CRF1 and CRF2 receptors in the central nervous system and anterior pituitary (34). The CRF1 receptor mediates anxiety and depression behaviors and the stress response. The role of CRF2 is not known, but has been hypothesized to counter the actions of CRF1. Alternatively, it may be that CRF1 is activated by escapable stressors and CRF2 is activated by inescapable stressors. It is a major regulator of basal and stress-induced release of proopiomelanocortin (POMC) and POMC-derived peptides, such as adrenocorticotrophic hormone (ACTH) and beta-endorphin, from the anterior pituitary. ACTH acts on the adrenal cortex to promote synthesis and release of cortisol and other glucocorticoids. Glucocorticoids inhibit subsequent release of CRF and ACTH. Gamma-aminobutyric acid (GABA) inputs from the hippocampus inhibit the stress response by decreasing CRF synthesis in the central nucleus of the amygdala (cnAmy) (35). Serotonin, norepinephrine, and acetylcholine inputs from the amygdala and hippocampus stimulate secretion of ACTH. Serotonin neurons terminate on inhibitory GABA neurons to block GABA inhibition of CRF synthesis (36). Dampened GABAergic tone in rats exposed to maternal separation enhances CRF expression in the amygdala and activation of the NE system (37). Thus, it appears that GABA might play a tonic regulatory role on the HPA axis.

The mechanisms underlying disturbance in the HPA axis include increased secretion of any or all of the hormones in the cascade or decreased sensitivity to negative feedback at any or all levels of the axis (38). CRF antagonists reduce stress-induced increases in plasma catecholamines, tyrosine hydroxylase mRNA in the locus coeruleus (LC), and CRF mRNA and Type 1 CRF receptor mRNA in the paraventricular nucleus (PVN) (39), giving evidence of a tonic regulatory role of CRF in specific brain regions in animal models.

Cortisol is elevated over 24-h periods in severely depressed patients (40) consistent with increased stress as part of the syndrome. Dexamethasone, a synthetic glucocorticoid, suppresses ACTH release in most healthy individuals at a standard dose (41, 42). Depressed patients have a significantly higher rate of nonsuppression than controls, although rates of nonsuppression are still not that high (43). This is one example of considerable overlap between patients with and without depression in a measure that distinguishes some, but not most, patients meeting the broad criteria for the diagnosis of depression.

CRF, which is increased in cerebral spinal fluid (CSF) and plasma in some depressed patients, activates the sympathetic nervous system and inhibits gastric emptying as well as gastric acid secretion. CRF also inhibits the secretion of growth hormone (35). After injection of CRF, the amount of ACTH released is less in depressed patients than in normal subjects (44, 45). This blunted ACTH secretion suggests that there is increased central CRF release (46, 47), since, in animals, stress and adrenalectomy lead to hypersecretion of CRF and downregulation of receptors in the anterior pituitary (48).

HPA Axis, Anxiety, and Stress

Acute stress leads to release of CRF, ACTH, and cortisol (HPA axis activation). With continued stress, adaptive changes occur. Most studies to date have focused on various animal models of stress. These reveal feedback inhibition by glucocorticoid receptors in the hippocampus and pituitary, downregulation of postsynaptic norepinephrine receptors as well as upregulation of inhibitory autoreceptors and heteroreceptors on presynaptic NE neurons.

In some types of anxiety, adaptive changes during chronic stress lead to lower levels of corticosterone and ACTH than seen acutely (49). In other types of anxiety, there are enhanced increases in corticosterone (50), and prior stress experience can lead to augmentation of subsequent stress response. The multiple forms of stress and anxiety that can be associated with depression and multiple inter-related possible physiological responses render any simple generalizations inappropriate. For instance, some relatively time-limited stressors lead to long-term HPA axis effects. Severe prenatal stress or early maternal deprivation stress leads rats to have higher corticosteroid concentrations with exaggerated glucocorticoid responses to stress persisting to adulthood (51, 52). A review of how this may account for the great impact of early neglect and abuse as well as its potential role in the etiology of depression is available elsewhere (20).

Limbic-Cortical-Striatal-Pallidal-Thalamic (LCSPT) Tract, Stress, and Depression

The LCSPT tract consists of several extensively interconnected brain structures: hippocampus, amygdala, caudate nucleus, putamen, and frontal cortex. These regions have glucocorticoid receptors (53, 54) and thus may be affected by variations in glucocorticoid concentrations. Most imaging studies, e.g., 3D MRI, show measurable, but relatively small, changes in volumes of LCSPT tract structures between depressed and control subjects; and postmortem brain studies have also noted volume loss. The hippocampus, the most studied of these structures, most consistently shows volume loss. Since these LCSPT brain structures are interconnected, they mutually influence each other; and effects, such as volume loss, in one structure might be expected to be reflected in structural or functional changes in the other structures (33).

Nevertheless, evaluation of volume reduction in the other LCSPT structures has lacked consistency with volume loss observed in some, but not all, studies. The lack of consistent findings in such studies has led to hypotheses related to subsets of patients who have reduction in structure volume rather than the alternative hypothesis that there is a significant overlap of LCSPT tract size between depressed and normal subjects. It should also be noted that compensatory changes, such as the presence of increased neurons in the paraventricular nucleus (PVN) of the hypothalamus (55, 56), may possibly obscure detection of volume loss. It has been noted that there is an apparent association of greater hippocampal atrophy with depression subtypes that are more likely to have hypercortisolemia (57). MRI studies have shown that the magnitude of hippocampal loss is associated with frequency of depressive episodes and the duration of symptoms prior to treatment (58). Another possibility that might have led to the lack of consistency in findings across studies is that the volume loss is small and may not be detectable using the techniques and technologies utilized by all evaluators. It should also be noted that volume loss does not necessarily imply cell loss which, when observed, may involve glia rather than neurons (see below).

The cause of the reported hippocampal volume loss is unknown. Various proposals include the following: (1) Depression susceptibility is associated with stress-related volume loss, precedes the onset of depression, and is central to the development of depression (22, 25). (2) Neuronal loss occurs secondary to exposure to hypercortisolemia (59). (3) Glial cell loss results in increased vulnerability to glutamate neurotoxicity since glia are responsible for most glutamate removal from the synapse and the production of brain-derived neurotrophic factor (BDNF). Thus, glial loss results in increases in synaptic glutamate and decreases in BDNF in the LCSPT tract, both potentially resulting in neuronal loss. (4) Stress results in reduction in neurotrophic factors (60), such as BDNF and glial-derived neurotrophic factor which tonically suppress apoptosis, the latent biochemical (suicide pathway) leading to cell death (61). (5) Stress results in reduced neurogenesis (62, 63). (6) Genetic polymorphisms decreasing activity-dependent release of BDNF, perhaps working synergistically with a polymorphism of the gene encoding the serotonin transporter and stress combine to produce depression (16).

Animal models provide support for the ability of many, but not all antidepressants to induce adult hippocampus neurogenesis, and when this effect is blocked, the signs of antidepressant response in rodent models are reversed. On the other hand, several rodent models of stress reduce hippocampal neurogenesis and that alone is insufficient for production of depressive-like signs. Considering these contradictory findings, it has been proposed that antidepressants act through neurogenesis-dependent and neurogenesis-independent processes (64). Furthermore, most evidence suggests that the reduction in adult hippocampal neurogenesis is not responsible for volume reductions in depression, although may be responsible for cognitive deficits observed in clinical depression. There is an increasing focus on the ventral hippocampus, which has connections to the prefrontal cortex and limbic system. The ventral hippocampus has hilar mossy cells and interneurons that are modulated by dopamine, serotonin, and norepinephrine, possibly linking structure and function in depression.

Additional evidence supporting a role for the LCSPT tract in depression is that late-onset depression is more common in age-associated medical and neurological disorders that cause damage to the LCSPT tract (65). Prolonged maturation and stabilization of neural elements and synapses in the prefrontal cortex (PFC) continues into adulthood. This neural plasticity may make the PFC more susceptible to reductions in neuronal density (66).

If the state of depression produces or increases reductions in critical brain structures, then the ability of antidepressants to increase neurotrophic factors such as BDNF may prove therapeutically important for the relief of symptoms. Some but not all antidepressants increase BDNF and neurogenesis, suggesting that this may be one of several therapeutic mechanisms of antidepressants.

Hippocampus: Possible Pivotal Role Among LCSPT Tract Structures?

During stress, normal feedback mechanisms in the HPA axis fail to operate, leading to damage to hippocampal neuronal cells (67). Stress is associated with damage to the hippocampus in animals (60). Sustained fetal social stress in vervet monkeys causes neuronal degeneration of the CA3 region (68). Chronic restraint stress in rats causes atrophy of apical dendrites of CA3 pyramidal neurons which could lead to decreased volume without loss of neurons themselves (69). Cold water immersion stress in rats causes structural damage to the CA2 and CA3 fields and decreases CRF in hippocampus (70, 71). Chronic exposure to corticosterone also leads to loss of CA3 region neurons (59, 72) and decreased dendritic branching and length of hippocampus (73). For example, in Cushing's syndrome, an endocrinopathy manifest by overproduction of cortisol leads to reduced hippocampal volume (74).

In man, those studies reporting hippocampal volume loss show it to persist over years and after depression has resolved. The amount of volume loss appears best related to the total lifetime duration of depression, not the age of the patient (57, 75). Whether or not hypercortisolemia is related to findings of decreased hippocampal volume remains, however, to be demonstrated. The close relationship that might have been predicted from preclinical studies has not, to date, been established.

Nonetheless, other lines of evidence point to linkages between glucocorticoids and hippocampal volume. For instance, hippocampal lesions lead to increased release of glucocorticoids during stress (76, 77), and this release may lead to further damage of the hippocampus (71). Hippocampal atrophy may result in impaired cognition, a feature of depression. Patients with hippocampal atrophy may be more treatment resistant (78); however, because the amount of hippocampal atrophy tends to be related to the duration of depression, hippocampal atrophy may be a surrogate marker for earlier onset and more frequent recurrence. This brings us back to the potential of restorative processes that may prove important in the long-term treatment and management of depression.

Neuronal Plasticity and Brain-Derived Neurotrophic Factor (BDNF)

BDNF is a downstream target of the c-AMP pathway. It regulates neuronal survival and synaptic plasticity both during development and in adult brain (79). Stress is associated with decreased BDNF (80). Serum BDNF concentrations have been reported to be decreased in depression and continue to be explored as a potential biomarker of the depressed state (81). When BDNF is infused into the midbrain, it produces an antidepressant-like effect in two behavioral models of depression, learned helplessness and forced swim tests, suggesting that BDNF may be involved in depression (82).

Consistent with this possibility, the cascade of events which follow antidepressant treatment can produce increased BDNF according to a series of studies in animal models, although many other studies have failed to replicate these findings. Chronic antidepressant treatment increases G_s coupling to adenyl cyclase which results in increased cyclic adenosine monophosphate (c-AMP) which increases Ca^{2+}-dependent protein kinases and leads to increased expression of the transcriptional regulator c-AMP response element binding protein (CREB) (83, 84) which increases both BDNF expression in limbic structures, including hippocampus, and the BDNF receptor, TrkB (85). Chronic administration of antidepressants and electroconvulsive seizures increases proliferation and survival of new neurons consistent with the effects shown after activation of the cAMP-CREB cascade or incubation with BDNF which increases differentiation of new cells into neurons (86). Taken together, these findings suggest that some treatments of depression enhance neurotrophic factor activity in specific brain regions (22, 24).

How Strong Is the Case for a Major Role of Stress and the HPA Axis in Depression?

As reviewed above, multiple lines of preclinical and clinical evidence argue that depression is associated with functional and/or structural alterations in the brain which are consistent with HPA dysfunction. Furthermore, whatever the primary biochemical effects of antidepressant treatments, pathways exist whereby long-term effects impinge on components of the HPA axis (87). What is not addressed by recent formulations is the failure to translate the finding of hypercortisolemia in depression reported three decades ago (40) into a convincing diagnostic tool and/or predictor of treatment response despite diverse and sustained efforts (41). As more sensitive methods have become available to document region-specific changes in structure or in function in the brains of patients with depression or effects of antidepressants on glucocorticoid receptor function in preclinical models, there has been a new wave of circumstantial evidence to support statements such as "...disturbed regulation of CRF neuronal circuitry plays a causative role in producing cardinal signs and symptoms of depression..." (88). The problem for the clinician or neuroscientist focused on providing or developing the best treatments is that no measure or combination of biochemical and physiological measures has allowed for a stable, reasonably replicable, and robust means of distinguishing a depressed from a normal individual, or for predicting an individual patient's response to different classes of antidepressants.

A primary focus on the HPA axis and, more recently, LCSPT tract risks subsuming findings of alterations in other measures as merely secondary. As will be succinctly reviewed in what follows, investigators have reported that other neuroendocrine or neurotransmitter systems are just as consistently dysregulated in depression as the "primary" HPA one. As cataloged in Table 1 and conceptualized in Figs. 1 and 2, these constitute a multitude of complex and potentially inter-related findings relevant to the pathophysiology and treatment of unipolar depression(s). As noted at the outset, trying to fit manic-depressive illness and unipolar depression into a common pathophysiologic model is an even more difficult task, particularly when one considers the differences in spectrum of efficacy between putative mood stabilizers and antidepressants. We will, therefore, continue to restrict our focus and only occasionally refer to those studies on bipolar disorder that help to elucidate investigations of unipolar depression.

Given the complexity of findings, even within the broad category of patients with unipolar depression and the spectrum of marketed antidepressants with highly variable efficacy, it is not surprising that researchers look for unifying hypotheses. Unfortunately, those that have been proposed and tested such as definable norepinephrine or serotonergic types of depression have not been supported and those, such as the primacy of HPA axis dysfunction, have not been testable in the absence

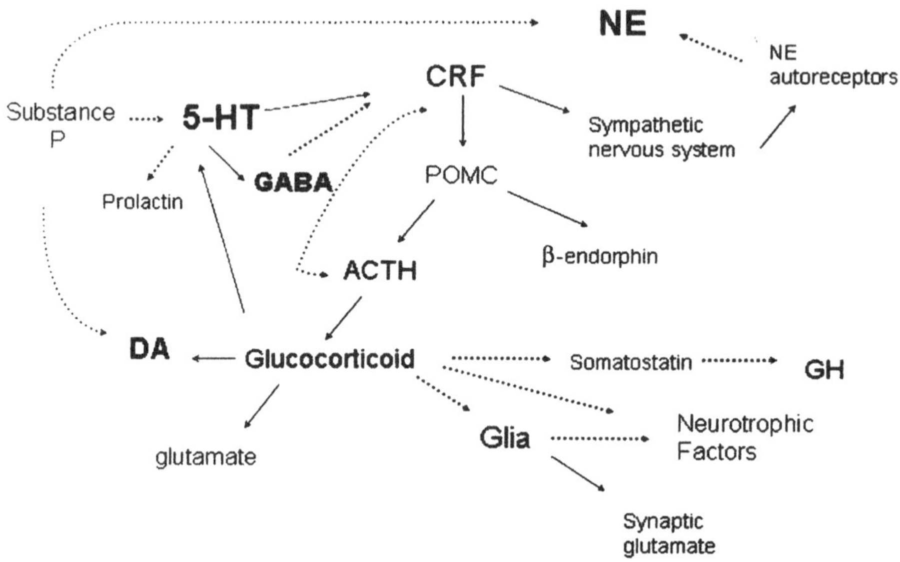

Fig. 1 Interaction of neuroendocrine system involved in the depression cascade

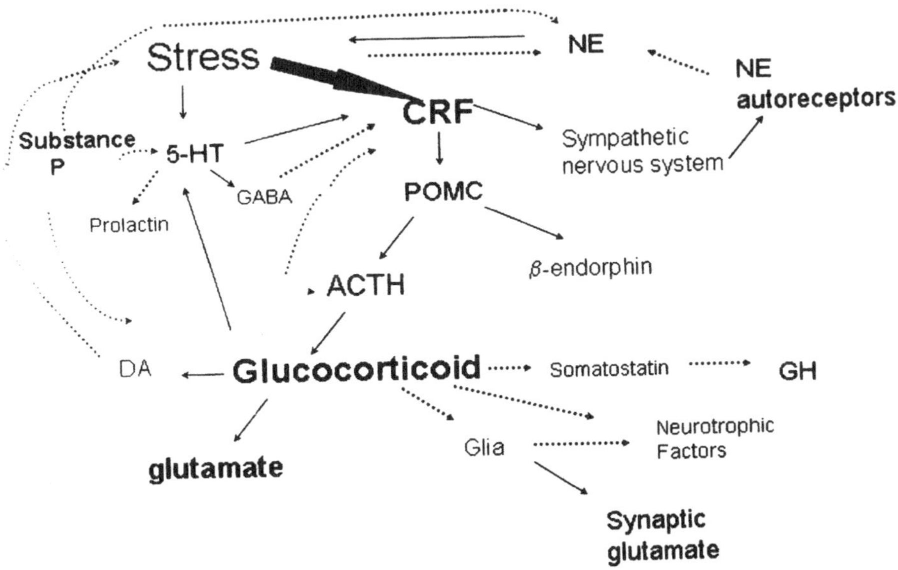

Fig. 2 Depression cascade. Hormones and neurotransmitters that have *larger fonts* tend to have increased concentration and those with *smaller fonts* tend to have reduced concentration

of appropriate pharmacologic agents. Reasoning that we should remain open to all lines of evidence, we will highlight reports of many other classes of abnormalities in depression that may or may not ultimately prove to be related to those of the HPA axis. In the absence of a compelling scientific case to narrow one's focus, we may best achieve therapeutic advances by targeting each of the systems implicated in depression and evaluating the potential advantage of selective interventions either alone or in combination (see below).

The Hypothalamus–Pituitary–Thyroid (HPT) Axis, Growth Hormone, Somatostatin, and Prolactin in Depression

It has been noted for many decades that many behavioral symptoms of hypothyroidism –dysphoria, anxiety, fatigue, and irritability – overlap those of depression. This observation plus the clinical finding that small doses of thyroid may potentiate the effects of antidepressants (89) has sustained an interest in the relevance of this system to depression. Thyrotropin-releasing hormone (TRH) released from hypothalamus stimulates TRH receptors in the pituitary to release TSH which stimulates specific receptors in the pituitary to release triiodothyroxine (T3) and thyroxine (T4) hormones. A subset of depressed patients show a blunted TSH response to TRH, others symptomless autoimmune thyroiditis (46), and still others an exaggerated

TSH response to TRH (88). Preclinical studies on the modulation of multiple neurotransmitter functions in the brain coupled with clinical observations on rates of mood switches in bipolar disorder point to the possibility that to understand certain forms of depression, it will be necessary to understand altered function of components of the HPT axis (90).

Growth hormone (GH) and somatostatin, the hypothalamic GH suppressing factor, regulation have also been found to be altered in depression. A change in the diurnal rhythm of GH may be reflected by increased plasma concentrations (91), a finding that is opposite in direction to what would be provided if CRF were exerting control (see below). It is here worth recalling that cortisol abnormalities are also best described in terms of the diurnal pattern with elevations only observed at certain times of the day (92). GH increases to α_2 agonists (e.g., clonidine) are blunted in depressed patients (93, 94). This blunted GH response has been consistently replicated and complemented by findings of blunted responses to uptake inhibitors, such as desmethylimipramine, which increase the intrasynaptic concentrations of the endogenous α_2 agonist norepinephrine (95).

Interestingly, somatostatin concentrations are reported to be reduced in the CSF of depressed patients compared with controls, although this finding is not specific to depression and may be related to elevated cortisol concentrations (44, 96, 97). A reduction of the inhibitory factor is also consistent with the previously described elevation of GH in blood but not the blunted response to α_2 stimulation. The latter is most consistent with several lines of evidence implicating altered α_2 function in depression (98). The complex inter-relationships of neuroendocrine and monoamine function are not well enough understood to allow us to test for primary causality of any single abnormality.

Another highly replicated neuroendocrine abnormality in depression is that of blunted prolactin responses to serotonergic stimulation. For instance, there is a blunted release of prolactin to a fenfluramine challenge in depressed patients (99, 100). Prolactin responses to intravenous tryptophan, a precursor of serotonin (101), or clomipramine, a serotonin uptake inhibitor (102, 103), are also blunted. Since abnormalities of unstimulated prolactin have not been reported, these responses would appear to best reflect altered serotonin function.

As already noted, the inter-relatedness of catecholamine and serotonin systems in the brain with modulation of neuroendocrine function makes it difficult to address cause vs. effect as reflected in the above examples. An additional issue is that many of the observed abnormalities involve a circadian component, which, in other words, may only show differences at certain times of day, which leads to an interest in a pathophysiologic role of altered circadian regulation (104), particularly in terms of seasonal affective disorder (105). Melatonin secretion varies over the 24 h period in a circadian pattern related to light and darkness. Its secretion is partly under norepinephrine control and exogenous melatonin and/or using light to shift the phase of endogenous melatonin may have a role in the treatment of circadian disorders under which seasonal affective disorder can be subsumed (105). It has also been suggested that blunted circadian variation in natural killer cell activity in depression may reflect some underlying chronobiological rhythm (106).

All these reports of altered neuroendocrine and possible circadian regulation in depression need to be considered in light of the extensive work on the monoamine neurotransmitters in brain which have been shown to be involved in the action of established antidepressant treatments. Despite the theoretical attractiveness of other approaches, no intervention derived from neuroendocrine or circadian hypotheses has yet led to a treatment which, by itself (e.g., light therapy), shows sustained efficacy in a substantial proportion of patients diagnosed with depression. Considerable effort has gone into identifying CRF antagonists which will ultimately allow for a test of whether excess CRF tone plays a pathologic role in patients with evidence of hypercortisolemia. Disappointingly, the most recent large study with a CRF antagonist in depression was negative (107), although it is not known whether the doses employed significantly altered function in the brain or the extent to which CRF1 receptors were blocked.

Classic Neurotransmitters and the Monoamine Hypothesis of Depression

Although agents that modify neurotransmitter action have become the primary therapies for depression and although numerous abnormalities in neurotransmitters have been uncovered in depression, the attempt to establish primacy of any single neurotransmitter or of neurotransmitters over hormones has been unsuccessful. As emerging technologies permit further examination of new systems, additional perturbations have been noted, but findings and formulations of hypotheses have necessarily reflected methods available at the time.

For over four decades, tricyclic antidepressants and monoamine oxidase inhibitors have been known to be effective treatments and show serotonergic, norepinephrinergic, and/or dopaminergic activities. These observations provide the so-called pharmacological bridge to the monoamine hypothesis of depression (108), which has guided much research to elucidate the role of the monoamine neurotransmitters, serotonin (5-HT), norepinephrine (NE), and dopamine (DA), in the pathophysiology of depression. Further development of more specific agents including selective serotonin reuptake inhibitors (SSRIs), norepinephrine reuptake inhibitors (NERI), and dopaminergic reuptake inhibitors, has reinforced the importance of monoamine systems for the treatment of depression. Thus, the monoamine hypothesis continues to encourage investigation of the biological basis of depression. Such, investigations are now focusing on additional components of monoamine action such as postsynaptic receptors, presynaptic autoreceptors and heteroreceptors, second messengers, and gene transcription factors. For example, several antidepressants have been noted to downregulate 5-HT_{1A} receptor activity reducing negative feedback of 5-HT_{1A} in the raphe nuclei resulting in greater 5-HT release (109). Such findings support the possibility of adding a 5-HT_{1A} antagonist to an SSRI to potentiate antagonist effects (110). Alternatively, it has been argued that postsynaptic 5-HT_{1A} receptors may be a target for antidepressant therapy although existing evidence suggests that full agonists may have too narrow a therapeutic index in humans to test the hypothesis (111).

In addition to their independent effects, the monoamines interact with all of the systems described here and elsewhere in this paper. For example, the glia have postsynaptic 5-HT and NE receptors on their cell bodies and processes (112, 113) that could be expected to affect concentrations of glutamate and neurotrophic factors. In addition, substance P is co-expressed with 5-HT in ascending dorsal raphe neurons (114) and substance P modulates mesolimbic DA activity and is involved in stress-induced activation of the ascending norepinephrine projection from the locus coeruleus (115). For the sake of clarity, we will briefly consider each monoamine by itself, recognizing that in vivo there are, among them, complex regional and structure-specific interactions.

Serotonin

A role for 5-HT in depression was established with the use of SSRIs in its treatment. That SSRIs really do depend on 5-HT has been elegantly tested by showing that depletion of tryptophan, a precursor of 5-HT synthesis, leads to return of depressive symptoms in patients with recent response to SSRIs (116). Women have lower rates of 5-HT synthesis and thus may show even greater relapse rates in response to depletion than men (117).

Evidence of reduced serotonergic function has been found in untreated depressed patients. Investigators have assessed [3H] imipramine and [3H] paroxetine binding in platelets from depressed and healthy subjects as a possible peripheral marker of the brain serotonin transporter (SERT) with some, but not all, studies showing reductions in depressed patients (118, 119). Postmortem studies show similarly decreased SERT binding in hypothalamus (120) as have imaging studies (121). One might expect more consistent findings in postmortem samples from suicides, since low serotonin metabolite concentrations in cerebrospinal fluid may be associated with reduced impulse control that might predispose depressed subjects to commit suicide (122). On the other hand, there is no obvious causal relationship between a measure of 5-HT turnover in cerebrospinal fluid and density of the transporter.

Mechanistically, 5-HT and the HPA axis are linked. Figure 1 shows the normal interaction of 5-HT, NE, and DA with the endocrine system. 5-HT can stimulate CRF release mediated by 5-HT_2, 5-HT_{1A}, and 5-HT_{1C} receptors. Glucocorticoids tend to enhance 5-HT function, possibly as a compensatory effect in chronic stress. The extent to which this input exerts major influences in humans remains to be established. Nonetheless, preclinical studies point to several potentially important relationships. For instance, acute stress increases 5-HT release transiently, but continued stress leads to 5-HT depletion. Chronic stress may also increase production of 5-HT_{1A} autoreceptors that further reduce 5-HT transmission. 5-HT_{1A} knockout mice demonstrate increased stress-like behaviors indicative of "increased anxiety" (123, 124). These mice show increased mobility in response to stressors which is used as a model for antidepressant drugs (125). These data provide a basis for the association of anxiety symptoms with depressed mood.

Imaging studies have investigated the relationship of 5-HT and hippocampal atrophy. Positron emission tomography studies of 5-HT_{2A} binding of [(18)F] altanserin has, however, led to disparate findings (121). It is to be anticipated that development of additional and more selective imaging ligands will clarify many of the suggestive, but variable, findings in depression that tend to overlap with both normal populations and those with other conditions (e.g., Alzheimer's disease).

Norepinephrine

The role of NE has also been demonstrated in clinical trials as well as in depletion studies. Alpha-methyl paratyrosine (AMPT), which blocks NE synthesis, does not alter the rating on the Hamilton Depression Rating Scale (HAMD) in normal subjects, but produces a depressive relapse (increases the HAMD rating) in patients who remitted to an NE antidepressant such as desipramine or mazindol (126). In contrast, there was no return of depression after AMPT in patients who had remitted on a serotonergic antidepressant (126).

NE neurons in the locus coeruleus (LC) project to almost all major brain regions and serve an important role in regulating and focusing additional and other responses to external stimuli (127, 128). Not surprisingly, NE systems are involved in responses to stress since there are multiple interactions between the HPA axis and NE. For instance, under experimental conditions, CRF secretion increases LC neuronal firing, resulting in enhanced NE release. NE release stimulates CRF secretion in the paraventricular nucleus (PVN) which leads to ACTH secretion. Increased ACTH leads to increased cortisol which provides a negative feedback to decrease CRF and NE in the PVN.

During behavioral stress, LC neuronal firing is increased (129) in association with increased release of NE. This LC responsiveness is enhanced with a novel stress after chronic or prior stress. When stress exposures are repeated in situations that prevent the animal from escaping, the animal exhibits learned helplessness which is associated with the depletion of NE (130). It is thought that this depletion is due to inability of the animal to synthesize sufficient NE to replace that which is released (131). Whether such depletion occurs in human brain following the chronic stress of depression is not known.

Various approaches to evaluating NE function in depression have been pursued over the last three decades from quantifying its metabolites in urine to radiolabel isotope dilution techniques to track its "spillover" in plasma (132). Taken together, there is evidence of a shift toward elevated turnover and release in unipolar depression, although values overlap with those observed in age and gender-matched healthy volunteers. One hypothesis to explain these increases emerges from consideration of reports on altered sensitivity of the platelet α_2 receptor in depression. Subsensitivity of α_2 receptors and/or their coupling mechanism to downstream intracellular events could be responsible for the exaggerated release of NE observed in depressed patients subjected to acute physiological or psychological manipulation (reviewed in Manji and Potter (133)).

Despite some evidence for an association of elevated HPA and NE function, relevant and consistent relationships have not yet been established among the available peripheral (blood and urine) measures. It is conceivable that availability of appropriate methods to simultaneously quantify CRF and NE in all brain regions would lead to demonstration of tight relationships. It is equally conceivable that elevations of CRF and NE can occur relatively independently as a function of different subtypes of depression. The result that emerges from such studies will have implications for the treatment and understanding of depression pathophysiology.

As noted above, antidepressant treatment, including that with NE and 5-HT uptake inhibitors, has effects on the NE signal transduction pathway and increases BDNF by blocking stress-induced decreases of BDNF in the hippocampus (134). Furthermore, stimulation of 5-HT_{2A} receptors increases BDNF mRNA (135, 136). Consequently, various elements along the NE and 5-HT pathways, including α receptors, G proteins, cyclic adenosine monophosphate (c-AMP), c-AMP regulatory element binding protein (CREB), and brain-derived neurotropic factor (BDNF), are being evaluated as targets for antidepressant medications (67). As an example, focused on the NE cascade, chronic administration of norepinephrine antidepressants, such as desipramine and reboxetine, causes desensitization of the β-adrenoceptor–coupled adenylate cyclase system. Nuclear phosphorylated CREB (CREB-P) decreases in rat frontal cortex after chronic administration and in fibroblasts after incubation, suggesting that norepinephrine antidepressants exert direct effects beyond β-adrenoceptors. This would be consistent with deamplification of the NE-mediated signal transduction cascade, resulting in "normalization" of increased norepinephrine activity, which is an evolving hypothesis (137).

Dopamine

Deficiencies in DA have been tied to depression and DA is tied to the regulation of the endocrine system. Moreover, there is a long-standing case for a role of enhancing DA function in the treatment of depression, particularly that not relating to monotherapy, as reflected in the special role of MAOIs or bupropion as an adjunctive therapy (138–140). CSF levels of homovanillic acid (HVA), a major DA metabolite (141–143), and urinary dihydroxyphenylacetic acid (DOPAC), another major DA metabolite (142), are reduced in a proportion of depressed patients. Consistent with the tendency for depressed patients to have decreased DA metabolites, imaging (single photon emission computed tomography, SPECT, with the high affinity D_2 ligand ^{123}I-iodobenzamide) studies of D_2 receptor binding have demonstrated 10% more basal ganglion activity in depressed patients than in controls. This may be due to decreased dopaminergic transmission since decreased intrinsic D_2 occupancy would tend to lead to upregulation of D_2 receptors (144). When antidepressant treatment is instituted, the D_2 activity decreases in the striatum

(145, 146), consistent with this hypothesis. Most recently, decreased density of the DA transporter and increased density of $D_{2/3}$ receptors were found in the amygdala in a study of postmortem brain samples from subjects with depression (147). Finally, in some brain regions, DA is transported by the NE transporter into the presynaptic neuron (148). Therefore, in brain areas with NE nerve terminals, a norepinephrine reuptake inhibitor may act like a DA reuptake inhibitor and avoid the peripheral dopaminergic effects, as well as cocaine-like effects, that might be seen if the DA transporter itself were universally inhibited.

Increased glucocorticoid activity leads to altered or decreased prefrontal cortical DA metabolism (149, 150) and increased mesolimbic DA activity (149). DA is also known to be a prolactin (PRL) release-inhibiting factor since it is released by the arcuate nucleus of the hypothalamus where it binds to the D_2 receptor inhibiting the activity of the acidophilic cells of the anterior pituitary, thereby blocking PRL and also growth hormone release. Thus, the blunted PRL response to a serotonergic agent, seen in depressed patients, could involve a dopaminergic component, especially in light of well-known 5-HT–DA interactions (96).

Other Neuromodulators: Cytokines, Substance P, Glutamate, γ-Aminobutyric Acid, and Enkephalins

Cytokines are chemical mediators of the inflammatory response. Several studies have found that patients with major depression have increased levels of inflammatory markers in CSF and blood. There is substantial inconsistency in reports identifying specific markers, although some evidence supports increased interleukin (IL)-1, IL-6, tumor necrosis factor (TNF)-alpha and increases in acute phase proteins such as C-reactive protein and chemokines. A meta-analysis (151) found that levels of TNF-alpha and IL-6 proinflammatory cytokines were higher in major depressed patients than controls. A SNP of the IL1B gene has been associated with decreased response to antidepressants, altered function of the amygdala, and the anterior cingulate gyrus in patients with major depression (152).

Cytokines can exert their behavioral effects by altering neurotransmitter function (decreasing serotonin), endocrine function (decreasing glucocorticoid receptor sensitivity), neuronal plasticity (block neurogenesis, increase glutamate excitatory damage), and regional brain activity (altered function of amygdala and ACC). Both peripheral and brain cytokine systems can have central nervous system effects. Peripheral cytokines may enter the brain through a transporter system, penetration of the blood brain barrier, or by other unidentified mechanisms. The brain itself has its own cytokine network: glial cells, microglia, and astrocytes can synthesize cytokines and neurons have cytokine receptors. The implications for antidepressant medication development is the discovery of drugs that block cytokine pro-inflammatory actions, and some pre-clinical evidence from IL-6 knockout mice suggests that this deletion may convey protection to stress-induced behaviors.

Substance P receptors, particularly the neurokinin-1 (NK_1) receptors, are highly expressed in brain regions, including the amygdala, septum, hippocampus, thalamus, and periaqueductal grey, that are critical to regulation of emotion and neurochemical responses to stress (153–155). Prostaglandin agonists and vanilloid receptor agonists, such as *N*-arachidonyl-dopamine, induce substance P release (156, 157). NK_1 antagonists may exert a significant part of their effects through the monoamines. Substance P and 5-HT are co-expressed in ascending raphe neurons in human brain (114). Sustained administration of an NK_1 antagonist increased spontaneous firing of dorsal raphe 5-HT neurons associated with reduction in 5-HT_{1A} autoreceptor responsiveness (158). This suggests that NK_1 antagonists enhance 5-HT receptor activation. In addition, glutamate receptor antagonists can block the effect of NK_1 agonists on firing of 5-HT neurons. This effect is blocked by NK_1 antagonists and an AMPA/kainate glutamate receptor antagonist, suggesting that the neurokinins may act by exciting glutamate neurons that input on 5-HT neurons (159).

Similarly, substance P is involved in stress-induced activation of the ascending norepinephrine projection from the LC. An NK_1 antagonist increased NE in the dialysate of frontal cortex in moving rats and increased the firing rate of adrenergic perikarya in the LC (160). Substance P antagonists attenuate stress responses and block anxiety behaviors in animal tests such as the social interaction test (161), maternal separation-elicited vocalization (162, 163), immobilization stress (164), and inescapable foot shock (165).

Since substance P activates NK_2 and NK_3, as well as NK_1 receptors, these too need to be considered. To date only NK_1 antagonists have been reported to be potentially relevant to depression. NK_2 antagonists also block anxiety behavior in the elevated plus maze and the marmoset threat test (166). Anxiolytic and antidepressant drugs downregulate substance P biosynthesis (163). The NK_2 antagonist SR48968 also mediates LC firing and NE release in prefrontal cortex (115). There has been at least one placebo controlled study of an antagonist in depression, in this case specific for NK_1, that showed a significant therapeutic effect (162) providing evidence in humans for a role of substance P in depression. Extensive subsequent studies, however, at doses shown to fully antagonize the NK_1 receptor in human brain, failed to replicate the earlier finding (167). There is no current evidence supporting a role of NK_1 antagonism, at least as monotherapy, as a viable treatment for depression.

Glutamate also is involved in depression. Both stress and glucocorticoids increase glutamate concentrations in the hippocampus. Glutamate may also be involved in hippocampal neuron death associated with stress (168). Normally glutamate is removed from the synapse through reuptake by the presynaptic neuron and the glia. Glia convert glutamate to glutamine which gets transported to the presynaptic neuron that converts it back to glutamate. Glucocorticoids impair glutamate removal from the synapse due to disruption of the energetic effects by glucocorticoid which inhibits glucose transport resulting in depletion of hippocampal ATP concentrations, increases free cytosolic calcium by impairing calcium extrusion from postsynaptic cytoplasm, and blunts compensatory increased activity of antioxidant enzymes compromising the ability of neurons to respond to an insult.

Of these effects, the effects on calcium, reducing calcium conductance and calcium ATPase pump activity, are likely to be most significant (68). Thus, it appears that glucocorticoids, when increased, impair the ability of neurons to survive coincident insults, such as hypoxia, metabolic poisons, hypoglycemia, oxygen radical generators, and seizure-related neurotoxicity. Suicide victims have been noted to have desensitization of *N*-methyl-aspartate (NMDA) receptors in the PFC as evidence that glutamate transport might be impaired in depression (169). In addition, NMDA antagonists are active in the forced swim test (170–173). Subanesthetic doses of the NMDA antagonist ketamine were found to produce rapid, but time limited, relief of depression in patients with major depression a decade ago (172), a finding that continues to be of interest with a recent extension to treatment-resistant depression (174).

Stress and depression are associated with increased number of 5-HT_{2A} receptor binding sites (175), resulting in increased glutamate release. Glutamate release is suppressed by μ-opioid, metabotropic glutamate (mGlu2), and monoamine β_2-adrenergic and 5-$HT_{1B/1D}$ and, possibly, 5-HT_7 receptors (113). Thus, combined use of both an SSRI and a 5-HT_{2A} antagonist, such as mirtazapine or olanzapine, may synergistically suppress glutamate release.

Repeated ECT and chronic antidepressant therapy desensitize NMDA-glutamatergic receptors in rat cortex (170). Antidepressant drugs directly or indirectly reduce *N*-methyl-D-aspartate (NMDA) glutamate function (176). It has been proposed that polymorphisms or mutations in the glutamate receptor genes, in particular the NMDA receptor complex, might alter susceptibility for development of depression (177).

Gamma-aminobutyric acid (GABA) has been reported to be decreased in plasma in many patients with symptomatic depression (178) in depression. $GABA_B$ is coupled to Ca^{2+} channels and may enhance c-AMP responses to NE and enhance β-adrenergic downregulation in response to tricyclic antidepressants (179, 180). Imaging studies indicate that depression is associated with reductions in cortical GABA concentrations. This effect may be tied to the 5-HT system. Both a GABA-A antagonist and a selective 5-HT_{2A} receptor antagonist reduced the inhibitory postsynaptic currents in the dorsal raphe nucleus, indicating that 5-HT_{2A} receptors activate GABA inhibitory inputs to 5-HT neurons in the DNR (181). Since antidepressant medications raise GABA concentrations, ameliorating GABA deficits associated with depression, GABA agents have been proposed as useful treatments in depression.

Opiates have effects on mood and interact with other neurotransmitters. Opiates are sometimes used to augment the effects of other treatments in refractory depression (182). Activation of μ-opioid receptors suppresses 5-HT_{2A}–induced excitatory postsynaptic currents, suggesting that μ-opioids suppress glutamate release through the 5-HT system (113). Chronic opiate exposure also upregulates the c-AMP–signaling pathway and increases expression of tyrosine hydroxylase, indicating a noradrenergic effect (183). Endogenous opioids may be involved in the effect of placebo on mood and behavior of patients (184). For example, the use of naloxone in analgesic trials can ablate the placebo response (185).

Alterations in Physiological Function: Circardian Rhythms, Sleep, Pain Perception, and Appetite

Given that depression is associated with perturbations of most endocrine and neurotransmitter systems, it is not surprising that depression alters physiologic function. The neurobiology of depression needs to account for these. In addition, it is apparent that the location of the insults in the particular individual can account for the specific symptoms of that individual and that the specific treatments used for restoring normal mood would influence the impact of those therapies on specific physiologic functions.

Diurnal, nocturnal, and seasonal effects are generated by an endogenous circadian pacemaker, entrained by environmental cues, particularly light/dark cycles. These circadian effects of sleep, temperature, and neuroendocrine secretion are mediated by periodic gene expression originating in the hypothalamic suprachiasmatic nuclei (186). Mutations in clock genes accelerate and delay circadian cycles (187). Serotonergic neurons project to the suprachiasmatic nucleus in the hypothalamus help regulate circadian sleep–wake cycles, temperature, and the HPA axis.

As part of circadian effects, there are normal 24-h fluctuations in neuroendocrine secretion, especially cortisol, growth hormone, TSH, and melatonin, as already noted above. These hormonal systems are often disrupted in depression thought to be due to heightened arousal. With shorter daylight hours, some individuals who experience the aforementioned have recurring autumn and winter depression (seasonal affective disorder, SAD) thought to be related to phase delay in the sleep–wake cycle (186, 188).

Sleep is often disturbed in depression. Imaging studies using [18(F)] 2-fluoro-2-deoxy-D-glucose PET have noted changes in oxygen utilization consistent with abnormal arousal in depressed patients associated with increased glucose utilization in ventromedial prefrontal cortex (189) and blunted response in anterior paralimbic regions during REM sleep (190). Hyper-aroused patients demonstrate loss of delta sleep, loss of sleep continuity, and increased core body temperature during sleep. Changes in quantitative perfusion MRI have been noted in treatment responders (191).

Since sleep is related to endocrine function and depression, it is interesting that deep sleep has an inhibitory influence on the HPA axis. Activation of the HPA axis or administration of glucocorticoids can lead to arousal and sleeplessness. A 24-h increase of ACTH and cortisol secretion can result in insomnia, consistent with a disorder of CNS hyper-arousal (192). In addition, elevated CRF in depressed patients can cause a hyper-arousal in some brain regions that can be observed by evaluating brain glucose utilization, consistent with the imaging findings. Sleep deprivation can produce temporary remission of depression in many patients with major depression, perhaps through effects on the HPA axis.

Sleep also is influenced by neurotransmitters. 5-HT neurons project from the dorsal raphe nuclei to the cholinergic cells of the pons to tonically inhibit rapid eye movement (REM) sleep. Depletion of 5-HT duplicates the findings of increased REM sleep time, decreased time to onset of first REM sleep (REM latency), and decreased amount of slow wave sleep that are seen in nearly 50% of depressed patients and 10% of controls. Depletion of 5-HT and NE shortens REM latency and increases REM sleep. REM rebound is an aspect of antidepressant rebound (193).

Painful physical symptoms are also common complaints in depression (194). This may in part be related to the shared 5-HT and NE pathways in depression and pain (195) since 5-HT and NE modulate pain through the descending pain pathways. Serotonergic projections descend through the rostral ventral medulla and the pontine raphe into the spinal cord where they modulate pain. Norepinephrine neurons also project through the dorsolateral pons, locus coeruleus, medial and lateral parabrachial nuclei, and associated areas into the spinal cord to modulate pain. The effects of 5-HT and NE are synergistic in this system. Thus, dual reuptake inhibitors are effective in relieving the physical symptoms associated with depression (196). Recent functional imaging studies indicate that the presence of anxiety may accentuate pain perception (197).

Depressed patients also frequently complain about altered appetite. Both the endocrine systems and neurotransmitters are involved in appetite control. The monoamines that are often perturbed during depression also have effects on appetite. DA modulates sensory feedback and appetite (198, 199). NE in the hypothalamus increases meal size and stimulates carbohydrate intake through α_2-adrenergic receptors (200). This effect shows rapid tolerance. Corticosterone upregulates α_2-adrenoreceptors. 5-HT acts through the 5-HT_{2C} receptor to affect eating rate and through the 5-HT_{1B} receptor to affect meal size (198). CRF is a potent anorectic when injected in cerebral ventricles or paraventricular nucleus. Thus, when present, elevated CRF associated with depression may contribute to anorexia.

Conclusion

Although our understanding of the biology of depression is far from complete, there appears to be a convergence of disparate research inquiries such that a more integrated biology of depression explaining the inter-relationship of both the emotional and physical components of depression is now emerging. The neuroendocrine effects of stress and the neurotransmitter effects of depression are now recognized to interact in a tightly linked system that offers a homeostatic mechanism for responding to stress. In addition, the neuronal pathways for the emotional and physical symptoms have common nuclei and pathways.

Many possibilities emerge from combining observations in patients and animals. Although the validity of extrapolating from animals to humans has not been demonstrated, numerous potential treatments can be proposed based upon the testable hypotheses of the mechanistic basis of depression. One relatively simple construct is that of depression as a cascade of neuroendocrine effects.

Stress in susceptible individuals results in HPA axis stimulation as an early step leading to depletion of the monoamines 5-HT, NE, and DA near the start of the cascade. If these monoamines are reduced in other ways, they can potentially induce the development of depression in the absence of HPA axis stimulation. Additional systems are influenced by the HPA axis and the monoamines. This interaction can be considered a depression cascade. Based upon this hypothetical construct, treatments closer to the initiating factors or early steps in the cascade or those that act at multiple branches of the cascade would be more effective than treatments that act only on a single branch. As one moves down, the cascade additional systems are enlisted depending on the individual's susceptibilities. Various branches of the cascade are responsible for some of the symptomatology of depression. Interventions that act on a single unique downstream target (e.g., a single postsynaptic 5-HT receptor) and efforts to identify subsets in which such selective interventions might be effective are likely to fail without validated biomarkers to identify the appropriate subjects.

Conversely, the tricyclics and combined 5-HT and NE reuptake inhibitors operating at two possible branches would be expected to have greater activity than an antidepressant that acts at only one path (201–203). Some speculate that a component of the glutamate system which was intimately involved in responses to stress and modulation of multiple transmitters could play a role near the start of the cascade. An insult further down the cascade might have significant consequences, but might also be limited in its production of symptomatology. For treatments, mechanisms of action further down the cascade are more likely to benefit a limited group of symptoms although as noted above, there are significant interactions among the many systems involved in depression. In addition, an adjunctive therapy that acts at additional branches from the primary therapy would be expected to be more effective than an adjunctive medication acting at the same branch as the primary medication.

The molecular basis of the liability to depression including the number of susceptibility and resistance genes involved in the development of depression is unknown (204), but such studies hold additional promise of furthering our understanding of the biology underlying this common illness by breaking out of the cycle of defining and refining our information of the underlying effects based upon knowledge of an antidepressant effect. Defining the roles of antidepressant therapy-induced genes in neural plasticity may prove useful in understanding the biological basis of depression (205). It is through such technology that the uncovering of triggers of the cascade above the HPA axis and the monoamines will be accomplished.

References

1. Fawcett J, Kravitz HM. Anxiety syndromes and their relationship to depressive illness. J Clin Psychiatry. 1983;44(8 Pt 2):8–11.
2. Gerber PD, Barrett JE, Barrett JA, Oxman TE, Manheimer E, Smith R, et al. The relationship of presenting physical complaints to depressive symptoms in primary care patients. J Gen Intern Med. 1992;7(2):170–3.
3. Posse M, Hallstrom T. Depressive disorders among somatizing patients in primary health care. Acta Psychiatr Scand. 1998;98(3):187–92.
4. Kroenke K, Price RK. Symptoms in the community. Prevalence, classification, and psychiatric comorbidity. Arch Intern Med. 1993;153(21):2474–80.

5. Kendler KS, Aggen SH. Time, memory and the heritability of major depression. Psychol Med. 2001;31(5):923–8.
6. Wurtman RJ. Genes, stress, and depression. Metabolism. 2005;54(5 Suppl 1):16–9.
7. Caspi A, Sugden K, Moffitt TE, Taylor A, Craig IW, Harrington H, et al. Influence of life stress on depression: moderation by a polymorphism in the 5-HTT gene. Science. 2003;301(5631):386–9.
8. Lesch KP, Bengel D, Heils A, Sabol SZ, Greenberg BD, Petri S, et al. Association of anxiety-related traits with a polymorphism in the serotonin transporter gene regulatory region. Science. 1996;274(5292):1527–31.
9. Hariri AR, Tessitore A, Mattay VS, Fera F, Weinberger DR. The amygdala response to emotional stimuli: a comparison of faces and scenes. Neuroimage. 2002;17(1):317–23.
10. Caspi A, Hariri AR, Holmes A, Uher R, Moffitt TE. Genetic sensitivity to the environment: the case of the serotonin transporter gene and its implications for studying complex diseases and traits. Am J Psychiatry. 2010;167(5):509–27.
11. Binder EB, Salyakina D, Lichtner P, Wochnik GM, Ising M, Putz B, et al. Polymorphisms in FKBP5 are associated with increased recurrence of depressive episodes and rapid response to antidepressant treatment. Nat Genet. 2004;36(12):1319–25.
12. Horstmann S, Binder EB. Pharmacogenomics of antidepressant drugs. Pharmacol Ther. 2009;124(1):57–73.
13. Levinson DF. The genetics of depression: a review. Biol Psychiatry. 2006;60(2):84–92.
14. Warner V, Weissman MM, Fendrich M, Wickramaratne P, Moreau D. The course of major depression in the offspring of depressed parents. Incidence, recurrence, and recovery. Arch Gen Psychiatry. 1992;49(10):795–801.
15. Hammen C, Burge D, Burney E, Adrian C. Longitudinal study of diagnoses in children of women with unipolar and bipolar affective disorder. Arch Gen Psychiatry. 1990;47(12):1112–7.
16. Krishnan V, Nestler EJ. The molecular neurobiology of depression. Nature. 2008;455(7215):894–902.
17. Kendler KS, Walters EE, Neale MC, Kessler RC, Heath AC, Eaves LJ. The structure of the genetic and environmental risk factors for six major psychiatric disorders in women. Phobia, generalized anxiety disorder, panic disorder, bulimia, major depression, and alcoholism. Arch Gen Psychiatry. 1995;52(5):374–83.
18. Holmes SJ, Robins LN. The influence of childhood disciplinary experience on the development of alcoholism and depression. J Child Psychol Psychiatry. 1987;28(3):399–415.
19. Magarinos AM, Deslandes A, McEwen BS. Effects of antidepressants and benzodiazepine treatments on the dendritic structure of CA3 pyramidal neurons after chronic stress. Eur J Pharmacol. 1999;371(2–3):113–22.
20. Kaufman J, Plotsky PM, Nemeroff CB, Charney DS. Effects of early adverse experiences on brain structure and function: clinical implications. Biol Psychiatry. 2000;48(8):778–90.
21. Lopez JF, Akil H, Watson SJ. Neural circuits mediating stress. Biol Psychiatry. 1999;46(11):1461–71.
22. Duman RS, Charney DS. Cell atrophy and loss in major depression. Biol Psychiatry. 1999;45(9):1083–4.
23. Duman RS, Malberg J, Nakagawa S, D'Sa C. Neuronal plasticity and survival in mood disorders. Biol Psychiatry. 2000;48(8):732–9.
24. Malberg JE, Eisch AJ, Nestler EJ, Duman RS. Chronic antidepressant treatment increases neurogenesis in adult rat hippocampus. J Neurosci. 2000;20(24):9104–10.
25. Rajkowska G. Postmortem studies in mood disorders indicate altered numbers of neurons and glial cells. Biol Psychiatry. 2000;48(8):766–77.
26. Sheline YI. 3D MRI studies of neuroanatomic changes in unipolar major depression: the role of stress and medical comorbidity. Biol Psychiatry. 2000;48(8):791–800.
27. Mayberg HS, Liotti M, Brannan SK, McGinnis S, Mahurin RK, Jerabek PA, et al. Reciprocal limbic-cortical function and negative mood: converging PET findings in depression and normal sadness. Am J Psychiatry. 1999;156(5):675–82.

28. Drevets WC, Price JL, Simpson JR, Jr., Todd RD, Reich T, Vannier M, et al. Subgenual prefrontal cortex abnormalities in mood disorders. Nature. 1997;386(6627):824–7.
29. Siegle GJ, Thompson W, Carter CS, Steinhauer SR, Thase ME. Increased amygdala and decreased dorsolateral prefrontal BOLD responses in unipolar depression: related and independent features. Biol Psychiatry. 2007;61(2):198–209.
30. Matthews SC, Strigo IA, Simmons AN, Yang TT, Paulus MP. Decreased functional coupling of the amygdala and supragenual cingulate is related to increased depression in unmedicated individuals with current major depressive disorder. J Affect Disord. 2008;111(1):13–20.
31. Mayberg HS, Lozano AM, Voon V, McNeely HE, Seminowicz D, Hamani C, et al. Deep brain stimulation for treatment-resistant depression. Neuron. 2005;45(5):651–60.
32. Bewernick BH, Hurlemann R, Matusch A, Kayser S, Grubert C, Hadrysiewicz B, et al. Nucleus accumbens deep brain stimulation decreases ratings of depression and anxiety in treatment-resistant depression. Biol Psychiatry. 2010;67(2):110–6.
33. Drevets WC, Price JL, Furey ML. Brain structural and functional abnormalities in mood disorders: implications for neurocircuitry models of depression. Brain Struct Funct. 2008; 213(1–2):93–118.
34. Hauger RL, Risbrough V, Brauns O, Dautzenberg FM. Corticotropin releasing factor (CRF) receptor signaling in the central nervous system: new molecular targets. CNS Neurol Disord Drug Targets. 2006;5(4):453–79.
35. Owens MJ, Nemeroff CB. Physiology and pharmacology of corticotropin-releasing factor. Pharmacol Rev. 1991;43(4):425–73.
36. Koenig JI. Pituitary gland: neuropeptides, neurotransmitters and growth factors. Toxicol Pathol. 1989;17(2):256–65.
37. Francis DD, Caldji C, Champagne F, Plotsky PM, Meaney MJ. The role of corticotropin-releasing factor – norepinephrine systems in mediating the effects of early experience on the development of behavioral and endocrine responses to stress. Biol Psychiatry. 1999;46(9):1153–66.
38. McAllister-Williams RH, Ferrier IN, Young AH. Mood and neuropsychological function in depression: the role of corticosteroids and serotonin. Psychol Med. 1998;28(3):573–84.
39. Jezova D, Ochedalski T, Glickman M, Kiss A, Aguilera G. Central corticotropin-releasing hormone receptors modulate hypothalamic-pituitary-adrenocortical and sympathoadrenal activity during stress. Neuroscience. 1999;94(3):797–802.
40. Sachar EJ, Hellman L, Roffwarg HP, Halpern FS, Fukushima DK, Gallagher TF. Disrupted 24-hour patterns of cortisol secretion in psychotic depression. Arch Gen Psychiatry. 1973;28(1):19–24.
41. Carroll BJ. Use of the dexamethasone suppression test in depression. J Clin Psychiatry. 1982;43(11 Pt 2):44–50.
42. Carroll BJ, Curtis GC, Mendels J. Neuroendocrine regulation in depression. II. Discrimination of depressed from nondepressed patients. Arch Gen Psychiatry. 1976;33(9):1051–8.
43. Arana GW, Baldessarini RJ, Ornsteen M. The dexamethasone suppression test for diagnosis and prognosis in psychiatry. Commentary and review. Arch Gen Psychiatry. 1985;42(12):1193–204.
44. Nathan KI, Musselman DL, Schatzberg AS, Nemeroff CB. Biology of mood disorders. In: Schatzberg AF, Nemeroff CB, editors. The American Psychiatric Press Textbook of Psychopharmacology. Washington, DC: The American Psychiatric Press; 1995. p. 439–78.
45. Nemeroff CB, Widerlov E, Bissette G, Walleus H, Karlsson I, Eklund K, et al. Elevated concentrations of CSF corticotropin-releasing factor-like immunoreactivity in depressed patients. Science. 1984;226(4680):1342–4.
46. Gold MS, Pottash AL, Extein I. "Symptomless" autoimmune thyroiditis in depression. Psychiatry Res. 1982;6(3):261–9.
47. Gold PW, Loriaux DL, Roy A, Kling MA, Calabrese JR, Kellner CH, et al. Responses to corticotropin-releasing hormone in the hypercortisolism of depression and Cushing's disease. Pathophysiologic and diagnostic implications. N Engl J Med. 1986;314(21):1329–35.

48. Luo X, Kiss A, Rabadan-Diehl C, Aguilera G. Regulation of hypothalamic and pituitary corticotropin-releasing hormone receptor messenger ribonucleic acid by adrenalectomy and glucocorticoids. Endocrinology. 1995;136(9):3877–83.
49. Kant GJ, Leu JR, Anderson SM, Mougey EH. Effects of chronic stress on plasma corticosterone, ACTH and prolactin. Physiol Behav. 1987;40(6):775–9.
50. Irwin J, Ahluwalia P, Zacharko RM, Anisman H. Central norepinephrine and plasma corticosterone following acute and chronic stressors: influence of social isolation and handling. Pharmacol Biochem Behav. 1986;24(4):1151–4.
51. Stanton ME, Gutierrez YR, Levine S. Maternal deprivation potentiates pituitary-adrenal stress responses in infant rats. Behav Neurosci. 1988;102(5):692–700.
52. Levine S, Atha K, Wiener SG. Early experience effects on the development of fear in the squirrel monkey. Behav Neural Biol. 1993;60(3):225–33.
53. McEwen BS. Protective and damaging effects of stress mediators: central role of the brain. Prog Brain Res. 2000;122:25–34.
54. Lopez JF, Chalmers DT, Little KY, Watson SJ. A.E. Bennett Research Award. Regulation of serotonin1A, glucocorticoid, and mineralocorticoid receptor in rat and human hippocampus: implications for the neurobiology of depression. Biol Psychiatry. 1998; 43(8):547–73.
55. Purba JS, Hoogendijk WJ, Hofman MA, Swaab DF. Increased number of vasopressin- and oxytocin-expressing neurons in the paraventricular nucleus of the hypothalamus in depression. Arch Gen Psychiatry. 1996;53(2):137–43.
56. Raadsheer FC, van Heerikhuize JJ, Lucassen PJ, Hoogendijk WJ, Tilders FJ, Swaab DF. Corticotropin-releasing hormone mRNA levels in the paraventricular nucleus of patients with Alzheimer's disease and depression. Am J Psychiatry. 1995;152(9):1372–6.
57. Sheline YI, Wang PW, Gado MH, Csernansky JG, Vannier MW. Hippocampal atrophy in recurrent major depression. Proc Natl Acad Sci U S A. 1996;93(9):3908–13.
58. MacQueen GM, Campbell S, McEwen BS, Macdonald K, Amano S, Joffe RT, et al. Course of illness, hippocampal function, and hippocampal volume in major depression. Proc Natl Acad Sci U S A. 2003;100(3):1387–92.
59. Sapolsky RM, Krey LC, McEwen BS. Prolonged glucocorticoid exposure reduces hippocampal neuron number: implications for aging. J Neurosci. 1985;5(5):1222–7.
60. Bremner JD. Does stress damage the brain? Biol Psychiatry. 1999;45(7):797–805.
61. Ohgoh M, Kimura M, Ogura H, Katayama K, Nishizawa Y. Apoptotic cell death of cultured cerebral cortical neurons induced by withdrawal of astroglial trophic support. Exp Neurol. 1998;149(1):51–63.
62. Gould E, Tanapat P. Stress and hippocampal neurogenesis. Biol Psychiatry. 1999;46(11): 1472–9.
63. Eriksson PS, Perfilieva E, Bjork-Eriksson T, Alborn AM, Nordborg C, Peterson DA, et al. Neurogenesis in the adult human hippocampus. Nat Med. 1998;4(11):1313–7.
64. Sahay A, Hen R. Adult hippocampal neurogenesis in depression. Nat Neurosci. 2007;10(9):1110–5.
65. Alexopoulos GS, Young RC, Meyers BS, Abrams RC, Shamoian CA. Late-onset depression. Psychiatr Clin North Am. 1988;11(1):101–15.
66. Koenderink MJ, Uylings HB, Mrzljak L. Postnatal maturation of the layer III pyramidal neurons in the human prefrontal cortex: a quantitative Golgi analysis. Brain Res. 1994; 653(1–2):173–82.
67. Young LT. Postreceptor pathways for signal transduction in depression and bipolar disorder. J Psychiatry Neurosci. 2001;26(Suppl):S17–22.
68. Uno H, Tarara R, Else JG, Suleman MA, Sapolsky RM. Hippocampal damage associated with prolonged and fatal stress in primates. J Neurosci. 1989;9(5):1705–11.
69. Watanabe Y, Gould E, McEwen BS. Stress induces atrophy of apical dendrites of hippocampal CA3 pyramidal neurons. Brain Res. 1992;588(2):341–5.
70. Endo Y, Nishimura JI, Kobayashi S, Kimura F. Chronic stress exposure influences local cerebral blood flow in the rat hippocampus. Neuroscience. 1999;93(2):551–5.

71. Sapolsky RM, Krey LC, McEwen BS. The neuroendocrinology of stress and aging: the glucocorticoid cascade hypothesis. Endocr Rev. 1986;7(3):284–301.
72. Sapolsky RM, Uno H, Rebert CS, Finch CE. Hippocampal damage associated with prolonged glucocorticoid exposure in primates. J Neurosci. 1990;10(9):2897–902.
73. Woolley CS, Gould E, McEwen BS. Exposure to excess glucocorticoids alters dendritic morphology of adult hippocampal pyramidal neurons. Brain Res. 1990;531(1–2):225–31.
74. Starkman MN, Gebarski SS, Berent S, Schteingart DE. Hippocampal formation volume, memory dysfunction, and cortisol levels in patients with Cushing's syndrome. Biol Psychiatry. 1992;32(9):756–65.
75. Bremner JD, Narayan M, Anderson ER, Staib LH, Miller HL, Charney DS. Hippocampal volume reduction in major depression. Am J Psychiatry. 2000;157(1):115–8.
76. Herman JP, Schafer MK, Young EA, Thompson R, Douglass J, Akil H, et al. Evidence for hippocampal regulation of neuroendocrine neurons of the hypothalamo-pituitary-adrenocortical axis. J Neurosci. 1989;9(9):3072–82.
77. Feldman S, Conforti N. Participation of the dorsal hippocampus in the glucocorticoid feedback effect on adrenocortical activity. Neuroendocrinology. 1980;30(1):52–5.
78. Shah PJ, Ebmeier KP, Glabus MF, Goodwin GM. Cortical grey matter reductions associated with treatment-resistant chronic unipolar depression. Controlled magnetic resonance imaging study. Br J Psychiatry. 1998;172:527–32.
79. McAllister AK, Katz LC, Lo DC. Neurotrophins and synaptic plasticity. Annu Rev Neurosci. 1999;22:295–318.
80. Smith MA, Makino S, Kvetnansky R, Post RM. Stress and glucocorticoids affect the expression of brain-derived neurotrophic factor and neurotrophin-3 mRNAs in the hippocampus. J Neurosci. 1995;15(3 Pt 1):1768–77.
81. Hashimoto K. Brain derived neurotrophic factor as a biomarker for mood disorders: an historical overview and future directions. Psychiatry Clin Neurosci. 2010;64:341–57.
82. Shirayama Y, Chen AC, Nakagawa S, Russell DS, Duman RS. Brain-derived neurotrophic factor produces antidepressant effects in behavioral models of depression. J Neurosci. 2002;22(8):3251–61.
83. Dowlatshahi D, MacQueen GM, Wang JF, Young LT. Increased temporal cortex CREB concentrations and antidepressant treatment in major depression. Lancet. 1998; 352(9142):1754–5.
84. Nibuya M, Nestler EJ, Duman RS. Chronic antidepressant administration increases the expression of cAMP response element binding protein (CREB) in rat hippocampus. J Neurosci. 1996;16(7):2365–72.
85. Bayer TA, Schramm M, Feldmann N, Knable MB, Falkai P. Antidepressant drug exposure is associated with mRNA levels of tyrosine receptor kinase B in major depressive disorder. Prog Neuropsychopharmacol Biol Psychiatry. 2000;24(6):881–8.
86. Palmer TD, Takahashi J, Gage FH. The adult rat hippocampus contains primordial neural stem cells. Mol Cell Neurosci. 1997;8(6):389–404.
87. Sulser F. The role of CREB and other transcription factors in the pharmacotherapy and etiology of depression. Ann Med. 2002;34(5):348–56.
88. Holsboer F. Current theories on the pathophysiology of mood disorders. In: Montgomery SA, Halbreich U, editors. Pharmacology for Mood, Anxiety, and Cognitive Disorders. Washington, DC: The American Psychiatric Press; 2000. p. 13–35.
89. Prange AJ, Loosen PT, Wilson IC. The therapeutic use of hormones of the thyroid axis in depression. In: Post RM, Ballenger JC, editors. Neurobiology of Mood Disorders, Frontiers of Clinical Neuroscience. New York: Marcel Dekker; 1990. p. 311–20.
90. Bauer MS, Whybrow PC, Winokur A. Rapid cycling bipolar affective disorder. I. Association with grade I hypothyroidism. Arch Gen Psychiatry. 1990;47(5):427–32.
91. Mendlewicz J, Linkowski P, Kerkhofs M, Desmedt D, Golstein J, Copinschi G, et al. Diurnal hypersecretion of growth hormone in depression. J Clin Endocrinol Metab. 1985;60(3):505–12.

92. Powell LH, Lovallo WR, Matthews KA, Meyer P, Midgley AR, Baum A, et al. Physiologic markers of chronic stress in premenopausal, middle-aged women. Psychosom Med. 2002;64(3):502–9.
93. Siever LJ, Uhde TW, Jimerson DC, Lake CR, Silberman ER, Post RM, et al. Differential inhibitory noradrenergic responses to clonidine in 25 depressed patients and 25 normal control subjects. Am J Psychiatry. 1984;141(6):733–41.
94. Amsterdam JD, Maislin G, Skolnick B, Berwish N, Winokur A. Multiple hormone responses to clonidine administration in depressed patients and healthy volunteers. Biol Psychiatry. 1989;26(3):265–78.
95. Laakmann G, Hinz A, Voderholzer U, Daffner C, Muller OA, Neuhauser H, et al. The influence of psychotropic drugs and releasing hormones on anterior pituitary hormone secretion in healthy subjects and depressed patients. Pharmacopsychiatry. 1990;23(1):18–26.
96. Agren H, Mefford IN, Rudorfer MV, Linnoila M, Potter WZ. Interacting neurotransmitter systems. A non-experimental approach to the 5HIAA-HVA correlation in human CSF. J Psychiatr Res. 1986;20(3):175–93.
97. Rubinow DR, Gold PW, Post RM, Ballenger JC, Cowdry R, Bollinger J, et al. CSF somatostatin in affective illness. Arch Gen Psychiatry. 1983;40(4):409–12.
98. Siever LJ, Davis KL. Overview: toward a dysregulation hypothesis of depression. Am J Psychiatry. 1985;142(9):1017–31.
99. Mitchell P, Smythe G. Hormonal responses to fenfluramine in depressed and control subjects. J Affect Disord. 1990;19(1):43–51.
100. O'Keane V, Dinan TG. Prolactin and cortisol responses to D-fenfluramine in major depression: evidence for diminished responsivity of central serotonergic function. Am J Psychiatry. 1991;148(8):1009–15.
101. Price LH, Charney DS, Delgado PL, Heninger GR. Serotonin function and depression: neuroendocrine and mood responses to intravenous L-tryptophan in depressed patients and healthy comparison subjects. Am J Psychiatry. 1991;148(11):1518–25.
102. Golden RN, Hsiao JK, Lane E, Ekstrom D, Rogers S, Hicks R, et al. Abnormal neuroendocrine responsivity to acute i.v. clomipramine challenge in depressed patients. Psychiatry Res. 1990;31(1):39–47.
103. Golden RN, Ekstrom D, Brown TM, Ruegg R, Evans DL, Haggerty JJ, Jr., et al. Neuroendocrine effects of intravenous clomipramine in depressed patients and healthy subjects. Am J Psychiatry. 1992;149(9):1168–75.
104. Kripke DF. Critical interval hypotheses for depression. Chronobiol Int. 1984;1(1):73–80.
105. Lewy AJ. Circadian phase sleep and mood disorders. In: David KL, Charney DS, Coyle JT, Nemeroff CB, editors. Neuropsychopharmacology, The Fifth Generation of Progress. New York: Lippincott Williams & Wilkins; 2002. p. 1879–93.
106. Petitto JM, Folds JD, Ozer H, Quade D, Evans DL. Abnormal diurnal variation in circulating natural killer cell phenotypes and cytotoxic activity in major depression. Am J Psychiatry. 1992;149(5):694–6.
107. Binneman B, Feltner D, Kolluri S, Shi Y, Qiu R, Stiger T. A 6-week randomized, placebo-controlled trial of CP-316,311 (a selective CRH1 antagonist) in the treatment of major depression. Am J Psychiatry. 2008;165(5):617–20.
108. Schildkraut JJ. The catecholamine hypothesis of affective disorders: a review of supporting evidence. Am J Psychiatry. 1965;122(5):509–22.
109. Blier P, de Montigny C. Clarifications on the effects of 5-HT1A agonists and selective 5-HT reuptake inhibitors on the 5-HT system. Neuropsychopharmacology. 1996;15(2):213–6.
110. Artigas F, Romero L, de Montigny C, Blier P. Acceleration of the effect of selected antidepressant drugs in major depression by 5-HT1A antagonists. Trends Neurosci. 1996;19(9):378–83.
111. Levine LR, Potter WZ. The 5HT1A receptor: an unkept promise? Curr Opin CNS Invest Drugs. 1999;1:448–52.
112. Griffith R, Sutin J. Reactive astrocyte formation in vivo is regulated by noradrenergic axons. J Comp Neurol. 1996;371(3):362–75.

113. Marek GJ. A novel approach to the identification of psychiatric drugs; serotonin-glutamate interactions in the prefrontal cortex. CNS Drug Rev. 2000;6:206–18.
114. Baker KG, Halliday GM, Hornung JP, Geffen LB, Cotton RG, Tork I. Distribution, morphology and number of monoamine-synthesizing and substance P-containing neurons in the human dorsal raphe nucleus. Neuroscience. 1991;42(3):757–75.
115. Steinberg R, Alonso R, Griebel G, Bert L, Jung M, Oury-Donat F, et al. Selective blockade of neurokinin-2 receptors produces antidepressant-like effects associated with reduced corticotropin-releasing factor function. J Pharmacol Exp Ther. 2001;299(2):449–58.
116. Delgado PL, Price LH, Miller HL, Salomon RM, Aghajanian GK, Heninger GR, et al. Serotonin and the neurobiology of depression. Effects of tryptophan depletion in drug-free depressed patients. Arch Gen Psychiatry. 1994;51(11):865–74.
117. Nishizawa S, Benkelfat C, Young S. Differences between male and female in rates of serotonin synthesis in human brain. Proc Natl Acad Sci U S A. 1997;94:5308–13.
118. Ellis PM, Salmud C. Is platelet imipramine binding reduced in depression? A meta-analysis. Biol Psychiatry. 1994;36:292–9.
119. Stockmeier CA, Dilley GE, Shapiro LA, Overholser JC, Thompson PA, Meltzer HY. Serotonin receptors in suicide victims with major depression. Neuropsychopharmacology. 1997;16(2):162–73.
120. Staley KJ, Longacher M, Bains JS, Yee A. Presynaptic modulation of CA3 network activity. Nat Neurosci. 1998;1(3):201–9.
121. Fujita M, Charney DS, Innis RB. Imaging serotonergic neurotransmission in depression: hippocampal pathophysiology may mirror global brain alterations. Biol Psychiatry. 2000;48(8):801–12.
122. Linnoila VM, Virkkunen M. Aggression, suicidality, and serotonin. J Clin Psychiatry. 1992;53(Suppl):46–51.
123. Ramboz S, Oosting R, Amara DA, Kung HF, Blier P, Mendelsohn M, et al. Serotonin receptor 1A knockout: an animal model of anxiety-related disorder. Proc Natl Acad Sci USA. 1998;95(24):14476–81.
124. Julius D. Serotonin receptor knockouts: a moody subject. Proc Natl Acad Sci USA. 1998;95(26):15153–4.
125. Heisler LK, Chu HM, Brennan TJ, Danao JA, Bajwa P, Parsons LH, et al. Elevated anxiety and antidepressant-like responses in serotonin 5-HT1A receptor mutant mice. Proc Natl Acad Sci U S A. 1998;95(25):15049–54.
126. Miller HL, Delgado PL, Salomon RM, Heninger GR, Charney DS. Effects of alpha-methyl-para-tyrosine (AMPT) in drug-free depressed patients. Neuropsychopharmacology. 1996;14(3):151–7.
127. Woodward DJ, Moises HC, Waterhouse BD, Hoffer BJ, Freedman R. Modulatory actions of norepinephrine in the central nervous system. Fed Proc. 1979;38(7):2109–16.
128. Aston-Jones G. Norepinephrine. In: David K, Charney DS, Coyle JT, Nemeroff CB, editors. The Fifth Generation of Progress. New York: Lippincott Williams & Wilkins; 2002. p. 47–58.
129. Abercrombie ED, Jacobs BL. Single-unit response of noradrenergic neurons in the locus coeruleus of freely moving cats. I. Acutely presented stressful and nonstressful stimuli. J Neurosci. 1987;7(9):2837–43.
130. Hellhammer DH, Hingtgen JN, Wade SE, Shea PA, Aprison MH. Serotonergic changes in specific areas of rat brain associated with activity – stress gastric lesions. Psychosom Med. 1983;45(2):115–22.
131. Lehnert H, Reinstein DK, Strowbridge BW, Wurtman RJ. Neurochemical and behavioral consequences of acute, uncontrollable stress: effects of dietary tyrosine. Brain Res. 1984;303(2):215–23.
132. Rosenblatt S, Chanley JD, Leighton WP. The investigation of adrenergic metabolism with 7H3-norepinephrine in psychiatric disorders. II. Temporal changes in the distribution of urinary tritiated metabolites in affective disorders. J Psychiatr Res. 1969;6(4):321–33.
133. Potter WZ, Manji HK. Catecholamines in depression: an update. Clin Chem. 1994; 40(2):279–87.

134. Nibuya M, Morinobu S, Duman RS. Regulation of BDNF and TrkB mRNA in rat brain by chronic electroconvulsive seizure and antidepressant drug treatments. J Neurosci. 1995;15(11):7539–47.
135. Vaidya VA, Marek GJ, Aghajanian GK, Duman RS. 5-HT2A receptor-mediated regulation of brain-derived neurotrophic factor mRNA in the hippocampus and the neocortex. J Neurosci. 1997;17(8):2785–95.
136. Rajkowska G. Histopathology of the prefrontal cortex in major depression: what does it tell us about dysfunctional monoaminergic circuits? Prog Brain Res. 2000;126:397–412.
137. Manier DH, Shelton RC, Sulser F. Noradrenergic antidepressants: does chronic treatment increase or decrease nuclear CREB-P? J Neural Transm. 2002;109(1):91–9.
138. Osman O, Potter W. Potentiation of dopamine in the treatment of refractory depression. In: Amsterdam JD, editor. Advances in Neuropsychiatry and Psychopharmacology: Refractory Depression. New York: Raven; 1991. p. 41–52.
139. Wilner P. Dopaminergic mechanisms in depression and mania. In: Bloom F, Kupfer D, editors. Psychopharmacology: The Fourth Generation of Progress. New York: Raven; 1995. p. 921–31.
140. Rush AJ, Ryan N. Current and emerging therpeutics for depression. In: Davis K, Harney D, Coyle J, Nemeroff CB, editors. Neuropsychopharmacology: The Fifth Generation of Progress. Philadelphia, PA: Lippincott Williams & Wilkins; 2002. p. 1081–95.
141. Garlow S, Musselman D, Nemreoff C. The neurochemistry of mood disorders: clinical studies. In: Davison R, Post R, editors. Neurobiology of Mental Illness. New York: Oxford Press; 1999. p. 348–64.
142. Roy A, Pickar D, Douillet P, Karoum F, Linnoila M. Urinary monoamines and monoamine metabolites in subtypes of unipolar depressive disorder and normal controls. Psychol Med. 1986;16(3):541–6.
143. Reddy PL, Khanna S, Subhash MN, Channabasavanna SM, Rao BS. CSF amine metabolites in depression. Biol Psychiatry. 1992;31(2):112–8.
144. D'Haenen H A, Bossuyt A. Dopamine D2 receptors in depression measured with single photon emission computed tomography. Biol Psychiatry. 1994;35(2):128–32.
145. Ebert D, Feistel H, Loew T, Pirner A. Dopamine and depression – striatal dopamine D2 receptor SPECT before and after antidepressant therapy. Psychopharmacology (Berl). 1996;126(1):91–4.
146. Larish R, Klimke A, Vosberg H, Gaebel W, Mueller-Gaertner HW. Cingulate function in depression. Neuroreport. 1997;8(15):i–ii.
147. Klimek V, Schenck JE, Han H, Stockmeier CA, Ordway GA. Dopaminergic abnormalities in amygdaloid nuclei in major depression: a postmortem study. Biol Psychiatry. 2002; 52(7):740–8.
148. Wong DT, Bymaster FP. Dual serotonin and noradrenaline uptake inhibitor class of antidepressants potential for greater efficacy or just hype? Prog Drug Res. 2002;58:169–222.
149. Lindley SE, Bengoechea TG, Schatzberg AF, Wong DL. Glucocorticoid effects on mesotelencephalic dopamine neurotransmission. Neuropsychopharmacology. 1999;21(3): 399–407.
150. Lyons DM, Lopez JM, Yang C, Schatzberg AF. Stress-level cortisol treatment impairs inhibitory control of behavior in monkeys. J Neurosci. 2000;20(20):7816–21.
151. Dowlati Y, Herrmann N, Swardfager W, Liu H, Sham L, Reim EK, et al. A meta-analysis of cytokines in major depression. Biol Psychiatry. 2010;67(5):446–57.
152. Baune BT, Dannlowski U, Domschke K, Janssen DG, Jordan MA, Ohrmann P, et al. The interleukin 1 beta (IL1B) gene is associated with failure to achieve remission and impaired emotion processing in major depression. Biol Psychiatry. 2010;67(6):543–9.
153. Mantyh PW, Hunt SP, Maggio JE. Substance P receptors: localization by light microscopic autoradiography in rat brain using [3H]SP as the radioligand. Brain Res. 1984;307(1–2):147–65.
154. Arai H, Emson PC. Regional distribution of neuropeptide K and other tachykinins (neurokinin A, neurokinin B and substance P) in rat central nervous system. Brain Res. 1986;399(2):240–9.

155. Hokfrlt T, Johansson O, Holets VR, Meister B, Melander T. Distribution of neuropeptides with special reference to their coexistence with clasical transmitters. In: Meltzer H, editor. Psychopharmacology: The Third Generation of Progress. New York: Raven Press; 1987. p. 401–16.
156. Chang HM, Wang L, Zhang XP, Kream RM, Yeh ET. Modulation of substance P release in primary sensory neurons by misoprostol and prostaglandins. Am J Ther. 1996;3(4):276–9.
157. Huang SM, Bisogno T, Trevisani M, Al-Hayani A, De Petrocellis L, Fezza F, et al. An endogenous capsaicin-like substance with high potency at recombinant and native vanilloid VR1 receptors. Proc Natl Acad Sci U S A. 2002;99(12):8400–5.
158. Haddjeri N, Blier P. Sustained blockade of neurokinin-1 receptors enhances serotonin neurotransmission. Biol Psychiatry. 2001;50(3):191–9.
159. Liu R, Ding Y, Aghajanian GK. Neurokinins activate local glutamatergic inputs to serotonergic neurons of the dorsal raphe nucleus. Neuropsychopharmacology. 2002;27(3):329–40.
160. Millan MJ, Lejeune F, De Nanteuil G, Gobert A. Selective blockade of neurokinin (NK) (1) receptors facilitates the activity of adrenergic pathways projecting to frontal cortex and dorsal hippocampus in rats. J Neurochem. 2001;76(6):1949–54.
161. File SE. Anxiolytic action of a neurokinin 1 receptor antagonist in the social interaction test. Pharmacol Biochem Behav. 1997;58(3):747–52.
162. Kramer MS, Cutler N, Feighner J, Shrivastava R, Carman J, Sramek JJ, et al. Distinct mechanism for antidepressant activity by blockade of central substance P receptors. Science. 1998;281(5383):1640–5.
163. Rupniak NM, Carlson EC, Harrison T, Oates B, Seward E, Owen S, et al. Pharmacological blockade or genetic deletion of substance P (NK(1)) receptors attenuates neonatal vocalisation in guinea-pigs and mice. Neuropharmacology. 2000;39(8):1413–21.
164. Takayama H, Ota Z, Ogawa N. Effect of immobilization stress on neuropeptides and their receptors in rat central nervous system. Regul Pept. 1986;15(3):239–48.
165. Bannon MJ, Deutch AY, Tam SY, Zamir N, Eskay RL, Lee JM, et al. Mild footshock stress dissociates substance P from substance K and dynorphin from Met- and Leu-enkephalin. Brain Res. 1986;381(2):393–6.
166. Walsh DM, Stratton SC, Harvey FJ, Beresford IJ, Hagan RM. The anxiolytic-like activity of GR159897, a non-peptide NK2 receptor antagonist, in rodent and primate models of anxiety. Psychopharmacology (Berl). 1995;121(2):186–91.
167. Keller M, Montgomery S, Ball W, Morrison M, Snavely D, Liu G, et al. Lack of efficacy of the substance p (neurokinin1 receptor) antagonist aprepitant in the treatment of major depressive disorder. Biol Psychiatry. 2006;59(3):216–23.
168. Sapolsky RM. The possibility of neurotoxicity in the hippocampus in major depression: a primer on neuron death. Biol Psychiatry. 2000;48(8):755–65.
169. Nowak G, Ordway GA, Paul IA. Alterations in the *N*-methyl-D-aspartate (NMDA) receptor complex in the frontal cortex of suicide victims. Brain Res. 1995;675(1–2):157–64.
170. Paul IA, Nowak G, Layer RT, Popik P, Skolnick P. Adaptation of the *N*-methyl-D-aspartate receptor complex following chronic antidepressant treatments. J Pharmacol Exp Ther. 1994;269(1):95–102.
171. Skolnick P, Miller R, Young A, Boje K, Trullas R. Chronic treatment with 1-aminocyclopropanecarboxylic acid desensitizes behavioral responses to compounds acting at the *N*-methyl-D-aspartate receptor complex. Psychopharmacology (Berl). 1992;107(4):489–96.
172. Berman RM, Cappiello A, Anand A, Oren DA, Heninger GR, Charney DS, et al. Antidepressant effects of ketamine in depressed patients. Biol Psychiatry. 2000;47(4):351–4.
173. Rogoz Z, Skuza G, Maj J, Danysz W. Synergistic effect of uncompetitive NMDA receptor antagonists and antidepressant drugs in the forced swimming test in rats. Neuropharmacology. 2002;42(8):1024–30.
174. Zarate CA, Jr., Singh JB, Carlson PJ, Brutsche NE, Ameli R, Luckenbaugh DA, et al. A randomized trial of an *N*-methyl-D-aspartate antagonist in treatment-resistant major depression. Arch Gen Psychiatry. 2006;63(8):856–64.

175. Yates M, Leake A, Candy JM, Fairbairn AF, McKeith IG, Ferrier IN. 5HT2 receptor changes in major depression. Biol Psychiatry. 1990;27(5):489–96.
176. Delgado PL, Miller HL, Salomon RM, Licinio J, Krystal JH, Moreno FA, et al. Tryptophan-depletion challenge in depressed patients treated with desipramine or fluoxetine: implications for the role of serotonin in the mechanism of antidepressant action. Biol Psychiatry. 1999;46(2):212–20.
177. Shiffer HH. Glutamate receptor genes: susceptibility factors in schizophrenia and depressive patients. Mol Biol. 2002;25:191–212.
178. Petty F. GABA and mood disorders: a brief review and hypothesis. J Affect Disord. 1995;34(4):275–81.
179. Lloyd KG, Thuret F, Pilc A. Upregulation of gamma-aminobutyric acid (GABA) B binding sites in rat frontal cortex: a common action of repeated administration of different classes of antidepressants and electroshock. J Pharmacol Exp Ther. 1985;235(1):191–9.
180. Kimber JR, Cross JA, Horton RW. Benzodiazepine and GABAA receptors in rat brain following chronic antidepressant drug administration. Biochem Pharmacol. 1987;36(23):4173–5.
181. Liu R, Jolas T, Aghajanian G. Serotonin 5-HT(2) receptors activate local GABA inhibitory inputs to serotonergic neurons of the dorsal raphe nucleus. Brain Res. 2000;873(1):34–45.
182. Stoll AL, Rueter S. Treatment augmentation with opiates in severe and refractory major depression. Am J Psychiatry. 1999;156(12):2017.
183. Akbarian S, Rios M, Liu RJ, Gold SJ, Fong HF, Zeiler S, et al. Brain-derived neurotrophic factor is essential for opiate-induced plasticity of noradrenergic neurons. J Neurosci. 2002;22(10):4153–62.
184. Sher L. The placebo effect on mood and behavior: the role of the endogenous opioid system. Med Hypotheses. 1997;48(4):347–9.
185. Amanzio M, Pollo A, Maggi G, Benedetti F. Response variability to analgesics: a role for non-specific activation of endogenous opioids. Pain. 2001;90(3):205–15.
186. Cardinali DP. The human body circadian: how the biologic clock influences sleep and emotion. Neuro Endocrinol Lett. 2000;21(1):9–15.
187. Bunney WE, Bunney BG. Molecular clock genes in man and lower animals: possible implications for circadian abnormalities in depression. Neuropsychopharmacology. 2000;22(4):335–45.
188. Lewy AJ, Bauer VK, Cutler NL, Sack RL, Ahmed S, Thomas KH, et al. Morning vs evening light treatment of patients with winter depression. Arch Gen Psychiatry. 1998;55(10):890–6.
189. Nofzinger EA, Price JC, Meltzer CC, Buysse DJ, Villemagne VL, Miewald JM, et al. Towards a neurobiology of dysfunctional arousal in depression: the relationship between beta EEG power and regional cerebral glucose metabolism during NREM sleep. Psychiatry Res. 2000;98(2):71–91.
190. Nofzinger EA, Mintun MA, Wiseman M, Kupfer DJ, Moore RY. Forebrain activation in REM sleep: an FDG PET study. Brain Res. 1997;770(1–2):192–201.
191. Clark CP, Frank LR, Brown GG. Sleep deprivation, EEG, and functional MRI in depression: preliminary results. Neuropsychopharmacology. 2001;25(5 Suppl):S79–84.
192. Vgontzas AN, Chrousos GP. Sleep, the hypothalamic-pituitary-adrenal axis, and cytokines: multiple interactions and disturbances in sleep disorders. Endocrinol Metab Clin North Am. 2002;31(1):15–36.
193. Benca RM, Obermeyer WH, Thisted RA, Gillin JC. Sleep and psychiatric disorders. A meta-analysis. Arch Gen Psychiatry. 1992;49(8):651–68; discussion 69–70.
194. Simon GE, VonKorff M, Piccinelli M, Fullerton C, Ormel J. An international study of the relation between somatic symptoms and depression. N Engl J Med. 1999;341(18):1329–35.
195. Stahl SM. Does depression hurt? J Clin Psychiatry. 2002;63(4):273–4.
196. Goldstein DJ, Lu Y, Detke MJ, Wiltse C, Mallinckrodt C, Demitrack MA. Duloxetine in the treatment of depression: a double-blind placebo-controlled comparison with paroxetine. J Clin Psychopharmacol. 2004;24(4):389–99.
197. Petrovic P, Ingvar M. Imaging cognitive modulation of pain processing. Pain. 2002; 95(1–2):1–5.

198. Yu J, Smith GP. Affinity maturation of phage-displayed peptide ligands. Methods Enzymol. 1996;267:3–27.
199. Gamaro GD, Manoli LP, Torres IL, Silveira R, Dalmaz C. Effects of chronic variate stress on feeding behavior and on monoamine levels in different rat brain structures. Neurochem Int. 2003;42(2):107–14.
200. Kalra SP, Dube MG, Pu S, Xu B, Horvath TL, Kalra PS. Interacting appetite-regulating pathways in the hypothalamic regulation of body weight. Endocr Rev. 1999;20(1):68–100.
201. Danish University Antidepressant Group. Paroxetine: a selective serotonin reuptake inhibitor showing better tolerance, but weaker antidepressant effect than clomipramine in a controlled multicenter study. J Affect Disord. 1990;18(4):289–99.
202. Nelson JC, Mazure CM, Bowers MB, Jr., Jatlow PI. A preliminary, open study of the combination of fluoxetine and desipramine for rapid treatment of major depression. Arch Gen Psychiatry. 1991;48(4):303–7.
203. Entsuah AR, Huang H, Thase ME. Response and remission rates in different subpopulations with major depressive disorder administered venlafaxine, selective serotonin reuptake inhibitors, or placebo. J Clin Psychiatry. 2001;62(11):869–77.
204. Malhi GS, Moore J, McGuffin P. The genetics of major depressive disorder. Curr Psychiatry Rep. 2000;2(2):165–9.
205. Yamada M, Higuchi T. Functional genomics and depression research. Beyond the monoamine hypothesis. Eur Neuropsychopharmacol. 2002;12(3):235–44.

Clinical Pharmacology and Therapeutics of Antidepressants

Domenic A. Ciraulo, Richard I. Shader, and David J. Greenblatt

Introduction

An understanding of the clinical pharmacology of antidepressant agents is essential to optimal prescribing. The following chapter outlines general principles that influence prescribing, and then discusses specific subgroups of antidepressants. There is no generally accepted classification scheme for antidepressants, and current groupings reflect marketing, the history of development, and pharmacologic effects. We use the following terminology in our discussion: selective serotonin reuptake inhibitors (SSRIs), tricyclic antidepressants (TCAs), cyclic antidepressants, mixed action agents, selective norepinephrine reuptake inhibitors (SNRIs), monoamine oxidase inhibitors (MAOIs), and alternative (non-traditional) antidepressants. Readers should keep in mind that there is no classification scheme that accurately reflects the actions of all the drug classes, and we have chosen a compromise classification system that is based on terms commonly used in clinical settings.

General Principles

Pharmacokinetics and Pharmacodynamics

There are several concepts that clinicians must be familiar with to understand the importance of different pharmacological characteristics among various antidepressants. These are broadly divided into pharmacokinetic and pharmacodynamic properties. Pharmacokinetics refers to drug absorption, distribution, and elimination. Pharmacodynamics refers to actions at the receptor and the cascade of events that follow.

D.A. Ciraulo (✉)
Department of Psychiatry, Boston University School of Medicine,
720 Harrison Avenue, Suite 914, Boston, MA, USA
e-mail: dciraulo@bu.edu

D.A. Ciraulo and R.I. Shader (eds.), *Pharmacotherapy of Depression*,
DOI 10.1007/978-1-60327-435-7_2,

Some examples of the important clinical pharmacokinetic considerations in prescribing involve the presence of active metabolites, how long it takes for a drug to reach steady state, or how quickly it is eliminated. Drugs that are slowly eliminated, or have long-acting metabolites, may present less of a problem if a patient misses a dose and are less likely to be associated with a discontinuation syndrome. On the other hand, if toxicity or drug–drug interactions develop with such drugs, symptoms will persist after drug administration has ceased.

The clinical importance of pharmacodynamics is illustrated by receptor actions that influence therapeutic response and adverse effect profile. Clinicians should be cautious about using in vitro binding studies to make inferences about clinical effects; however, in many cases, there is a good correlation between binding and adverse effects. The relative potencies at the receptors that mediate antidepressant response provide a rationale for choosing medications, especially when faced with a poor response to initial therapy. Table 1 presents receptor binding data of commonly used antidepressants.

Table 1 Relative potencies at transporters

	Relative potencies		
	Serotonin transporters	Norepinephrine transporters	Dopamine transporters
Nefazodone	++	++	–
Hydroxynefazodone	+	+	–
Triazole-dione	–	–	–
mCPP	++	+	–
Trazodone	++	–	–
Amitriptyline	+++	++	–
Desipramine	++	++++	–
Paroxetine	++++	++	–
Sertraline	++++	+	±
Citalopram	++++	–	–
Fluoxetine	+++	+	–
Fluvoxamine	+++	+	–
Venlafaxine	++	+	±
Desmethylvenlafaxine	++	+	–
Chloroimipramine	ND	++++	–
Nortriptyline	++	+++	–
Imipramine	+++	++	–
Norfluoxetine	+++	+	–
Desmethylsertraline	++	+	–

Metabolites are italicized

– none; ± uncertain; +, ++, +++, ++++ weak, mild, moderate, strong; *ND* not determined

Pharmacogenetics

Genetics influences both the metabolism and receptor effects of antidepressants. Genetic influences on metabolism are most important for antidepressants that have a low therapeutic index. Tricyclic antidepressants, for example, may cause toxic anticholinergic, cardiac, and CNS effects at plasma levels that are only two times therapeutic levels. Four different levels of CYP2D6 activity have been identified, and some leading laboratories now report seven levels from ultra rapid to poor (for a review see (1)). The clinical literature suggests that approximately 7–10% of Caucasians are slow metabolizers through CYP2D6 and toxic levels of imipramine, desipramine, and other agents metabolized via this pathway may result from standard therapeutic doses. Poor metabolizers of drugs that utilize the CYP2C19 may also develop adverse effects at standard doses. Although the SSRI have a large therapeutic index, so that most patients are able to tolerate wide fluctuations in plasma levels due to pharmacokinetic interactions, several are potent inhibitors of the CYP450 system (fluoxetine, fluvoxamine, paroxetine) and can affect toxicity of coadministered drugs that are metabolized via this system.

The activity level of specific cythochromes is determined both by genetics and by drug inhibition of their function. In the instance of genetic determinants, there is great variability in the allele frequencies among seemingly homogeneous populations with a history of migrations, isolation, and other factors. Although some centers advise genotyping all patients receiving antidepressants, we believe that if the usual dosing guidelines are followed, therapeutic levels can be achieved and toxicity avoided. Plasma levels are a reasonable, lest costly alternative to genotyping at this time. On the other hand, genotyping may be appropriate for drugs that have a low therapeutic index, drugs that are associated with serious toxicity at levels close to therapeutic level, or high-risk patients, for whom high levels may be dangerous. For non-responders, it seems easier to examine plasma or serum levels to determine if adequate doses are being prescribed.

P-glycoprotein is a transmembrane transporter protein that has several functions, one of which is to transport xenobiotics out of the brain across the blood–brain barrier against a concentration gradient (2). Genetic variants of the gene encoding for P-glycoprotein (MDR1 or ABCB1 gene) may influence brain concentrations of several antidepressants, including citalopram, sertraline, venlafaxine, amitriptyline, nortriptyline, doxepin, and trimipramine, but not mirtazapine, fluoxetine, or bupropion. It is also located in intestinal epithelial cells, hepatocytes, and proximal tubular epithelial cells of the kidney. In most cases, pharmacogenetic testing is not required; however, in treatment-resistant depressions, these analyses may be helpful. Uhr et al. (3) reported that polymorphisms of ABCB1 were associated with outcome for citalopram, venlafaxine, and paroxetine. Drugs that are substrates of P-glycoprotein have higher rates of antidepressant response with these polymorphisms, suggesting that there is decreased efficiency of the transporter that removes drugs from the brain. One research group has suggested that antidepressants that inhibit P-glycoprotein increase cortisol in the brain, resulting in increased glucocorticoid-mediated negative feedback on the HPA axis, and normalization of the glucocorticoid receptor resistance associated with major depression (4, 5).

Pharmacodynamic genetic studies have focused on hypothesis-driven approaches to genes encoding for receptors thought to be the target of antidepressants or altered in major depressive disorders. The most extensively studied gene is SLC6A4, which encodes for the serotonin transporter. Most studies have focused on a functional polymorphism in the 5 promoter region (5-HTTLPR). This polymorphism produces a short (S) allele and a long (L) allele (although rare long and extra long alleles have been reported in Asians and African Americans). There are a number of other variants reported, but for the purposes of drug response, we can focus on the S and L alleles, which have been linked to basal activity of the transporter and response to antidepressants. Although findings differ, the majority of studies show a poor response to SSRI in individuals with the S allele compared to LL subjects. The STAR*D study was able to replicate this finding only in a White, non-Hispanic subgroup. Other studies have found that the LL group responds better to placebo and sleep deprivation compared to the S allele group. At this time, genetic subtyping of the SLC6A4 gene is not clinically useful.

As described in chapter "Biological Theories of Depression and Implications for Current and New Treatments," substantial evidence suggests that overactivity of the HPA axis is a key neuropathological finding underlying unipolar major depression. Many authorities in the field believe that the core action of antidepressants is to normalize the HPA axis by reversing impaired activity of the glucocorticoid receptor. The genetic focus has been on FKBP5 which decreases binding affinity of the glucocorticoid receptor for cortisol. On the other hand, when FKBP4 replaces FKBP5, the receptor complex has high affinity for cortisol. Three polymorphisms in FKBP5 (rs 1360780, rs 4713916, and rs 3800373) have been associated with response to antidepressants (6). Homozygotes for the rare allele had a more rapid response to antidepressants (10 days earlier) than the other two genotypes. Perhaps most importantly, it was not limited to treatment with any specific antidepressant (2). Some support for these findings comes from the STAR*D study (7, 8), in which weak associations were found between rs 4713916 and response in a subgroup of the population identified as White, non-Hispanic. Other studies have found weaker associations than the original report (9) and the GENDEP study (10) with a cohort of 760 did not replicate the finding, nor did smaller Spanish and Korean studies (11, 12). The same alleles associated with a rapid antidepressant response are risk alleles for major depression, bipolar disorder, and PTSD. As explained by Horstmann and Binder (2), these alleles result in glucocorticoid receptor insensitivity by inducing FKBP5 mRNA and increased FKBP5, which in turn leads to prolonged elevated cortisol in response to stress (6, 13).

Given the central role of serotonin in the action of antidepressants, many studies have focused on genes coding for serotonin receptors. Promising findings come from studies of the HTR2A gene that codes for the 5-HT_{2A} receptor. The initial studies focused on two SNPs: (1) 102T/C, rs 6313 in exon 1 and (2) 1438 A/G, rs 6311 in the promoter region. While many have found an association between these SNPs and antidepressant response, many other larger studies could not replicate the finding. Other variants of this gene have been associated with positive antidepressant response. STAR*D found that rs 7997012 was the only SNP associated with citalopram response (14, 15). When combined with a SNP located within the glutamate receptor inotropic kainite 4 (GRIK4) gene, namely rs 1954787, encoding for a high affinity kainite receptor improves prediction of response. Homozygotes for both GRIK4 and HTR2A alleles were 23% less likely to be non-responders compared to subjects not carrying these alleles. Similar other studies have found that a single SNP accounts for less than 3% of the variance, but when the investigators combined their three strongest predictors: 5HTR2A, GRIK4, and FKBP5 SNPs, thirteen percent of the variance was explained (16). Still other variants of the 5HTR2A gene may be associated with antidepressant response (10, 17). Using a genomewide association pharmacogenomic approach to antidepressant response, Ising et al. (18) did not find any single SNP predicted response. However, when individuals were characterized by the binary variable of high versus low number of response alleles, the model predicted antidepressant response. Patients with comorbid anxiety and a low number of response alleles had the worst outcomes. Research on pharmacogentics is advancing rapidly; however, at the present time, routine use in clinical practice is premature.

Practical Aspects of Treatment

Prior to initiation of antidepressant treatment, clinicians should be confident that a medical condition, medication therapy, or substance use disorder is not the primary cause of depressed mood (see Tables 2 and 3). Some medical conditions, such as hypothyroidism, are so common that patients should be routinely screened. Others, such as diabetes, anemia, and vitamin deficiencies (folate, B12), are less common, but easily tested, and also should be ruled out. Some medical illnesses are common but more difficult to diagnose, such as autoimmune disorders, fibromyalgia, and chronic pain syndromes; fortunately, mood symptoms associated with these disorders often respond to antidepressants. Cushing's syndrome and polycystic ovary disease are commonly associated with mood disorders. Neurological conditions associated with depression include Parkinsonism, epilepsy, multiple sclerosis, cerebrovascular disease and stroke, dementia, and Huntington's disease. An association of depression and infectious disease is found with HIV and perhaps other viral illnesses. The association between depression and carcinoma is controversial, but if depression is the presenting complaint, there are usually symptoms that provide clues to the etiology (e.g., weight loss, pallor, fatigue that is worse in evening). In cases of depression associated with medical illness, treatment of the underlying disease is paramount, but antidepressants are often necessary. Superior efficacy for a particular antidepressant has not been established, so a reasonable approach is to use a medication that is unlikely to interact with drugs prescribed for the primary illness.

A meta-analysis found that mirtazapine, escitalopram, venlafaxine, and sertraline were more efficacious for MDD than duloxetine, fluvoxamine, paroxetine, and

Table 2 Medical illness with prominent psychiatric symptoms

Vitamin B deficiencies	Serum folate may be low in presence of normal tissue levels. RBC folate less subject to dietary changes. Clinically significant folate deficiency is associated with macrocytosis and megaloblastic anemia. Depressive symptoms associated with folate deficiency	Etiology is decreased dietary intake, alcoholism, pregnancy. Less common are malignancy, liver disease, hemolytic disorders	Testing requires levels of folate, B12. Also, in folate deficiency, homocysteine levels are elevated and methylmalonic acid levels normal. In B12 deficiency, both homocysteine and methylmalonic acid are elevated
Diabetes mellitus	Routine screening in depressed patients with risk factors is recommended. Fasting blood glucose over 120, hypertension, obesity, polycystic ovary disease, acute coronary syndrome, high triglycerides, low HDL-C. Classic symptoms of polyuria, polydipsia, polyphagia, weight loss, paresthesias, yeast infections, blurred vision	Genetic predisposition, high caloric intake, low energy expenditure. Secondary causes are ingestion of glucocorticoids, atypical antipsychotics, diseases that decrease insulin sensitivity (Cushing's, pheochromocytoma, acromegaly)	Fasting plasma glucose of 126 mg/dl or greater on two occasions. Random glucose greater than 200 mg/dl with symptoms of diabetes, HbA1c of 6.5% or higher
Thyroid disease	Hypothyroidism: weakness, fatigue, lethargy, cold intolerance, dry skin, decreased sweating, headache, edema, impaired cognition, depression, weight gain, paresthesias, arthralgias, muscle cramps, constipation	Hashimoto's thyroiditis, iodine deficiency, pituitary damage, irradiation, drugs (lithium, glucocorticoids, L-dopa, dopamine, iodide, sulfonylureas, phenylbutazone, phenytoin, salicylates, propylthiouracil, propranolol, amiodarone)	Measure free T3 and free T4 in serum (decreased in hypothyroidism). TSH increased in hypothyroidism. TSH-immunometric assay distinguishes between normal and reduced levels of TSH. Persistent high TSH after treatment may indicate pituitary adenoma. Consider Hashimoto's thyroiditis and Grave's disease (thyroid microsomal antibodies present in both 95 and 55%, respectively). Thyroglobulin antibodies with 60% of Hashimoto patients. Graves disease has antibodies against TSH receptor

Fibromyalgia	Chronic diffuse pain in muscles and joints, multifocal and migratory, stiffness, poor sleep, daytime lethargy, cognitive dysfunction, depression, anxiety, dizziness	Genetic contribution, altered serotonin function, toxins, HPA axis hyperactivity, more common in women	Labs to rule out other disorders (hypothyroidism, rheumatoid arthritis, systemic lupus erythematosis, etc)
Cushing's syndrome	Typical pattern of weight gain, purple stretch marks, skin thinning, easy bruising, proximal muscle weakness, in women menstrual irregularities, in men loss of libido and impotence, hypertension, diabetes mellitus, osteoporosis, depression, emotional lability, cognitive impairment	Exogenous steroid administration, pituitary adenoma, adrenal adenoma, oat cell or small cell carcinoma of lung. Carcinoid tumors	Urinary free cortisol, serum and salivary cortisol, dexamethasone-CRH test
Polycystic ovary disease	Depression, menstrual abnormalities, infertility, hyperandrogenism (excess hair in male pattern, acne, enlarged clitoris), obesity, acanthosis nigricans, diabetes mellitus, sleep apnea	Abnormalities in regulation of androgens and estrogens	Labs to rule out acromegaly, thyroid disease, Cushing's, and hyperprolactinemia
Pituitary adenomas	May produce a variety of psychiatric symptoms depending on hormones involved. If large may have mass effects. Symptoms may include those associated with thyroid disease, elevated prolactin levels, Cushing syndrome, somatotropin (acromegaly)	Diagnosed by hormone levels of LH, FSH, estradiol, adrenocorticotropin, cortisol, growth hormone, testosterone, prolactin, thyrotropin, thyroxine, insulin-like growth factor-1, and α subunit glycoprotein. Challenge tests are also used (e.g., TRH challenge and others)	Treatment usually surgical with adjunctive medication

(continued)

Table 2 (continued)

Multiple sclerosis	Multiple sclerosis May be relapsing and remitting or progressive. Weakness of limbs, optic neuritis, sensory defects, cognitive decline. T1 hypointensities, brain, spinal cord atrophy, fatigue cognitive slowing, depression, central vertigo, nystagmus, urinary incontinence, bipolar, dementia, high suicide rate	Diagnosis: elevated IgG in plasma cells and CSF. Elevated IgG index, T2 hyperintensities in white matter, inflammation and degeneration of gray matter and cortical atrophy-associated potentials, visual and somatosensory-evoked potentials, histology indicating perivascular infiltration of inflammatory cells, but other findings common. Expression of HLA, interferon γ, IL-12, B7 molecules increased early in disease	Treatment: β interferons and drug treatment of associated symptoms (e.g., for depression, spasticity, tremors, fatigue, etc)
Parkinson's disease	Early symptoms: daytime sleepiness, constipation, loss of smell. REM behavior disorder. Motor signs begin with asymmetrical resting tremor in upper extremity, progresses to clumsiness in hand, bradykinesia, rigidity, gait disturbance. Tremors may progress to lower extremities, tongue, lips. Dementia late	Diagnosis is clinical. No characteristic laboratory. PET scans show decrease of labeled dopa in putamen	Treatment includes selegiline, rasagiline (MAO-B inhibitors) are used early in disease. Dopamine prodrugs are primary agents (levodopa/carbidopa); other agents include dopamine agonists, anticholinergics, NMDA inhibitors, COMT inhibitors.Surgical intervention is deep brain stimulation
Dementia	All types may have prominent depressive symptoms and may be difficult to distinguish from severe depression with neurovegetative signs		
Epilepsy	Depression is common co-morbidity		

Porphyria	Porphyria, acute intermittent: abdominal pain, psychiatric symptoms—depression is common, motor neuropathies (can mimic Guillain–Barre' syndrome)	Caused by genetic impaired functioning of porphobilinogen-deaminase and exposure to substances that increase heme synthesis (e.g., estrogens, barbiturates, sulfonamides, alcohol (see websiteU of Queensland) Diagnosed by urine porphyrin elevation (especially coporphobilinogen, some labs do not routinely include porphobilinogen and must be specifically ordered—this is the sine qua non of AIP, if porphobilinogen is not elevated AIP diagnosis eliminated. During attack may have hyponatremia, SIADH	Other types of porphyria: (1) CHESTER: Genetic etiology with symptoms of AIP but reduction in activity of both porphobilinogen deaminase (as in AIP) and protoporphyrinogen. This subtype does not have cutaneous symptoms or photosensitivity. Labs indicate increased urine for porphyrins. May be confirmed by genetic testing. (2) Hereditary coproporphyria: Prominent psychiatric symptoms that mimic depression, mania, psychotic disorders, delirium seizures, peripheral neuropathy. Severe abdominal pain that is colicky in nature and lasts for several days, constipation, vomiting. Blisters develop in sun-exposed areas, and may lead to scarring. May have excessive hair growth in sun-exposed areas. Diagnosed by clinical features and elevated stool coproporphyrins 10–20 times above normal, urine levels may also be elevated. (3) ALA dehydratase deficiency
Huntington's disease	Usually choreiform movement are initial presentation, with dementia and psychiatric symptoms appearing late	Genetic etiology	
Systemic lupus erythematosis	Fatigue, fever, arthralgia, malar rash, discoid rash, photosensitivity, alopecia, renal disease (50% clinically significant)seizures, psychosis, delirium, depression, optic neuropathy, cognitive deficits	Diagnosed by clinical presentation and laboratory ENA panel, consisting of ANA titers, Anti-dsDNA, complement, Anti-Sm. Anti-SSA, Anti-SSB, Anti-ribosomal P, Anti-RNP, Anticardiolipin, Inflammatory markers, and others	

(continued)

Table 2 (continued)

Mixed connective tissue disease	Arthralgia, arthritis, edema of hands, Raynaud's phenomenon, myositis, esophageal hypomotility, rash, leucopenia, pulmonary hypertension, pleuritis, pericarditis. Depression and anxiety common	Laboratory shows high-titer speckled pattern fluorescent antinuclear antiboidy (FANA) may be present, not specific; High levels of anti-RNP antibodies and anti-U1-70 kd small nuclear ribonucleoprotein	NSAIDS, corticosteroids, plaquenil, cyclophosphamide, and symptomatic treatment
Fibromyalgia	Depression, anxiety, fatigue, and sleep disturbance present in most cases. Other symptoms include increased pain sensitivity, mainly in muscles, joints, but which include entire body. Pain is described as burning, of severe intensity, and may be migratory. The patient's complaint of having "pain all over" is often dismissed by inexperienced clinicians as hypochondriasis. Complaints of pain vary considerably and may include headache, pelvic pain, chest pain, dyspepsia, jaw pain, abdominal pain, and irritable bowel syndrome. Women often have urinary frequency and urgency. Syncope and shortness of breath may also be present. Cognitive function is impaired, especially memory	There is a genetic component to fibromyalgia, and studies have focused on SNP's of COMT, β-2-adrenergic receptor genes, and the serotonin transporter gene. HPA axis dysfunction and cytokine inflammatory factors have been implicated in the etiology of the illness	Antidepressants, such as duloxetine (Cymbalta), Milnacipram (Savella), and amitriptyline have been used with some success. Dosages required are not the same as antidepressant doses. Anticonvulsants, such as pregabalin (Lyrica) and gabapentin (Neurontin), are also helpful. Other agents include sedative hypnotics, muscle relaxants, and clonidine

Table 3 Drugs used for medical conditions that may induce depression

Medications	Comment
β-adrenergic blockers	In 1967, a letter to the British Medical Journal reported a case series of 89 patients treated with propranolol, of whom 30% developed depression. Two of these patients committed suicide (396). Subsequent pharmacoepidemiologic and meta-analyses studying patients on many different agents in the class have found no difference in depression compared to placebo (397). The likelihood of depression is highest for propranolol, which is lipophilic and readily enters the brain. Depression is most likely in individuals with a history of depression and occurred at dosage increases. Dose reduction or discontinuation results in resolution of depression (398). Lipophilic agents in this class may present greatest risk (propranolol, carvedilol, bucindolol)
ACE inhibitors	No direct evidence implicating ACE inhibitors in depression. Relationship based solely on a study that found antidepressant prescriptions higher in patients treated with ACE inhibitors than controls. Clinical experience does not support depression induced by this class of agents
Angiotensin II blockers	Case reports of depression, psychosis, and delirium associated with valsartan and losartan. There is insufficient evidence to establish this adverse reaction; however, clinicians should be aware of a potential psychiatric adverse effect
Calcium channel blockers	Case reports have implicated nifedipine, diltiazem, and verapamil in drug-induced depression. Larger studies did not confirm this (399), although one did report the risk of suicide was 1.1 suicides per 1,000 person-years, higher than other cardiovascular agents (400). We believe evidence supporting this adverse event is weak
Diuretics	Thiazides are not associated with depression, although neuropsychiatric symptoms may develop in the context of hypernatremia and hypercalcemia. Furosemide is not associated with new onset depression, but long-term use leads to thiamine deficiency and Wernicke's syndrome. Acetazolamide, a carbonic anhydrase inhibitor, can produce, fatigue, malaise, lethargy, and delirium most likely related to drug-induced acidosis
Corticosteroids	Clinical experience is extensive. There is substantial variability among patients, but depression, hypomania, mania, paranoia, psychosis. Risk factors unknown
Leukotriene inhibitors	Montelukast-induced depression recognized by WHO and FDA. May be associated with aggressive behavior, agitation. Abnormal dreams, hallucinations, insomnia, suicidal ideation, and suicide. Risk not known at present time
Inteferons	α Interferons induce depression in about 30% of patients. β Interferons have a much lower likelihood of causing depression, but are not without risk
Varenicline	There is a substantial risk of new onset suicidal ideation and depression within days to 6 weeks of starting treatment (there are insufficient data to establish the true period of risk). Anxiety and abnormal dreams also possible
Levonorgestrol (norplant)	One of the most common reasons for discontinuation of drug is onset of depression. Major depression usually develops within 1–3 months of starting the drug and resolves 1–2 months after the implant is removed
Isoretinoin	There is an established relationship between the drug and new onset of depression and suicide. FDA warning
Finasteride	Men treated for alopecia may develop moderate to severe depression with an onset during the first few months of therapy. Mechanism may be reduction in neurosteroid allopregnanolone

reboxetine (19). Escitalopram and sertraline demonstrated the best acceptability, suggesting that these agents may be the best initial treatments for major depression, although interpretation of the results is confounded by the absence of data on dose, duration, patient adherence, and other methodological problems.

Once the diagnosis of a primary depression is established, it is important to consider the following subtypes: unipolar, bipolar, psychotic features, melancholia (some prefer the term "endogenous"), retarded, agitated, anxious, and atypical depressions. As will be described in various sections below, many (but certainly not all) studies indicate that these subtypes predict response to different antidepressants. Anxious depression, co-morbid substance abuse, and chronic severe depressions are less responsive to pharmacotherapy than first-episode depressions.

A controversial meta-analysis suggests that the greatest benefit from antidepressant treatment occurs in the most severe depressions (20), although other studies and clinical experience suggest that moderate depression also responds to antidepressants (21, 22). Therefore, in clinical practice, the decision to start an antidepressant depends not only on severity but also on chronicity and resistance to behavioral treatments. Despite the aforementioned meta-analysis, superior efficacy of a particular antidepressant has not been established, and the selection of an antidepressant for initial treatment is based on avoiding certain adverse effects and taking advantage of others. For example, in depressed patients with insomnia, a sedating antidepressant is helpful, but daytime administration should be avoided. Similarly, highly anticholinergic agents would be a poor first choice in an elderly patient because of the potential for urinary retention and memory problems. With the exceptions of citalopram, escitalopram, and sertraline, many of the SSRIs produce clinically significant inhibition of cytochrome P450 enzymes, and are usually not the first choice in patients who are taking other prescribed medications that are metabolized by this system. In the reality of clinical practice, the choice of a specific agent or combination of drugs is restricted by algorithms developed by formulary committees, decisions that are based primarily on comparative cost of agents with established efficacy.

Once an antidepressant is selected, a trial of adequate doses for at least 8–12 weeks is recommended (23). Many experienced psychopharmacologists believe that if a partial response is not achieved by 3 weeks, a change in drug should be instituted. The goal of treatment is a complete remission, although many patients will have only partial response of their symptoms. When a partial response is observed during this time period, dosage adjustments or augmentation with other agents is recommended. If the patient can tolerate an increase in dose, this is the most straightforward approach and is supported by clinical studies (24). An alternative strategy is to use another medication in combination with the antidepressant to achieve full remission. The usual strategies in partial or non-responders are to increase dose, augmentation with another medication, or switch to another agent. There is no evidence that establishes the superiority of any one of these approaches.

Although there was an intriguing finding in the STAR*D trial, suggesting that in non-responders augmentation response rates were higher than response rates to switching drugs, a valid comparison cannot be made because of bias inherent in the study design. The specific problem with the design was that a subject's decision to switch or augment after failure of citalopram treatment was not randomized. Several atypical antipsychotics, including olanzapine, aripiprazole, and quetiapine are FDA approved for augmentation of partial antidepressant response, and a combination product of olanzapine/fluoxetine (Symbyax) is marketed for treatment-resistant depression and depressive episodes associated with Bipolar I disorder.

Once full response is achieved, continuation therapy is based on the natural course of depression. On average, the course of an untreated depression is about 1 year, after which 40% of patients achieve spontaneous recovery, 40% stay depressed, and 20% have dysthymia (25). Some clinicians find it useful to describe three treatment phases, an acute phase of 6–12 weeks with the goal of full remission, a continuation phase that lasts up to a year, and a maintenance phase of 1 year or longer. For first episodes of unipolar major depression, treatment of the episode is continued for at least 1 year. In cases of recurrent depressions, severe single episodes, onset of the first episode before the age of 20 years, and a family history of serious depression, antidepressant therapy may continue indefinitely. Even with successful treatment, the risk of recurrence of major depression is substantial. It has been estimated at 50% after one episode, 70% after two episodes, and 90% after three episodes (25). Fifty percent of patients with a major depression will experience only one episode, while 30% become chronically depressed, and 20% have a recurrent episodic course.

There are two commonly used terms to describe improvement during antidepressant treatment: *response* and *remission*. Response is defined as a 50% or greater reduction from baseline score on a standardized depression scale (most commonly Hamilton Depression Scale (HDRS), the Montgomery Asberg Depression Rating Scale (MADRS), or the Quick Inventory of Depressive Symptomatology (QIDS)). Remission is defined as achieving a specific score on one of these scales. For example, commonly used scores indicating remission are a score of 7 or lower on the HDRS-17, a score of 10 or lower on the MADRS (7, 8), or a score of 5 or lower on the QIDS 16. The STAR*D study, which simulated typical clinical practice, reported a remission rate of about 30% with citalopram treatment. Approximately half of these remissions occurred within 6 weeks of beginning the drug (26). The response rate (50% reduction on the QIDS-SR16) was 47%. Predictors of poor response were mixed anxiety and depression, melancholic or atypical features, poor quality of life, lower socio-economic level, and minority status. Distinguishing response and remission has clinical implications. Patients who achieve full remission are less likely to relapse than responders. The responder group experiences longer periods of depression and greater impairment in social functioning over a 10-year follow-up period compared to patients who achieved full remission (27–29).

SSRIs

History

The first selective serotonin reuptake inhibitor (SSRI), fluoxetine, was introduced to the American market in 1988 (30). Other SSRIs, sertraline, paroxetine, and fluvoxamine, followed closely. Although widely used in Europe for some time, it was not until the late 1990s that another SSRI, citalopram, became available to American clinicians; and later, its enantiomer, escitalopram, was introduced. By the early 1990s, the SSRIs became first-line antidepressants in clinical practice and accounted for more than half of all antidepressant prescriptions. They enjoyed unprecedented marketing success (31), had great exposure in popular literature and news, and at first were thought to be orders of magnitude superior to already existing antidepressant drugs. Indeed, SSRI compounds have a more favorable side effect profile, simpler dosing strategies, better tolerability, and thus better adherence than older antidepressants. Their relative safety in overdose, minimal cardiovascular effects, and lower anticholinergic activity make them especially appealing as first-line agents.

As clinical experience with SSRIs has grown, it has become apparent that they have their own share of adverse effects. Also, the equivalence of SSRIs' efficacy to TCAs' has been challenged, and still remains a matter of some controversy. Even with these concerns, SSRIs are widely used and are effective in a wide range of psychiatric disorders other than depression, such as anxiety disorders, obsessive-compulsive disorder (OCD), panic disorder, bulimia nervosa, social phobia, post-traumatic stress disorder (PTSD), premenstrual dysphoric syndrome (PMDS), dysthymia, and seasonal affective disorder. SSRIs are the most widely prescribed antidepressants in America and worldwide (32).

Six SSRIs are available in the United States: *citalopram (Celexa)*, *escitalopram (Lexapro)*, *fluoxetine (Prozac)*, *fluvoxamine (Luvox)*, *paroxetine (Paxil)*, and *sertraline (Zoloft)*. All except fluvoxamine are approved by the U.S. Food and Drug Administration for use in depression; fluvoxamine is FDA approved for treatment of OCD but not depression (33). In Europe, however, fluvoxamine has been used as an antidepressant for many years (34). Table 4 lists the FDA-approved indications at the time of the writing of this chapter.

Pharmacokinetics

The pharmacokinetic properties and the cytochrome inhibiting properties of the SSRIs (with some comparison antidepressants) are shown in Tables 5 and 6. Of clinical importance is the fact that fluoxetine, paroxetine, and fluvoxamine do not exhibit linear kinetics or dose proportionality. That means that as the dose increases, there is not a proportional increase in plasma levels due to autoinduction of

Table 4 FDA-approved indications for commonly used antidepressants

Citalopram (Celexa)	MDD
Escitalopram (Lexapro)	MDD, GAD
Fluoxetine (Prozac)	MDD, OCD, bulimia nervosa, panic disorder with or without agoraphobia
Fluvoxamine (Luvox)	OCD
Paroxetine (Paxil CR)	MDD, OCD, panic disorder with or without AG, social anxiety disorder, GAD, PTSD
Sertraline (Zoloft)	MDD, acute and maintenance OCD. PD with or without agoraphobia PTSD. PMDD, social anxiety
VenlafaxineXR (Effexor XR)	MDD, GAD, social anxiety disorder, panic disorder with or without agoraphobia
Desvenlafaxine (Pristiq)	MDD
Mirtazapine (Remeron)	MDD
Bupropion (Wellbutrin)	MDD
Nefazodone	MDD
Trazodone	MDD with or without anxiety
Clomipramine (Anafranil)	OCD
Duloxetine (Cymbalta)	MDD, GAD, diabetic peripheral neuropathic pain, fibromyalgia
Milnacipram (Savella)	Fibromyalgia (not FDA approved for treatment of depression)
Selegeline (EMSAM)	MDD
Tranylcypromine (Parnate)	MDD without melancholia
Phenelzine (Nardil)	Depression characterized as atypical, nonendogenous, neurotic
Isocarboxazid (Marplan)	Major depression, especially with anxious mood, panic, and phobic symptoms

enzymes that metabolize these drugs. Citalopram, escitalopram, and sertraline differ in this regard, showing linear kinetics at the usual therapeutic doses.

Stereochemistry influences pharmacological activity and the pharmacokinetics of SSRIs. Fluoxetine and citalopram are racemic mixtures of the parent compound (30, 35). Although the S- and R-enantiomers of fluoxetine are approximately equivalent in their ability to inhibit serotonin reuptake, their metabolites, S- and R-norfluoxetine, respectively, are not. R-norfluoxetine is not active in terms of serotonin inhibition, while S-norfluoxetine is a more potent serotonin reuptake inhibitor than the parent drug (36). Furthermore, plasma levels of the S-enantiomer of norfluoxetine can be twice that of the R-enantiomer. S-norfluoxetine, but not R-norfluoxetine, is metabolized via cytochrome P450 2D6; therefore, individual variations in CYP 2D6 or drug interactions have the potential to affect clinical response. Paroxetine and sertraline are marketed as the most serotonergically potent forms of their two isomers. Citalopram's S-enantiomer, escitalopram, is the most active of citalopram's isomers and metabolites; it is a more potent and a more selective serotonin reuptake inhibitor than citalopram itself (37). These stereochemical differences may be one reason why it has been so difficult to establish therapeutic plasma concentrations for SSRIs, and could explain some interindividual differences in antidepressant response and adverse effects.

Another factor influencing the pharmacokinetics of antidepressants is the activity of membrane transport proteins. P-glycoprotein, a member of the ATP-binding

Table 5 Pharmacology of SSRIs

	Fluoxetine (Prozac®) (Sarafem®)	Fluvoxamine (Luvox®)	Paroxetine (Paxil CR®)	Sertraline (Zoloft®)	Citalopram (Celexa®)	Escitalopram (Lexapro®)
Time to peak plasma level after oral dose (h)	6–8	5	6–10	4.5–8.4	2–4	4–5
Protein binding (%)	94.5	77	93–95	98	50	56
Elimination half-life	Parent 1–3 days acute 4–6 days chronic metabolite 4–16 days (acute or chronic)	15 h	15–20 h	26 h (parent) 62–104 h (metabolite)	33 h	27–532 h (parent) 50–54 (metabolite)
Active metabolite	Norfluoxetine	No	No clinically important metabolites	Desmethyl-serrtaline (limited activity)	Desmethyl -citalopram	*S*-desmethyl citalopram. Not clinically important

Adapted with permission from Ciraulo et al. (401)

Table 6 Inhibition of human cytochromes P450 by selected antidepressants

Cytochrome P450 inhibition							
	1A2	2C9	2C19	2D6	2E1	3A	2B6
Fluoxetine	+	++	+ to ++	+++	–	+	+
Norfluoxetine	+	++	+ to ++	+++	–	++	0
Sertraline	+	+	+ to ++	+	–	+	+
Desmethyl-sertraline	+	+	+ to ++	+	–	+	0
Paroxetine	+	+	+	+++	–	+	+++
Fluvoxamine	+++	++	+++	+	–	+	+
Citalopram	+	0	0	0	0	0	0
Monodesmethyl-citalopram	0	0	0	+	0	0	0
Escitalopram	0	0	0	+	0	0	0
Nefazodone	0	0	0	0	–	+++	0
Triazole-dione	0	0	0	0	–	+	0
Hydroxy nefazodone	0	0	0	0	–	+++	0
Duloxetine	0	0	0	++	0	0	0
Venlafaxine	0	0	0	0/+	–	0	0
Desmethyl-venlafaxine	0	0	0	+	–	0	0
Mirtazapine	0	0	0	0	0	0	0
Bupropion	0	0	0	++	0	0	+

Adapted with permission from Greenblatt et al. (402)
Metabolites are italicized
0 Minimal or zero inhibition; +, ++, +++ mild, moderate, or strong inhibition; *Dash (–)* indicates no data available

cassette family of membrane transport proteins, is an important functional component of the blood–brain barrier and the intestinal epithelial cells (38). Alterations in P-glycoprotein can thus affect drug entry into the brain as well as bioavailability. Some evidence indicates that paroxetine and venlafaxine may be P-glycoprotein substrates, while animal studies suggest that amitriptyline, fluoxetine, and norfluoxetine are not (39). With respect to inhibition of P-glycoprotein activity, sertraline and paroxetine have the potential to do so, but only at concentrations of 250–500-fold higher than found clinically. One study found citalopram brain concentrations higher in mice without P-glycoprotein activity (40). Nefazodone is an inhibitor of P-glycoprotein activity in clinically relevant doses (41). P-glycoprotein inhibition has been proposed as a possible therapeutic mechanism of antidepressants, not only allowing higher brain AD levels but also resulting in higher corticosteroid levels to counteract the insensitivity of the GR receptor.

Dosages (Table 7)

There is not a consensus on the optimal dosing of SSRIs. One authority has suggested that adequate trials of SSRIs would consist of at least 4-week treatment with sertraline, at least 100 mg daily, fluoxetine or paroxetine or citalopram, at least

Table 7 SSRI doses (33, 34)

SSRI	Dose range (mg/day)	Initial dose (333)	Usual range (333)	Available formulations
Citalopram	10–80	10–20	20–40	Tablets 20, 40 mg; oral solution 10 mg/5 ml
Escitalopram	10–20	10	10	Tablets 10, 20 mg
Fluoxetine	10–80	10–20	20–60	Capsules 10, 20, 40 mg[a]; tablets 10 mg; oral solution 20 mg/5 ml
Fluvoxamine	50–300	25–50	150–200	Tablets 25, 50, 100 mg
Paroxetine	10–50	10–20	20–40	Tablets 10, 20, 30, 40 mg; oral suspension 10 mg/5 ml
Sertraline	50–200	25–50	100–200	Tablets 25, 50, 100 mg; oral concentrate 20 mg/ml

[a]Fluoxetine is also available as a "Prozac Weekly." The formulation is a delayed release, enteric-coated capsule containing 90 mg; it was calculated to achieve a blood concentration equivalent to a standard daily dose of 10–20 mg. The formulation has been shown to be as effective an antidepressant as daily doses of 20 mg fluoxetine, with similar adverse effects and similar tolerability (403–405). Adherence to the dosing schedule for patients on Prozac Weekly is a bit higher than daily dosing: 87.5 and 79–85% patients on daily dosing, respectively, although the difference appears modest (403, 405, 406). Since fluoxetine and norfluoxetine have long elimination half-lives, occasional non-adherence or skipping a dose is rarely clinically significant with the standard formulation. Fluoxetine is also marketed as Sarafem for prementsrual dysphoric disorder. Administered daily or 14 days before menstruation and through first day of menses. Repeat each cycle

20 mg daily, or fluvoxamine, at least 100 mg daily (34). We would recommend higher doses and an 8-week trial although full remission may take 12 weeks or longer in some patients (42). In most patients, some improvement should occur after 2–3 weeks. If the depression severity remains unchanged by 4 weeks, it is unlikely that an additional 2–4 weeks of treatment with the same drug at the same dose will be successful. Unfortunately, plasma levels do not appear helpful in guiding dosage; therapeutic plasma levels have not been established for any SSRI.

Mechanism of Action

Prevailing theories on the mechanism of action of antidepressant agents center around their aminergic effects, despite recent data suggesting other mechanisms may be important (see chapter "Biological Theories of Depression and Implications for Current and New Treatments," this volume). All SSRIs, although differ structurally, have the same mechanisms of action: as the name implies, these compounds selectively inhibit the serotonin transporter (43). While the degree of selectivity varies depending on the in vitro model used, all agents are potent inhibitors of the serotonin reuptake transporter. In addition, paroxetine may have relatively greater inhibitory potential at the norepinephrine transporter, and sertraline at the dopamine transporter, based on in vitro studies, and fluoxetine may be a 5-HT_{2C} agonist, although the clinical implications of these differences are not established (44). Further complicating the matter is the presence of heteroreceptors, serotonin receptors that modulate activity via their location on non-serotonergic neurons, including GABA interneurons, and glutamate, dopamine, noradrenergic, and cholinergic neurons. Thus, there is great danger in assuming that in vitro binding studies will provide a reliable guide to clinical differences between SSRIs. As with other antidepressants, the onset of full antidepressant action of SSRI is usually delayed for weeks.

Acute administration of SSRIs inhibit the 5-HT reuptake pump (SERT) of the presynaptic serotonin neuron, resulting in an increased concentration of serotonin around the somatodendritic area of the neuron, and to a lesser degree in the synapse itself (45). Early effects on serotonin probably account for adverse effects, while therapeutic actions depend on subsequent neuronal events. It is only after some time of continuous SSRI administration (usually 2 or more weeks), the lasting high concentrations of 5-HT in the somatodendritic area of the neuron cause desensitization of the somatodendritic 5-HT_{1A} autoreceptors, which are responsible for inhibition of 5-HT release. The result is increased 5-HT in the synapse and desensitization of postsynaptic serotonin receptors. In addition, various SSRIs and other antidepressants have differing activities at serotonin receptor subtypes. The existence of serotonin receptor isoforms is also likely, further complicating our understanding of how these drugs exert their antidepressant effect. Downstream actions that affect signal transduction and gene expression are likely to be responsible for the actual therapeutic action and delayed onset, linking the aminergic changes to other mechanisms such as synthesis of brain-derived neurotrophic factor and other neuronal growth factors. In addition, the HPA axis and the serotonin system are functionally linked; serotonin stimulates CRH release which is mediated by 5-HT_2, 5-HT_{1A}, and 5-HT_{1C} receptors. As a result, the mechanism of action of SSRI may be to normalize activity of glucocorticoid receptors. Decreased function of glucocorticoid and/or mineralocorticoid receptors (GR, MR) has been linked to lower 5-HT_{2A} protein levels in the hippocampus, decreased 5-HT_{2A} receptor binding in frontal areas, and lower serotonergic innervations of frontal cortex in animal models. The role of serotonin receptor subtypes remains unclear, but activity of several subtypes is associated with neurogenesis in the limbic region. For example, agonists of the 5-HT_{1A} heteroreceptor increase neurogenesis in the sublenticular zone (SZ) and the subgranular zone of the dentate gyrus (SGL/DG), agonists of the 5-HT_{2A} are more selective, increasing growth only in the SGL/DG, while agonists of 5-HT_{2C} act on the SZ (46). Another study found that 5-HT_{1A} activation promotes the growth factor VEGF in the hippocampus, and that fluoxetine-induced neurogenesis can be blocked by 5-HT_{1A} antagonists (47).

A novel theory is that SSRIs increase brain levels of the neurosteroid, allopregnanolone, which enhances GABA function in the brain (48). Supporting this mechanism is the fact that depressed patients have low levels of CSF allopregnanolone, which normalize with treatment with fluoxetine and fluvoxamine and correlate with improvement assessed by the HDRS.

Some evidence suggests that a loss of SERT-binding sites occurs with long-term SSRI administration (49). This occurs only after 10–15 days of drug exposure, the time frame of antidepressant response. Recent theories have extended the mechanism of antidepressant response to signal transduction pathways. Under one such model, antidepressants are believed to decrease the activity of protein kinase C (PKC) which catalyzes phosphorylation, whereby they may directly affect the SERT and/or serotonin receptors. Other studies support a role for activation of protein kinase A and calcium calmodulin-dependent protein kinase II (CaMKII). PKA-mediated phosphorylation results in changes in neurotransmission and gene expression. CaMKII, also through the process of phosphorylation, may facilitate neurotransmitter activity. Phosphorylation of CREB influences gene expression, such as those for BDNF and its receptor trkB. Since BDNF is able to promote neurogenesis, it may reverse the neuronal atrophy in the brain, believed by some to be the fundamental pathology of depression.

Although there is not universal consensus on the role of the presynaptic 5-HT_{1A} receptor (the autoreceptor), it is believed that after a week or two of SSRI administration desensitization of this receptor must occur to turn of the feedback inhibition of serotonin release. Attempts to hasten or augment SSRI antidepressant response have been examined in studies with pindolol. Pindolol, a β-adrenergic blocker that also antagonizes the 5-HT_{1A} autoreceptor, has been extensively studied as a possible SSRI augmenting strategy (50–55). It has been hypothesized that pindolol used concomitantly with SSRIs blocks the presynaptic somatodendritic 5-HT_{1A} autoreceptors in the dorsal raphe nucleus more rapidly than an SSRI alone.

Clinical studies are contradictory, complicated by the variability among SSRIs in the potency of 5-HT_{1A} blockade, low doses of pindolol and study design differences. Doses of pindolol that have been used do not produce complete blockade of the receptor (56). In addition, genetic polymorphism of the 5-HT_{1A} receptor (57, 58) and the mixed enantiomer formulations of pindolol complicate interpretation of existing studies (59). In some studies, pindolol augmented the antidepressant effect of concomitantly administered SSRIs and shortened the time necessary for achieving a full therapeutic response (50, 51, 53, 60, 61). These findings have encouraged the study of antagonists of other serotonin receptors such as 5-$HT_{2A/C}$ that inhibit serotonin release. The ultimate goal would be to synthesize a compound that inhibited SERT and 5-$HT_{2A/C}$.

Attempts that have been made to link actions of SSRI on serotonin receptor subtype are interesting but in the early stages in clinical studies. Of importance is that we know that the antidepressants share some but not all of the actions at these receptor types. This could explain why switches within class of SSRI are often successful, and why there might be significant differences in clinical effects based on the postsynaptic receptor activity.

Receptor subtypes also contribute to adverse effects, e.g., 5-HT_3 to gastrointestinal discomfort, although the role of other subtypes remains uncertain. Generally, in vitro studies indicate that SSRIs have very low affinity for other neuroreceptors such as alpha, histaminic, and muscarinic receptors, which is consistent with their adverse effect profile (30, 43).

Paroxetine is the only SSRI antidepressant which has been shown to inhibit norepinephrine uptake. A study comparing norepinephrine and serotonin transporter function in human transporter transfected cells in serum from patients assigned to either desipramine or paroxetine (44) found that both drugs acted as mixed serotonin/norepinephrine uptake inhibitors, especially at doses of 40 mg or higher of paroxetine. Sertraline is the only SSRI to show dopamine reuptake inhibition in in vitro models. These data also support the notion that SSRIs are not homogeneous in their mechanisms of action.

Drug Interactions/P450 Metabolism

SSRIs are predominantly metabolized by the hepatic cytochrome P450 system and may inhibit their own metabolism or that of other drugs (Table 6). Among SSRIs, sertraline, citalopram, and escitalopram possess minimal interactions within the P450 system; this quality makes them the antidepressants of choice in medically ill patients requiring coadministration of other medications.

The inhibitory action of SSRIs may give rise to multiple drug–drug interactions with other medications; these interactions when the drugs are coadministered may lead to no effect, intoxication, or even improving a drug's therapeutic response via a rise in its plasma concentration. Generally, SSRIs that inhibit the CYP 450 systems will impair metabolism of other medications (P450 enzyme substrates), thus prolonging their elimination half-life and increasing their blood level. For example, the SSRI inhibition of cytochrome P450 activity may lead to elevated levels of concurrently administered TCAs which are metabolized by CYP 2D6 and 3A4 isoenzymes (62). This may lead to side effects, but it may also permit clinicians to use a low-dose TCA to augment or potentiate the SSRI. Citalopram does not alter TCA levels (62). On the other hand, fluvoxamine inhibits the CYP 1A2 isoenzyme and can produce toxic levels of medications that are usually metabolized by this isoenzyme, namely tacrine, warfarin, theophylline, propranolol, and many others.

Since SSRIs are also substrates for the hepatic cytochrome system, medications such as carbamazepine, rifampin, dexamethasone, which induce CYP 450 isoenzymes, accelerate SSRI metabolism if coadministered. Medications such as quinidine, cimetidine, and diltiazem inhibit CYP 450; they will delay SSRI clearance and may produce toxic levels of SSRI (34, 63, 64). Comprehensive lists of drug interactions with SSRI antidepressants can be accessed at http://www.drugfactsandcomparisons.com, *The Medical Letter: Adverse Drug Interactions Program*, or other computer databases (35, 63–67).

Adverse Effects

Overview

Although generally well tolerated, SSRIs may produce anxiety, sleep disturbances, and gastrointestinal discomfort, especially at the initiation of therapy. These can usually be managed by lowering the dose, slowing dose escalation, or temporarily treating the target symptom (e.g., ondansetron for nausea, lorazepam for insomnia). More troublesome and persistent are sexual adverse effects, including anorgasmia, decreased libido, ejaculation disturbances, and erectile dysfunction. Transient adverse effects are likely the result of acute stimulation of postsynaptic serotonin receptors; however, efforts to link these symptoms to specific receptor subtypes are speculative. Table 8 lists common adverse effects associated with SSRIs, and options for clinical management.

Table 8 Common adverse effects associated with SSRIs

Symptom	Approximate incidence in clinical practice	Management
Headache	Common initially, especially with fluoxetine	Dosage reduction, slow/stop dose increases, NSAIDS, or change to another antidepressant
Nervousness	Common initially, highest with fluoxetine, sertraline, but can occur with others	Dosage reduction, slow/stop dose increases, lorazepam, or change to another antidepressant
Insomnia	Less common with paroxetine	Dosage reduction, slow/stop dose increases, add lorazepam, "Z" drug hypnotic, or sedative antidepressant, or change to another antidepressant
Drowsiness	More common with paroxetine	Dosage reduction, slow/stop dose increases; some clinicians recommend temporary stimulant (methylphenidate) addition
Nausea	Common for all agents generally at initiation of therapy	Antiemetic agents (5-HT_3 blockers such as ondansetron are preferred by some clinicians) or mirtazapine
Sexual dysfunction	30–60%, paroxetine slightly higher than others, but difference probably not clinically significant	Dosage reduction, slow/stop dose increases, sildenafil (Viagra), or change to another antidepressant, bupropion
Anorexia	Only early in treatment	Time limited
Dizzy/lightheaded	5–10% fluoxetine at low end	Dosage reduction, slow/stop dose increases, or change to another antidepressant
Tremor	Common early in treatment for all agents	Dosage reduction, slow/stop dose increases, or change to another antidepressant
Diarrhea	More common with sertraline and less common with paroxetine	Dosage reduction, slow/stop dose increases, loperamide, add low dose of an anticholinergic antidepressant, or change to another antidepressant
Constipation	Most common with paroxetine	Dosage reduction, slow/stop dose increases, temporary laxatives/stool softener, or change antidepressant

Gastrointestinal

The most common gastrointestinal adverse effect experienced by patients is nausea, occurring in 15–35% of all patients on SSRIs (68, 69). Some patients may also experience vomiting and/or diarrhea (33). These tend to decrease over time, in most cases after a few weeks of treatment. For some patients, these symptoms may be quite troublesome and interfere with adherence. In these cases, if lowering the dose is unsuccessful, we recommend specific therapy. Ondansetron or other 5-HT_3 blockers (mirtazapine) are very effective for nausea; ranitidine may be helpful for dyspepsia; loperamide may be used to reduce diarrhea. Occasionally, a medication change is required. For example, if diarrhea is problematic, changing the medication to paroxetine may be helpful.

Very rare cases of hepatotoxicity in the form of either cholestatic or hepatocellular injury have been reported with fluoxetine, sertraline, and paroxetine (70–72). The incidence of such cases is quite low; sertraline, for example, has been associated with hepatotoxicity at a rate of 1.28 cases per 100,000 patient-years (72).

CNS

Both tension headaches and migraines have been reported to worsen when SSRIs are started (33), although improvement has also been noted. In some cases, headaches tend to increase in frequency over time (69). Sedation or activation with insomnia is known to occur, especially at the initiation of treatment, although this is somewhat variable depending on the SSRI. Some patients report increased dreaming, vivid dreams, and nightmares. Some authorities believe that fluoxetine has the highest incidence among SSRIs of insomnia, nervousness, restlessness, and anxiety (68). Decreasing the dose and titrating slowly and adding eszopiclone are usually effective management.

Tremors, increased anxiety, anger attacks, and akathisia have been observed with SSRI treatment in a small proportion of patients (73, 74). In general, the incidence of extrapyramidal side effects (EPS) such as Parkinsonism, dystonia, and akathisia is quite low but does occur (73, 75).

SSRIs may induce a switch to mania, with some experts estimating rates as high as 10–20% (34) but most others suggest rates of under 5% (76). Rates of manic switch in bipolar patients on placebo are 4%, and in patients taking TCAs it is estimated at 11% (76). The evidence for inducing mania or hypomania in unipolar depression is mostly anecdotal; the rate of manic switch in these patients is estimated at less than 1% (76). Some believe that antidepressant-induced manic episodes are generally milder and of shorter duration than spontaneous manic episodes experienced by bipolar patients (77).

Behavioral toxicity may also occur with SSRIs. The "apathy syndrome" may occur in patients who have been successfully treated for depression but develop loss of motivation, passivity, and lethargy, often described by patients as "flatness." This condition can be differentiated from the patient's depressive state as there is lack of prevailing sadness, tearfulness, decreased concentration, hopelessness/helplessness, and suicidality. In these patients, decreasing the SSRI dose and/or adding a stimulant is recommended. Bupropion and mirtazapine have also been used in combination with SSRI-induced apathy. It is often necessary to switch to another antidepressant of a different class.

Suicidality

In the early 1990s, reports of treatment emergent suicidal ideation in patients treated with fluoxetine appeared (78). Subsequent studies, however, did not confirm greater risk of de novo suicidal ideation in patients on SSRI treatment. A study of more than 1,000 outpatients in Boston centers failed to find a relationship between increased suicidality and fluoxetine treatment (79). A meta-analysis of 17 double-blind studies comparing fluoxetine, tricyclics, and placebo, evaluating a total of 3,065 patients with major depression failed to detect any increased risk of emergence of suicidal ideation with fluoxetine when compared to either placebo controls or patients treated with tricyclic antidepressants; moreover, the suicidal ideation was found significantly less in patients on fluoxetine than in patients on placebo (80). Another concluded that even though a small percentage of patients experienced increased anxiety, anger attacks, and akathisia during SSRI treatment, there was no evidence of a direct link between SSRI use and violent or suicidal behavior (74). Case reports and litigation have claimed an association between suicidal ideation and paroxetine, especially in children and young adults. The FDA has issued a black box warning for all antidepressants. It states "Antidepressants increased the risk compared to placebo of suicidal thinking and behavior (suicidality) in children, adolescents, and young adults in short-term studies of major depressive disorder (MDD) and other psychiatric disorders. Anyone considering the use of any antidepressant in a child, adolescent, or young adult must balance this risk with the clinical need. Short-term studies did not show an increase in the risk of suicidality with antidepressants compared to placebo in adults beyond age 24; there was a reduction in risk with antidepressants compared to placebo in adults aged 65 and older. Depression and certain other psychiatric disorders are themselves associated with increases in the risk of suicide. Patients of all ages who are started on antidepressant therapy should be monitored appropriately and observed closely for clinical worsening, suicidality, or unusual changes in behavior. Families and caregivers should be advised of the need for close observation and communication with the prescriber."

Some clinicians remain convinced of an association even if extremely uncommon. According to some, the rare cases of suicidal ideation can be explained by the adverse somatic effects of the SSRI. One possibility is that the activating properties of SSRIs energize some patients to act on pre-existing suicidal plans (81). Also suggested by some is that SSRIs induce akathisia and severe insomnia, which is associated with self-destructive or aggressive impulses (81). Emergence of akathisia-like effects may activate suicidal thoughts or impulses in especially susceptible patients (82).

It has been noted that the association between SSRIs and suicidality, even if it truly exists, may be lost in larger epidemiologic studies (81). Similarly, most clinical trials exclude suicidal patients from participation, thus undermining the generalizability of pooled data analyses (81). In any event, the findings do not alter the usual clinical practice of close monitoring of all depressed patients for emergence of suicidal ideation, especially early in treatment. Frequent visits are necessary for children and young adults, who may have a greater risk than adults.

Serotonin Syndrome

Serotonin syndrome is a potentially fatal condition resulting from excessive serotonergic activity, usually the result of coadministration of similarly acting medications. It can occur when SSRIs are combined with MAOIs (83) or with other drugs that increase CNS serotonergic activity, such as other SSRIs, other antidepressants, especially clomipramine, but also nefazodone, venlafaxine, trazodone, amitriptyline, imipramine, and also other drugs such as tramadol, meperidine, amphetamine, cocaine, and tryptophan (84). Unfortunately, this syndrome often is not recognized in a timely manner due to varied, nonspecific symptoms (84). Diagnostic criteria for serotonin syndrome have been proposed by Sternbach (83). In general, patients with serotonin syndrome will present with cognitive changes such as confusion, disorientation, behavioral changes such as agitation or restlessness, neuromuscular problems of ataxia, hyperreflexia, myoclonus, and/or problems with autonomic nervous function such as fever, shivering, diaphoresis or diarrhea (83). Others have suggested more stringent criteria that require a triad of pyrexia, neuromuscular symptoms, and mental status changes (84), although the most important issue is that clinicians should always be alert for the development of the serotonin syndrome when prescribing SSRI. Fatalities have been associated with the syndrome (33, 83, 84). The therapy for serotonin syndrome is discontinuation of the offending agents and supportive patient care. Dantrolene and bromocriptine have been used with mixed results.

It should be noted that even reversible MAOIs such as moclobemide can produce the serotonin syndrome when given with an SSRI (e.g., citalopram) (85). It may also occur as a result of pharmacokinetic drug–drug interactions. Five suspected cases of serotonin syndrome were reported in HIV-infected patients taking fluoxetine concomitantly with their antiretroviral therapy (protease inhibitors and nonnucleoside reverse transcriptase inhibitors) (86). The symptoms were attributed to the antiretroviral drug inhibition of the P450 enzymes and elevation of SSRI levels, resulting in enhanced serotonergic tone. The patients recovered completely after SSRIs were either stopped or their doses adjusted.

Endocrine System

The endocrine effects of SSRIs are still not fully elucidated. The picture is complicated by neuroendocrine disturbances in depression. It has been postulated that the hypothalamus–pituitary–adrenal (HPA) axis is activated in depressed patients, possibly in an attempt to normalize neuroendocrine function (87). Plasma ACTH was reduced but cortisol and vasopressin remained at the same levels during treatment of depressed patients with fluoxetine (88). A possible explanation is that SSRIs restore glucocorticoid negative feedback on ACTH levels and return the HPA axis to a normal state (88).

SSRIs, like all antidepressants, can cause the syndrome of inappropriate antidiuretic hormone secretion (SIADH) (34). The risk of developing the syndrome seems to be related to older age, female sex, concomitant use of hyponatremia-inducing medications and increasing the SSRI doses (89). On geriatric psychiatry units, this is a common adverse effect that precipitates hospitalization. SSRIs have also been reported to produce galactorrhea and increase prolactin levels (33).

Weight loss may occur in patients with initiation of fluoxetine treatment (90, 91); but these effects are transient (an exception may be in some elderly patients). Fluoxetine as well as paroxetine and citalopram have actually been known to cause weight gain in patients on long-term treatment (91, 92). The rate of emergence of significant weight gain (defined as 7% increase from baseline patient weight) during long-term treatment has been estimated as 6.8% for fluoxetine and 4.2% for sertraline. Paroxetine may be associated with the greatest weight gain, estimated at 25.5% (92).

Hematologic

There have been some reports of serotonergically mediated platelet dysfunction and abnormal bleeding associated with SSRIs (93). This effect is more likely to occur with high doses of SSRI medications. Fluoxetine, paroxetine, sertraline are the SSRIs most commonly associated with bleeding and abnormal hematological tests (94). Hemostatic markers that may be abnormal in SSRI-treated patients include decreased platelet aggregation and prolongation of bleeding time, although changes in platelet count, PT, and PTT are less common. In addition to the three SSRI mentioned above, other antidepressants, such as fluvoxamine, venlafaxine, mirtazapine and the tricyclic agents, amitriptyline, and imipramine may affect hemostasis. There is substantial evidence that abnormal bleeding is causally related to antidepressant treatment, and that potent serotonergic reuptake inhibition is the mechanism involved. Gastrointestinal bleeds occur at twice the rate in SSRI-treated patients compared to patients taking other antidepressants. Blood transfusions during surgery were more common in patients taking SSRI than other antidepressants. The prescription of drugs that are associated with increased bleeding, such as NSAIDs or aspirin, should be avoided whenever possible (34).

Sexual

Among the sexual side effects most commonly associated with SSRIs are decreased or absent libido, difficulties with sexual arousal, erectile dysfunction, delayed ejaculation, painful orgasm, and anorgasmia (95–99). These effects of SSRIs appear to be dose related (100). Most experts agree that SSRIs cause significantly more sexual dysfunction than either TCAs or MAOIs (96). Studies differ as to the incidence of these findings. For example, the percentage of patients developing anorgasmia is reported to be from 8.3 (101) to 75% (102) with fluoxetine. A review article concluded that 30–40% of patients on an SSRI will experience some degree of sexual dysfunction (103). A well-designed multicenter prospective study of 344 patients of both genders found that the frequency of adverse sexual effects was highest on paroxetine (65%), followed by fluvoxamine (59%), sertraline (56%), and fluoxetine (54%) (100). None of the patients in this study had sexual problems prior to initiation of SSRI antidepressant therapy; none had a medical illness or additional psychiatric disorders. The study used systematic inquiry of sexual dysfunction, performed by a physician, but was somewhat limited by lack of randomization of treatment and concurrent medications.

The frequency of SSRI-induced sexual dysfunction is still unknown; however, it is significantly higher than previously reported in pre-marketing studies and in product labeling of the SSRI (97, 98). A possible explanation for this underestimation of the incidence may be due to a lack of a structured assessment of sexual dysfunction (98) as well as to underreporting by patients (96).

SSRI-induced sexual dysfunction is a serious problem that often leads to drug discontinuation if not properly managed. There are several approaches to management: including dose reduction, waiting for tolerance to develop, switching to a different antidepressant, drug holiday, or addition of other medications (99). Medications that have been studied include α_2-adrenergic antagonist yohimbine, nefazodone, serotonin antagonist cyproheptadine, granisetron, mirtazapine, amantadine and pramipexole, methylphenidate, buproprion, the herb ginko biloba, and sildenafil and related phosphodiesterase Type 5 inhibitors (96, 98, 99).

Sildenafil citrate has been an effective agent to treat SSRI-induced sexual dysfunction. A small open study of sildenafil showed improved erectile dysfunction in patients with antidepressant-induced sexual side effects (104). Another open-label trial of 10 female patients, who had developed sexual dysfunction as a result of ongoing antidepressant treatment, reported that all patients who took sildenafil as instructed experienced a "complete or very significant reversal" of their sexual dysfunction (105). And finally, a review of sildenafil's efficacy in erectile dysfunction analyzed the results of 3 randomized, placebo-controlled trials and data from 10 earlier clinical trials (106). The authors concluded that sildenafil is an effective first-line treatment for either SSRI-induced or depression-related erectile dysfunction.

Another strategy is the addition or switch to bupropion (107). Some also recommend weekend drug holidays of 3-day duration (Thursday noon to Sunday noon), which was shown to improve sexual functioning in 30 outpatients who were maintained on an SSRI after recovering from a depressive episode and who had SSRI-induced sexual dysfunction (108). None of the patients experienced return of depressive symptoms, nor were there any significant increases in mean HAM-D scores after SSRI holidays. Patients who were taking sertraline and paroxetine reported improvement; patients taking fluoxetine reported no change, which may relate to the long half-life of this drug and its metabolite (108). We recommend periodic use of sildenafil (Viagra®) 50–100 mg, vardenafil (Levitra®) 2.5–20 mg, or tadalafil (Cialis®) 5–20 mg, as needed to treat SSRI-induced sexual dysfunction.

SSRI Discontinuation/Withdrawal Syndrome

Serotonin withdrawal syndrome, also known as SSRI discontinuation syndrome, can develop when an SSRI drug is stopped abruptly after a long-term use. The symptoms are "flu-like"; patients describe nausea, diarrhea, general malaise, myalgias and paresthesias, dizziness, vertigo, headache, and insomnia (109, 110). Vivid dreams, anxiety, and irritability may also be present (33). The criteria proposed for the diagnosis of SSRI discontinuation syndrome require two or more of the following symptoms developing within 1–7 days of discontinuation or reduction in dosage of an SSRI after at least 1-month use and not accounted for by medical illness: dizziness, lightheadedness, vertigo, paresthesia, anxiety, diarrhea, fatigue, gait instability, headache, insomnia, irritability, nausea or emesis, tremors, and visual disturbances (110).

The syndrome was first noted with paroxetine (111); however, all antidepressants can lead to a discontinuation syndrome if they are not gradually tapered. Fluoxetine, with its active metabolite's long half-life, was at first thought to be free of this effect due to presumed self-tapering of serum levels; however, the syndrome still may appear after long-term fluoxetine treatment. It had been reported that the withdrawal symptoms occur an average of 6.4 days after fluoxetine discontinuation as compared with 2–4 days after fluvoxamine, sertraline, or paroxetine discontinuation (30). In our experience, it is still much less common and not as severe with fluoxetine as with other SSRIs, such as paroxetine. The treatment for the SSRI discontinuation syndrome is drug reinstitution and then gradual tapering of the offending antidepressant (109), or a substitution of fluoxetine for shorter acting SSRI, followed by the taper of fluoxetine.

Safety

Safety in Overdose

SSRIs are perhaps the safest antidepressants on the market with respect to overdose risks, having a very high therapeutic index (32, 69). A study of SSRI overdoses analyzed published cases, data from the American Association of Poison Control Centers, and reports to the U.S. Food and Drug Administration adverse event database (112). This analysis concluded that SSRI antidepressants were far safer than the TCAs in overdose. There was also no difference among SSRIs with respect to morbidity or mortality. In general, mild to moderate overdoses of up to 30 times the usual daily dose were asymptomatic or associated with mild symptoms, and patients recovered fully without sequelae. Larger overdoses, of up to 75 times the prescribed daily dose, were associated with drowsiness, tremor, nausea, and vomiting. More serious consequences were associated with the largest overdoses and included seizures and ECG changes. There have been fatalities with overdoses of more than 150 times the usual daily dose. Almost all fatalities occurred in patients who took SSRIs and other substances, usually alcohol, benzodiazepines, or other drugs (112).

Reporting of overdoses is sporadic, making it impossible to accurately calculate the true incidence of morbidity and mortality. There are more data available on fluoxetine and citalopram because they have been in clinical use for a longer time. Some evidence has suggested higher overdose toxicity of citalopram compared to other SSRIs. Six fatalities from a citalopram overdose have been reported (113). However, as was pointed out by Glassman (114), 5 of the reported deaths involved citalopram taken with either alcohol or sedative drugs and the amounts of drugs ingested were quite high. In the only reported case of overdose with citalopram taken alone, the patient had taken 4,000 mg of the drug, which at the usual daily dose of 20 mg, is a 6-month supply. On the other hand, the didesmethyl metabolite of citalopram, which has demonstrated cardiotoxicity in animals, may reach high enough levels in overdose to cause morbidity.

Safety in Pregnancy and Lactation (See Also Chapter "Diagnosis and Treatment of Depression During Pregnancy and Lactation")

The treatment of depression during pregnancy and the postpartum period are discussed in detail in Chapter "Diagnosis and Treatment of Depression During Pregnancy and Lactation." Briefly, untreated major depression during pregnancy poses a risk to both mother and fetus. Both psychosocial and pharmacologic treatments have been used to treat pregnant women. When psychotherapeutic interventions are unsuccessful, clinicians and patients are faced with difficult decision regarding the safety of antidepressant therapy. Even the most competent clinician can be overwhelmed by the conflicting safety data generated by many studies. The first practical point is that there are not sufficient data to ensure the safety of any antidepressant. For adverse effects that are as rare as teratogenicity, very large sample sizes are required to avoid a Type II error (not finding an effect that would be evident with larger samples). There are no studies large enough to differentiate the risk of specific antidepressants on the fetus. Paroxetine has been associated with cardiac malformations and resulted in a change in product labeling and an FDA advisory, although other studies have not replicated the finding. A prospective multicenter controlled cohort study to assess risk of SSRI teratogenicity studied infants of 267 women exposed to SSRIs (fluvoxamine, paroxetine, and sertraline) during pregnancy and the infants of 267 controls (115). Investigators did not find increased risk for major malformations or higher rates of miscarriage, stillbirth, or prematurity in infants born to mothers treated with SSRIs during pregnancies. There were no detectable differences in infant birth weights or gestational ages at delivery among the groups, although the sample size was probably too small. An additional three studies were larger (116–118) and did not find cardiac abnormalities with paroxetine exposure. In the large studies, the malformations included ventricular and atrial septal defects, with one study reporting a 4% risk with paroxetine compared to a 2% risk with other antidepressants. The risks from other SSRIs are not known, but there is some evidence to suggest that the risk of teratogenicity for tricyclic antidepressants and bupropion appears lower than SSRI, with the exception of clomipramine.

The risk of spontaneous abortion may be increased with antidepressant use during pregnancy, although the rate in the general population is high and studies do not always support increased risk with antidepressant treatment. Studies have also found an increased rate of preterm birth in women who took SSRIs during pregnancy, although this finding is complicated by the failure to control for depression severity. One study found a six fold increase in persistent pulmonary hypertension in newborns of women who took SSRIs during the second half of the pregnancy (119), although the finding has not been consistently replicated.

Most studies have not found developmental delays in infants whose mothers took antidepressants during pregnancy although one study (118) found gross motor delays and delays in attention in children whose mothers had taken SSRIs in the second or third trimester compared to a control group of women who were depressed during pregnancy and not taking antidepressants. Scores remained within the normal range for the exposed group, and the clinical significance of these findings was uncertain. A withdrawal syndrome is sometimes seen in neonates whose mothers took antidepressants up to the time of delivery. Symptoms include jitteriness, poor muscle tone, weak or absent cry, respiratory distress, hypoglycemia, seizures, and low Apgar scores. It is possible to avoid this by a slow taper prior to delivery; however, the clinician should be cautious about recurrence of depression in the mother.

In summary, the clinician is faced with making decisions about antidepressant therapy in pregnancy without a consistent database to inform the discussion with the patient. Our approach is to discuss the rates of pregnancy complications with the patient and present the potential increased risk of antidepressant therapy based on our best evaluation of the data. If the rate of a specific anomaly in the general population is 2%, and the risk of a specific drug-induced anomaly is doubled, we present the information as percentages – 2 chances out of 100 compared to 4 out of 100. Even this approach overstates the chances, because it does not account for the severity of depression and associated hyperactivity of the HPA axis and other physiologic changes associated with depression alone that may contribute to adverse fetal effects.

Efficacy

As a class, SSRIs have been proven effective in a wide range of psychiatric disorders; mood disorders including dysthymia (120), obsessive-compulsive disorder (OCD)

(121, 122), panic disorder (123), social phobia (124–126), eating disorders (127), premenstrual dysphoric disorder (128), and GAD (129).

In his review article of available pharmacological treatments for PTSD, Davidson cites evidence from large long-term clinical trials of SSRI antidepressants' efficacy in patients with this disorder (130). In chronic PTSD, we have found that the combination of SSRIs and atypical antipsychotics produces the best effects (see also Chapter "Antidepressants in the Treatment of PTSD").

SSRI may be the preferred class of antidepressants in depression associated with medical illness. Fluoxetine proved significantly better than placebo in the treatment of depression in patients with HIV and AIDS, diabetes mellitus, or strokes (131). The long half-life of fluoxetine and norfluoxetine, as well as their potential for interactions with other medications via P450 isoenzymes are potential limitations for use in medically ill patients. Sertraline and escitalopram would appear to be better choices in the medically ill, due to a lower likelihood of pharmacokinetic interactions (132) (see Chapter "Treatment of Depression in the Medically Ill").

SSRIs are being studied as possible treatment for alcohol-induced depression and appear most effective when used in combination with naltrexone (see also Chapter "Substance Abuse and Depression") (133, 134). At present, there are no widely accepted typologies that predict SSRI response in alcohol-dependent subjects.

Equivalent efficacy between SSRIs and TCAs is a matter of some debate. A meta-analysis of approximately 300 double-blind randomized controlled clinical trials found that most antidepressants have similar efficacy, and that MAOIs, SSRIs, and TCAs all have response rate of 60–68%, as defined by 50% improvement in the HAM-D or the Montgomery Asberg Depression Rating Scale (MADRS) (135). This concurs with another study where SSRIs were deemed not more efficacious or faster acting than TCAs in MDD (68). In another study, fluoxetine appeared to be no better than imipramine for treatment of atypical depression (136). These results held true in many reviews of specific SSRIs and in other studies (69, 137). One study found that sertraline but not other SSRIs were as efficacious as TCAs in patients with melancholic depression (138), although this remains a controversial issue. A 1-year, double-blind study of suicidal behavior in patients with repeated suicide attempts found that paroxetine significantly reduced suicidal behavior (139), although the issue of suicidality remains controversial. Others have questioned the equivalency of SSRIs and TCAs (see TCA section).

SSRIs may lose their efficacy during maintenance treatment. A recent study found return of depressive symptoms in 9–57% of the patients during maintenance treatment; most of these patients were treated with an SSRI (140). Another double-blind study reported relapse in depression in 26 out of 77 patients on a maintenance dose of 20 mg daily of fluoxetine (141). In these cases, increasing the dose, switching to a different class of antidepressant, or adding an augmenting agent is recommended.

To summarize, the SSRI antidepressants remain the first-line treatment for major depression, dysthymia, generalized anxiety disorder, panic disorder, obsessive-compulsive disorder, social phobia, PTSD, and bulimia. They have a favorable side effect profile as compared to older antidepressants, better patient tolerability, ease of administration, and well-proven safety in overdose. The drug interactions of some SSRIs may be significant and it is prudent to use the SSRI with least potential for drug–drug interactions (citalopram, escitalopram, sertraline) when treating patients with other medical or other psychiatric comorbidities. Information on interactions mediated by induction or inhibition of transporters, such as P-glycoprotein, is incomplete, but should be considered as potential confounders of clinical effects and toxicity.

Cyclic Antidepressants

History

Imipramine was the first tricyclic antidepressant (TCA) used in clinical practice. After unsuccessful trials as a potential antihistamine and antipsychotic (31), in 1957, Roland Kuhn in Switzerland reported its efficacy in the treatment of depression (142). Some years later, Klerman and Cole demonstrated superiority of imipramine to placebo in depressed patients by analyzing pooled data from 23 published studies; 65% of patients from those studies improved clinically on imipramine compared to only 31% improvement among placebo patients (143). For three decades, TCAs were the first-line agents for the treatment of depression.

Desipramine is the demethylated metabolite of imipramine, and like its parent drug, it has antidepressant action. Amitriptyline was also introduced in the 1960s, and later its secondary amine metabolite, nortriptyline, was marketed. The TCAs offer advantages over monoamine oxidase inhibitor (MAOI) antidepressants, having less risk of drug–drug interactions and requiring no food restrictions, but they have troublesome adverse effects in many patients. They also have a low therapeutic index, which can present problems in patients with suicidal risk. Heterocyclic and other types of antidepressants were introduced to the market over the past 20 years, but none have demonstrated superior efficacy to the TCAs.

Currently, the following tricyclic and heterocyclic compounds are FDA approved for treatment of depression in the United States: *amitriptyline* (Elavil, Vanatrip), *amoxapine* (Asendin), *clomipramine* (Anafranil), *desipramine* (Norpramin), *doxepin* (Sinequan, Zonalon), *imipramine* (Tofranil), *maprotiline* (Ludiomil), *nortriptyline* (Aventyl, Pamelor), *protriptyline* (Vivactil), and *trimipramine* (Surmontil). Among these, amoxapine and maprotiline are less commonly used.

Pharmacology

The basic tricyclic structure is similar to that of chlorpromazine and related phenothiazines, which have a 6-member central ring joining two benzene rings, resulting in a planar molecule. Most classifications of TCAs distinguish between tertiary and secondary amines. The tertiary amine tricyclics, such as imipramine and amitriptyline, are made up of two benzene rings linked by a central imino ring. The 7-member central ring distorts the molecule and it becomes non-planar. Imipramine and amitriptyline are tertiary amines as three carbon substituents are located on the terminal nitrogen of their side chains. Desipramine is a demethylated metabolite of imipramine and thus a secondary amine; it has two carbons on the terminal nitrogen of the side chain. Similarly, nortriptyline is the demethylated metabolite of amitriptyline.

Doxepin, trimipramine, and protriptyline all have the three-ring structure of imipramine with some minor differences. Drugs in this family that were developed subsequently had a different molecular structure (tetracyclic, heterocyclic, or even structurally unrelated compounds). Amoxapine, a drug introduced in 1980, for example, has the three-ring structure of imipramine but has a fourth ring as a side structure. Maprotiline is a tetracyclic compound, with the central portion consisting of four rings. However, both amoxapine and maprotiline are often classified as TCA-like, because they share the same action, efficacy, and side effect profile (144). Thus, the term "TCA," which is still commonly used in clinical practice and literature to denote all drugs in this family, is inaccurate, and terms such as "cyclic," "atypical," and "mixed action" are sometimes used. Other classification schemes use terms such as "nonselective serotonin and norepinephrine reuptake inhibitors (NSNRI)" and "selective norepinephrine reuptake inhibitors (SNRI)" to maintain consistency with the SSRI terminology. None of these approaches is entirely satisfactory or precise. As we approach the era of triple reuptake inhibitors and drugs that promote reuptake inhibition and also mixed receptor agonist/antagonist properties, we expect that the current nomenclature will be radically revised.

Pharmacokinetics

TCAs are highly lipophilic, well absorbed from the gastrointestinal tract with large volumes of distribution, and relatively long half-lives (145). TCAs are bound to α_1-acid glycoprotein and albumin. Since they are highly protein bound, they are subject to drug interactions that are caused by displacement from protein binding sites and factors such as medical illnesses, which alter the amounts or activity of binding proteins may change the free fraction of active drug that enters the brain, at least transiently. Metabolism of TCAs occurs in the liver via demethylation and/or hydroxylation, followed by glucuronide conjugation (145). Metabolism may also occur within the brain. There is wide interindividual variation in the hepatic metabolism of TCAs. The presence of active metabolites complicates the interpretation of the therapeutic and adverse effects of these agents. Metabolites differ from the parent compound in their pharmacokinetic characteristics and effects on different neurotransmitter systems. Among tertiary amines, imipramine is demethylated to desipramine and hydroxylated to 2-hydroxyimipramine and 2-hydroxydesipramine. Imipramine is 86–93% protein bound and has an elimination half-life of 15–30 h. The metabolism of amitriptyline is complex, since its hydroxy metabolites, and those of its demethylated metabolite nortriptyline, exist as isomers. Amitriptyline is 95% protein bound with an elimination half-life of 9–25 h. Desipramine is

85–90% protein bound with an elimination half-life of 12–36 h. Nortriptyline is 92% protein bound with an elimination half-life of 18–33 h. During treatment with either amitriptyline or nortriptyline, the *E*-10-OH-nortiptyline reaches greater plasma and cerebrospinal fluid concentrations than the parent drug (145). In contrast, 2-OH-desipramine plasma levels are less than half that of the parent drug during desipramine administration (146). Hydroxy metabolites pass the blood–brain barrier and contribute to pharmacodynamic effects. Clinical doses of non-SSRIs and their cytochrome substrates are shown in Tables 9 and 10.

The pharmacokinetic properties of TCAs have several clinical implications: (1) Within the usual therapeutic range, increases in dose will produce proportional increases in plasma levels; (2) correlation between clinical outcome and plasma levels has been difficult to establish, in part due to a failure of some studies to consider metabolites, free concentration of drug, activity of transporter proteins, such as P-glycoprotein, and failure to assay for isomers; however, many clinicians believe that nortriptyline response is optimal in a therapeutic window of plasma levels between 50 and 150 ng/ml, while other TCAs such as desipramine require a minimal plasma concentration, exhibiting the classical sigmoidal response curve; (3) first-pass metabolism by the liver is genetically determined and is the major factor leading to large interindividual variability in plasma levels; (4) metabolites contribute to the therapeutic and toxic effects and may reach higher levels than the parent compound; (5) renal clearance is an important route of elimination for hydroxylated metabolites, and factors such as age and disease may impair excretion; (6) impaired elimination in the young and elderly is believed to be related to renal function; (7) gender differences in metabolism have not been consistently found; however, increased metabolism and plasma volume during pregnancy may require dosage adjustments.

Cyclic antidepressants are subject to pharmacokinetic drug–drug interactions as a consequence of metabolism via the hepatic cytochrome P450 system. Pharmacokinetic drug–drug interactions of TCAs can be anticipated with knowledge of the cytochromes that are involved in metabolism and familiarity with drugs that induce or inhibit these enzymes. The most commonly encountered clinical situations involve combined therapy of antidepressants with inhibitors or inducers of the cytochromes involved in antidepressant metabolism. It is also possible to encounter an interaction with other drugs that are substrates for the same cytochromes if the latter have higher affinity for binding sites. An example of this is the ability of some TCAs to compete for CYP2C19 and alter phenytoin metabolism. The discussion that follows focuses on the most common pharmacokinetic interactions of the TCA. It is meant to outline some of the principles of these interactions, not serve as an exhaustive list of all interactions.

Whereas *N*-demethylation of TCAs is catalyzed by CYP1A2, CYP2C19, and CYP3A4, the contribution of active hydroxy metabolites makes the hydroxylation step, mediated by CYP2D6, extremely important. Approximately 7–10% of Caucasians are poor CYP2D6 metabolizers (147), whereas less than 1% of Asians are PM. Several antipsychotics, SSRI antidepressants (see SSRI section), and moclobemide (an MAOI marketed outside of the United States) are the most common psychotropic agents to impair CYP2D6-mediated metabolism. Some other drugs that impair CYP2D6 are cimetidine, ranitidine, methadone, metclopramide,

Table 9 Adult doses and formulations of antidepressants

Tertiary amines	Usual starting dose[a]	Maximal dose[a]	Formulation	Available dosages
Amitriptyline	25 mg t.i.d.	300 mg q.d.	Suspension, tablet	Suspensions: 10 mg/ mlTablets: 10, 25, 50, 75, 100, 150 mg
Imipramine	25 mg t.i.d.	300 mg q.d.	Tablet, capsule	Tablets: 10, 25, 50 mgCapsule: 75, 100, 125, 150 mg
Clomipramine	25 mg q.d.	250 mg q.d.	Capsule	25, 50, 75 mg
Trimipramine	75 mg q.d.	300 mg q.d.	Capsule	25, 50, 100 mg
Secondary amines				
Nortriptyline	25 mg q.d.	150 mg q.d. (monitor plasma levels)	Capsule, solution	Capsule: 10, 25, 50, 75 mgSolution: 2 mg/ml
Desipramine	25 mg b.i.d.	250–300 mg q.d.	Tablet	10, 25, 50, 75, 100, 150 mg
Protriptyline	15 mg q.d.	60 mg q.d.	Tablet	5, 10 mg
Amoxapine	50 mg b.i.d. or t.i.d.	120–300 mg q.d.	Tablet	25, 50, 100, 150 mg
Aminoketones				
Buproprion	100 mg b.i.d. (IR)150 mg q.d. (SR)	150 mg t.i.d. (IR)200 mg b.i.d. (SR)	Tablet, SR tablet	Tablet: 75, 100 mg SR Tablet: 100, 150 mg
Tetracyclics				
Mirtazapine	15 mg q.h.s.	45 mg q.d.	Tablets, dissolving tablets	15, 30, 45 mg
Maprotiline	75 mg q.d.	225 mg q.d.	Tablet	25, 50, 75 mg
Phenylethamine				
Venlafaxine XR	75 mg b.i.d.	375 mg q.d.	Tablet, SR capsule	Tablet: 25, 37.5, 50, 75, 100 mgSR Capsule: 37.5, 75, 150 mg
Desvenlafaxine	50 mg q.d.	+	XR tablet	50, 100 mg
Triazolopyridine				
Trazodone	50 mg t.i.d.	400–600 mg	Tablet	50, 100, 150, 300 mg
Phenylpiperazine				
Nefazodone	100 mg b.i.d.	600 mg q.d.	Tablet	50, 100, 150, 200, 250 mg
Thiophenepropylamine				
Duloxetine	40–60 mg	120 mg	Delayed release tablets	20, 30, 60 mg

Used in clinical trials
+ No additional benefit noted at doses higher than 50 mg daily, although doses up to 400 mg daily
[a]Lower doses should be used in the elderly

Table 10 Selected non-SSRI antidepressant metabolites

Tertiary amines	Metabolites	Cytochrome substrates
Amitriptyline	Nortriptyline 10-OH nortriptyline (cis, trans, +, –), 10-OH amitriptyline (cis, trans, +, –)	1A2, 2C19, 2C9, 2D6, 3A4
Imipramine	Desipramine 2-OH desipramine 2-OH imipramine	2C19, 2C9, 1A2, 3A4, 2D6
Clomipramine	Desmethylclomipramine 8-OH clomipramine 8-OH desmethylclomipramine	3A4, 2D6 (also inhibits 2D6), 2C19
Trimipramine	Desmethyltrimipramine Didesmethyltimipramine 2-OH trimipramine 2-OH desmethyltrimipramine	2C19, 1A2, 3A4, 2D6
Doxepin	Desmethyldoxepin	2C19, 3A4, 1A2, 2C9
Secondary amines		
Nortriptyline	10-OH nortriptyline (cis, trans, +, –)	2D6
Desipramine	2-OH desipramine	2D6
Protriptyline	2-OH protriptyline desmethylprotriptyline *N*-acetylprotriptyline	?2D6
Aminoketones		
Bupropion	Hydroxybupropion Threohydrobupropion Erythrohydrobupropion	2B6 (also inhibits 2B6), 2D6 (also inhibits 2D6)
Tetracyclics		
Mirtazapine	Desmethylmirtazapine (8-OH mirtazapine) (mirtazapine N-oxide)	3A, 2D6, 1A2
Maprotiline	Desmethylmaprotiline	2D6, 1A2
Phenylethylamine		
Venlafaxine	*O*-desmethylvenlafaxine	2D6
Desvenlafaxine	None clinically significant	Conjugation (UGP), 3A4 minor
Triazolopyridine		
Trazodone	*m*-CPP	3A4
Phenylpiperazine		
Nefazodone	Hydroxynefazodone Meta-chlorophenylpiperazine (*m*-CPP) Triazole-dione	3A4 (also inhibits 3A4), 2D6
Thiophenepropylamine		
Duloxetine	4-hydroxy duloxetine glucuronide , 5-hydroxy, 6-methoxy, duloxetine sulfate (do not contribute to clinical actions)	CYP1A2, CYP2D6 Conjugation (UGP)

amiodarone, celecoxib, and ritonavir. Ritonavir and other antivirals (indinavir, nelfinavir, saquinavir, delaviridine), antifungals (ketoconazole, itraconozole), macrolide antibiotics (erythromycin, clarithromycin), ciprofloxacin, and the calcium channel blocker diltiazem inhibit CYP3A4. Fluoroquinolines inhibit CYP1A2. Enzyme inducers, such as modafinil (1A2), barbiturates (3A, 2B6, 2C9), rifampin

(2D6, 3A, 2C19, 2B6), carbamazepine (2C19, 3A), tamoxifen (3A), and chronic ethanol may all lower plasma levels of cyclic antidepressants. Some foods, such as grapefruit juice, may also reduce CYP3A4 and CYP1A2 activity.

Mechanism of Action

The antidepressant action of TCAs is thought to be due to their inhibition of norepinephrine (NE) and serotonin (5-HT) reuptake, thus leading to increased concentrations of these monoamines in the synaptic cleft. Down-regulation of postsynaptic receptors and subsequent changes in gene expression (see SSRI section and Chapter "Biological Theories of Depression and Implications for Current and New Treatments") are ultimately responsible for the antidepressant action. TCAs inhibit NE and 5-HT in different proportions. In general, secondary amines such as desipramine and nortriptyline are much more selective and preferentially block NE reuptake. Thus, desipramine, nortripytyline, and also protriptyline, are primarily NE reuptake inhibitors, with only some 5-HT reuptake inhibition. Conversely, clomipramine inhibits 5-HT reuptake much more than it does NE reuptake. Imipramine, amitriptyline, doxepin, and trimipramine inhibit NE and 5-HT reuptake equally, although one must also take into consideration the effect of their metabolites, which together with the parent compound produce a mixed noradrenergic–serotonergic effect. Nortriptyline, amitriptyline, and clomipramine are also antagonists at the 5-HT_{2A} receptor, although the clinical significance of this effect is not known.

Adverse effects of TCAs are due to their actions as agonists at α_1-adrenergic (orthostatic hypotension), H_1-histaminic (sedation, weight gain), and anticholinergic receptors (dry mouth, urinary retention, constipation, blurred vision, memory problems). All of the TCAs have clinically significant anticholinergic effects, although the two with the least among them are desipramine and nortriptyline. Nortriptyline has the lowest α_1-adrenergic antagonism, with desipramine having somewhat more, but still less than the tertiary amines. Amitritpyline, doxepin, and trimipramine have the strongest histaminergic (H_1) antagonism among the group.

Adverse Effects

TCAs have strong anticholinergic (antimuscarinic) activity, which may cause constipation, dry mouth, urinary hesitancy/retention, blurred vision, dyspepsia, and confusion (32, 148). In elderly patients, more severe side effects, such as tachycardia, confusion, agitation, or even delirium may occur at therapeutic doses (149). Although rare, these severe complications may occur when a patient has been taking another anticholinergic drug concomitantly with a TCA; neuroleptics, anti-Parkinsonian agents, antihistamines, antispasmodics and over the counter sleeping pills are commonly involved.

Initial management of mild to moderate symptoms should include decreasing the TCA dose or slowing dosage escalation. In patients who still have troublesome symptoms, oral bethanechol 25–50 mg 3 or 4 times per day may relieve peripheral cholinergic symptoms. Central nervous system symptoms may be reversed by intravenous physostigmine; however, this should be done by an experienced clinician, because it can be associated with tremors, vomiting, and seizures if given too rapidly or at too high a dose. Some clinicians recommend 4% pilocarpine eye drops for blurred vision and a 1% solution for dry mouth; however, we have found bethanechol as effective and more convenient for patients. If a patient cannot tolerate the anticholinergic effects, switching classes is the best approach.

Cardiovascular: Orthostatic Hypotension

Direct peripheral α-adrenergic receptor blockade causes orthostatic hypotension, dizziness, and drowsiness (150, 151). This effect does not directly correlate with the patient's age or dose of TCA, although the consequence can be disastrous in the elderly or cardiac impaired patient. Following the onset of orthostatic hypotension, further dosage increases do not produce greater declines in blood pressure (150). In many patients, the severity of orthostatic hypotension will prohibit TCA use; up to 10% of otherwise medically healthy patients and up to 25–50% of patients with pre-existing cardiac disease will require alteration of dose or discontinuation of the medication (152). Orthostatic hypotension is of special concern in the elderly, in whom falls may result in physical injuries such as fractures or significant lacerations. Injuries resulting from falls may occur at a rate of up to 4% of patients treated with imipramine (150). Nortriptyline may offer some advantages over other TCAs. Lack of postural effect was reported in a study of 32 patients, two-thirds of whom were taking nortriptyline (153). Nortriptyline was found to be significantly less likely to cause orthostatic hypotension than imipramine, desipramine, clomipramine, or amitriptyline. This property makes it the TCA of choice in the elderly population (153, 154).

Cardiovascular: Conduction Effects

One of the most serious adverse effects of TCAs is a consequence of their effects on cardiac conduction. ECG changes are well known and consist of T wave flattening, lengthening of the P-R interval, and the QRS complex (153). TCAs slow cardiac atrioventricular conduction, lengthen the QT interval, and are associated with arrhythmias, especially in overdose and in patients with pre-existing cardiac disease (155). TCAs are class 1A antiarrhythmics (similar to quinidine), which exert their clinical effect by slowing conduction through the His–Purkinje system and myocardium (155). This class of antiarrhythmics can actually produce arrhythmias after myocardial infarction. Cardiac mortality associated with TCA use is a matter of some controversy. Studies prior to the introduction of antidepressants indicated that there was higher mortality in severely depressed patients compared to the general population, with cardiovascular mortality 8 times more likely (156). Witchel and associates (155) have proposed that TCA-induced prolongation of the QT_c interval (greater than 440 ms) may be responsible for proarrhythmic effects and sudden death. Drawing comparisons to genetic forms of long QT syndrome (LQTS), these investigators suggest that TCAs may induce QT prolongation by direct effects on ion channels within the myocardium fibers. Identification of genes encoding for these ion channels and defective functioning of these channels in LQTS led to the hypothesis that TCAs (and other drugs) may produce altered function, especially in individuals who have "silent mutations." These authors also stress that the multiple additional effects of TCAs such as monoamine reuptake inhibition, anticholinergic activity, antihistamine effects, as well as blockade of Ca and K channels influence the risk of prolonged QT_c (155). In cases of TCA overdose, the TCA-induced QT interval prolongation has been linked to *torsades de pointes* (TdP), complete heart block, and sudden cardiac death. The risk of arrhythmia is especially high in patients with pre-existing cardiovascular disease or conduction abnormalities, those on high doses of TCA medications, and in overdose (see discussion below) (152).

Although cardiac toxicity in overdose was well known during early clinical use of TCAs (157), prevailing clinical opinion has been that there were a few cardiovascular side effects from TCA treatment if patients did not have pre-existing cardiovascular pathology (150). As noted above, in some cases, the TCAs proved to have antiarrhythmic properties, suppressing ectopic pacemakers and suppressing premature ventricular contractions (158). On the other hand, it was also recognized that these drugs should not be used in patients with a known cardiac illness, such as pre-existing conduction delays second-degree heart block, bifascicular heart block, sick sinus syndrome heart failure, or bundle branch disease (159). The risks of TCA-induced impairment of left ventricular function remain unresolved (160).

The Cardiac Arrhythmia Suppression Trial (CAST) evaluated the effect of antiarrhythmic therapy in patients with either mildly symptomatic or asymptomatic ventricular arrhythmias after myocardial infarction. The CAST study was stopped prematurely when a significantly higher death rate in the groups treated with either encainide or flecainide (and eventually moricizine) versus placebo group was found (161, 162). The results indicated that both class 1C and 1A antiarrhythmics, the latter of which includes TCAs, had a proarrhythmic effect post-MI. When cardiac tissue becomes anoxic or ischemic, the class 1 antiarrhythmics become pro-arrhythmic (151). Thus, SSRI are the preferred antidepressants for these patients. Most cyclic antidepressants are associated with arrhythmia risk, including amitriptyline, amoxapine, clomipramine, desipramine, doxepin, imipramine, maprotiline, and nortriptyline. Doxepin, once thought to be safer in patients with cardiac disease, has cardiac risk comparable to other drugs of this class (163).

Sexual Dysfunction

Sexual dysfunction has not been well studied in TCAs, but it is generally believed that they are associated with decreased libido, erectile or ejaculatory dysfunction, delayed orgasm, anorgasmia, and less commonly, impotence (95–97). There are no reliable data that indicate how often these occur, and many studies refer only to a "decrease or impaired sexual function." Several studies have used clomipramine, a strong serotonergic TCA, as a comparator to SSRI and found equivalent rates of sexual dysfunction. Clomipramine was associated with anorgasmia in approximately 90% of patients in a study in patients with OCD (164). The most often quoted numbers for depressed patients who experience decreased sexual function and libido while being treated with clomipramine are 14% for females and 26% for males (97); however, women may be less likely to report sexual side effects (96). On the other hand, an increase in libido with imipramine and amoxapine has been known to occur (97). These disparate findings highlight the difficulty in separating sexual dysfunction associated with depression and that resulting from drug therapy.

Other Adverse Effects

Other common adverse effects include tremors, mycolonus, and perspiration. Maprotiline has been associated with seizures at high therapeutic doses. All TCAs lower the seizure threshold, but this is usually only a problem in patients with a seizure disorder or in overdose. Amoxapine has been associated with extrapyramidal symptoms.

Overdose

TCAs have a relatively low therapeutic index and serious consequences in overdose. For most TCAs, the therapeutic dose is about 3–4 mg/kg/day and a potentially lethal dose is 15–20 mg/kg/day. The potentially fatal dose is only a 5-day supply of medication. This creates an obvious problem in the treatment of depressed patients, many of whom have suicidal ideation. The epidemiological data from the 1970s to mid-1980s, prior to the SSRIs' entry into the market, provide the richest data on TCA overdose. During that period, the annual incidence of TCA overdose in United States was estimated at 500,000 (144). Approximately 1,500–2,000 patients a year committed suicide with TCAs (150). TCAs became the most commonly ingested drugs among suicidal patients and the third most common cause of drug-related death, following closely deaths from alcohol–drug combinations and heroin overdoses (165). In 1983 and 1984, TCAs were the most common drug involved in overdose deaths, and 70% of patients taking TCAs in suicides died before reaching the hospital (144) and a substantial number died within 5–6 h of admission to a hospital (165). More recently, some have opined that the risk of overdose has been exaggerated. For example, it has been argued that only 5% of suicidal patients use their prescribed antidepressant medications for that purpose (81); however, most clinicians are unwilling to take any risk as long as safer alternatives are available.

The clinical presentation of TCA overdose is an extension of their pharmacodynamic actions. Frommer and associates (144) describe the initial symptoms as primarily anticholinergic, including mydriasis, blurred vision, urinary retention, dry mucous membranes, decreased peristalsis, tachycardia, general CNS excitation with increased reflexes, hyperactivity, and insomnia. CNS toxicity includes confusion, agitation, hallucinations, and seizures. CNS depression may begin as drowsiness or lethargy and progress rapidly to coma and respiratory arrest in the most severe cases (144). Cardiac abnormalities may include hypotension and arrhythmias, such as sinus tachycardia, supraventricular and ventricular tachycardia, prolongation of PR, QRS, and QT intervals, bundle branch or second- and third-degree blocks, or sudden death (32). Death is caused by intractable myocardial depression or cardiac arrhythmias such as ventricular tachycardia or fibrillation (144). Generalized seizures are associated with increased mortality and often occur immediately prior to cardiac arrest. The progression from mild symptoms to death can be extremely rapid, and often does not follow a predictable pattern.

In terms of individual differences among cyclic antidepressants, amoxapine has been associated with least cardiotoxicity in large overdoses (144, 166); however, it has significant CNS toxicity, and has been known to cause status epilepticus and coma with overdose (166, 167). Maprotiline, a tetracyclic compound, was reported to possess greater cardiac and CNS toxicity (seizures) than other agents (168).

Treatment of a TCA overdose includes administration of activated charcoal lavage, fluids, and supportive measures. Several authors have proposed specific therapies for hypotension, seizures, and arrhythmias; however, there are substantial variations in approach. Regardless of the specific approaches used, all patients should be hospitalized in a cardiac or intensive care unit. Some clinicians advise administration of physostigmine, but this may precipitate seizure and cardiac arrhythmias in some instances (168).

Clinical Use

A study published in 1993 analyzed data on antidepressant use from three National Ambulatory Medical Care Surveys for years 1980, 1985, and 1989 (169) and found that TCAs were the most widely prescribed type of antidepressant in an office-based practice throughout 1980s, and were still widely used at the time of that publication. TCAs have now become second-line agents in the United States, but in other countries, they remain first-line agents. This is especially true for European psychiatrists, many of whom believe in the superior efficacy of tertiary amines such as clomipramine and amitriptyline over other antidepressants (32). In the United States, however, newer antidepressants, such as SSRIs, have replaced the TCAs as first-line agents, primarily due to the belief of equivalent efficacy, greater safety, improved tolerability, and ease of dosing compared to TCAs.

Most clinicians believe that data support the equivalent efficacy of all the TCA, although some argue for the superior effectiveness of clomipramine. Estimates indicate that up to 80% of heterogeneous depressed patients will experience clinically significant improvements in depression when treated with adequate doses of TCAs (148).

There remains disagreement on the issue of superior efficacy of TCAs compared to SSRI. In a review of 186 randomized controlled trials that compared amitriptyline with other antidepressants, including SSRIs, heterocyclics, and other tricyclics, Barbui and Hotopf (170) concluded that amitriptyline was more efficacious in the treatment of depression than SSRIs, heterocyclics, or other TCAs. A small, but statistically significant, higher response rate was found with amitriptyline (170). Boyce and Judd (171) have argued that not only are the TCAs more effective in melancholic depression and inpatients with depression but also the tolerability and safety of SSRI have been overstated.

There is support for the position that TCAs should remain a first-line treatment for patients with severe depression (sometimes referred to as endogenous or melancholic depression). The Danish University Antidepressant Group found that clomipramine was superior in efficacy to citalopram, paroxetine, and moclobemide (172). In another study, nortriptyline was found superior to fluoxetine, for treating depression in hospitalized elderly patients, especially for those patients with a melancholic subtype of depression (173). In a review of 6 controlled trials, Perry (174) concluded that TCAs are more effective agents in the treatment of "endogenous depression or major depression with melancholic features" compared to SSRIs. On the other hand, clinicians should be aware that there are many studies that have found the two classes "equivalent," although most of these have not differentiated melancholic subtypes of depression. Equivalency studies are notorious for Type II errors, i.e., having a sample size that is too small to detect significant group differences.

TCAs have a broad spectrum of efficacy. In addition to major depression and dysthymia, they are effective in panic disorder, social phobia, other anxiety disorders, bulimia nervosa, PTSD, ADHD, and, in young children, enuresis. Toxicity of TCAs in children has been the matter of some controversy. Some reports have linked desipramine to sudden death in children; however, a review by a leading authority in the area did not find an association (175). As a precaution, ECG should be monitored in children taking TCAs. Clomipramine is approved for treatment of obsessive-compulsive disorder. Adult as well as childhood ADHD responds well to treatment with TCAs, with most data available for imipramine and desipramine (176, 177). TCAs are sometimes used for chronic pain syndromes and migraine headaches, but more effective medications (duloxetine, milnacipram, gabapentin, pregabalin) have largely supplanted their use in these illnesses.

Gender differences in therapeutic response to TCAs have been studied but have produced inconsistent findings. A 12-week, double-blind, randomized prospective study found that depressed men were significantly more likely to show a favorable response to imipramine, a TCA, than to sertraline, a SSRI, while the reverse was true for women. This difference was most apparent in premenopausal women; postmenopausal women had equal rates of response to the two agents (178). In general, women had a slower antidepressant response to imipramine and poor tolerability of the TCA. The reasons for the gender differences are unclear but may include the presence of SSRI-responsive subtypes of depression in women (e.g., atypical, premenstrual dysphoric disorder) and/or an interaction between antidepressants and female sex hormones. Complicating the interpretation of this study are high dropout rates for women taking imipramine and for men taking sertraline (179).

A retrospective study analyzed data for 1,746 patients treated with TCAs (imipramine, desipramine), SSRIs (fluoxetine), MAOIs (phenelzine, tranylcypromine, *l*-deprenyl), or placebo over a 20-year period (180). The authors found no difference in response rates to TCAs and fluoxetine between male and female patients of all studied ages, but women had a statistically significant superiority in their response to MAOI antidepressants. The authors also failed to find a clinically relevant difference in treatment response of female patients in older age groups, suggesting a lack of influence by menopausal status.

Other Antidepressants

A number of antidepressants were introduced after SSRIs. *Venlafaxine* is a nonselective serotonin and norepinephrine reuptake inhibitor. *Desvenlafaxine*, the primary metabolite of venlafaxine, has a similar profile to its parent compound, but dosing may be easier. *Duloxetine* is also a nonselective serotonin and norepinephrine reuptake inhibitor, but has greater potency than venlafaxine (181). Neither compound has significant anticholinergic or antihistaminic effects. *Mirtazapine* is a noradrenergic α_2 antagonist at auto- and heteroreceptors, enhancing serotonin release and a 5-HT_{2A} and 5-HT_3 antagonist. *Nefazodone* and *trazodone* are phenylpiperazine derivatives. Nefazodone is a 5-HT_{2A} antagonist and serotonin reuptake inhibitor. *Bupropion* is an aminoketone that in vivo may block norepinephrine reuptake via its active metabolite hydroxybupropion and also increase dopamine activity by an unknown mechanism. *Reboxetine* is a selective norepinephrine reuptake inhibitor that is currently used to treat mood disorders in Canada and Europe but is not available in the United States. These newer antidepressants offer some advantages in tolerability over the older agents and perhaps more importantly have different mechanisms of action, which may provide alternatives for patients who do not respond to other antidepressants.

Bupropion

Bupropion is an aminoketone compound that was introduced in the United States in 1989 amid concerns about its seizure-inducing potential, a factor that delayed its marketing from the original FDA approval in 1985. A large study in the interim period established that the seizure risk from bupropion at usual therapeutic doses was similar to the cyclic antidepressants. Bupropion has three active metabolites: hydroxybupropion, threobupropion, and erythrobupropion. The relative contributions of the metabolites to clinical or adverse effects are unclear; however, they reach higher plasma levels than the parent compound. Bupropion's plasma half-life after chronic dosing is about 20 h and it is 80% protein bound. The half-life of hydroxybupropion is longer, about 22 h, and it is a norepinephrine reuptake inhibitor (182).

Bupropion is believed to exert its antidepressant action by inhibiting norepinephrine reuptake and enhancing dopamine activity. It has no serotonergic, anticholinergic, or antihistaminergic effects, nor does it interact with monoamine oxidase (182). There is still some ambiguity concerning its mechanism of action which arises from differences in bupropion's actions in vivo and in vitro. Bupropion is a potent dopamine reuptake inhibitor as well as a moderate norepinephrine reuptake inhibitor in vitro. In vivo, the drug is twice as potent in its norepinephrine reuptake inhibition compared to its dopamine reuptake inhibition (183). Although bupropion has demonstrated dopamine uptake inhibition using in vitro models, the concentrations required may not have clinical relevance. In addition, even though homovanillic acid is increased during bupropion treatment (an indication of enhanced dopamine activity), these levels are not associated with a positive antidepressant response. Hydroxybupropion is associated with down-regulation of postsynaptic β-adrenergic receptors in animal models.

Bupropion IR (immediate release) carries a relatively higher risk of lowering seizure threshold compared to SSRIs. Bupropion IR has a risk of seizures of 0.4% at doses up to 450 mg/day, which is about 2–4 times higher than the incidence of seizures associated with SSRI treatment (0.1–0.2%) (184). Seizure risk is strongly related to dose and the rate of dosage escalation. Even with modest increases of the dose to 450–600 mg/day seizure risk increases tenfold. An extended release formulation has lowered the risk of seizures to a level comparable to other antidepressant classes. A seizure rate of 0.1% was associated with bupropion SR (sustained release) at doses of 300 mg/day and 0.4% at 400 mg/day (184). Clinicians should be aware that Wellbutrin® and Zyban® are both bupropion, and inadvertent overdoses have occurred when both have been prescribed for the same patient to treat depression and for smoking cessation.

Because of bupropion's dopaminergic and adrenergic actions, it can be activating and may cause overstimulation, agitation, nausea, nervousness, and insomnia as well as tremors and palpitations (182, 184, 185); however, in our experience, it is usually very well tolerated. It has the potential to induce mania in bipolar patients; however, bupropion-induced mania tends to be milder and have a shorter course than either spontaneous mania or mania elicited in patients by tricyclic or SSRI antidepressants (77). Bupropion has a favorable cardiovascular profile and does not cause orthostatic hypotension or conduction delay. Some patients may have elevated blood pressure with bupropion, but in our experience is not as frequent a problem as with venlafaxine.

Since bupropion does not interact with serotonergic receptors, it has an extremely low incidence of sexual side effects which are common with SSRIs and most other antidepressants (97, 184, 185). Bupropion is a reasonable alternative to SSRI when sexual adverse effects limit their use. Bupropion is not associated with weight gain.

Dermatologic adverse effects of bupropion are rare but may also include urticarial and pruritic rashes and very rarely extreme dermatologic reactions (186).

Because of its unique mechanism of action and good tolerability it has become one of the first choices for SSRI augmentation for many clinicians.

Venlafaxine

Venlafaxine is a bicyclic phenylethylamine derivative marketed as a racemic mixture of its R- and S-enantiomers; the R-enantiomer is more potent of the 2 (187). Venlafaxine is only 27% protein bound and has a half-life of 4–5 h. It undergoes first-pass metabolism to *O*-demethylvenlafaxine, ODV, which is active and just as potent as its parent compound, and has an elimination half-life 11 h. Clearance of both venlafaxine and ODV is decreased by 55% in patients with severe renal disease and by 33% in patients with cirrhosis (188). Venlafaxine XR (extended release) formulation has become the preferred agent, and the immediate release formulation is rarely used in the US. Pharmacologically, the XR it is quite similar to the original venlafaxine IR (immediate release); the differences are increased time to peak plasma concentration as well as lower plasma concentrations of the XR drug (189).

Venlafaxine acts on both serotonergic and norepinephrine reuptake at higher therapeutic doses (225 mg or higher), but at lower doses, it affects mainly serotonin, making it comparable to SSRI. However, as the dose is increased, it becomes a potent inhibitor of the synaptic reuptake of norepinephrine (182, 187, 188). At low doses, inhibition of serotonin reuptake is about three to fivefold higher than that of norepinephrine reuptake (32, 188). Venlafaxine also possesses weak affinity toward the dopamine receptor (188). It rapidly down-regulates β-adrenergic receptors, a property that some contend supports those studies that have found a more rapid onset of antidepressant effect with venlafaxine compared to other agents. It has minimal or no interaction with muscarinic, histaminic, or α-adrenergic receptors, which accounts for its low incidence of adverse effects (187). It is an effective antidepressant and antianxiety agent.

Most common adverse effects include those associated with SSRI, such as nausea, vomiting, sexual dysfunction, somnolence, and sweating (182, 185, 190). The incidence of sexual dysfunction is thought by some to be lower than SSRI (103, 185, 191).

Of most concern has been elevated blood pressure which occurs at higher doses of venlafaxine (between 101 and 300 mg daily) that returns to normal after drug discontinuation (69, 182). Blood pressure changes are dose related, with an incidence of about 5% at doses under 200 mg daily and 13% at doses greater than 300 mg daily. Pre-existing hypertension does not appear to be a risk factor for this effect. If the dose cannot be reduced, blood pressure should be treated pharmacologically, using standard drug algorithms.

Discontinuation syndromes upon abruptly stopping venlafaxine have been reported (192). The most common symptoms are dizziness or lightheadedness, excessive sweating, irritability, dysphoria, and insomnia, which is similar to the SSRI discontinuation syndrome (192). A slow taper of the medication usually prevents the occurrence of this syndrome. On rare occasions, it may be necessary to reinstitute the medication or switch to a long-acting SSRI, such as fluoxetine.

Venlafaxine is one of the few antidepressants that has been studied in pregnancy. A recent prospective study of 150 pregnant women receiving venlafaxine found no significant differences between women taking venlafaxine during pregnancy and those taking either SSRI antidepressants or known non-teratogenic drugs (193). The rates of major neonatal malformations in all groups were the same as baseline rate for the general population of 1–3%. It should be noted that the sample size is too small to detect rare occurrences of adverse effects, such as teratogenic risk.

Desvenlafaxine is the major active metabolite of the SNRI antidepressant venlafaxine formulated as an extended-release tablet for once-daily, oral administration. It inhibits the neuronal reuptake of both serotonin and norepinephrine and, to a lesser degree, dopamine. It is approximately tenfold more potent at inhibiting serotonin uptake than norepinephrine uptake. Desvenlafaxine lacks monoamine oxidase inhibitory activity and shows no affinity for muscarinic cholinergic, H_1-histaminergic, or α_1-adrenergic receptors in vitro.

Desvenlafaxine is well absorbed after oral administration (80% bioavailability) but somewhat slowly, with a T_{max} of 7–8 h. It has a mean terminal half-life (t½) of approximately 9–15 h. Metabolism is primarily through phase II glucuronidation and, to a minor extent, through CYP3A4. It has linear pharmacokinetics through supratherapeutic doses, with very small differences between subjects. It does not inhibit CYP2D6 to a clinically significant extent. Desvenlafaxine plasma binding is approximately 30% and independent of drug concentration. There are no active metabolites, and it is excreted by the kidney as unchanged desvenlafaxine and the glucuronide conjugate.

Several studies have established the efficacy of desvenlafaxine in major depression and it is FDA approved for that indication. Despite an active research program in the area, studies do not yet support the efficacy and safety of desvenlafaxine for vasomotor symptoms associated with menopause, such as hot flushes, night sweats, and associated sleep disruptions.

Similar to its parent compound, discontinuation symptoms are observed after cessation of desvenlafaxine treatment in both short-term and long-term MDD studies. The most common symptoms reported by patients after discontinuation of short-term desvenlafaxine treatment were dizziness, nausea, irritability, and diarrhea, which are characteristic of the serotonin reuptake inhibitor discontinuation syndrome. Symptoms associated with treatments of 6-month duration include fatigue, abnormal dreams, anxiety, and hyperhidrosis. About half of patients taking desvenlafaxine have some discontinuation symptoms, but they are relatively few and mild compared to short-acting SSRI withdrawal syndromes. At the recommended dose of 50 mg daily, discontinuation symptoms appear shortly after abrupt discontinuation and resolve within a week.

In summary, desvenlafaxine offers a few advantages over venlafaxine, although among them are ease of dosing—a single dose of 50 mg for initiation and maintenance, lower potential for pharmacokinetic drug interactions, and apparently a less severe discontinuation syndrome.

Duloxetine

Duloxetine is an antidepressant that inhibits both serotonin and norepinephrine reuptake. Although similar to venlafaxine, duloxetines's greater potency at noradrenergic reuptake is thought to contribute to its greater efficacy in pain treatment than venlafaxine. It is approved by the FDA for use in major depression, generalized anxiety disorder, diabetic neuropathic pain, and fibromyalgia. The recommended therapeutic doses range from 40-60 mg daily, but lower doses (20-30 mg daily) should be used for the first week of treatment to avoid adverse effects. Although clinical studies do not support doses higher than 60 mg daily, our experience suggests that higher doses are usually necessary for pain syndromes related to fibromyalgia and other autoimmune diseases. Common adverse effects are nausea, decreased appetite, constipation, headache, dry mouth, insomnia, and somnolence. Men, but not women, treated with duloxetine experience more difficulty achieving orgasm compared to placebo. Increases in both systolic and diastolic blood pressure of approximately 2 mm Hg and an increase in heart rate of 3-4 beats per minute. Some patients experience palpitations but clinically significant changes in electrocardiograms were not different in duloxetine and placebo groups in premarketing studies. The drug is among a class of agents that increase urethral resistance, which may lead to urinary hesitation. Duloxetine has an elimination half-life ranging from 8-17 hours, with hepatic metabolism by P450 isozymes CYP1A2 and CYP2D6. Numerous metabolites are produced, but it is believed that the primary therapeutic effect is from the parent compound.

Nefazodone and Trazodone

Nefazodone and *trazodone* are two closely related antidepressants. Nefazodone is a phenylpiperazine derivative of trazodone with lower α_1 activity. Trazodone is a triazolopyridine derivative developed in early 1980s as an alternative to TCAs, but its efficacy has always been questioned, and its most common use today is to promote sleep. Its antidepressant properties are believed to be related to its 5-HT_2 receptor antagonism and only partially from its weak serotonin reuptake inhibition (32, 187). Aside from its therapeutic actions, trazodone is a weak to moderate histamine H_1 receptor antagonist as well as α_1-adrenergic antagonist, which makes it similar to TCAs in terms of the undesired side effects (187).

Nefazodone has three pharmacologically active metabolites: hydroxynefazodone (OHN), triazole-dione, and *m*-chlorophenylpiperazine (mCPP). Both triazole-dione and OHN contribute to the antidepressant effect of nefazodone. Like nefazodone, OHN is a very potent inhibitor of 5-HT_{2A} receptors as well as serotonin reuptake. The triazole-dione metabolite has weak 5-HT_{2A} antagonism. mCPP is an agonist at the 5-$HT_{1A,1B,1C,1D}$ and 5-HT_{2C} receptors but is not considered to have a significant impact on nefazodone's overall actions (182, 189). Nefazodone antagonizes and down-regulates postsynaptic 5-HT_{2A} receptors, which in turn leads to enhanced 5-HT_{1A} receptor-meditated postsynaptic neurotransmission (194). It is a moderate presynaptic serotonin reuptake inhibitor (194). Nefazodone also inhibits presynaptic norepinephrine reuptake, but to a much lesser degree, and this probably does not contribute to its therapeutic actions (182). Nefazodone is a weak α_1-adrenergic antagonist and has very little if any α_2-adrenergic, antihistaminic, or dopamine receptor interactions (187, 195).

As discussed above, trazodone is a histamine H_1 receptor antagonist, as well as an α_1-adrenergic antagonist, which makes it similar to TCA drugs in terms of the undesired side effects (187). Despite isolated case reports of conduction delay and arrhythmias with trazodone (especially in overdoses), studies have not found this effect even in patients with pre-existing cardiac disease. Anticholinergic and antihistamine effects are negligible (182, 187). Due to its α_1-adenoreceptor blocking properties, trazodone may cause orthostatic hypotension (69). The most serious adverse effect of trazodone therapy in male patients is priapism, a urologic emergency (196). The incidence of trazodone-induced priapism is unknown with estimates ranging from 1 in 1,000 to 1 in 10,000 patients. It tends to occur early in treatment, usually within the first month, but has also been reported after 18 months of treatment. It can occur at doses as low as 50 mg daily. Approximately one-third of patients require surgical intervention. Priapism is believed to be due to α-adrenergic blockade.

Nefazodone has weak α_1 and cholinergic receptor antagonism and virtually no α_2-adrenergic, dopamine, or histaminic blockade (182, 190). Nefazodone does not cause sexual dysfunction, and it is a reasonable alternative to SSRI when this effect is of concern (97, 103). It has not been associated with priapism, despite its structural similarity to trazodone (34, 69). The most frequent side effects of nefazodone as compared to placebo in patients in clinical trials are nausea (21 vs. 14%), somnolence (19 vs. 13%), dry mouth (19 vs. 13%), dizziness (12 vs. 6%), constipation (11 vs. 7%), lightheadedness (10 vs. 4%), and blurred vision (6 vs. 3%) (195). It should be noted that occurrence of nausea and gastrointestinal distress in patients taking nefazodone or trazodone is usually less than that produced by either SSRI or venlafaxine treatment (185).

A study of hepatotoxicity of the newer antidepressants using the Spanish Pharmacovigilance System database reported a high incidence of hepatotoxicity with nefazodone, with 28.96 cases per 100,000 patient-years, compared to 1.28 for sertraline and 4.0 for clomipramine (72). The Canadian Adverse Drug Reaction Monitoring Program found 32 cases of hepatotoxicity associated with nefazodone, with 26 classified as severe (197). Patients were between 30 and 69 years old and were taking doses of 100–600 mg daily. Sixty-eight and eight-tenths percent were women; 88% developed toxicity within 6 months of beginning the drug. Toxicity is hepatocellular in such cases, with high serum aminotransferase levels and increased total bilirubin. Withdrawal of nefazodone may lead to improvement in liver function; however, deaths have also been reported (72, 198). It is likely that both pharmacovigilance studies suffer from underreporting (72). If this is so, the incidence of hepatotoxicity associated with nefazodone may be even higher. In the United States, nefazodone now carries a "black box" warning concerning hepatotoxicity, and some countries have removed it from the market. It retains a niche market in the U.S. for anxious and depressed patients, often with substance abuse, who have not responded to several other agents.

Mirtazapine

Mirtazapine, is a 6-aza-analogue of mianserin but has a different pharmacologic profile (199). Mirtazapine is a less-potent noradrenergic reuptake blocker and 5-HT_2 antagonist than mianserin (199). Mirtazapine is an effective antidepressant and antianxiety agent, and some authorities believe it has a more rapid onset than other antidepressants.

Mirtazapine's mechanism of antidepressant action is believed to be related to enhancement of serotonin and norepinephrine neurotransmission through potent and direct blockade of α_2-adrenergic autoreceptors and heteroreceptors (199, 200). This action results in increased noradrenergic transmission which stimulates α_1-adrenergic receptors on the serotonergic cell body. Blockade of the α_2-adrenergic heteroreceptor on the serotonin nerve terminal prevents this receptor from "turning off" the increased serotonin activity (199, 200). Mirtazapine is also a weak agonist of the 5-HT_{1A} serotonin receptor and causes some enhancement of 5-HT_{1A}–mediated serotonergic transmission through this mechanism (200). Another major action of mirtazapine is inhibition of 5-HT_2 and 5-HT_3 receptors postsynaptically, which may limit the adverse effects that are usually associated with increased serotonin activity and may also contribute to mirtazapine's anxiolytic and hypnotic effects. Because it has a unique pharmacodynamic profile, it is among the first agents used for augmentation and combination therapy with SSRI.

Mirtazapine is marketed as a racemate of R- and S-enantiomers (187). The R-enantiomer is more active, reaches higher plasma concentrations, and has a longer half-life than the S-enantiomer. Mirtazapine is rapidly absorbed from the gastrointestinal tract after oral administration with high bioavailability. It is 85% plasma protein bound and has an elimination half-life of 20–40 h (201). Mirtazapine's major metabolite is demethylmirtazapine, which has only weak activity compared to the parent compound. Hepatic and renal impairment may cause a 30 and 50% decrease in oral mirtazapine clearance, respectively, necessitating a dose adjustment in some patients (201).

Mirtazapine is associated with dry mouth, drowsiness, and sedation in about 25% of patients (199, 202). Because of its antihistaminic activity, this drug may also cause weight gain in approximately 10–20% of patients. A similar percentage of patients have elevated cholesterol and somewhat fewer have elevated triglycerides. Mirtazapine has low incidence of sexual side effects among antidepressants (103).

A causal association of mirtazapine with severe neutropenia (absolute neutrophil count less than 500/ml^3) has been reported in three cases. Of these, 2 patients developed agranulocytosis. All 3 patients recovered upon discontinuation of the drug. It is therefore recommended that mirtazapine be stopped if any signs of infection with a low white cell count occur (201).

Overdose

As a group, the antidepressants introduced since 1985 appear to be safer in overdose compared to the cyclic antidepressants. Although reports of mortality in overdose can be found for most of these agents, fatal overdoses usually occur when they are combined with other agents. One review of venlafaxine reported 16 overdoses of up to 6,750 mg of venlafaxine, either alone or with other medications and/or alcohol without any deaths (201). The most common problems were somnolence and sinus tachycardia. On the other hand, a cohort study of 538 deliberate antidepressant overdoses found that both venlafaxine and SSRIs were more likely to cause serotonin syndromes, but less likely to cause coma, compared to TCAs (203). That study also found that 7 of 51 (14%) venlafaxine patients had seizures. There were no deaths reported. A study from the United Kingdom calculated fatal toxicity from antidepressants using the number of deaths per million prescriptions (204). A rate of 13.2 was reported for venlafaxine, which placed it at the low end of TCA death rates (5.5–200), but higher than SSRI death rates (0.7–3.0). These data must be interpreted with caution because they do not take into account selection bias. For example, patients with high suicide risk may be prescribed drugs that clinicians believe are safer (such as venlafaxine and SSRIs) or used preferentially in severe depression (dual action agents), and avoid those with a low therapeutic index (such as TCAs) or those that may not be as effective in endogenous depression (such as SSRIs).

Data on *mirtazapine*'s safety in overdose are limited. One review reported 8 patients in clinical trials who overdosed on mirtazapine either alone in doses from 100 to 315 mg, or with benzodiazepines, or "pain killers" (190). No fatalities or ECG changes occurred. Another study analyzed 6 cases of overdose with mirtazapine, including overdoses in a 3-year-old child and a 90-year-old man, which occurred during postmarketing surveillance and in clinical trials (205). Again, no serious sequelae were reported. Mirtazapine safety in overdose appears to be comparable to SSRI.

Seven overdose cases of *nefazodone*, with or without co-ingestion of other medications or alcohol, have been reported (195). The symptoms of overdose included nausea, vomiting, and somnolence. All of the patients recovered with general supportive care (195). The American Association of Poison Control Centers reported on 1,338 cases of nefazodone poisoning that were not associated with other drug use (206). There were no deaths, and the most serious effect was hypotension in 1.6% of cases. More common symptoms included drowsiness (17.3%), nausea (9.7%), and dizziness (9.5%), which resolved within 24 h.

A fatal case of *trazodone* overdose had been reported in European literature. The patient sustained arrhythmias (torsades de pointes and complete AV block) and multiple organ failure and died within 24 h after admission to emergency department (207).

Buproprion has been associated with fatalities when ingested with other medications or at very high doses. An overdose of 23 g resulted in death (208). In another report, a patient recovered after grand mal seizures, and sinus tachycardia occurred following intentional ingestion of 9 g of bupropion (209). A 3-year, multicenter, retrospective study of bupropion overdoses reported to poison control centers described 58 cases of bupropion ingestion alone and 9 cases of ingestion of bupropion and a benzodiazepine (210). There were no fatal outcomes among these patients, but many had sinus tachycardia, hypotension, hypokalemia, lethargy, tremors, and seizures (210). The seizure risk of bupropion increases with dose (184), and higher seizure rates are seen in bulimic patients, with approximately one-third of overdoses with bupropion IR resulting in seizures in these individuals (34).

The Role of Mixed Action Antidepressants in Therapeutics

Recently marketed non-SSRI antidepressants are considered by most clinicians as second-line therapeutic options for treatment refractory patients or as augmenting agents. Since these antidepressant medications act on different neuronal systems, they are a rational choice in non-responders (182). They are also used as adjunctive agents to augment SSRIs in partial responders. Their overall efficacy as antidepressants is comparable to that of the standard antidepressant classes such as SSRIs, TCAs, and MAOIs, and some data indicate superiority compared to SSRI in depression with melancholic or endogenous features. They are second-line agents because the SSRI are easier to dose, are available in generic form, and have few medically serious adverse effects.

In addition to the efficacy of non-SSRI agents in depression, studies support efficacy in anxiety disorders (especially venlafaxine, mirtazapine, nefazodone) and ADHD (venlafaxine, bupropion). Bupropion's role in smoking cessation is well recognized (211) but it has also been used to treat neuropathic pain (212). Duloxetine and milnacipram are the preferred antidepressant agents in fibromyalgia. Bupropion and mirtazapine have become the agents of choice if SSRI-induced sexual dysfunction limits continued treatment with that class of drugs.

Trazodone has a limited role, but may be useful in promoting sleep in patients taking energizing antidepressants, or as an augmentation agent. Nefazodone is a very effective antidepressant but its use has declined since reports of hepatotoxicity have appeared. Mirtazapine is also an effective antidepressant and antianxiety agent that is frequently used in combination with other antidepressants as an augmentation strategy and to improve sleep, although with higher doses its hypnotic actions are eliminated.

The possibility of a more rapid onset of clinical effect for agents that have mixed actions, mirtazapine and venlafaxine in particular, has been the subject of much debate. At present, there are insufficient data to support such a claim.

Antidepressants Without United States FDA Approval

Reboxetine

Reboxetine is a selective norepinephrine reuptake inhibitor approved for use as an antidepressant in Canada and Europe, but not yet available in the United States. It is a racemic mixture of two stereoisomers, consisting of (S,S)-(+)- and

(R, R)-(−)-reboxetine; the (S,S) enantiomer is more potent as an antidepressant and has greater affinity to the norepinephrine receptor (213, 214).

Women have a 30% higher S, S to R, R ratio than men (215). Reboxetine downregulates β-adrenergic receptors (213). Although it is somewhat less potent as a norepinephrine reuptake inhibitor than desipramine and nortriptyline (187), it has very low affinity for α-adrenergic and muscarinic cholinergic receptors, and no affinity for serotonergic or dopaminergic receptors (213).

Reboxetine has linear pharmacokinetics with either single or multiple oral doses. Its elimination half-life is approximately 12–13 h; absolute bioavailability is 94.5%. Reboxetine is rapidly absorbed; it reaches its maximal concentration in 2 h after administration (213, 214). It is 97% bound to plasma proteins, particularly α_1-acid glycoprotein (213, 214). The suggested dosage for reboxetine is 8–10 mg/day in divided dose (216). It has no active metabolites. Plasma concentrations of reboxetine are increased in patients who are elderly or have hepatic or renal insufficiency (213, 214). The recommended dose for such patients is 4–6 mg/day. Reboxetine is metabolized hepatically by cytochrome P450 CYP 3A4 but has no known inhibitory or inducing effect on any of the CYP isoforms.

Adverse Effects

Clinical trials have established its safety (216, 217). The most frequent adverse effects include dry mouth, constipation, increased diaphoresis, insomnia, and urinary retention (187, 218–220). Most of these appear to be dose related (216, 219). Clinically insignificant orthostatic hypotension has been reported (218). Also, headache, palpitations, tachycardia, decreased appetite, dizziness, and abnormal sensation in the genitals have been reported with reboxetine use; the incidence of all side effects, except tachycardia, was dose related (219).

Reboxetine did not alter cardiac conduction in healthy volunteers in a randomized, open-label, placebo-controlled study, which was specifically designed to test reboxetine's effect on cardiac repolarization at different plasma concentrations, including those exceeding the normal therapeutic range (219). Subjects' ECGs were used to assess the QTc, PR, and QRS intervals; no changes in these parameters as a result of reboxetine treatment were reported (219). However, reboxetine resulted in heart rate increases of 8–11 beats per minute at doses of ≥8 mg/day (219).

Efficacy

Several double-blind, randomized clinical trials, conducted mostly outside the United States, showed superiority of reboxetine to placebo and/or to established antidepressants such as fluoxetine in patients suffering from moderate to severe MDD. In a 6-week randomized, double-blind, placebo-controlled study of reboxetine, hospitalized patients with MDD found that both the improvement in the mean HAM-D-21 total score and the response rate (defined as percentage of patients achieving ≥50% reduction in HAM-D-21 total score) were significantly greater in the reboxetine group than those in the placebo group (218).

In an 8-week double-blind, randomized, placebo- and active treatment-controlled, multisite clinical trial of 381 inpatients and outpatients with MDD and baseline HAM-D-17 scores 22 or higher, reboxetine, at daily doses of 8–10 mg, was shown to be as effective as fluoxetine, at 20–40 mg/day (as judged by a similar percentage of patients achieving ≥50% reduction in HAM-D scores) (220). Both active drugs were shown to be significantly superior to placebo (220). Efficacy in severe depression was also found and replicated by Montgomery and associates (221). Some investigators have found reboxetine to have a faster onset of action than other antidepressants, improving patients' HAM-D scores as soon as 10 days after initiating treatment (217).

In general, however, the perception is that reboxetine has weak efficacy in MDD. An intriguing study found that a single 4 mg dose reduced negative information processing that is commonly seen in patients with mood and anxiety disorders (222). Reboxetine may share some actions with cognitive behavioral therapies. A related study found that reboxetine and citalopram (SSRI) both modulated information processing in depressed patients, although different brain areas were affected (223). These findings provide support for individualized assessment of depressed patients based on activity of specific brain regions assessed by fMRI. At present, it appears that an SSRI and an SNRI affect different brain regions that are important in emotional processing.

Mifepristone

Mifepristone is a progesterone-receptor antagonist and glucocorticoid antagonist, which in preliminary studies has been effective as short-term monotherapy for patients with psychotic major depression (PMD) at doses of 600–800 mg daily (224, 225). Adverse effects include fatigue, anorexia, and nausea. A maculopapular erythematous cutaneous eruption has also been reported (224, 225). Caution must be exercised when used in women because this agent induces abortion.

Substance P

Recent studies have examined compounds that inhibit substance P (SP)-neurokinin-1 (NK_1) receptor pathways as potential antidepressants (226). SP and NK_1 receptors are located in brain regions that regulate mood and are associated with neurotransmitter pathways thought to play a role in depression. In one postmortem study, higher concentrations of SP were found in the cerebrospinal fluid of depressed patients compared to controls (227). Aprepitant and compound A, SP-NK_1 antagonists, have a high affinity and selectivity for the NK_1 receptor, but have not been shown to inhibit other depression-related neurotransmitters. Both compounds have been studied for the treatment of depression with disappointing results.

Melantonergic Agents

Agomelatine is an agonist at melatonin MT_1, and MT_2 receptors, an antagonist at 5-HT_{2C} receptors, and has very weak affinity for 5-HT_{1A}, and 5-HT_{2B} receptors. It is approved in Europe and marketed as Valdoxan. It has shown equivalency to sertraline and venlafaxine. It improves sleep without producing daytime drowsiness (228).

Sigma Agonists

Some currently marketed antidepressants such as fluvoxamine and sertraline, but not paroxetine, are sigma 1 agonists. The sigma agonist igmesine has shown efficacy and safety in early human studies (229).

MAOIs

History

Monoamine oxidase inhibitors (MAOIs) were the first antidepressants used in clinical practice. Iproniazid, the isopropyl derivative of isoniazid, was developed by Herbert Fox at Roche Laboratories in 1951 for the treatment of tuberculosis (230). The drug proved ineffective for tuberculosis, but did have a mood elevating effect in some patients (231). Its antidepressant properties are believed to be the result of the inhibition of monoamine oxidase (MAO), the enzyme that catalyzes oxidative deamination of monoamines such as dopamine, epinephrine, norepinephrine, and serotonin among others, thus rendering these amines inactive (31, 232–234). Inhibition of the enzyme results in increased availability of these biogenic amines by preventing their breakdown. Unfortunately, most United States clinicians who have entered practice over the last two decades have little experience using MAOIs for the treatment of depression. The efficacy of SSRI in atypical and mixed depression accounts in part for this phenomenon. However, as described below, the pharmacological actions of MAOIs are unique and should still be considered as alternative agents when other antidepressants are not effective.

In 1950s and 1960s, MAOIs became a primary treatment for depression. At their peak, there were five hydrazines (isocarboxazid, nialamide, mebanazine, phenelzine, and pheniprazine) which are structurally similar to iproniazid, one indole (etryptamine), and one cyclopropylamine (tranylcypromine) in clinical use. The first MAOI, iproniazid, and then pheniprazine were withdrawn from the market due to hepatotoxicity (31). As clinical experience grew, the serious adverse effects of MAOIs combined with the introduction of safer antidepressants led to a decline in MAOI use. Currently, only four MAOIs are approved by the FDA for treatment of depression in the United States. They are *phenelzine (Nardil)*, *tranylcypromine (Parnate)*, *isocarboxazide (Marplan)*, and *selegiline (EMSAM)*.

Pharmacology

A clinically relevant classification of MAOIs is based on three characteristics: (1) hydrazine vs. non-hydrazine structure; (2) selectivity for MAO-A or MAO-B; (3) reversibility of MAO inhibition. Phenelzine and isocarboxazid are hydrazines. The non-hydrazine MAOIs, tranylcypromine and selegeline, are arylalkamines. Hydrazine derivatives may be associated with hepatotoxicity, requiring monitoring of liver enzymes during treatment.

Monoamine oxidase is an enzyme located principally on the outer membrane of mitochondria. Its role is oxidative deamination of monoamines, many of which modulate mood states. The development of substrate selective MAOIs in the 1960s provided evidence for the existence of two forms of the enzyme: MAO-A and MAO-B. MAO-A selectively deaminates serotonin, norepinephrine, and epinephrine, whereas MAO-B selectively metabolizes tyramine, phenylethylamine, phenylethanolamine, and benzylamine. Both forms are involved in tyramine, tryptamine, and dopamine metabolism, although dopamine is the preferred substrate for MAO-B. Both MAO-A and MAO-B are widely distributed in the human body, with some cells containing both forms while others contain only one. The human brain MAO is 70–95% MAO-B; however, in other species, such as rodents, MAO-A may predominate in the brain. In humans, gut and platelet MAO is primarily Type A.

Although *selegiline* (referred to as *l*-deprenyl in the older research literature) has selectivity for MAO-B at low doses, as the dose increases, it affects both forms of the enzyme. The oral formulation is approved for use as an anti-Parkinson agent, but has also shown promise as an antidepressant at higher doses than used for Parkinsonism. The transdermal formulation of selegiline (EMSAM) is approved for the treatment of depression and offers less risk of food interactions than the antidepressant doses of oral selegiline. Pargyline, a drug that is no longer marketed, but was once used as an antihypertensive, is selective for MAO-B. All other clinically available MAOIs inhibit both MAO-A and MAO-B. An interesting compound is TV-3326, which is a cholinesterase inhibitor affecting both MAO-A and MAO-B, but it differentially inhibits Type A in the brain and does not inhibit Type A in the gut of rabbits (235). The reason for the selectivity is unclear, but possibly related to metabolites. It suggests that it may be possible to develop irreversible MAOIs that do not induce hypertensive crises with tyramine-containing foods. Another intriguing strategy to avoid the tyramine hypertensive reaction has been the development of a transdermal delivery system for selegiline that permits high brain concentrations of the drug to block both Type A and Type B MAO in the brain, but has no effect on intestinal MAO-A. Inhibition of Type A in the brain is necessary for antidepressant effects, whereas gut inhibition causes the tyramine reaction.

Other drugs have been developed that produce reversible MAO inhibition may be reversible, such as moclobemide and brofaromine, neither of which are marketed in the United States. This class of MAOIs is referred to as RIMA (reversible inhibitors of monoamine oxidase-A). The advantages of the reversible agents are fewer risks of tyramine-containing food interactions, because tyramine is able to displace RIMA from MAO-binding sites. In contrast, the agents available in the United

States are classified as irreversible or "suicide enzyme inhibitors" because they form covalent bonds at specific sites on the enzyme. Phenelzine inactivates the flavin group and phenelzine the sulfhydryl group. There is some evidence to suggest that MAO activity may return more quickly following discontinuation of tranylcypromine (3–5 days) compared to phenelzine. There is considerable variability among patients; therefore, most clinicians follow the manufacturer's guideline of a 10- to 14-day interval after discontinuing an MAOI prior to starting a drug that has the potential for an adverse interaction.

The pharmacological properties of available agents have not been well studied, although there has been renewed interest in the area (236). Phenelzine (Nardil) is rapidly absorbed after oral administration, with maximum concentrations occurring 2–4 h post-dose and it has a short elimination half-life (1.5–4 h). On the other hand, the pharmacodynamic effects are long lasting, the result of irreversible MAO inhibition. The pathways of metabolism (236) are not well known; however, phenelzine is both a substrate and inhibitor of MAO, and this pathway may lead to the production of phenylacetic acid. Intermediate metabolites may be phenylethylidene hydrazine and 1-2-phenylehtyldiazene, also resulting from the action of MAO. Another metabolite is believed to be phenylethylamine (PEA). Substantial levels of phenylethylamine may derive both from metabolism of phenelzine and from inhibition of endogenous metabolism (PEA is a substrate of MAO). Another pathway probably involves ring-hydroxylation leading to the formation of *p*-hydroxyphenelzine and via MAO to *p*-hydroxyphenylacetic acid. Contrary to early studies, it is now generally believed that despite its structural similarity to isoniazid, phenelzine acetylation is only a minor pathway, but low levels of *N*-acetyl phenelzine have also been reported. The contributions of the metabolites to clinical effects are not known.

Tranylcypromine (Parnate) is also rapidly absorbed with peak plasma levels occurring 1–2 h after an oral dose. It too is rapidly eliminated, with a $t_{1/2}$ of less than 2 h; however, a single 10 mg dose can produce MAO inhibition lasting as long as 1 week. Human metabolic pathways remain uncertain. Perhaps the most controversy has centered on the issue of whether tranylcypromine is metabolized to amphetamine, which was detected in the plasma of a patient who took an overdose of tranylcypromine (237). More recent studies have not detected amphetamine after any dose of tranylcypromine in humans or animals (238, 239). Most of the information on tranylcypromine metabolites is derived from animal studies, and their clinical relevance is not established. Tranylcypromine is marketed as a racemic mixture and studies indicate that S-tranylcypromine is absorbed more rapidly, metabolized more slowly, and reaches higher levels than R-tranylcypromine (240, 241). R-tranylcypromine is a more potent inhibitor of MAO, but is less potent in inhibiting catecholamine reuptake than S-tranylcypromine (236).

We are unaware of published studies on the human pharmacokinetics of isocarboxazid (Marplan).

Selegiline (Eldepryl) has antidepressant effects at oral doses of 40–60 mg daily, although it is not approved by the FDA for this use. Its absorption is increased by food, and its elimination half-life is 2 h after a single dose, but 10 h at steady state. With oral administration, there is wide variability in selegiline metabolism among individuals. Its primary metabolite, desmethylselegiline, possesses MAO-B inhibiting activity; although it is less potent than the parent compound, it is present in higher concentrations. Other metabolites include L-amphetamine and L-methamphetamine; however, the concentrations of these metabolites are thought to be too low to contribute to the drug's therapeutic effects. Even at the 10 mg oral dose used to treat Parkinsonism, MAO-B selectivity is not absolute, and hypertensive reactions after ingestion of tyramine have occasionally been observed. As the dose increases, selectivity is lost, and although the exact dose at which selectivity is lost varies, at doses over 30 mg daily, tyramine restrictions should be instituted.

Emsam™ is FDA approved for major depressive disorder. Elimination half-life of selegiline with this transdermal delivery system ("patch") is 18 h in single dosing, and 22–30 h with chronic dosing. Time to reach steady state with the patch is 4–5 days. The Emsam™ patch is applied to dry, intact skin with a starting dose of 6 mg/24 h. If dose increases are indicated, they should occur in increments of 3 mg/24 h, up to a maximal dose of 12 mg/24 h at 2-week intervals. A tyramine-restricted diet is required with doses of 9 mg/24 h or higher and must be continued for 2 weeks after stopping the drug. As with other MAOIs, serious drug–drug interactions occur especially with serotonergic agents which can lead to a serotonin syndrome. Emsam™ should not be coadministered with other antidepressants, tramadol, methadone, meperidine, or drugs that have MAOI activity. It is not approved for use in children and has the same FDA black box warning concerning suicide as other antidepressants. The drug is generally well tolerated with the most common side effect being a skin reaction at the application site.

Reversible inhibitors of monoamine oxidase Type A (RIMAs) include moclobemide and brofaromine. Moclobemide and brofaromine both have proven antidepressant efficacy and are considered as effective and better tolerated than the tricyclic antidepressants (TCAs) (69, 242–244). RIMAs are also thought to have a much improved side effect profile due to their reversibility and selectivity. Although not entirely free of risk, they may be less likely to be associated with the serotonin syndrome based on significantly smaller number of reported cases compared to the traditional MAOIs (245). At this time, brofaromine is not being developed as an antidepressant for reasons unrelated to its adverse effects or efficacy. It had been studied as a possible treatment for panic disorder, and clinical improvements in anxiety symptoms and subsequent reduction in agoraphobic avoidance were found (246).

Moclobemide is widely used throughout much of the world except the United States (31, 247). Moclobemide was found to be comparable to the SSRIs in both efficacy and tolerability (243). It was also found to be better tolerated with an earlier onset of antidepressant activity when compared to clomipramine in a UK-based study (244).

Conventional explanations of the mechanism of MAOIs' antidepressant action are consistent with the biogenic amine hypothesis of depression, attributing their effects to inactivation of an enzyme responsible for catabolic metabolism of these amines which results in increased concentration of norepinephrine, dopamine, serotonin, and trace amines in the brain (31). In turn, these effects lead ultimately to changes in gene expression (see SSRI section, and Chapter "Biological Theories of Depression and Implications for Current and New Treatments", this volume). Although an integrative theory has appeal, it should not be misinterpreted to mean that all MAOIs act identically. There are at least three related mechanisms that have been identified that may contribute to the therapeutic actions MAOIs: (1) inhibition of metabolism of brain biogenic amines, including trace amines such as phenylethlylamine, tyramine, and octopamine; (2) enhanced neurotransmitter release, blockade of synaptic reuptake, and/or direct receptor effects; and (3) inhibition of other enzymes, altering other neurotransmitters.

Both phenelzine and tranylcypromine have direct effects on reuptake of dopamine, noradrenaline, and to a lesser extent serotonin. They have been reported to down-regulate β_1, β_2, and α_2 adrenoreceptors, and down-regulate the serotonin somatodendritic autoreceptor. Tryptamine receptors are reduced in rat cortex after chronic tranylcypromine administration, and 5-HT_2 receptors are decreased. Phenelzine and/or its metabolites inhibit γ-aminobutyric acid and alanine transaminases (leading to elevation in brain GABA and alanine), dopamine-β-hydroxylase, tryptophan pyrolase, aromatic amino acid decarboxylase, and tyramine amino transaminase.

Clinical Use

MAOIs are now considered third or fourth-line agents in depression due to the potential for drug–drug and drug–food interactions. They have established efficacy in atypical depression, bipolar depression, and dysthymia, and some studies have even found them superior to other established antidepressants (244, 246, 248–252). MAOIs have also been effective in the treatment of depression in the elderly (253). MAOIs were as effective as the tricyclics in all recent controlled studies of depressed patients with either typical (unipolar) or atypical depression. Phenelzine's superiority to imipramine, for example, was demonstrated in atypical depression (254). Other studies support MAOI's advantages for treatment of patients with atypical depression (249, 250). Some have argued that higher than usual doses of MAOI may be needed in severely depressed patients and those who failed treatment with a TCA (255).

The use of MAOIs in patients who failed trials with other antidepressants is well supported (250, 255–257). In a double-blind crossover trial, phenelzine was effective in up to 67% of depressed outpatients who were not responding to treatment with imipramine (248). Tranylcypromine in combination with lithium was effective in treating depression in 12 treatment refractory patients (256). Tranylcypromine was found more effective than imipramine for bipolar depression and is often used to treat patients in the depressive phases of the illness (258). In bipolar patients, who developed manic states associated with antidepressant treatment, those treated with MAOIs experienced milder and shorter manic episodes than patients treated with SSRIs or TCAs (77).

MAOIs are also effective in dysthymia, anxiety, and phobic disorders (251). There are also some reports of efficacy in PTSD and personality disorders, although the data are conflicting (130, 259–261).

Adverse Effects

The older MAOIs have been limited in use as a consequence of their potential for toxicity. Of greatest concern have been drug–drug interactions with sympathomimetic amines and the food–drug interaction with tyramine, both of which may cause a hypertensive crisis. Another serious adverse effect is the serotonin syndrome, which can occur when MAOIs are coadministered with SSRIs (83). Other significant side effects include dizziness, hypotension, liver toxicity, dry mouth with GI upset, blurred vision, urinary retention/hesitancy, headache, fatigue late in the day, skin rashes, weight gain, pedal edema, and paresthesias. Muscle pain and paresthesias may respond to 100 mg of vitamin B6 (pyridoxine). Phenelzine is known to cause sedation, especially late in the day; tranylcypromine can cause insomnia. Hypotension, particularly orthostatic hypotension, is a major concern in treating elderly patients as this increases their risk for falls and fractures. We have not found a consistently effective way to manage orthostatic hypotension, although some clinicians recommend increased fluid and salt intake, fludrocortisone 0.3–0.8 mg daily dose, and support hose.

Sexual dysfunction such as decreased libido, erectile dysfunction, and inhibition of ejaculation in males and anorgasmia in females has been reported (97). These are common problems and have been shown to occur with all of MAOIs. Some of these are known to resolve over time; for example, spontaneous remission of MAOI-induced anorgasmia has been reported (262). It is also worth noting that rates of sexual effects with MAOIs seem to be equivalent to those of TCA drugs and significantly lower than those with SSRIs (96).

Hypertensive Crises

In the 1960s, there were several case reports of a sudden emergence of hypertension in patients taking MAOIs who were exposed to aged cheese. The name "cheese reaction" was coined by Asatoor et al. in 1963 who hypothesized that the combination of MAOIs with the pressor tyramine in cheese was responsible (263). Dietary precautions limiting ingestion of tyramine-containing foods have greatly increased the safety of MAOI treatment. It is generally accepted that greater than 10 mg of tyramine must be ingested to produce a clinically significant interaction. Symptoms may include severe headache, nausea, neck stiffness, diaphoresis, mydriasis, neuromuscular irritability, occasionally cardiac arrhythmias, and severe hypertension (263–265). Hypertensive crises are managed with intravenous phentolamine in closely monitored medical settings. Some clinicians advise patients to take oral nifedipine (10 mg) if hypertension develops.

Our dietary recommendations are shown in Table 11.

Table 11 Dietary restrictions with MAOI therapy (see (407, 408) for tyramine content of specific foods)

Contraindicated	Moderate restrictions	Relative restrictions	Unnecessary to restrict
Aged cheese (English Stilton, Blue Cheese, 3-year-old white, Old Cheddar and others)	*Bottled or canned beer* (highest contents have 1–1.5 mg tyramine per serving)	*Red or white wine* (most have less than 0.5 mg tyramine per serving)	*Bananas*
Marmite yeast	*Pizza* (caution patients about different types of cheeses that may be used)	*Banana peel or overripe bananas* (1.4 mg tyramine per peel)	*Chocolate*
Sauerkraut		*Distilled spirits* (most do not contain tyramine, but some MAOI inhibit acetaldehyde metabolism creating a potential for a disulfiram-like effect)	*Fresh/mild cheeses*
Some aged/cured meats (salami contains 5.6 mg, mortadella 5.5 mg, air-dried sausage 3.8 mg tyramine/30 g)			*Fresh meat*
Tap beer			*Pickled/smoked fish*
Improperly stored meats or fish			*Yeast extracts, except Marmite*
Soy sauce (tyramine content is highly variable)			*Chicken liver* (little evidence unless not fresh, by day 5 contains 1.5 mg tyramine/30 g, while undetectable at day 1)
Soybean			
Tofu			
Fava Beans (reactions not related to tyramine content, which is negligible)			

Drug–Drug Interactions

The "serotonin syndrome" has been reported with concurrent administration of MAOI and drugs that increase serotonin activity. Most common drug interactions associated with serotonin syndrome were combinations of an MAOI and L-tryptophan (removed from the US market because of an independent association with eosinophilia-myalgia syndrome), and fluoxetine (83). There is also a report of the development of serotonin syndrome in patients who were started on clomipramine 4 weeks after discontinuation of clorgyline (MAO-A inhibitor) (83, 266). A fatal case of serotonin syndrome occurred after combined moclobemide and citalopram intoxication in a Belgian patient with history of depression and prior suicide attempts (85). The serotonin syndrome consists of confusion or hypomania, agitation or restlessness, tremor, hyperreflexia, myoclonus, fever, diaphoresis, diarrhea, incoordination, and shivering. In general, the treatment for the serotonin syndrome should be immediate withdrawal of the offending agent and supportive measures.

Sympathomimetic amines, often contained in cold remedies, weight control products, and dietary supplements, can cause hypertensive reactions with MAOIs. Both indirect-acting sympathomimetics (more dangerous) as well as direct-acting (less dangerous) sympathomimetics may cause a hypertensive crisis when administered with MAOIs. The following indirect-acting vasopressors produce their pressor effects through the release of bound intraneuronal stores of norepinephrine and dopamine: amphetamine, methamphetamine cyclopentamine, ephedrine, pseudoephedrine, L-dopa, dopamine, mephentermine, phentermine, metaraminol, methylphenidate, phenylpropanolamine, and tyramine. The indirect-acting agents are generally believed to be more dangerous than direct-acting amines, with the indirect agents, ephedrine, pseudoephedrine, and phenylpropanolamine, being especially hazardous (267). An additional concern is the use of MAOI antidepressants with drugs used for medical conditions that also inhibit monoamine oxidase, e.g., the antibiotic linexolid (Zyvox).

Overdose

MAOIs are dangerous in overdose, and suicidal patients may exploit the inherent toxicity to commit suicide (268). A fatal dose is considered to be 4–6 mg/kg body weight (69). The onset of symptoms usually occurs 6–12 h after ingestion of a toxic dose, but has been known to be delayed by 24 h. Clinical presentation of a patient who overdosed with an MAOI may include fainting, anxiety, flushing and sweating, headachy, tachycardia, and tremor in early stages; this will progress to agitation, coma, seizures, severe hypotension, and possible cardiac arrest (69). Also, physical tolerance and dependence has been reported with tranylcypromine, with one patient taking doses as high as 440 mg daily (269).

Augmentation Strategies

Combinations of Antidepressants

Some clinicians make a distinction between "combination" and "augmentation" therapies, with the former referring to the use of antidepressants in combination, and the latter referring to the use of drugs that are not antidepressants to augment-approved antidepressants. In our view, this is an artificial distinction, and prefer the term "augmentation" to refer to any combination of medications used to enhance antidepressant response. We recognize that a growing segment of clinical pharmacologists are recommending augmentation therapy at the initiation of treatment, with a rationale that the "best" treatment should be initiated at the start of treatment. This reflects, in part, that primary care providers provide initial pharmacotherapy for depression, and referral to psychiatrists occurs only after monotherapy with antidepressants have failed. The problem with this approach is that there are no augmentation therapies that have superior efficacy.

We recommend augmentation approaches only after monotherapy with two different antidepressants has failed, an opinion based on the observation that at least 50% of out-of-class switches result in treatment response (270–272). In instances of partial responders who have been taking adequate doses for sufficient time, we are inclined to follow an augmentation strategy. Once a decision has been made to augment, a number of options are available. The most common augmentation strategy is to combine antidepressants from different classes. With SSRI, our current practice is to add mirtazapine in doses of 15–30 mg, a strategy that is supported by the somewhat limited literature on the topic (273–275). Alternatively, we employ bupropion augmentation which has a small body of evidence supporting its efficacy in augmentation of SSRIs (276–278) and survey data that indicate it is the most popular SSRI augmentation strategy among clinicians (279). Addition of low doses of a TCA, such as desipramine or nortriptyline, has yielded mixed results (280–283).

Lithium has moderately strong evidence supporting its efficacy as an augmentation agent; however, it is less commonly used than other approaches. The STAR*D study found poor tolerability compared to T3 augmentation. Studies in the early 1980s found that the addition of lithium to TCAs in non-responding patients with unipolar depression resulted in improvement in depression (284, 285) and was comparable to thyroid (T3) supplementation, both of which were better than placebo (286). Other investigators reported similar results, including efficacy in potentiating MAOIs, although lack of efficacy and toxicity has also been reported (287–289). Most but not all studies have found that lithium is also effective in augmentation of SSRIs (281, 290–292). We suspect that the reasons for less frequent use of lithium are its low therapeutic index and the necessity for monitoring serum levels. Typical augmentation doses are 600–1,200 mg daily to produce a target serum level of 0.6–0.9 mEq/L.

Atypical Antipsychotic Augmentation of SSRI

The strongest efficacy data for augmentation of partial antidepressant response to SSRI is the growing clinical trial data on atypical antipsychotics. Despite the strong data for efficacy, it is rarely our first choice for augmentation because there are several unanswered questions regarding optimal dosing and long-term adverse effects. One of us (DAC) began using risperidone in doses of 0.5–1.0 mg as an adjunct to SSRI, and occasionally as a monotherapy in treatment-resistant depression following reports suggesting the effectiveness of this approach (293, 294). We limited it to patients with a partial SSRI response and those who demonstrated depressive features that had symptoms that were resistant to psychotherapy. These included guilt out of proportion to realistic events, inability to engage in introspection, perseveration of ideas of wrongdoing that were exaggerated, and recognition that their beliefs were not a reflection of reality (in other words, maintained capacity for introspection). While these symptoms resembled psychotic depression, the quality of their interpersonal relationships and level of impairment was not consistent with that diagnosis. Following the Ostroff and Nelson (1999) report, we used low doses of risperidone to treat depressive symptoms. To our surprise, the results were a dramatic improvement in symptoms, and since then we have used both risperidone and quetiapine with very good success. Aripiprazole would probably have produced similar results. Since that time, there is increasing evidence that four atypical antipsychotics are effective in augmentation of SSRI: olanzapine, quetiapine, aripiprazole, and risperidone (295–299). The combination product of olanzapine and fluoxetine, marketed under the trade name of Symbax, is approved by the US FDA for use in treatment-resistant depression (defined as failure to respond to treatment with two trials of antidepressants at adequate doses for sufficient time). Aripiprazole is approved by the FDA for adjunctive treatment of major depressive disorder "who had an inadequate response to antidepressant therapy during the current episode."Quetiapine is also approved for use as an adjunct to SSRI, but there is strong evidence of its efficacy as monotherapy of depression, where it has a more rapid onset than duloxetine with fewer adverse effects leading to discontinuation (300).

The mechanism of antidepressant effect of atypical antipsychotics has not been established. The action of aripiprazole as a partial agonist at D2 and D3, 5-HT_{1A} receptors, and an antagonist at 5-HT_2 receptors is consistent with an antidepressant action. Quetiapine has moderate antagonism of D2 and serotonin 5-HT_{1A}, 5-HT_{2A} receptors and its metabolite norquetiapine inhibits the norepinephrine transporter. The antidepressant effects of risperidone may be due to its high affinity for α-2-adrenergic receptors which could enhance norepinephrine neuronal firing and release (301).

It appears that lower doses should be used for atypical antipsychotics when they are used as antidepressants as opposed to antipsychotic agents. For example, 300 mg of quetiapine, 0.5–2.0 mg risperidone, and 10 mg aripiprazole appear to be the optimal antidepressant doses. The combination product of olanzapine and fluoxetine (Symbyax) recommends doses of olanzapine of 6–18 mg of olanzapine with 25–75 mg of fluoxetine.

Despite strong data for efficacy, adequate dose response studies have not been done, long-term efficacy has not been studied, and antipsychotics as a class have been associated with serious adverse effects such as metabolic syndrome and extrapyramidal syndromes (although EPS are of a less concern with atypicals, they can occur).

Buspirone

Conflicting data exist concerning the efficacy of buspirone augmentation. Many open trials have suggested efficacy as an augmentation strategy (302–305); however, placebo-controlled trials have not fully supported the clinical reports. In a study of 102 outpatients with MDD who did not have an adequate response to 6 weeks of treatment with fluoxetine or citalopram, buspirone (doses of 10–30 mg b.i.d.) or placebo was added after a 2-week placebo wash-in period (306). Although buspirone was superior to placebo on the MADRS after 1 week, no difference was found at 6 weeks, except in patients with baseline MADRS scores greater than 30. In another study of 119 patients who failed to respond to paroxetine or placebo after a minimum of 4 weeks, buspirone or placebo was added for an additional 4 weeks (307). Although the combinations were well tolerated, there was no difference between groups, with both showing substantial improvement on the Clinical Global Impression Scale (50.9% buspirone, 46.7% placebo). An open-label, 2-week, follow-up phase with buspirone augmentation produced a response rate of 69.4%. Despite the lack of strong support for efficacy, we have found that the addition of buspirone in doses of 30–50 mg daily produces dramatic results in some patients; however, we recognize that this may be a placebo effect.

Psychostimulants

Methylphenidate is a secondary amine stimulant that exists as four isomers, with the marketed preparation containing the *d,l*-threo racemate, with *d*-threo believed to be responsible for therapeutic activity. The major metabolite is ritalinic acid (approximately 70%), with smaller amounts of *p*-hydroxyritalinic acid (1%) and 6-oxoritalinic acid (2%) also produced. It is believed that only the parent compound contributes to therapeutic effects. In its standard preparation, methylphenidate reaches peak plasma concentrations in 1–2 h and has an elimination half-life of 2–3 h, and exhibits dose proportionality through the therapeutic range (308). Newer preparations of methylphenidate include *d*-methylphenidate (Focalin®), and long-acting preparations (Metadate CD®, Concerta®, Ritalin-SR®). Dextroamphetamine is available as Dexedrine® and Dexedrine Spansule®. Adderall® and Adderall-XR® contain a mixture of *d*-amphetamine and *l*-amphetamine. Lisdexamfetamine (Vyvanse) is a prodrug of dextroamphetamine.

The pharmacologic actions of both methylphenidate and dextroamphetamine are complex. Both drugs affect dopamine and norepinephrine reuptake, although there may be subtle differences in the mechanism. Also, both drugs promote release of monoamines, but methylphenidate acts on reserpine-sensitive storage pools, while dextroamphetamine releases them from newly synthesized stores. Both drugs affect α-adrenergic receptors. Effects of stimulants on acetylcholine, serotonin, glutamate, and GABA result from the influence of dopamine on these systems and in some cases, from direct actions at receptors. Their actions in the brain during PET studies also suggest differences among stimulants.

There has been a long history of stimulant therapy in depression, both as monotherapy in the medically ill and as an augmenting agent (309–315). In the Boston area, it is not uncommon for stimulants to be prescribed as sole agents, or in combination with antidepressants. The scientific literature supporting the practice is weak, but clinical experience, as well as survey data of psychiatrists in the United States and Canada, provides support for the practice. The body of research in this area appears to be growing (316, 317).

In clinical practice, methylphenidate can be started at 10 mg doses and increased gradually up to 80 mg daily. We use approximately half that dose for dextroamphetamine therapy. Frequent patient monitoring, both for adverse effects and misuse, is necessary. Once the proper dose is achieved, response is rapid. Modafinil (Provigil®), a medication for the treatment of narcolepsy, has also been used in doses of 100–200 mg daily to augment and hasten antidepressant response (318, 319).

Thyroid Hormone

A series of studies of thyroid augmentation of antidepressant response have been reported by Prange and associates (320). In their first study, 20 euthyroid patients (16 women and 4 men) most of whom were diagnosed as unipolar retarded depression, were given imipramine (150 mg) plus 25 μg of triiodothyronine (T3). Reductions in HAM-D scores were greater and occurred more rapidly in the T3 group. Other studies from the same research group found that women with nonretarded depressions also responded to T3 augmentation but men did not. In a study of T3 augmentation of amitriptyline, patients who were treated with 40 μg of T3 with amitriptyline (100 mg) improved more rapidly than those on 20 μg of T3 or placebo; women had better responses than men (321). An open trial using clomipramine had similar results (322). Several other studies have also found that patients who were unresponsive to tricyclic antidepressants improved with the addition of T3 in doses of 25–50 μg (323–326). SSRI augmentation with T3 appears to be efficacious and well tolerated (327–329). On the other hand, some studies indicate a lack of efficacy (330) or efficacy only for those patients with elevated TSH response to TRH (331). It is not clear whether T3 augmentation is superior to thyroxine (T4) or lithium augmentation. One small study suggested that T4 augmentation should precede lithium augmentation

(332). The weight of the evidence suggests that T3 is more effective than T4 augmentation; however, some studies suggest that it may be necessary to administer high doses of T4 for long periods of time to obtain maximum benefit. An open-label study that administered T4 at a mean dose of 482 μg/day for 8 weeks reported a substantial improvement in depression in over half of the sample (333).

A meta-analysis of 6 double-blind, placebo-controlled clinical trials evaluating coadministration of T3 and tricyclic antidepressants concluded that adjunctive T3 led to a more rapid clinical response (334). Women were more likely to benefit from the administration of T3 than men (334). The mechanism of action is believed to be related to correction of underlying subsyndromal thyroid dysfunction or direct effects on adrenergic activity.

In clinical practice, T3 (Cytomel) is begun in doses ranging from 12.5 to 25 μg and may be increased weekly up to 50 μg/day. One to 4 weeks is considered an adequate trial of T3 augmentation. It should be used with caution in patients with arrhythmias, hypertension, and cardiac disease. Some practioners believe that the best response occurs in women, patients with mild thyroid abnormalities, and individuals with severe or retarded depression.

Testosterone

Testosterone supplementation may improve depressive symptoms for a subset of male patients with low or borderline testosterone levels suffering from refractory depression. A randomized, double-blind, placebo-controlled trial in 23 patients with a low or borderline serum testosterone level (range 100–350 ng/dl; normal range is 270–1,070 ng/dl) who met the DSM-IV criteria for current MDD and were being treated with antidepressant medications prior to and during the trial received either testosterone gel (1% gel, 10 g/day) or placebo for 8 weeks (335). There was significantly greater improvement in HAM-D scores in the testosterone-treated group compared to placebo in both the vegetative and affective symptom subscales of the HAM-D Scale. Overall, the testosterone gel was well tolerated. One patient in the study experienced exacerbation of benign prostatic hyperplasia, which may be attributed to testosterone supplementation and was withdrawn from the study, although the relationship of testosterone supplementation to prostate cancer has been challenged. The mechanism of testosterone's antidepressant action is not known.

Estrogen

The increased prevalence of depression in women during perimenopause and postmenopause has led to several studies examining estrogen replacement and augmentation therapy for women during these stages of life. Perimenopause is the phase before menopause, which continues until menstruation has ceased for 12 consecutive months. Common symptoms include hot flashes, decreased libido, sleep disruption, and depression. In one study, perimenopausal women with major depression, dysthymic disorder, or minor depressive disorder received transdermal patches of 17[β]-estradiol (100 μg) or placebo in a 12-week study (336). Sixty-eight percent of women treated with estradiol had remission of depression compared to 20% in the placebo group (336). An earlier study also found that estrogen was superior to placebo in reducing depressive symptoms in perimenopausal women (337). A small study of 16 perimenopausal women found that estrogen replacement therapy was effective in treating depression (338). Other studies have found that both transdermal patches and sublingual estradiol improved mood in women with premenstrual dysphoric disorder and postpartum depression (339–341). Other studies have not found efficacy of estrogen replacement therapy for depression (342–344). In a review of the literature, Epperson and associates (345) reported that five studies found estrogen replacement therapy more effective than placebo in a mixed group of perimenopausal and postmenopausal women and 5 found it as effective as placebo. One study (346) found that estrogen was superior to placebo in perimenopausal, but not postmenopausal women. In an early study, estrogen 5–25 mg/day, which is 5–25 times the replacement dose, was more effective than placebo in the treatment of women with depression that were unresponsive to antidepressants (347). A more recent study in postmenopausal Chinese women did not find differences between 1 and 2 mg of oral estradiol and placebo on symptoms of anxiety and depression (348).

In addition to estrogen replacement as a monotherapy, it has also been used as an augmentation strategy in women with menopausal depression. Fluoxetine in combination with estrogen replacement therapy proved superior to fluoxetine alone in a single study (349). On the other hand, Oppenheim and colleagues did not find estrogen augmentation effective when administered with imipramine (345, 350).

In summary, data are conflicting regarding the efficacy of estrogen replacement therapy in perimenopausal or postmenopausal women with depression. Some investigators have attributed inconsistent findings to the use of poorly bioavailable oral preparations, failure to use laboratory measures to confirm menopausal status, and wide variability of diagnostic and outcome measures (336). The mechanism of action of estrogen is unknown; however, a substantial body of evidence indicates that it influences monoamine and GABA systems. There is little evidence to support the use of estrogen augmentation with cyclic antidepressants, although some evidence supports its value in combination with fluoxetine. Its use as an augmentation agent is also limited by the risks of toxicity when used in combination with imipramine, which is most likely a consequence of a pharmacokinetic interaction. Increased risk of carcinoma and cardiovascular disease may be associated with estrogen replacement (351–354).

Amantadine

A small series of patients with a partial response to imipramine, SSRI, and mixed action antidepressants improved after amantadine was added to the antidepressant (355, 356). Larger controlled studies are required to replicate this finding; however, amantadine is a NMDA antagonist and promotes increased dopamine, which provides a rationale for studying this combination in adequately designed trials.

Alternative and Non-Traditional Antidepressants

St John's Wort

St John's Wort (*Hypericum perforatum*, available commercially as Hypericum alcohol extract standardized by level of hypericin) has been used as a traditional herbal medicine for more than 2,000 years. Pharmacologically, the plant contains naphthodianthrones (such as hypericin and pseudohypericin), phloroglucinols (such as hyperforin and adhyperforin), flavonoids, phenylpropanes, proanthocyanidins, xanthones, and amino acids (357–359). It remains uncertain which of these constituents are responsible for antidepressant effects. Although extracts have been standardized for hypericin content, this component may not cross the blood–brain barrier (359). Consequently, hyperforin has been the focus of recent research. It inhibits reuptake of serotonin, dopamine, norepinephrine, GABA, and glutamate (360). It also has affinity for opioid receptors and 5-HT_6 and 5-HT_7 receptors. It may also have a direct effect on ion channels. Adhyperforin has similar effects on monoamine reuptake. Pseudohypericin inhibits dopamine-β-hydroxylase. Flavonoids and xanthones inhibit MAO-A and the former also inhibit catechol-*O*-methyl-transferase (COMT). Amentoflavone binds to the benzodiazepine receptor. Similar to synthetic antidepressants, chronic administration of St John's wort down-regulates β-receptors in animal models.

Several standardized extracts are available in Europe; however, preparations available in the United States may vary in concentrations of active constituents. Of particular importance is that most preparations used in clinical trials have not been standardized to hyperforin. Typical doses range from 900 to 1,800 mg/day of the herb administered in 2 or 3 divided doses. Initial does are typically one-third of that with weekly increases as needed to the maximum dose (296, 357, 358, 361, 362).

Adverse Effects

Extracts of St John's wort have been well tolerated under the conditions of physician supervision, monotherapy, and controlled doses of standardized extracts used in clinical trials (358, 361–363). The most common adverse effects reported in clinical trials are headache, dry mouth, gastrointestinal upset, nausea, dizziness, sedation, fatigue, and insomnia (296, 364, 365). Among the more serious adverse effects, which are very rare, are photosensitivity and possible induction of manic symptoms (362). A serotonin syndrome due to St John's wort had been reported in patients using St John's wort together with an SSRI or other antidepressants such as nefazodone and venlafaxine (358, 366, 367).

Drug–Drug Interactions

Due to its induction of P-glycoprotein (a transporter protein in the blood–brain barrier and intestine) (38, 368) and its induction of P450 cytochromes 3A4, 1A2, and possibly 2C9, St John's wort has the potential to interact with other medications (358, 369). St John's wort can decrease plasma levels of many prescribed drugs, such as anticoagulants, oral contraceptives, and antiviral agents. An interaction between St John's wort and cyclosporine (metabolized by 3A4) resulted in cyclosporine's reduced activity and organ rejection after transplantation (370, 371). Interactions have resulted in decreased international normalized ratio (INR) in patients on warfarin (metabolized by CYP2C9 [S-warfarin] and CYP1A2 [R-warfarin]) (358, 372, 373), and decreased digoxin levels when these drugs are administered with St John's wort (374). Bioavailability of indinavir, cyclosporine, and digoxin may be altered as a result of P-glycoprotein induction (368).

In the United Kingdom and Sweden, where St John's wort is used extensively for medicinal purposes along with other herbal remedies, clinical interactions between St John's wort and other licensed medications were deemed serious enough to warrant a change in product labeling of the involved medications and to warn health care practitioners and patients about potential for such interactions (369).

Efficacy

Numerous European clinical trials examined efficacy of St John's wort. Most of these studies have found St John's wort more effective than placebo and at least as effective as a reference antidepressant for short-term treatment of mild to moderate depression (361, 363, 365).

A randomized, double-blind, multicenter clinical trial studied 263 German outpatients with the diagnosis of moderate depression according to International Classification of Diseases, 10th revision (ICD-10), who were randomized to either placebo, imipramine, 100 mg/day or St John's wort extract 1,050 mg/day, for 8 weeks (361). The investigators concluded that the standardized St John's wort extract was more effective than placebo and as effective as imipramine in reducing HAM-D scores, Hamilton Rating Scale for Anxiety (HAM-A) scores, and Clinical Global Impression (375) scores (361). The authors themselves note the study limitation of suboptimal dosing of imipramine (361).

Several meta-analyses and systematic reviews have supported efficacy of St John's wort in mild depression (364, 376, 377). Linde et al (376) conducted a meta-analysis of 23 randomized clinical trials of acceptable methodologic quality that included a total of 1,757 outpatients with mild to moderate depression. They found that St John's wort extract was significantly superior to placebo and as effective as a standard antidepressant (imipramine, amitriptyline, or maprotiline).

Gaster and Holroyd (364) identified eight randomized, controlled, double-blind trials that were of acceptable methodological quality. They concluded that St John's wort is more effective than placebo in the treatment of mild to moderate depression. The investigators also noted that there were insufficient data to assess the efficacy of St John's wort in severe depression or to compare its efficacy to other antidepressants.

Kasper and Dienel (377) performed a meta-analysis on the original published data of three double-blind, randomized multicenter trials. In these trials, a total of 544 patients with mild to moderate depression based on DSM-IV diagnostic criteria received 900 mg/day of St John's wort (WS 5570 or WS 5572 standardized extracts) or placebo for 6 weeks. The authors found that St John's wort was significantly superior to placebo for treating mild to moderate depression and was especially effective in reducing the core symptoms of depression.

Serious methodological flaws exist in most published clinical trials (296, 364, 376, 377). Common problems are failure to use standardized diagnostic instruments or rating scales, short study duration, and administration of ratings by inexperienced investigators (296, 364, 376, 377). The earliest studies were limited by their small size, short duration, lack of either placebo or active reference drug arm, differences in preparation of the extract, failure to describe randomization and blinding methods, to measure compliance, or to report or explain the dropout rate (358, 378). In those studies using a well-established antidepressant for comparison, results may have been skewed by underdosing the reference drug. Doses such as 100 mg/day or less of imipramine or amitriptyline were used without plasma level monitoring to insure compliance or adequate dosing (296, 376). In many studies, the blind may have been transparent if care was not taken to mask the peculiar taste of St John's wort extract, or if a specific constellation of side effects allowed investigators to guess the treatment arm (296, 376).

The first major American randomized, double-blind, placebo-controlled clinical trial was conducted by Shelton et al. (296). While criticizing prior studies for methodological flaws and biases, these investigators succeeded in conducting a well-designed, large-scale, multicenter clinical trial. Two hundred patients were recruited through tertiary care centers associated with academic centers in the United States. Participants had a diagnosis of MDD according to DSM-IV criteria and a baseline HAM-D score of at least 20. Care was taken to assure similarity in outward appearance, taste, and smell of placebo and St John's wort preparations, protecting the blind. The study followed a 1-week, single-blind, run-in of placebo, done to minimize the effect of early placebo response, and the treatment arm lasted 8 weeks. The outcome measures were decrease in scores on HAM-D, Beck Depression Inventory (BDI), CGI, or HAM-A. The investigators failed to detect a significant difference in response rates between St John's wort and placebo after 8 weeks of the study; response rates were 26.5% for St John's wort and 18.6% for placebo. It was concluded that St John's wort was not effective in treating MDD.

The American and European study populations were quite different. Shelton and associates recruited subjects from tertiary care outpatient clinics affiliated with academic medical centers. Patients had a diagnosis of MDD and baseline HAM-D scores of at least 20, with an average duration of depression of more than 2 years (296). On the other hand, the population groups studied in Europe came mostly from primary care settings, were not suffering from chronic depression but had either first or recurrent episodes of "mild to moderate" depression with a lower baseline HAM-D scores (296, 377). All of these distinctions make the American patient sample quite different from the European populations studied previously; it may also explain lower response rate for both placebo and the studied compound. Kasper and Dienel (377) suggested that this difference of populations studied accounted for disparate findings of the American and European studies, noting that St John's wort may not be appropriate for treatment of chronic MDD.

A randomized controlled trial by the Hypericum Depression Trial Study Group of 340 adult outpatients, with major depression and a baseline HAM-D score of at least 20, did not support the use of St John's wort in the treatment of moderately severe major depression (379). The trial's two primary outcome measures showed that neither sertraline nor St John's wort differed significantly from placebo, which may have been due to the low sensitivity of the trial or inadequate doses of sertraline. The investigators indicated that St John's wort may be most effective in treating less severe major depression, but that this cannot be supported until there are additional efficacy trials.

Conclusion

The efficacy of St John's wort in major depression has not been established. There is evidence to suggest it may be effective in milder forms of depression. Its clinical use is limited by uncertainty concerning its active components, propensity for drug–drug interactions, and paucity of safety data. Currently, there is no available literature on using St John's wort in children and adolescents, in patients with major psychiatric comorbidities, or in pregnant or lactating women. The drug–drug interactions associated with St John's wort limit its use in patients with other medical or psychiatric comorbidities. Its efficacy is not established in moderate to severe major depression. Further research and well-designed clinical trials are needed to determine the efficacy of St John's wort in the treatment of mood disorders.

SAMe

*SAMe (S-adenosyl-*l*-methionine 1,4-butanedisulfonate)* is a dietary supplement that has been used as an antidepressant by European psychiatrists for approximately 30 years (380). It is a naturally occurring compound which acts as a methyl group donor to multiple substances in the Central Nervous System; thus, it is involved in synthesis of various neurotransmitters (dopamine, serotonin, and norepinephrine) as well as nucleic acids and proteins (380). SAMe is synthesized in the brain from L-methionine, an amino acid. Both folate and methylcobalamin (vitamin B12) are necessary for its production (380). Deficiencies in folate and vitamin B12 have been linked to some types of depression (380). When low plasma concentrations of SAMe are found in depressed patients, interventions that increase SAMe levels are associated with improved mood (381). Although supporting evidence is lacking, several mechanisms have been suggested to explain SAMe's effects in depression. Potentially, SAMe could increase neurotransmitter synthesis (e.g., serotonin or norepinephrine synthesis), increase neurotransmitter receptor responsiveness, or increase phospholipid production, which would enhance cell membrane fluidity.

Two meta-analyses of clinical trials of SAMe involving over 1,300 patients concluded that SAMe had superior efficacy compared to placebo and was equivalent to tricyclic antidepressants (382, 383). More recently, two multicenter studies were conducted in patients with major depression and HAM-D scores 18 or higher (384). The first study compared 1,600 mg orally of SAMe per day to 150 mg of imipramine per day orally in a double-blind design. The second study compared 400 mg of SAMe per day administered intramuscularly (SAMe has very poor oral availability) compared to 150 mg/day of oral imipramine. The primary efficacy measures were HAM-D scores and percent responders on clinical global impression scales. Secondary outcome measures were MADRS scores. Responders were defined as those patients demonstrating a decrease in HAM-D scores of 50% or greater from baseline (384). Responders in both studies ranged from 50 to 59% with no statistical difference between oral or intramuscular SAMe and imipramine (384). The failure to include a placebo control group limits these findings. An earlier study reported that 400 mg/day of SAMe administered intramuscularly produced an antidepressant effect at 7 and 15 days, which is more rapid than conventional antidepressants (385).

A recently published review of SAMe's use in the treatment of depression concluded that doses of oral or parenteral SAMe from 200 to 1,600 mg/day were a safe and effective alternative to tricyclics, with a faster possible onset of action and could have a role in augmentation of traditional antidepressants (380). Additional studies of the oral administration of SAMe are necessary to establish the efficacy of the oral formulation (386). Evidence to date supports efficacy for parenteral SAMe in depression; however, adoption of this route of administration will be difficult in mental health settings. Additional studies of SAMe augmentation are needed.

Omega-3 Fatty Acids

The rationale for the use of *omega-3 fatty acids (OFA)* in the treatment of depression is based on converging evidence from diverse theoretical perspectives that seems to link OFAs and mood disorders. First, the epidemiologic evidence suggests that populations with low intake of dietary OFAs (e.g., fish oils) have a higher prevalence of depression than populations consuming large amounts (387). Second, red blood cell membrane OFAs are lower in depression compared to healthy controls (388, 389) and are correlated with the severity of depression (390). Third, fatty acids are involved in signal transduction in the brain (391).

The OFAs in the brain consist of 6-OFAs (e.g., arachidonic acid) and 3-OFAs [e.g., decosapentaenoic acid (DPA) and docosahexaenoic acid (DHA) and eicosapentanoic acid (EPA)]. A preliminary study of 3-OFAs (a combination of 6.2 g EPA and 3.4 g DHA daily) as adjunctive therapy in bipolar patients found it superior to placebo in improving mood and preventing relapse (392–394). In another study of depressed patients who were not responding to antidepressant therapy, the addition of EPA 1 g/day improved HAM-D, MADRS, and BDI scores, whereas placebo and higher doses of ECA did not (391). Both studies found 3-OFAs were well tolerated, with common side effects including loose stools and breath "fish odor."

At the present time, the efficacy of OFAs in depression has not been established. Although preliminary evidence suggests that 1 g of EPA is effective as an adjunctive therapy, and most authorities believe that EPA is the active component for antidepressant response, neither OFA doses nor optimal composition of fatty acids have been established. There are ongoing clinical trials comparing the efficacy of DHA and EPA (395). In our clinical practice, we have not been impressed with the clinical response to OFAs, even as an adjunct. Many of our patients have been taking OFAs for the cardiac effects, and we have not observed significant changes in mood at the initiation of OFAs or when patients discontinue them. On the other hand, OFAs are unlikely to be associated with severe adverse effects and may be beneficial in preventing cardiovascular disease.

Conclusion

Appropriate clinical use of antidepressants relies on the ability of clinicians to make an accurate diagnosis, rule out medical conditions or substance-induced mood disorders, and differentiate subtypes of depression (e.g., unipolar and bipolar subtypes). Further, the ability to integrate knowledge of the pharmacology of specific drugs and the neuropathophysiology of depression forms the basis of rational prescribing.

Several multisite clinical trials have established approximate equivalent efficacy of all marketed antidepressants, with the clinically relevant differences related to adverse effects, ease of dosing, and safety. SSRIs remain the first-line agents under most circumstances, with mixed action, TCAs, heterocyclics, and MAOIs additional options. Antidepressants are effective across a range of disorders including depression, PTSD, anxiety, and chronic pain. Combination and augmentation therapies have been developed for depressions that are resistant to monotherapy, although evidence to date does not favor a specific approach. Novel treatments, whether developed from herbal preparations or new chemical compounds, are an exciting area for further research, but data supporting their efficacy and safety are limited. Combinations of antidepressants with Transcranial Magnetic Stimulation offers another potential augmentation strategy, however there is a paucity of data addressing this approach.

Acknowledgments The authors would like to acknowledge the contributions of Lucy Tsirulnik-Barts, MD, who was a co-author on this chapter for the first edition.

References

1. Mrazek D. Psychiatric pharmacogenomics. Oxford: Oxford University Press; 2010.
2. Horstmann S, Binder EB. Pharmacogenomics of antidepressant drugs. Pharmacol Ther. 2009;124(1):57–73.
3. Uhr M, Tontsch A, Namendorf C, Ripke S, Lucae S, Ising M, et al. Polymorphisms in the drug transporter gene ABCB1 predict antidepressant treatment response in depression. Neuron. 2008;57(2):203–9.
4. Pariante CM. Glucocorticoid receptor function in vitro in patients with major depression. Stress. 2004;7(4):209–19.
5. Pariante CM. The role of multi-drug resistance p-glycoprotein in glucocorticoid function: studies in animals and relevance in humans. Eur J Pharmacol. 2008;583(2–3):263–71.
6. Binder EB, Salyakina D, Lichtner P, Wochnik GM, Ising M, Putz B, et al. Polymorphisms in FKBP5 are associated with increased recurrence of depressive episodes and rapid response to antidepressant treatment. Nat Genet. 2004;36(12):1319–25.
7. Zimmerman M, Posternak MA, Chelminski I. Derivation of a definition of remission on the Montgomery-Asberg depression rating scale corresponding to the definition of remission on the Hamilton rating scale for depression. J Psychiatr Res. 2004;38(6):577–82.
8. Hawley CJ, Gale TM, Sivakumaran T. Defining remission by cut off score on the MADRS: selecting the optimal value. J Affect Disord. 2002;72(2):177–84.
9. Kirchheiner J, Lorch R, Lebedeva E, Seeringer A, Roots I, Sasse J, et al. Genetic variants in FKBP5 affecting response to antidepressant drug treatment. Pharmacogenomics. 2008;9(7):841–6.
10. Uher R, Huezo-Diaz P, Perroud N, Smith R, Rietschel M, Mors O, et al. Genetic predictors of response to antidepressants in the GENDEP project. Pharmacogenomics J. 2009;9(4):225–33.
11. Papiol S, Arias B, Gasto C, Gutierrez B, Catalan R, Fananas L. Genetic variability at HPA axis in major depression and clinical response to antidepressant treatment. J Affect Disord. 2007;104(1–3):83–90.
12. Tsai SJ, Hong CJ, Chen TJ, Yu YW. Lack of supporting evidence for a genetic association of the FKBP5 polymorphism and response to antidepressant treatment. Am J Med Genet B Neuropsychiatr Genet. 2007;144B(8):1097–8.
13. Ising M, Depping AM, Siebertz A, Lucae S, Unschuld PG, Kloiber S, et al. Polymorphisms in the FKBP5 gene region modulate recovery from psychosocial stress in healthy controls. Eur J Neurosci. 2008;28(2):389–98.
14. Laje G, Perlis RH, Rush AJ, McMahon FJ. Pharmacogenetics studies in STAR*D: strengths, limitations, and results. Psychiatr Serv. 2009;60(11):1446–57.
15. Paddock S, Laje G, Charney D, Rush AJ, Wilson AF, Sorant AJ, et al. Association of GRIK4 with outcome of antidepressant treatment in the STAR*D cohort. Am J Psychiatry. 2007;164(8):1181–8.
16. Horstmann S, Lucae S, Menke A, Hennings JM, Ising M, Roeske D, et al. Polymorphisms in GRIK4, HTR2A, and FKBP5 show interactive effects in predicting remission to antidepressant treatment. Neuropsychopharmacology. 2010;35(3):727–40.
17. Perlis RH, Patrick A, Smoller JW, Wang PS. When is pharmacogenetic testing for antidepressant response ready for the clinic? A cost-effectiveness analysis based on data from the STAR*D study. Neuropsychopharmacology. 2009;34(10):2227–36.
18. Ising M, Lucae S, Binder EB, Bettecken T, Uhr M, Ripke S, et al. A genomewide association study points to multiple loci that predict antidepressant drug treatment outcome in depression. Arch Gen Psychiatry. 2009;66(9):966–75.

19. Cipriani A, Furukawa TA, Salanti G, Geddes JR, Higgins JP, Churchill R, et al. Comparative efficacy and acceptability of 12 new-generation antidepressants: a multiple-treatments meta-analysis. Lancet. 2009;373(9665):746–58.
20. Fournier JC, DeRubeis RJ, Hollon SD, Dimidjian S, Amsterdam JD, Shelton RC, et al. Antidepressant drug effects and depression severity: a patient-level meta-analysis. JAMA. 2010;303(1):47–53.
21. Dunner DL. Acute and maintenance treatment of chronic depression. J Clin Psychiatry. 2001;62(Suppl 6):10–6.
22. Stewart JW, McGrath PJ, Quitkin FM. Can mildly depressed outpatients with atypical depression benefit from antidepressants? Am J Psychiatry. 1992;149(5):615–9.
23. Fava M, Rush AJ, Trivedi MH, Nierenberg AA, Thase ME, Sackiem HA, et al. Background and rationale for the sequenced treatment alternatives to relieve depression (STAR*D) study. Psychiatr Clin North Am. 2003;26(2):457–94.
24. Fava M, Davidson KG. Definition and epidemiology of treatment-resistant depression. Psychiatr Clin North Am. 1996;19(2):179–200.
25. Kupfer DJ. Long-term treatment of depression. J Clin Psychiatry. 1991;52(Suppl):28–34.
26. Rush AJ, Warden D, Wisniewski SR, Fava M, Trivedi MH, Gaynes BN, et al. STAR*D: revising conventional wisdom. CNS Drugs. 2009;23(8):627–47.
27. Kennedy N, Abbott R, Paykel ES. Longitudinal syndromal and sub-syndromal symptoms after severe depression: 10-year follow-up study. Br J Psychiatry. 2004;184:330–6.
28. Kennedy N, Paykel ES. Residual symptoms at remission from depression: impact on long-term outcome. J Affect Disord. 2004;80(2–3):135–44.
29. Kennedy N, Paykel ES. Treatment and response in refractory depression: results from a specialist affective disorders service. J Affect Disord. 2004;81(1):49–53.
30. DeVane CL. Differential pharmacology of newer antidepressants. J Clin Psychiatry. 1998;59(Suppl 20):85–93.
31. Ban TA. Pharmacotherapy of depression: a historical analysis. J Neural Transm. 2001;108(6):707–16.
32. Feighner JP. Mechanism of action of antidepressant medications. J Clin Psychiatry. 1999;60(Suppl 4):4–11; discussion 2–3.
33. Sampson SM. Treating depression with selective serotonin reuptake inhibitors: a practical approach. Mayo Clin Proc. 2001;76(7):739–44.
34. Goldberg JF. New drugs in psychiatry. Emerg Med Clin North Am. 2000;18(2):211–31; viii.
35. Goodnick PJ, Goldstein BJ. Selective serotonin reuptake inhibitors in affective disorders. I. Basic pharmacology. J Psychopharmacol. 1998;12(3 Suppl B):S5–20.
36. Fuller RW, Snoddy HD, Krushinski JH, Robertson DW. Comparison of norfluoxetine enantiomers as serotonin uptake inhibitors in vivo. Neuropharmacology. 1992;31(10):997–1000.
37. Gorman JM, Korotzer A, Su G. Efficacy comparison of escitalopram and citalopram in the treatment of major depressive disorder: pooled analysis of placebo-controlled trials. CNS Spectr. 2002;7(Suppl 1):40–4.
38. Weiss J, Dormann SM, Martin-Facklam M, Kerpen CJ, Ketabi-Kiyanvash N, Haefeli WE. Inhibition of P-glycoprotein by newer antidepressants. J Pharmacol Exp Therap. 2003;305(1):197–204.
39. Uhr M, Steckler T, Yassouridis A, Holsboer F. Penetration of amitriptyline, but not of fluoxetine, into brain is enhanced in mice with blood-brain barrier deficiency due to mdr1a P-glycoprotein gene disruption. Neuropsychopharmacology. 2000;22(4):380–7.
40. Uhr M, Graucer MT. abc1ab P-glycoprotein is involved in the uptake of citalopram and trimipramine into the brain of mice. J Psychiatr Res. 2003;37:179–85.
41. Stormer E, von Moltke LL, Perloff MD, Greenblatt DJ. P-glycoprotein interactions of nefazodone and trazodone in cell culture. J Clin Pharmacol. 2001;41(7):708–14.
42. Quitkin FM, Petkova E, McGrath PJ, Taylor B, Beasley C, Stewart J, et al. When should a trial of fluoxetine for major depression be declared failed? Am J Psychiatry. 2003;160(4):734–40.
43. Goodwin GM. How do antidepressants affect serotonin receptors? The role of serotonin receptors in the therapeutic and side effect profile of the SSRIs. J Clin Psychiatry. 1996;57(Suppl 4):9–13.

44. Gilmor ML, Owens MJ, Nemeroff CB. Inhibition of norepinephrine uptake in patients with major depression treated with paroxetine. Am J Psychiatry. 2002;159(10):1702–10.
45. Blier P, de Montigny C, Chaput Y. Modifications of the serotonin system by antidepressant treatment: implications for the therapeutic response in major depression. J Clin Psychopharmacol. 1987;7:24S–35.
46. Banasr M, Hery M, Printemps R, Daszuta A. Serotonin-induced increases in adult cell proliferation and neurogenesis are mediated through different and common 5-HT receptor subtypes in the dentate gyrus and the subventricular zone. Neuropsychopharmacology. 2004;29(3):450–60.
47. Greene J, Banasr M, Lee B, Warner-Schmidt J, Duman RS. Vascular endothelial growth factor signaling is required for the behavioral actions of antidepressant treatment: pharmacological and cellular characterization. Neuropsychopharmacology. 2009;34(11):2459–68.
48. Pinna G, Costa E, Guidotti A. SSRIs act as selective brain steroidogenic stimulants (SBSSs) at low doses that are inactive on 5-HT reuptake. Curr Opin Pharmacol. 2009;9(1):24–30.
49. Benamansour S, Owens WA, Cecchi M, Morilak DA, Frazer A. Serotonin clearance in vivo is altered to a greater extent by antidepressant-induced downregulation of the serotonin transporter than by acute blockade of this transporter. J Neurosci. 2002;22(15):6766–72.
50. Artigas F, Perez V, Alvarez E. Pindolol induces a rapid improvement of depressed patients treated with serotonin reuptake inhibitors. Arch Gen Psychiatry. 1994;51(3):248–51.
51. Blier P, Bergeron R. Effectiveness of pindolol with selected antidepressant drugs in the treatment of major depression. J Clin Psychopharmacol. 1995;15(3):217–22.
52. Berman RM, Darnell AM, Miller HL, Anand A, Charney DS. Effect of pindolol in hastening response to fluoxetine in the treatment of major depression: a double-blind, placebo-controlled trial. Am J Psychiatry. 1997;154(12):37–43.
53. Perez V, Gilaberte I, Faries D, Alvarez E, Artigas F. Randomised, double-blind, placebo-controlled trial of pindolol in combination with fluoxetine antidepressant treatment. Lancet. 1997;349(9065):1594–7.
54. Maes M, Libbrecht I, van Hunsel F, Campens D, Meltzer HY. Pindolol and mianserin augment the antidepressant activity of fluoxetine in hospitalized major depressed patients, including those with treatment resistance. J Clin Psychopharmacol. 1999;19(2):177–82.
55. Stein MB, Sareen J, Hami S, Chao J. Pindolol potentation of paroxetine for generalized social phobia: a double-blind, placebo-controlled, crossover study. Am J Psychiatry. 2001;158(10):1725–7.
56. Rabiner EA, Bhagwagar Z, Gunn RN, Sargent PA, Bench CJ, Cowen PJ, et al. Pindolol augmentation of selective serotonin reuptake inhibitors: PET evidence that the dose used in clinical trials is too low. Am J Psychiatry. 2001;158(12):2080–2.
57. Wu S, Comings DE. A common C-1018G polymorphism in the human 5-HT_{1A} receptor gene. Psychiatr Genet. 1999;9(2):105–6.
58. Nishiguchi N, Shirakawa O, Ono H, Nishimura A, Nushida H, Ueno Y, et al. Lack of an association between 5-HT_{1A} receptor gene structural polymorphisms and suicide victims. Am J Med Genet. 2002;114(4):423–5.
59. Isaac MT, Tome MB. Pindolol-paroxetine combination. Am J Psychiatry. 1997; 154(12):1790–1.
60. Blier P, Bergeron R. The use of pindolol to potentiate antidepressant medication. J Clin Psychiatry. 1998;59(Suppl 5):16–23.
61. Bordet R, Thomas P, Dupuis B. Effect of pindolol on onset of action of paroxetine in the treatment of major depression: intermediate analysis of a double-blind, placebo-controlled trial. Reseau de Recherche et d'Experimentation Psychopharmacologique. Am J Psychiatry. 1998;155(10):1346–51.
62. Taylor D. Selective serotonin reuptake inhibitors and tricyclic antidepressants in combination. Interactions and therapeutic uses. Br J Psychiatry. 1995;167(5):575–80.
63. Ereshefsky L, Riesenman C, Lam YWF. Serotonin selective reuptake inhibitor drug interactions and the cytochrome P450 system. J Clin Psychiatry. 1996;57(Suppl 8):17–25.

64. Nemeroff CB, DeVane CL, Pollock BG. Newer antidepressants and the cytochrome P450 system. Am J Psychiatry. 1996;153(3):311–20.
65. Baumann P. Care of depression in the elderly: comparative pharmacokinetics of SSRIs. Int Clin Psychopharmacol. 1998;13(Suppl 5):S35–43.
66. Baker GB, Fang J, Sinha S, Coutts RT. Metabolic drug interactions with selective serotonin reuptake inhibitor (SSRI) antidepressants. Neurosci Biobehav Rev. 1998;22(2):325–33.
67. Johnson MD, Newkirk G, White JR, Jr. Clinically significant drug interactions. Postgrad Med. 1999;105(2):193–5, 200, 5–6 passim.
68. Rickels K, Schweizer E. Clinical overview of serotonin reuptake inhibitors. J Clin Psychiatry. 1990;51(Suppl B):9–12.
69. Frazer A. Antidepressants. J Clin Psychiatry. 1997;58(Suppl 6):9–25.
70. Benbow SJ, Gill G. Drug points: paroxetine and hepatotoxicity. Br Med J. 1997;314(7091):1387.
71. Cai Q, Benson MA, Talbot TJ, Devadas G, Swanson HJ, Olson JL, et al. Acute hepatitis due to fluoxetine therapy. Mayo Clin Proc. 1999;74(7):692–4.
72. Garcia-Pando A, Garcia del Pozo J, Sanchez A, et al. Hepatotoxicity associated with the new antidepressants. J Clin Psychiatry. 2002;63:135–7.
73. Lane RM. SSRI-induced extrapyramidal side-effects and akathisia: implications for treatment. J Psychopharmacol. 1998;12(2):192–214.
74. Walsh MT, Dinan TG. Selective serotonin reuptake inhibitors and violence: a review of the available evidence. Acta Psychiatr Scand. 2001;104(2):84–91.
75. Gill HS, DeVane CL, Risch SC. Extrapyramidal symptoms associated with cyclic antidepressant treatment: a review of the literature and consolidating hypotheses. J Clin Psychopharmacol. 1997;17(5):377–89.
76. Peet M. Induction of mania with selective serotonin re-uptake inhibitors and tricyclic antidepressants. Br J Psychiatry. 1994;164(4):549–50.
77. Stoll AL, Mayer PV, Kolbrener M, Goldstein E, Suplit B, Lucier J, et al. Antidepressant-associated mania: a controlled comparison with spontaneous mania. Am J Psychiatry. 1994;151(11):1642–5.
78. Teicher MH, Glod C, Cole JO. Emergence of intense suicidal preoccupation during fluoxetine treatment. Am J Psychiatry. 1990;147(2):207–10.
79. Fava M, Rosenbaum JF. Suicidality and fluoxetine: is there a relationship? J Clin Psychiatry. 1991;51:267–85.
80. Tollefson GD, Rampey AH, Jr., Beasley CM, Jr., Enas GG, Potvin JH. Absence of a relationship between adverse events and suicidality during pharmacotherapy for depression. Journal of Clinical Psychopharmacology. 1994;14(3):163–9.
81. Muller-Oerlinghausen B, Berghofer A. Antidepressants and suicidal risk. J Clin Psychiatry. 1999;60(Suppl 2):94–9; discussion 111–6.
82. Tueth MJ. Revisiting fluoxetine (Proxac) and suicidal preoccupations. J Emerg Med. 1994;12(5):685–7.
83. Sternbach H. The serotonin syndrome. Am J Psychiatry. 1991;148(6):705–13.
84. Lane R, Baldwin D. Selective serotonin reuptake inhibitor-induced serotonin syndrome: review. J Clin Psychopharmacol. 1997;17(3):208–21.
85. Dams R, Benijts TH, Lambert WE, Van Bocxlaer JF, Van Varenbergh D, Van Peteghem C, et al. A fatal case of serotonin syndrome after combined moclobemide and citalopram intoxication. J Anal Toxicol. 2001;25(2):147–51.
86. DeSilva KE, Le Flore DB, Marston BJ, Rimland D. Serotonin syndrome in HIV-infected individuals receiving antiretroviral therapy and fluoxetine. AIDS. 2001;15(10):1281–5.
87. Holsboer F. Neuroendocrinology of mood disorders. In: Bloom FE, Kupfer DJ, editors. Psychopharmacology: the fourth generation of progress. New York: Raven; 1995. p. 957–69.
88. Inder WJ, Prickett TC, Mulder RT, Donald RA, Joyce PR. Reduction in basal afternoon plasma ACTH during early treatment of depression with fluoxetine. Psychopharmacology (Berl). 2001;156(1):73–8.
89. Barclay TS, Lee AJ. Citalopram-associated SIADH. Ann Pharmacother. 2002;36:1558–63.

90. Michelson D, Amsterdam JD, Quitkin FM, Reimherr FW, Rosenbaum JF, Zajecka J, et al. Changes in weight during a 1-year trial of fluoxetine. Am J Psychiatry. 1999;156(8):1170–6.
91. Harvey BH, Bouwer CD. Neuropharmacology of paradoxic weight gain with selective serotonin reuptake inhibitors. Clin Neuropharmacol. 2000;23(2):90–7.
92. Fava M. Weight gain and antidepressants. J Clin Psychiatry. 2000;61(Suppl 11):37–41.
93. Alderman CP, Seshadri P, Ben-Tovim DI. Effects of serotonin reuptake inhibitors on hemostasis. Ann Pharmacother. 1996;30:1232–4.
94. Halperin D, Reber G. Influence of antidepressants on hemostasis. Dialogues Clin Neurosci. 2007;9(1):47–59.
95. Balon R, Yeragani VK, Pohl R, et al. Sexual dysfunction during antidepressant treatment. J Clin Psychiatry. 1993;54:209–12.
96. Gitlin MJ. Psychotropic medications and their effects on sexual function: diagnosis, biology, and treatment approaches. J Clin Psychiatry. 1994;55(9):406–13.
97. Margolese HC, Assalian P. Sexual side effects of antidepressants: a review. J Sex Marital Ther. 1996;22(3):209–17.
98. Rosen RC, Lane RM, Menza M. Effects of SSRIs on sexual function: a critical review. J Clin Psychopharmacol. 1999;19(1):67–85.
99. Fava M, Rankin MA. Sexual functioning and SSRIs. J Clin Psychiatry. 2002;63(Suppl 5): 13–6.
100. Montejo-Gonzalez AL, Llorca G, Izquierdo JA, Ledesma A, Bousono M, Calcedo A, et al. SSRI-induced sexual dysfunction: fluoxetine, paroxetine, sertraline, and fluvoxamine in a prospective, multicenter, and descriptive clinical study of 344 patients. J Sex Marital Ther. 1997;23(3):176–94.
101. Herman JB, Brotman AW, Pollack MH, Falk WE, Biederman J, Rosenbaum JF. Fluoxetine-induced sexual dysfunction. J Clin Psychiatry. 1990;51(1):25–7.
102. Patterson WM. Fluoxetine-induced sexual dysfunction. J Clin Psychiatry. 1993;54(2):71.
103. Rothschild AJ. Sexual side effects of antidepressants. J Clin Psychiatry. 2000;61(Suppl 11): 28–36.
104. Fava M, Rankin MA, Alpert JE, Nierenberg AA, Worthington JJ. An open trial of oral sildenfalin in antidepressant-induced sexual dysfunction. Psychother Psychosom. 1998;67(6):328–31.
105. Nurnberg HG, Lauriello J, Hensley PL, Parker LM, Keith SJ. Sildenafil for sexual dysfunction in women taking antidepressants. Am J Psychiatry. 1999;156(10):1664.
106. Nurnberg HG, Seidman SN, Gelenberg AJ, Fava M, Rosen R, Shabsigh R. Depression, antidepressant therapies, and erectile dysfunction: clinical trials of sildenafil citrate (Viagra) in treated and untreated patients with depression. Urology. 2002;60(2 Suppl 2):58–66.
107. Walker PW, Cole JO, Gardner EA, Hughes AR, Johnston JA, Batey SR, et al. Improvement in fluoxetine-associated sexual dysfunction in patients switched to bupropion. J Clin Psychiatry. 1993;54(12):459–65.
108. Rothschild AJ. Selective serotonin reuptake inhibitor-induced sexual dysfunction: efficacy of a drug holiday. Am J Psychiatry. 1995;152(10):1514–6.
109. Haddad P. The SSRI discontinuation syndrome. J Psychopharmacol. 1998;12(3):305–13.
110. Black K, Shea C, Dursun S, Kutcher S. Selective serotonin reuptake inhibitor discontinuation syndrome: proposed diagnostic critieria. J Psychiatr Neurosci. 2000;25(3):255–61.
111. DeBattista C, Schatzberg AF. Physical sysmptoms associated with paroxetine withdrawal [letters to the editor]. Am J Psychiatry. 1995;152(8):1235–6.
112. Barbey JT, Roose SP. SSRI safety in overdose. J Clin Psychiatry. 1998;59(Suppl 15):42–8.
113. Ostrom M, Eriksson A, Thorson J, Spigset O. Fatal overdose with citalopram. Lancet. 1996;348(9023):339–40.
114. Glassman AH. Citalopram toxicity. Lancet. 1997;350:818.
115. Kulin NA, Pastuszak A, Sage SR, Schick-Boschetto B, Spivey G, Feldkamp M, et al. Pregnancy outcome following maternal use of the new selective serotonin reuptake inhibitors: a prospective controlled multicenter study. JAMA. 1998;279(8):609–10.

116. Berard A, Ramos E, Rey E, Blais L, St-Andre M, Oraichi D. First trimester exposure to paroxetine and risk of cardiac malformations in infants: the importance of dosage. Birth Defects Res B Dev Reprod Toxicol. 2007;80(1):18–27.
117. Oberlander TF, Warburton W, Misri S, Riggs W, Aghajanian J, Hertzman C. Major congenital malformations following prenatal exposure to serotonin reuptake inhibitors and benzodiazepines using population-based health data. Birth Defects Res B Dev Reprod Toxicol. 2008;83(1):68–76.
118. Pedersen LH, Henriksen TB, Olsen J. Fetal exposure to antidepressants and normal milestone development at 6 and 19 months of age. Pediatrics. 2010;125(3):e600–8.
119. Chambers CD, Hernandez-Diaz S, Van Marter LJ, Werler MM, Louik C, Jones KL, et al. Selective serotonin-reuptake inhibitors and risk of persistent pulmonary hypertension of the newborn. N Engl J Med. 2006;354(6):579–87.
120. Ravindran AV, Guelfi JD, Lane RM, Cassano GB. Treatment of dysthymia with sertraline: a double-blind, placebo-controlled trial in dysthymic patients without major depression. J Clin Psychiatry. 2000;61(11):821–7.
121. Leonard HL. New developments in the treatment of obsessive-compulsive disorder. J Clin Psychiatry. 1997;58(Suppl 14):39–47.
122. Pigott TA, Seay SM. A review of the efficacy of selective serotonin reuptake inhibitors in obsessive-compulsive disorder. J Clin Psychiatry. 1999;60(2):101–6.
123. Oehrberg S, Christiansen PE, Behnke K, Borup AL, Severin B, Soegaard J, et al. Paroxetine in the treatment of panic disorder. A randomised, double-blind, placebo-controlled study. Br J Psychiatry. 1995;167(3):374–9.
124. Katzelnick DJ, Kobak KA, Greist JH, Jefferson JW, Mantle JM, Serlin RC. Sertraline for social phobia: a double-blind, placebo-controlled crossover study. Am J Psychiatry. 1995;152(9):1368–71.
125. Davidson JRT. Pharmacology of social anxiety disorder. J Clin Psychiatry. 1998;59(Suppl 17): 47–51.
126. Liebowitz MR, Stein MB, Tancer M, Carpenter D, Oakes R, Pitts CD. A randomized, double-blind, fixed-dose comparison of paroxetine and placebo in the treatment of generalized social anxiety disorder. J Clin Psychiatry. 2002;63(1):66–74.
127. Marcus MD, Wing RR, Ewing L, Kern E, McDermott M, Gooding W. A double-blind, placebo-controlled trial of fluoxetine plus behavior modification in the treatment of obese binge-eaters and non-binge-eaters. Am J Psychiatry. 1990;147(7):876–81.
128. Steiner M, Steinberg S, Stewart D, Carter D, Berger C, Reid R, et al. Fluoxetine in the treatment of premenstrual dysphoria. Canadian Fluoxetine/Premenstrual Dysphoria Collaborative Study Group. New Engl J Med. 1995;332(23):1529–34.
129. Pollack MH, Zaninelli R, Goddard A, McCafferty JP, Bellew KM, Burnham DB, et al. Paroxetine in the treatment of generalized anxiety disorder: results of a placebo-controlled, flexible-dosage trial. J Clin Psychiatry. 2001;62(5):350–7.
130. Davidson JRT. Biological therapies for posttraumatic stress disorder: an overview. J Clin Psychiatry. 1997;58(9):29–32.
131. Cheer SM, Goa KL. Fluoxetine: a review of its therapeutic potential in the treatment of depression associated with physical illness. Drugs. 2001;61(1):81–110.
132. Glassman AH, O'Connor CM, Califf RM, Swedberg K, Schwartz P, Bigger JT, Jr., et al. Sertraline treatment of major depression in patients with acute MI or unstable angina. JAMA. 2002;288(6):701–9.
133. Pettinati HM. The use of selective serotonin reuptake inhibitors in treating alcoholic subtypes. J Clin Psychiatry. 2001;62(Suppl 20):26–31.
134. Pettinati HM, Volpicelli JR, Luck G, Kranzler HR, Rukstalis MR, Cnaan A. Double-blind clinical trial of sertraline treatment for alcohol dependence. J Clin Psychopharmacol. 2001;21(2):143–53.
135. Davis JM, Wang Z, Janicak PG. A quantitative analysis of clinical drug trials for the treatment of affective disorders. Psychopharmacol Bull. 1993;129:175–81.

136. McGrath PJ, Stewart JW, Janal MN, Petkova E, Quitkin FM, Klein DF. A placebo-controlled study of fluoxetine versus imipramine in the acute treatment of atypical depression. Am J Psychiatry. 2000;157(3):344–50.
137. Kasper S, Fuger J, Moller HJ. Comparative efficacy of antidepressants. Drugs. 1992;43(Suppl 2): 11–23.
138. Amsterdam JD. Selective serotonin reuptake inhibitor efficacy in severe and melancholic depression. J Psychopharmacol. 1998;12(3 Suppl B):S99–111.
139. Verkes RJ, Van der Mast RC, Hengeveld MW, Tuyl JP, Zwinderman AH, Van Kempen GM. Reduction by paroxetine of suicidal behavior in patients with repeated suicide attempts but not major depression. Am J Psychiatry. 1998;155(4):543–7.
140. Byrne SE, Rothschild AJ. Loss of antidepressant efficacy during maintenance therapy: possible mechanisms and treatments. J Clin Psychiatry. 1998;59:279–88.
141. Fava M, Rappe SM, Pava JA, Nierenberg AA, Alpert JE, Rosenbaum JF. Relapse in patients on long-term fluoxetine treatment: response to increased fluoxetine dose. J Clin Psychiatry. 1995;56(2):52–5.
142. Kuhn R. The treatment of depressive states with G22355 (imipramine hydrochloride). Am J Psychiatry. 1958;115:459–64.
143. Klerman GL, Cole JP. Clinical pharmacology of imipramine and related antidepressant compounds. Pharmacol Rev. 1965;17:101–41.
144. Frommer DA, Kulig KW, Marx JA, Rumack B. Tricyclic antidepressant overdose. A review. JAMA. 1987;257(4):521–6.
145. Rudorfer MV, Potter WZ. Metabolism of tricyclic antidepressants. Cell Mol Neurobiol. 1999;19(3):373–409.
146. Wilens TE, Biederman J, Baldessarini RJ, Puopolo PR, Flood JG. Developmental changes in serum concentrations of desipramine and 2-hydroxydesipramine during treatment with desipramine. J Am Acad Child Adolesc Psychiatry. 1992;31(4):691–8.
147. Pettinati HM, Oslin DW, Kampman KM, Dundon WD, Xie H, Gallis TL, et al. A Double-Blind, Placebo-Controlled Trial combining sertraline and naltrexone for treating co-occurring depression and alcohol dependence. Am J Psychiatry. 2010;167:668–75.
148. Blackwell B. Adverse effects of antidepressant drugs; part 1: MAOIs and tricyclics. Drugs. 1981;21:201–19.
149. Nelson JC, Jatlow PI, Bock J, Quinlan DM, Bowers MB, Jr. Major adverse reactions during desipramine treatment: relationship to plasma drug concentrations, concomitant antipsychotic treatment, and patient characteristics. Arch Gen Psychiatry. 1982;39(9):1055–61.
150. Glassman AH, Bigger JT, Jr. Cardiovascular effects of therapeutic doses of tricyclic antidepressants. A review. Arch Gen Psychiatry. 1981;38(7):815–20.
151. Glassman AH. Cardiovascular effects of antidepressant drugs: updated. Int Clin Psychopharmacol. 1998;13(Suppl 5):S25–30.
152. Roose SP, Glassman AH. Antidepressant choice in the patient with cardiac disease: lessons from the Cardiac Arrhythmia Suppression Trial (CAST) studies. J Clin Psychiatry. 1994;55(Suppl A):83–7; discussion 8–9, 98–100.
153. Vohra J, Burrows GD, Sloman G. Assessment of cardiovascular side effects of therapeutic doses of tricyclic anti-depressant drugs. Aust N Z J Med. 1975;5(1):7–11.
154. Roose SP, Glassman AH, Siris SG, Walsh BT, Bruno RL, Wright LB. Comparison of imipramine- and nortriptyline-induced orthostatic hypotension: a meaningful difference. J Clin Psychopharmacol. 1981;1(5):316–9.
155. Witchel HJ, Hancox JC, Nutt DJ. Psychotropic drugs, cardiac arrhythmia, and sudden death. J Clin Psychopharmacol. 2003;23(1):58–77.
156. Maltzberg B. Mortality among patients with involutional melancholia. Am J Psychiatry. 1937;93:1231–8.
157. Williams RB, Jr., Sherter C. Cardiac complications of tricyclic antidepressant therapy. Ann Intern Med. 1971;74(3):395–8.
158. Bigger JT, Jr., Giardina EGV, Perel JM, Kantor SJ, Glassman AH. Cardiac antiarrhythmic effect of imipramine hydrochloride. N Engl J Med. 1977;296(4):206–8.

159. Roose SP, Glassman AH, Giardina EG, Walsh BT, Woodring S, Bigger JT. Tricyclic antidepressants in depressed patients with cardiac conduction disease. Arch Gen Psychiatry. 1987;44(3):273–5.
160. Dalack GW, Roose SP, Glassman AH. Tricyclics and heart failure. Am J Psychiatry. 1991;148(11):1601.
161. Cardiac Arrhythmia Suppression Trial (CAST) Investigators. Preliminary report: effect of encainide and flecainide on mortality in a randomized trial of arrhythmia suppression after myocardial infarction. N Engl J Med. 1989;321:406–12.
162. Cardiac Arrhythmia Suppression Trial II Investigators. Effect of the antiarrhythmic agent moricizine on survival after myocardial infarction. N Engl J Med. 1992;327:227–33.
163. Roose SP, Dalack GW, Glassman AH, Woodring S, Walsh BT, Giardina EG. Is doxepin a safer tricyclic for the heart? J Clin Psychiatry. 1991;52(8):338–41.
164. Monteiro WO, Noshirvani HF, Marks IM, Lelliott PT. Anorgasmia from clomipramine in obsessive-compulsive disorder. A controlled trial. Br J Psychiatry. 1987;151:107–12.
165. Callaham M, Kassel D. Epidemiology of fatal tricyclic antidepressant ingestion: implications for management. Ann Emerg Med. 1985;14:1–9.
166. Kulig K, Rumack BH, Sullivan JB, Jr., Brandt H, Spyker DA, Duffy JP, et al. Amoxapine overdose. Coma and seizures without cardiotoxic effects. JAMA. 1982;248(9):1092–4.
167. Litovitz TL, Troutman WG. Amoxapine overdose. Seizures and fatalities. JAMA. 1983;250(8):1069–71.
168. Knudsen K, Heath A. Effects of self poisoning with maprotiline. Br Med J (Clin Res Ed). 1984;288(6417):601–3.
169. Olfson M, Klerman GL. Trends in the prescription of antidepressants by office-based psychiatrists. Am J Psychiatry. 1993;150(4):571–7.
170. Barbui C, Hotopf M. Amitriptyline v. the rest: still the leading antidepressant after 40 years of randomized controlled trials. Br J Psychiatry. 2001;178:129–44.
171. Boyce P, Judd F. The place for the tricyclic antidepressants in the treatment of depression. Aust N Z J Psychiatry. 1999;33:323–7.
172. Vestergaard P, Gram LF, Kragh-Sorensen P, Bech P, Reisby N, Bolwig TG. Therapeutic potentials of recently introduced antidepressants. Danish University Antidepressant Group. Psychopharmacol Ser. 1993;10:190–8.
173. Roose SP, Glassman AH, Attia E, Woodring S. Comparative efficacy of selective serotonin reuptake inhibitors and tricyclics in the treatment of melancholia. Am J Psychiatry. 1994;151(12):1735–9.
174. Perry PJ. Pharmacotherapy for major depression with melancholic features: relative efficacy of tricyclic versus selective serotonin reuptake inhibitor antidepressants. J Affect Disord. 1996;39(1):1–6.
175. Biederman J, Thisted RA, Greenhill LL, Ryan ND. Estimation of the association between desipramine and the risk for sudden death in 5- to 14-year-old children. J Clin Psychiatry. 1995;56(3):87–93.
176. Spencer T, Biederman J, Wilens T, Harding M, O'Donnell D, Griffin S. Pharmacotherapy of attention-deficit hyperactivity disorder across the life cycle. J Am Acad Child Adolesc Psychiatry. 1996;35(4):409–32.
177. Wilens TE, Biederman J, Prince J, Spencer TJ, Faraone SV, Warburton R, et al. Six-week, double-blind, placebo-controlled study of desipramine for adult attention deficit hyperactivity disorder. Am J Psychiatry. 1996;153(9):1147–53.
178. Kornstein SG, Schatzberg AF, Thase ME, Yonkers KA, McCullough JP, Keitner GI, et al. Gender differences in treatment response to sertraline versus imipramine in chronic depression. Am J Psychiatry. 2000;157(9):1445–52.
179. Quitkin FM, Stewart JW, McGrath PJ. Gender differences in treatment response. Am J Psychiatry. 2001;158(9):1531–3.
180. Quitkin FM, Stewart JW, McGrath PJ, Taylor BP, Tisminetzky MS, Petkova E, et al. Are there differences between women's and men's antidepressant responses? Am J Psychiatry. 2002;159(11):1848–54.

181. Detke MJ, Lu Y, Goldstein DJ, Hayes JR, Demitrack MA. Duloxetine, 60 mg once daily, for major depressive disorder: a randomized double-blind placebo-controlled trial. J Clin Psychiatry. 2002;63(4):308–15.
182. Horst WD, Preskorn SH. Mechanisms of action and clinical characteristics of three atypical antidepressants: venlafaxine, nefazodone, bupropion. J Affect Disord. 1998;51(3):237–54.
183. Ascher JA, Cole JO, Colin JN, Feighner JP, Ferris RM, Fibiger GC, et al. Bupropion: a review of its mechanism of antidepressant activity. J Clin Psychiatry. 1995;56(9):395–401.
184. Settle EC, Jr. Bupropion sustained release: side effect profile. J Clin Psychiatry. 1998;59(Suppl 4): 32–6.
185. Preskorn SH. Comparison of the tolerability of bupropion, fluoxetine, imipramine, nefazodone, paroxetine, sertraline, and venlafaxine. J Clin Psychiatry. 1995;56(Suppl 6):12–21.
186. Lineberry TW, Peters GE, Jr., Bostwick JM. Bupropion-induced erythema multiforme. Mayo Clin Proc. 2001;76(6):664–6.
187. DeVane CL, Grothe DR, Smith SL. Pharmacology of antidepressants: focus on nefazodone. J Clin Psychiatry. 2002;63(Suppl 1):10–7.
188. Holliday SM, Benfield P. Venlafaxine. A review of its pharmacology and therapeutic potential in depression. Drugs. 1995;49(2):280–94.
189. Owen JR, Nemeroff CB. New antidepressants and the cytochrome P450 system: focus on venlafaxine, nefazodone, and mirtazapine. Depress Anxiety. 1998;7(Suppl 1):24–32.
190. Nelson JC. Safety and tolerability of the new antidepressants. J Clin Psychiatry. 1997;58(Suppl 6): 26–31.
191. Schweizer E, Feighner J, Mandos LA, Rickels K. Comparison of venlafaxine and imipramine in the acute treatment of major depression in outpatients. J Clin Psychiatry. 1994;55(3):104–8.
192. Fava M, Mulroy R, Alpert J, Nierenberg AA, Rosenbaum JF. Emergence of adverse events following discontinuation of treatment with extended-release venlafaxine. Am J Psychiatry. 1997;154(12):1760–2.
193. Einarson A, Fatoye B, Sarkar M, Lavigne SV, Brochu J, Chambers C, et al. Prenancy outcome following gestational exposure to venlafaxine: a multicenter prospective controlled study. Am J Psychiatry. 2001;158(10):1728–30.
194. Eison AS, Eison MS, Torrente JR, Wright RN, Yocca FD. Nefazodone: preclinical pharmacology of a new antidepressant. Psychopharmacol Bull. 1990;26(3):311–5.
195. Lader MH. Tolerability and safety: essentials in antidepressant pharmacotherapy. J Clin Psychiatry. 1996;57(Suppl 2):39–44.
196. Warner MD, Peabody CA, Whiteford HA, Hollister LE. Trazodone and priapism. J Clin Psychiatry. 1987;48(6):244–5.
197. Stewart DE. Hepatic adverse reactions associated with nefazodone. Can J Psychiatry. 2002;47(4):375–7.
198. Ehrentraut S, Rothenhausler HB, Gerbes AL, Rau HG, Thiel M, Schirren CA, et al. Acute liver failutre in nefazodone therapy? A case report [article in German]. Nervenarzt. 2002;73(7):686–9.
199. de Boer T, Maura G, Raiteri M, de Vos CJ, Wieringa J, Pinder RM. Neurochemical and autonomic pharmacological profiles of the 6-aza-analogue of mianserin, ORG 3770 and its enantiomers. Neuropharmacology. 1988;27(4):399–408.
200. de Boer T. The pharmacologic profile of mirtazapine. J Clin Psychiatry. 1996;57(Suppl 4): 19–25.
201. Kent JM. SNaRIs, NaSSAs, and NaRIs: new agents for the treatment of depression. Lancet. 2000;355(9207):911–8.
202. Stahl SM. Basic psychopharmacology of antidepressants, part 1: antidepressants have seven distinct mechanisms of action. J Clin Psychiatry. 1998;59(Suppl 4):5–14.
203. Whyte IM, Dawson AH, Buckley NA. Relative toxicity of venlafaxine and selective serotonin reuptake inhibitors in overdose compared to tricyclic antidepressants. QJM. 2003;86(5):369–74.

204. Buckley NA, McManus PR. Fatal toxicity of serotoninergic and other antidepressant drugs: analysis of United Kingdom mortality data. BMJ. 2002;325(7376):1332–3.
205. Bremner JD, Wingard P, Walshe TA. Safety of mirtazapine in overdose. J Clin Psychiatry. 1998;59:233–5.
206. Benson BE, Mathiason M, Dahl B, Smith K, Foley MM, Easom LA, et al. Toxicities and outcomes associated with nefazodone poisoning: an analysis of 1,338 exposures. Am J Emerg Med. 2000;18(5):587–92.
207. de Meester A, Carbutti G, Gabriel L, Jacques JM. Fatal overdose with trazodone: case report and literature review. Acta Clin Belg. 2001;56(4):258–61.
208. Harris CR, Gualtieri J, Stark G. Fatal bupropion overdose. J Toxicol Clin Toxicol. 1997;35(3):321–4.
209. Storrow AB. Bupropion overdose and seizure. Am J Emerg Med. 1994;12(2):183–4.
210. Spiller HA, Ramoska EA, Krenzelok EP, Sheen SR, Borys DJ, Villalobos D, et al. Bupropion overdose: a 3-year multi-center retrospective analysis. Am J Emerg Med. 1994;12(1):43–5.
211. Hays JT, Hurt RD, Rigotti NA, Niaura R, Gonzales D, Durcan MJ, et al. Sustained-release bupropion for pharmacologic relapse prevention after smoking cessation. a randomized, controlled trial. Ann Intern Med. 2001;135(6):423–33.
212. Semenchuk MR, Sherman S, Davis B. Double-blind, randomized trial of bupropion SR for the treatment of neuropathic pain. Neurology. 2001;57(9):1583–8.
213. Dostert P, Benedetti MS, Poggest I. Review of the pharmacokinetics and metabolism of reboxetine, a selective noradrenaline reuptake inhibitor. Eur Neuropsychopharmacol. 1997;7(Suppl 1):S23–35.
214. Fleishaker JC. Clinical pharmacokinetics of reboxetine, a selective norepinephrine reuptake inhibitor for the treatment of patients with depression. Clin Pharmacokinet. 2000;39(6):413–27.
215. Ohman D, Cherma MD, Norlander B, Bengstosson F. Determination of serum reboxetine enantiomers in patients on chronic medication with racemic reboxetine. Ther Drug Monit. 2003;25(2):174–82.
216. Burrows GD, Maguire KP, Norman TR. Antidepressant efficiancy and tolerability of the selective norepinephrine reuptake inhibitor reboxetine: a review. J Clin Psychiatry. 1998;59(Suppl 14):4–7.
217. Schatzberg AF. Clinical efficacy of reboxetine in major depression. J Clin Psychiatry. 2000;61(Suppl 10):31–8.
218. Versiani M, Amin M, Chouinard G. Double-blind, placebo-controlled study with reboxetine in inpatients with severe major depressive disorder. J Clin Psychopharmacol. 2000;20(1):28–34.
219. Fleishaker JC, Francom SF, Herman BD, Knuth DW, Azie NE. Lack of effect of reboxetine on cardiac repolarization. Clin Pharmacol Ther. 2001;70(3):261–9.
220. Andreoli V, Caillard V, Deo R, Rybakowski JK, Versiani M. Reboxetine, a new noradrenaline selective antidepressant, is at least as effective as fluoxetine in the treatment of depression. J Clin Psychopharmacol. 2002;22(4):393–9.
221. Montgomery S, Fuerguson JM, Schwartz GE. The antidepressant efficacy of reboxetine in patients with severe depression. J Clin Psychopharmacol. 2003;23(1):45–50.
222. Harmer CJ, O'Sullivan U, Favaron E, Massey-Chase R, Ayres R, Reinecke A, et al. Effect of acute antidepressant administration on negative affective bias in depressed patients. Am J Psychiatry. 2009;166(10):1178–84.
223. Bruhl AB, Kaffenberger T, Herwig U. Serotonergic and noradrenergic modulation of emotion processing by single dose antidepressants. Neuropsychopharmacology. 2010;35(2):521–33.
224. Belanoff JK, Flores BH, Kalezhan M, Sund B, Schatzberg AF. Rapid reversal of psychotic depression using mifepristone. J Clin Psychopharmacol. 2001;21(5):516–21.
225. Belanoff JK, Rothschild AJ, Cassidy F, DeBattista C, Baulieu EE, Schold C, et al. An open trial of C-1073 (mifepristone) for psychotic major depression. Biol Psychiatry. 2002;52(5):386–92.

226. Krishnan KR. Clinical experience with substance P receptor (NK_1) antagonists in depression. J Clin Psychiatry. 2003;63(Suppl 11):25–9.
227. Rimon R, Le Greves P, Nyberg F, Heikkila L, Salmela L, Terenius L. Elevation of substance P-like peptides in the CSF of psychiatric patients. Biol Psychiatry. 1984;19(4):509–16.
228. McAllister-Williams RH, Baldwin DS, Haddad PM, Bazire S. The use of antidepressants in clinical practice: focus on agomelatine. Hum Psychopharmacol. 2010;25(2):95–102.
229. Fishback JA, Robson MJ, Xu YT, Matsumoto RR. Sigma receptors: potential targets for a new class of antidepressant drug. Pharmacol Ther. 2010;127:271–82.
230. Fox H, Gibas J. Synthetic tuberculostats. VII. Monoalkyl derivatives of isonicotinylhydrazine. J Org Chem. 1953;18:994–1002.
231. Selikoff IJ, Robitzek EH, Orenstein GG. Treatment of pulmonary tuberculosis with hydrazine derivatives of isonicotinic acid. JAMA. 1952;150:973–80.
232. Loomers HP, Saunders JC, Kline NS. A clinical and pharmacodynamic evaluation of iproniazid as a psychic energizer. Psychiatr Res Rep. 1957;8:129–41.
233. Kline NS. Clinical experience with iproniazid (MARSILID). J Clin Exp Pyschopathol. 1958;19(Suppl 1):72–8.
234. Zeller EA, Barsky JR, Fouts W, et al. Influence of isonicotinic acid hydrazide (INH) and 1-isonicotinyl-2-isopropyl hydrazide (IIH) on bacterial and mammalian enzymes. Experientia. 1952;8:349–50.
235. Weinstock M, Gorodetsky E, Wang RH, Gross A, Weinreb O, Youdim MBH. Limited potentiation of blood pressure response to oral tyramine by brain-selective monoamine oxidase A-B inhibitor, TV-3326 in conscious rabbits. Neuropharmacology. 2002;43(6):999–1005.
236. Baker GB, Urichuk LJ, McKenna KF, Kennedy SH. Metabolism of monoamine oxidase inhibitors. Cell Mol Neurobiol. 1999;19(3):411–26.
237. Youdim MB, Aronson JK, Blau K, Green AR, Grahame-Smith DG. Tranylcypromine ('Parnate') overdose: measurement of tranylcypromine concentrations and MAO inhibitory activity and identification of amphetamines in plasma. Psychol Med. 1979;9(2):377–82.
238. Sherry-McKenna RL, Baker GB, Mousseau DD, Coutts RT, Dewhurst WG. 4-methyoxytranylcypromine, a monoamine oxidase inhibitor: effects on biogenic amines in rat brain following chronic administration. Biol Psychiatry. 1992;31(9):881–8.
239. Sherry RL, Rauw G, McKenna KF, Paetsch PR, Coutts RT, Baker GB. Failure to detect amphetamine or 1-amino-3-phenylpropane in humans or rats receiving the MAO inhibitor tranylcypromine. J Affect Disord. 2000;61(1–2):23–9.
240. Lang A, Geissler HE, Mutschler E. Determination and comparison of the plasma and urine concentrations in men given tranylcypromine stereoisomers [article in German]. Arzneimittelforschung. 1979;29(1):154–7.
241. Spahn-Langguth H, Hahn G, Mutschler E, Mohrke W, Langguth P. Enantiospecific high-performance liquid chromatographic assay with fluoroscence detection for the monoamine oxidase ihibitor tranylcypromine and its applicability in pharmacokinetic studies. J Chromatogr. 1992;584(2):229–37.
242. Livingston MG, Livingston HM. Monoamine oxidase inhibitors. An update on drug interactions. Drug Saf. 1996;14(4):219–27.
243. Lotufo-Neto F, Trivedi M, Thase ME. Meta-analysis of the reversible inhibitors of monoamine oxidase type A moclobemide and brofaromine for the treatment of depression. Neuropsychopharmacology. 1999;20(3):226–47.
244. Guelfi JD, Payan C, Fermanian J, Pedarriosse AM, Manfredi R. Moclobemide versus clomipramine in endogenous depression. A double-blind randomised clinical trial. Br J Psychiatry. 1992;160:519–24.
245. Hilton SE, Maradit H, Moller HJ. Serotonin syndrome and drug combinations: focus on MAOI and RIMA. Eur Arch Psychiatr Clin Neurosci. 1997;247(3):113–9.
246. van Vliet IM, Westenberg HG, Den Boer JA. MAO inhibitors in panic disorder: clinical effects of treatment with brofaromine. A double blind placebo controlled study. Psychopharmacology (Berl). 1993;112(4):483–9.

247. Haefely W, Burkard WP, Cesura AM, Kettler R, Lorez HP, Martin JR, et al. Biochemistry and pharmacology of moclobemide, a prototype RIMA. Psychopharmacology (Berl). 1992;106(Suppl):S6–14.
248. McGrath PJ, Stewart JW, Nunes EV, Ocepek-Welikson K, Rabkin JG, Quitkin FM, et al. A double-blind crossover trial of imipramine and phenelzine for outpatients with treatment-refractory depression. Am J Psychiatry. 1993;150(1):118–23.
249. Liebowitz MR, Quitkin FM, Stewart JW, McGrath PJ, Harrison WM, Markowitz JS, et al. Antidepressant specificity in atypical depression. Arch Gen Psychiatry. 1988;45(2):129–37.
250. McGrath PJ, Stewart JW, Harrison WM, Ocepek-Welikson K, Rabkin JG, Nunes EN, et al. Predictive value of symptoms of atypical depression for differential drug treatment outcome. J Clin Psychopharmacol. 1992;12(3):197–202.
251. Vallejo J, Gasto C, Catalan R, Salamero M. Double-blind study of imipramine versus phenelzine in melancholias and dysthymic disorders. Br J Psychiatry. 1987;151:639–42.
252. Himmelhoch JM, Thase ME, Mallinger AG, Houck P. Tranylcypromine versus imipramine in anergic bipolar depression. Am J Psychiatry. 1991;148(7):910–6.
253. Georgotas A, McCue RE, Hapworth W, Friedman E, Kim OM, Welkowitz J, et al. Comparative efficacy and safety of MAOIs versus TCAs in treating depression in the elderly. Biol Psychiatry. 1986;21(12):1155–66.
254. Quitkin FM, McGrath PJ, Stewart JW, Harrison W, Tricamo E, Wager SG, et al. Atypical depression, panic attacks, and response to imipramine and phenelzine. A replication. Arch Gen Psychiatry. 1990;47(10):935–41.
255. Thase ME, Trivedi MH, Rush AJ. MAOIs in the contemporary treatment of depression. Neuropsychopharmacology. 1995;12(3):185–219.
256. Price LH, Charney DS, Heninger GR. Efficacy of lithium-tranylcypromine treatment in refractory depression. Am J Psychiatry. 1985;142(5):619–23.
257. Roose SP, Glassman AH, Walsh BT, Woodring S. Tricyclic nonresponders: phenomenology and treatment. Am J Psychiatry. 1986;143(3):345–8.
258. Thase ME, Mallinger AG, McKnight D, Himmelhoch JM. Treatment of imipramine-resistant recurrent depression, IV: a double-blind crossover study of tranylcypromine for anergic bipolar depression. Am J Psychiatry. 1992;149(2):195–8.
259. Liebowitz MR, Schneier F, Campeas R, Hollander E, Hatterer J, Fyer A, et al. Phenelzine vs atenolol in social phobia. A placebo-controlled comparison. Arch Gen Psychiatry. 1992;49(4):290–300.
260. Stein G. Drug treatment of the personality disorders. Br J Psychiatry. 1992;161:167–84.
261. Cornelius JR, Soloff PH, Perel JM, Ulrich RF. Continuation pharmacotherapy of borderline personality disorder with haloperidol and phenelzine. Am J Psychiatry. 1993;150(12):1843–8.
262. Nurnberg HG, Levine PE. Spontaneous remission of MAOI-induced anorgasmia. Am J Psychiatry. 1987;144(6):805–7.
263. Asatoor AM, Levi AJ, Milne MD. Tranylcypromine and cheese (letters to the editor). Lancet. 1963;2:733–4.
264. Blackwell B, Marley E, Price J, et al. Hypertensive interactions between monoamine oxidase inhibitors and foodstuffs. Br J Psychiatry. 1967;113:349–65.
265. Hyman S. Toxic side effects of psychotropic medications and their management. In: Hyman S, Tesar G, editors. Manual of psychiatric emergencies. 3rd ed. Boston: Little Brown 1994. p. 204–17; 304–22.
266. Insel TR, Roy BF, Cohen RM, Murphy DL. Possible development of the serotonin syndrome in man. Am J Psychiatry. 1982;139(7):954–5.
267. Creelman WL, Ciraulo DA. Monoamine oxidase inhibitors (MAOIS). In: Ciraulo DA, Shader RI, Greenblatt DJ, Creelman WL, editors. Drug interactions in psychiatry. 2nd ed. Baltimore, MD: Williams & Wilkins; 1995. p. 430.
268. Linden CH, Rumack BH, Strehlke C. Monoamine oxidase inhibitor overdose. Ann Emerg Med. 1984;13(12):1137–44.

269. Vartzopoulos D, Krull F. Dependence on monoamine oxidase inhibitors in high dose. Br J Psychiatry. 1991;158:856–7.
270. Thase ME, Rush AJ. Treatment-resistant depression. In: Bloom FE, Kupfer DJ, editors. Psychopharmacology: the fourth generation of progress. New York: Raven; 1995. p. 1081.
271. Thase ME, Rush AJ. When at first you don't succeed: sequential strategies for antidepressant nonresponders. J Clin Psychiatry. 1997;58(Suppl 13):23–9.
272. Fava M. Management of nonresponse and intolerance: switching strategies. J Clin Psychiatry. 2000;61(Suppl 2):10–2.
273. Carpenter LL, Jocic Z, Hall JM, Rasmussen SA, Price LH. Mirtazapine augmentation in the treatment of refractory depression. J Clin Psychiatry. 1999;60(1):45–9.
274. Debonnel G, Gobbi G, Turcotte J, et al., editors. The α_2 antagonist mirtazapine combined with the SSRI paroxetine induces a greater antidepressant response: a double-blind controlled study. 39th Annual Meeting of the American College of Neuropsychopharmacology; 2000; San Juan, Puerto Rico.
275. Carpenter LL, Yasmin S, Price LH. A double-blind, placebo-controlled study of mirtazapine augmentation for refractory depression. Biol Psychiatry. 2002;51:183–8.
276. Marshall RD, Liebowitz MR. Paroxetine/bupropion combination treatment for refractory depression. J Clin Psychopharmacol. 1996;16:80–1.
277. Bodkin JA, Lasser RA, Wines JD, Jr., Gardner DM, Baldessarini RJ. Combining serotonin reuptake inhibitors and bupropion in partial responders to antidepressant monotherapy. J Clin Psychiatry. 1997;58(4):137–45.
278. Spier SA. Use of bupropion with SRIs and venlafaxine. Depress Anxiety. 1998;7:73–5.
279. Fredman SJ, Fava M, Kienke AS, White CN, Nierenberg AA, Rosenbaum JF. Partial response, nonresponse, and relapse with selective serotonin reuptake inhibitors in major depression: a survey of current "next-step" practices. J Clin Psychiatry. 2000;61(6):403–8.
280. Nelson JC, Mazure CM, Bowers MB, Jr., Jatlow PI. A preliminary, open study of the combination of fluoxetine and desipramine for rapid treatment of major depression. Arch Gen Psychiatry. 1991;48(4):303–7.
281. Fava M, Rosenbaum JF, McGrath PJ, Stewart JW, Amsterdam JD, Quitkin FM. Lithium and tricyclic augmentation of fluoxetine treatment for resistant major depression: a double-blind, controlled study. Am J Psychiatry. 1994;151(9):1372–4.
282. Rothschild BS. Fluoxetine-nortiptyline therapy of treatment-resistant major depression in a geriatric patient. J Geriatr Psychiatry Neurol. 1994;7(3):137–8.
283. Amsterdam JD, Garcia-Espana F, Rosenzweig M. Clomipramine augmentation in treatment-resistant depression. Depress Anxiety. 1997;5(2):84–90.
284. de Montigny C, Grunberg F, Mayer A, Deschenes JP. Lithium induces relief of depression in tricyclic antidepressant drug non-responders. Br J Psychiatry. 1981;138:252–6.
285. de Montigny C, Cournoyer G, Morissette R, Langlois R, Caille G. Lithium carbonate addition in tricyclic antidepressant-resistant unipolar depression. Correlations with the neurobiologic actions of tricyclic antidepresant drugs and lithium ion on the serotonin system. Arch Gen Psychiatry. 1983;40(12):1327–34.
286. Joffe RT, Singer W, Levitt AJ, MacDonald C. A placebo-controlled comparison of lithium and triiodothyronine augmentation of tricyclic antidepressants in unipolar refractory depression. Arch Gen Psychiatry. 1993;50(5):387–93.
287. Gray EG. Severe depression: a patient's thoughts. Br J Psychiatry. 1983;143:319–22.
288. Heninger GR, Charney DS, Sternberg DE. Lithium carbonate augmentation of antidepressant treatment. An effective prescription for treatment-refractory depression. Arch Gen Psychiatry. 1983;40(12):1335–42.
289. Graham PM. Drug combination for chronic depression. Br J Psychiatry. 1984;145:214.
290. Pope HG, Jr., McElroy SL, Nixon RA. Possible synergism between fluoxetine and lithium in refractory depression. Am J Psychiatry. 1988;145:1292–4.
291. Katona CL, Abou-Saleh MT, Harrison DA, Nairac BA, Edwards DR, Lock T, et al. Placebo-controlled trial of lithium augmentation of fluoxetine and lofepramine. Br J Psychiatry. 1995;166(1):80–6.

292. Bauer M, Zaninelli R, Muller-Oerlinghausen B, Meister W. Paroxetine and amitriptyline augmentation of lithium in the treatment of major depression: a double-blind study. J Psychopharmacol. 1999;19(2):164–71.
293. Peterson EA, Nelson K. How to meet your clients' spiritual needs. J Psychosoc Nurs Ment Health Serv. 1987;25(5):34–9.
294. Ostroff RB, Nelson JC. Risperidone augmentation of selective serotonin reuptake inhibitors in major depression. J Clin Psychiatry. 1999;60(4):256–9.
295. Nelson JC, Papakostas GI. Atypical antipsychotic augmentation in major depressive disorder: a meta-analysis of placebo-controlled randomized trials. Am J Psychiatry. 2009; 166(9):980–91.
296. Shelton RC, Keller MB, Gelenberg A, Dunner DL, Hirschfeld R, Thase ME, et al. Effectiveness of St John's wort in major depression: a randomized controlled trial. JAMA. 2001;285(15):1978–86.
297. Papakostas GI. Augmentation strategies in the treatment of major depressive disorder. Examining the evidence on augmentation with atypical antipsychotics. CNS Spectr. 2007;12(12 Suppl 22):10–2.
298. Berman RM, Marcus RN, Swanink R, McQuade RD, Carson WH, Corey-Lisle PK, et al. The efficacy and safety of aripiprazole as adjunctive therapy in major depressive disorder: a multicenter, randomized, double-blind, placebo-controlled study. J Clin Psychiatry. 2007;68(6):843–53.
299. Marcus RN, McQuade RD, Carson WH, Hennicken D, Fava M, Simon JS, et al. The efficacy and safety of aripiprazole as adjunctive therapy in major depressive disorder: a second multicenter, randomized, double-blind, placebo-controlled study. J Clin Psychopharmacol. 2008;28(2):156–65.
300. Cutler AJ, Montgomery SA, Feifel D, Lazarus A, Astrom M, Brecher M. Extended release quetiapine fumarate monotherapy in major depressive disorder: a placebo- and duloxetine-controlled study. J Clin Psychiatry. 2009;70(4):526–39.
301. Blier P, Szabo ST. Potential mechanisms of action of atypical antipsychotic medications in treatment-resistant depression and anxiety. J Clin Psychiatry. 2005;66(Suppl 8):30–40.
302. Jacobsen FM. A possible augmentation of antidepressant response by buspirone. J Clin Psychiatry. 1991;52:217–20.
303. Joffe RT, Schuller DR. An open study of buspirone augmentation of serotonin reuptake inhibitors in refractory depression. J Clin Psychiatry. 1993;54:269–71.
304. Bouwer C, Stein DJ. Buspirone is an effective augmenting agent of serotonin selective reuptake inhibitors in severe treatment-refractory depression. S Afr Med J. 1997;87(Suppl 4): 534–7.
305. Dimitriou EC, Dimitriou CE. Buspirone augmentation of antidepressant therapy. J Clin Psychopharmacol. 1998;18:465–9.
306. Appelberg BG, Syvalahti EK, Koskinen TE, Mehtonen OP, Muhonen TT, Naukkarinen HH. Patients with severe depression may benefit from buspirone augmentation of selective serotonin reuptake inhibitors: results from a placebo-controlled, randomized, double-blind, placebo wash-in study. J Clin Psychiatry. 2001;62(6):448–52.
307. Landen M, Bjorling G, Agren H, Fahlen T. A randomized, double-blind, placebo-controlled trial of buspirone in combination with an SSRI in patients with treatment-refractory depression. J Clin Psychiatry. 1998;59(12):664–8.
308. Patrick KS, Mueller RA, Gualtieri CT, Breese GR. Pharmacokinetics and actions of methylphenidate. In: Meltzer HY, editor. Psychopharmacology: the third generation of progress. New York: Raven; 1987. p. 1387–95.
309. Wharton RN, Perel JM, Dayton PG, Malitz SM. A potential clinical use for methylphenidate with tricyclic antidepressants. Am J Psychiatry. 1971;127:1619–25.
310. Fawcett JA, Kravitz HM, Zajecka JM, Schaff MR. CNS stimulant potentiation of monoamine oxidase inhibitors in treatment-refractory depression. J Psychopharmacol. 1991;11:127–32.
311. Stoll AL, Pillay SS, Diamond L, Workum SB, Cole JO. Methylphenidate augmentation of serotonin selective reuptake inhibitors: a case series. J Clin Psychiatry. 1996;57(2):72–6.

312. Bader GM, Hawley JM, Short DD. Venlafaxine augmentation with methylphenidate for treatment-refractory depression: a case report. J Clin Psychopharmacol. 1998;18(3):255–6.
313. Masand PS, Anand VS, Tanquary JF. Psychostimulant augmentation of second generation antidepressants: a case series. Depress Anxiety. 1998;7:89–91.
314. Postolache TT, Rosenthal RN, Hellerstein DJ, Aromin R, Kelton GM, Muran JC, et al. Early augmentation of sertraline with methylphenidate. J Clin Psychiatry. 1999;60(2):123–4.
315. Lavretsky H, Kumar A. Methylphenidate augmentation of citalopram in elderly depressed patients. Am J Geriatr Psychiatry. 2001;9(3):298–303.
316. Naranjo CA, Tremblay LK, Busto UE. The role of the brain reward system in depression. Prog Neuropsychopharmacol Biol Psychiatry. 2001;25:781–823.
317. Tremblay LK, Naranjo CA, Cardenas L, Herrmann N, Busto UE. Probing brain reward system function in major depressive disorder: altered response to dextroamphetamine. Arch Gen Psychiatry. 2002;59(5):409–16.
318. Menza MA, Kaufman KR, Castellanos A. Modafinil augmentation of antidepressant treatment in depression. J Clin Psychiatry. 2000;61(5):378–81.
319. Markovitz PJ, Wagner S. An open-label trial of modafinil augmentation in patients with partial response to antidepressant therapy [letter]. J Clin Psychopharmacol. 2003;23(2):207–9.
320. Prange AJ, Jr., et al. Hormonal alteration of imipramine response: a review. In: Sachar EJ, editor. Hormones, behavior, and psychopathology. New York: Raven; 1976.
321. Wheatley D. Potentiation of amitriptyline by thyroid hormone. Arch Gen Psychiatry. 1972;26:229–33.
322. Tsutsui S, Yamazaki Y, Namba T, Tsushima M. Combined therapy of T3, and antidepressants in depression. J Int Med Res. 1979;7(2):138–46.
323. Earle BV. Thyroid hormone and tricyclic antidepressants in resistant depressions. Am J Psychiatry. 1970;126(11):1667–9.
324. Ogura C, Okuma T, Uchida Y, Imai S, Yogi H. Combined thyroid (triodothyronine)-tricyclic antidepressant treatment in depressive states. Folia Psychiatr Neurol Jpn. 1974;28(3):179–86.
325. Goodwin FK, Prange A, Post R, Muscettola G, Lipton MA. Potentiation of antidepresant effects by L-triiodothyronine in tricyclic nonresponders. Am J Psychiatry. 1982;139(1):34–8.
326. Joffe RT, Levitt AJ, Bagby RM, MacDonald C, Singer W. Predictors of response to lithium and triiodothyronine: augmentation of antidepressants in tricyclic non-responders. Br J Psychiatry. 1993;163:574–8.
327. Crowe D, Collins JP, Rosse RB. Thyroid hormone supplementation of fluoxetine treatment [letter]. J Clin Psychopharmacol. 1990;10:150–1.
328. Gupta S, Masand P, Tanquary JF. Thyroid hormone supplementation of fluoxetine in the treatment of major depression. Br J Psychiatry. 1991;159:866–7.
329. Joffe RT. Triiodothyronine potentiation of fluoxetine in depressed patients. Can J Psychiatry. 1992;37:48–50.
330. Gitlin MJ, Weiner H, Farbanks L, Hershman JM, Friedfeld N. Failure of T3 to potentiate tricyclic antidepressant response. J Affect Disord. 1987;13(3):267–72.
331. Targum SD, Greenberg RD, Harmon RL, Kessler K, Salerian AJ, Fram DH. Thyroid hormone and the TRH stimulation test in refractory depression. J Clin Psychiatry. 1984;45(8):345–6.
332. Spoov J, Lahdelma L. Should thyroid augmentation precede lithium augmentation – a pilot study. J Affect Disord. 1998;49:235–9.
333. Bauer M, Hellweg R, Graf KJ, Baumgartner A. Treatment of refractory depression with high-dose thyroxine. Neuropsychopharmacology. 1998;18(6):444–55.
334. Altshuler LL, Bauer M, Frye MA, Gitlin MJ, Mintz J, Szuba MP, et al. Does thyroid supplementation accelerate tricyclic antidepressant response? A review and meta-analysis of the literature. Am J Psychiatry. 2001;158(10):1617–22.
335. Pope HG, Jr., Cohane GH, Kanayama G, Siegel AJ, Hudson JI. Testosterone gel supplementation for men with refractory depression: a randomized, placebo-controlled trial. Am J Psychiatry. 2003;160(1):105–11.

336. de Novaes Soares C, Almeida O, Joffe H, Cohen LS. Efficacy of estradiol for the treatment of depressive disorders in perimenopausal women: a double-blind, randomized, placebo-controlled trial. Arch Gen Psychiatry. 2001;58(6):529–34.
337. Schmidt PJ, Nieman L, Danaceau MA, Tobin MB, Roca CA, Murphy JH, et al. Estrogen replacement in perimenopause-related depression: a preliminary report. Am J Obstet Gynecol. 2000;183:414–20.
338. Rasgon NL, Altshuler LL, Fairbanks LA, Dunkin JJ, Davtyan C, Elman S, et al. Estrogen replacement therapy in the treatment of major depressive disorder in perimenopausal women. J Clin Psychiatry. 2002;63(Suppl 7):745–8.
339. Smith RN, Studd JW, Zamblera D, Holland EF. A randomised comparison over 8 months of 100 micrograms and 200 micrograms twice weekly doses of transdermal oestradiol in the treatment of severe premenstrual syndrome. Br J Obstet Gynaecol. 1995;102:475–84.
340. Gregoire AJ, Kumar R, Everitt B, Henderson AF, Studd JW. Transdermal oestrogen for treatment of severe postnatal depression. Lancet. 1996;347:930–3.
341. Ahokas A, Kaukoranta J, Aito M. Effect of oestradiol on postpartum depression. Psychopharmacology. 1999;146:108–10.
342. Campbell S, Whitehead M. Oestrogen therapy and the menopausal syndrome. Clin Obstet Gynecol. 1977;4:31–47.
343. Coope J. Is oestrogen therapy effective in the treatment of menopausal depression? J R Coll Gen Pract. 1981;31:134–40.
344. Pearce J, Hawton K, Blake F, Barlow D, Rees M, Fagg J, et al. Psychological effects of continuation versus discontinuation of hormone replacement therapy by estrogen implants: a placebo-controlled study. J Psychosom Res. 1997;42:177–86.
345. Epperson CN, Wisner KL, Yamamoto B. Gonadal steroids in the treatment of mood disorders. Psychosom Med. 1999;61(5):676–97.
346. Montgomery JC, Brincat M, Tapp A, Appleby L, Versi E, Fenwick PBC, et al. Effect of oestrogen and testosterone implants on psychological disorders in the climacteric. Lancet. 1987;1:297–9.
347. Kaliber EL, Broverman DM, Vogel W, Kobayashi Y. Estrogen therapy for severe persistent depressions in women. Arch Gen Psychiatry. 1979;36:550–4.
348. Haines CJ, Yim SF, Chung TKH, Lam CWK, Lau EWC, Ng MHL, et al. A prospective, randomized, placebo-controlled study of the dose effect of oral oestradiol on menopausal symptoms, psychological well being, and quality of life in postmenopausal Chinese women. Maturitas. 2003;44:207–14.
349. Schneider LS, Small GW, Hamilton SH, Bystritsky A, Nemeroff CB, Meyers BS. Estrogen replacement and response to fluoxetine in a multicenter geriatric depression trial. Am J Geriatr Psychiatry. 1997;5:97–106.
350. Sheline YI, Pieper CF, Barch DM, Welsh-Boehmer K, McKinstry RC, MacFall JR, et al. Support for the vascular depression hypothesis in late-life depression: results of a 2-site, prospective, antidepressant treatment trial. Arch Gen Psychiatry. 2010;67(3):277–85.
351. Gambacciani M, Monteleone P, Sacco A, Genazzani AR. Hormone replacement therapy and endometrial, ovarian and colorectal cancer. Best Pract Res Clin Endocrinol Metab. 2003;17(1):139–47.
352. Hodis HN, Mack WJ, Azen SP, Lobo RA, Shoupe D, Mahrer PR, et al. Hormone therapy and the progression of coronary-artery atherosclerosis in postmenopausal women. N Engl J Med. 2003;349(6):535–45.
353. Li CI, Malone KE, Porter PL, Weiss NS, Tang MT, Cushing-Haugen KL, et al. Relationship between long durations and different regimens of hormone therapy and risk of breast cancer. JAMA. 2003;289(24):3254–63.
354. Manson JE, Hsia J, Johnson KC, Rossouw JE, Assaf AR, Lasser NL, et al. Estrogen plus progestin and the risk of coronary heart disease. N Engl J Med. 2003;349(6):523–34.
355. Rogoz Z, Skuza G, Daniel WA, Wojcikowski J, Dudek D, Wrobel A. Amantadine as an additive treatment in patients suffering from drug-resistant unipolar depression. Pharmacol Rep. 2007;59(6):778–84.

356. Stryjer R, Strous RD, Shaked G, Bar F, Feldman B, Kotler M, et al. Amantadine as augmentation therapy in the management of treatment-resistant depression. Int Clin Psychopharmacol. 2003;18(2):93–6.
357. Schultz V, Haensel R, Tyler VE, editors. Rational phytotherapy. 3rd ed. Berlin: Springer; 1998.
358. Assemi M. Herbs affecting the central nervous system: gingko, kava, St. John's wort, and valerian. Clin Obstet Gynecol. 2001;44(4):824–35.
359. De Smet P. Herbal remedies. N Engl J Med. 2002;347(25):2046–56.
360. Bilia AR, Gallori S, Vincieri FF. St. John's wort and depression: efficacy, safety and tolerability-an update. Life Sci. 2002;70(26):3077–96.
361. Philipp M, Kohnen R, Hiller KO. Hypericum extract versus imipramine or placebo in patients with moderate depression: randomised multicentre study of treatment for eight weeks. BMJ. 1999;319(7224):1534–8.
362. Ernst E. The risk-benefit profile of commonly used herbal therapies: Ginkgo, St. John's Wort, Ginseng, Echinacea, Saw Palmetto, and Kava. Ann Intern Med. 2002;136(1):42–53.
363. Woelk H. Comparison of St John's wort and imipramine for treating depression: randomised controlled trial. BMJ. 2000;321(7260):536–9.
364. Gaster B, Holroyd J. St John's wort for depression: a systematic review. Arch Intern Med. 2000;160(2):152–6.
365. Lecrubier Y, Clerc G, Didi R, Kieser M. Efficacy of St. John's wort extract WS 5570 in major depression: a double-blind, placebo-controlled trial. Am J Psychiatry. 2002;159(8):1361–6.
366. Lantz MS, Buchalter E, Giambanco V. St. John's wort and antidepressant drug interactions in the elderly. J Geriatr Psychiatr Neurol. 1999;12(1):7–10.
367. Prost N, Tichadou L, Rodor F, Nguyen N, David JM, Jean-Pastor MJ. [St. Johns wort-venlafaxine interaction]. Presse Med. 2000;29(23):1285–6.
368. Perloff MD, von Moltke LL, Stormer E, Shader RI, Greenblatt DJ. Saint John's wort: an in vitro analysis of P-glycoprotein induction due to extended exposure. Br J Pharmacol. 2001;134(8):1601–8.
369. Henderson L, Yue QY, Bergquist C, Gerden B, Arlett P. St John's wort (Hypericum perforatum): drug interactions and clinical outcomes. Br J Clin Pharmacol. 2002;54(4):349–56.
370. Barone GW, Gurley BJ, Ketel BL, Lightfoot ML, Abul-Ezz SR. Drug interaction between St. John's wort and cyclosporine. Ann Pharmacother. 2000;34(9):1013–6.
371. Barone GW, Gurley BJ, Ketel BL, Abul-Ezz SR. Herbal supplements: a potential for drug interactions in transplant recipients. Transplantation. 2001;71(2):239–41.
372. Yue QY, Bergquist C, Gerden B. Safety of St John's wort (Hypericum perforatum). Lancet. 2000;355(9203):576–7.
373. Wang Z, Gorski JC, Hamman MA, Huang SM, Lesko LJ, Hall SD. The effects of St John's wort (Hypericum perforatum) on human cytochrome P450 activity. Clin Pharmacol Ther. 2001;70(4):317–26.
374. Johne A, Brockmoller J, Bauer S, Maurer A, Langheinrich M, Roots I. Pharmacokinetic interaction of digoxin with an herbal extract from St John's wort (*Hypericum perforatum*). Clin Pharmacol Ther. 1999;66(4):338–45.
375. Mayberg HS, Liotti M, Brannan SK, McGinnis S, Mahurin RK, Jerabek PA, et al. Reciprocal limbic-cortical function and negative mood: converging PET findings in depression and normal sadness. Am J Psychiatry. 1999;156(5):675–82.
376. Linde K, Ramirez G, Mulrow CD, Pauls A, Weidenhammer W, Melchart D. St John's wort for depression--an overview and meta-analysis of randomised clinical trials. BMJ. 1996;313(7052):253–8.
377. Kasper S, Dienel A. Cluster analysis of symptoms during antidepressant treatment with Hypericum extract in mildly to moderately depressed out-patients. A meta-analysis of data from three randomized, placebo-controlled trials. Psychopharmacology (Berl). 2002;164(3):301–8.
378. Spira JL. Comparison of St John's Wort and imipramine. Study design casts doubt on value of St John's wort in treating depression. BMJ. 2001;322(7284):493; author reply 4.

379. Hypericum Depression Trial Study Group. Effect of Hypericum perforatum (St John's wort) in major depressive disorder: a randomized controlled trial. JAMA. 2002;287(14):1807–14.
380. Mischoulon D, Fava M. Role of S-adenosyl-L-methionine in the treatment of depression: a review of the evidence. Am J Clin Nutr. 2002;76(5):1158S–61S.
381. Bell KM, Potkin SG, Carreon D, Plon L. S-adenosylmethionine blood levels in major depression: changes with drug treatment. Acta Neurol Scand Suppl. 1994;154:15–8.
382. Bressa GM. S-adenoxyl-methionine (SAMe) as antidepressant: metanalysis of clinical studies. Acta Neurol Scand. 1994;154:7–14.
383. Pancheri P, Racagni G, Delle Chiaie R, Popoli M. Recent experimental and clnical findings on the efficacy and safety of ademetionine in the pharmacological treatment of depression. G Ital Psicopat. 1997;3:1–23.
384. Delle Chiaie R, Pancheri P, Scapicchio P. Efficacy and tolerability of oral and intramuscular S-adenosyl-L-methionine 1,4-butanedisulfonate (SAMe) in the treatment of major depression: comparison with imipramine in 2 multicenter studies. Am J Clin Nutr. 2002;76(5):1172S–6S.
385. Fava M, Giannelli A, Rapisarda V, Patralia A, Guaraldi GP. Rapidity of onset of the antidepressant effect of parental S-adenosyl-L-methionine. Psychiatr Res. 1995;56:295–7.
386. Papakostas GI. Evidence for S-adenosyl-L-methionine (SAM-e) for the treatment of major depressive disorder. J Clin Psychiatry. 2009;70(Suppl 5):18–22.
387. Hibbeln JR. Fish consumption and major depression. Lancet. 1998;351(9110):1213.
388. Maes M, Smith R, Christophe A, Cosyns P, Desnyder R, Meltzer H. Fatty acid composition in major depression: decreased omega 3 fractions in cholesteryl esters and increased C20: 4 omega 6/C20:5 omega 3 ratio in cholesteryl esters and phospholipids. J Affect Disord. 1996;38(1):35–46.
389. Edwards R, Peet M, Shay J, Horrobin D. Omega-3 polyunsaturated fatty acid levels in the diet and in red blood cell membranes of depressed patients. J Affect Disord. 1998;48(2–3):149–55.
390. Adams PB, Lawson S, Sanigorski A, Sinclair AJ. Arachidonic acid to eicosapentaenoic acid ratio in blood correlates positively with clinic symptoms of depression. Lipids. 1996;31(Suppl):157–61.
391. Peet M, Horrobin DF. A dose-ranging study of the effects of ethyl-eicosapentaenoate in patients with ongoing depression despite apparently adequate treatment with standard drugs. Arch Gen Psychiatry. 2002;59:913–9.
392. Calabrese JR, Rapport DJ, Shelton MD. Fish oils and bipolar disorder: a promising but untested treatment [commentary]. Arch Gen Psychiatry. 1999;56(5):413–4.
393. Stoll AL, Severus WE, Freeman MP, Rueter S, Zboyan HA, Diamond E, et al. Omega 3 fatty acids in bipolar disorder: a preliminary double-blind, placebo-controlled trial. Arch Gen Psychiatry. 1999;56:407–12.
394. Stoll AL, Marangell LB. In reply [commentary]. Arch Gen Psychiatry. 1999;56(5):415–6.
395. Freeman MP. Omega-3 fatty acids in major depressive disorder. J Clin Psychiatry. 2009;70(Suppl 5):7–11.
396. Waal HJ. Propranolol-induced depression. Br Med J. 1967;2(5543):50.
397. Ko DT, Hebert PR, Coffey CS, Sedrakyan A, Curtis JP, Krumholz HM. Beta-blocker therapy and symptoms of depression, fatigue, and sexual dysfunction. JAMA. 2002;288(3):351–7.
398. Steffensmeier JJ, Ernst ME, Kelly M, Hartz AJ. Do randomized controlled trials always trump case reports? A second look at propranolol and depression. Pharmacotherapy. 2006;26(2):162–7.
399. Dunn NR, Freemantle SN, Mann RD. Cohort study on calcium channel blockers, other cardiovascular agents, and the prevalence of depression. Br J Clin Pharmacol. 1999;48(2):230–3.
400. Hallas J. Evidence of depression provoked by cardiovascular medication: a prescription sequence symmetry analysis. Epidemiology. 1996;7(5):478–84.
401. Ciraulo DA, Shader RI, Greenblatt DJ, Creelman WL, editors. Drug interactions in psychiatry. 2nd ed. Baltimore, MD: Williams & Wilkins; 1995.

402. Greenblatt DJ, von Moltke LL, Harmatz JS, Shader RI. Human cytochromes and some newer antidepressants: kinetics, metabolism, and drug interactions. J Clin Psychopharmacol. 1999;19(5 Suppl 1):23S–35S.
403. Burke WJ, McArthur-Miller DA. Exploring treatment alternatives: weekly dosing of fluoxetine for the continuation phase of major depressive disorder. J Clin Psychiatry. 2001;62(Suppl 22): 38–42.
404. Dinan TG. Efficacy and safety of weekly treatment with enteric-coated fluoxetine in patients with major depressive disorder. J Clin Psychiatry. 2001;62(Suppl 22):48–52.
405. Wagstaff AJ, Goa KL. Once-weekly fluoxetine. Drugs. 2001;61(15):2221–30.
406. de Klerk E. Patient compliance with enteric-coated weekly fluoxetine during continuation treatment of major depressive disorder. J Clin Psychiatry. 2001;62(Suppl 22):43–7.
407. Shulman KI, Walker SE, MacKenzie S, Knowles S. Dietary restriction, tyramine, and the use of monoamine oxidase inhibitors. J Clin Psychopharmacol. 1989;9(6):397–402.
408. Shulman KI, Walker SE. Refining the MAOI diet: tyramine content of pizzas and soy products. J Clin Psychiatry. 1999;60(3):191–3.

Antidepressant Treatment of Geriatric Depression

Domenic A. Ciraulo, James A. Evans, Wei Qiao Qiu, Richard I. Shader, and Carl Salzman

Epidemiology

The aging of the world's population has resulted in a new demographic phenomenon: a significant increase in the percentage of elderly compared with the general population. Between 1960 and 1990, the general population in the U.S. increased by less than 50%, while those over 65 increased by almost 100%, and those over 85 years of age increased by almost 250% (1).

Known as the "oldest-old," those over 85 are the fastest growing segment of our population. They are more likely to be female, experience more poverty, to have less education, and to need far greater Medicare and Medicaid services. Life expectancy at age 65 is currently 15.5 years for men and 19.1 years for women, so reaching age 80 has become the norm. For those currently 80 years old or older, life expectancy is greater in the U.S. than in Sweden, France, England, or Japan, and is increasing (2–4). The inevitable result of this demographic shift is the need to confront the common disorders of the elderly, including depression, dementia, and delirium.

Various studies have investigated the prevalence of depression in the geriatric population and their results vary. There have been few large population-based studies, and many studies exclude those with comorbid medical or psychiatric disorders or those living in institutions. The results range from a point prevalence of 1.6% in one large U.S. study (5) to other studies with ranges between 12 and 15% (6, 7). A large (n=2,640) study of depression in older people in the community living in England found the prevalence of depression to be 8.7% increasing to 9.7% if those with concurrent dementia were included. Depression was more common in women than men (10.4 vs. 6.5%) and was associated with functional disability, comorbid medical issues, and social isolation (8). A study from Singapore looking at 2,611 community-dwelling Chinese aged 55 and older showed a prevalence of depressive symptoms (Geriatric Depression Scale, GDS ≥5) of 13.3% in those with comorbid medical illness

D.A. Ciraulo (✉)
Department of Psychiatry, Boston University School of Medicine, 720 Harrison Avenue, Suite 914, Boston, MA 02118, USA
e-mail: dciraulo@bu.edu

D.A. Ciraulo and R.I. Shader (eds.), *Pharmacotherapy of Depression*,
DOI 10.1007/978-1-60327-435-7_3, © Springer Science+Business Media, LLC 2011

and 7.5% in those not reporting chronic illness. Particular illnesses independently associated with depressive symptoms were asthma/COPD, gastric problems, arthritis, and heart failure (9). For the physically ill or institutionalized, the prevalence of depression is thought to be upwards of 24–30% (10). Counter-intuitively, a Netherlands study showed a decline in the prevalence of depressive symptoms in individuals in a nursing home study, from 41.3 to 28.9% during 6 months, raising the question of adaptation of residents to the nursing home environment (11). Several studies have suggested that the prevalence of depressive disorders decreases after age 65, but these studies included few individuals older than 80 years; other reports that include the old–old suggest that the prevalence of depression may increase after age 80 (5).

An English study of subjects between 80 and 90 years old living alone in the community showed a prevalence rate of 21% with an annual incidence of 12.4%, showing the particular vulnerability of our isolated elderly (12). The Leiden 85-plus Study also supports the frequency and persistence of depression in the oldest old in the community, finding a prevalence of 15% and an annual risk for the emergence of depression of 6.8%, with poor functioning and institutionalization as predictors.

Whatever the true rate of depressive disorders, no one doubts that geriatric depression is undertreated (13) and becoming an issue of greater concern (14–16). Blazer has discussed the relationship of depression in later life to the broader concept of health, which includes both psychiatric and physical well-being (2). Patrick and Erickson (17) have described this as health-related quality of life, defined as "the value assigned to duration of life as modified by the impairments, functional states, perceptions and social opportunities that are influenced by disease, injury, treatment, or policy." Two Swedish studies found that only 27% of centenarians were diagnosed with dementia, 25% lived in their own homes, and 52% had little or no assistance managing their daily activities (18, 19). Function tends to decline with increasing age, but there is wide variation among individuals.

Yet, advanced age, even with good functioning, can mask an increasing vulnerability to a cascade of psychiatric and physical problems, which can be triggered by the onset of a single psychiatric or physical problem. This possible spiral of downward events reveals the interrelatedness of psychiatric issues, decline in functioning, medical comorbidity, and quality of life. In such a situation, depression is one piece of the puzzle and can either start a chain of events or be caused by them.

According to Blazer (2), after age 85, about half of those living in the community are frail despite their apparent functional well-being. Frailty is defined as a constellation of weight loss, weakness, fatigue, inactivity, decreased food intake, and depression. Medically, they may have muscle loss, balance and gait abnormalities, deconditioning, and decreased bone mass. "Failure to thrive" is the end stage of frailty and is characterized by further weight loss, muscle wasting, apathetic depression, anemia, decubitus ulcers, and results ultimately in death (2).

The interplay of depression, chronic medical illness, and disability is becoming clearer over time. Social and physical disabilities are shorter term outcomes of depression, and mortality is a longer term consequence of depression. Depression has a similar, and perhaps stronger, impact on disability than chronic illness. The reverse is also apparently true, that chronic illness and disability predicts the onset and persistence of depression (2).

In a large ($n = 652$) Netherlands study ,which looked at the temporal association between depression and disability in patients aged 55–85, a diagnosis of depression was associated with disability 5 months later. The association held whether the depression was major depression or a subsyndromal depression (20). A nursing home study in England showed that residents who died before a 5-month follow-up had higher depression scores than those who survived (21).

There is growing evidence in the literature that depression is either a risk factor (22–26) or pre-symptomatic of Alzheimer's disease (AD) (27–31). For each depressive symptom, assessed by the Center for Epidemiological Studies Depression Scale (CES-D), risk of developing AD increases by an average of 19% and risk of annual decline of global cognition increases by an average of 24% (30). The association between depression and AD remains after adjusting for subjective memory complaints, suggesting that the connection between depression and AD is not merely secondary to self-perceived cognitive difficulties (27). In a longitudinal study over a period of 14 years, pre-morbid depression significantly increases the risk for dementia, particularly AD, in men (32). Apolipoprotein E4 allele (ApoE4), the major risk factor of AD, is not found to be associated with late-onset depression (33). However, for subjects aged 80 and older, during the period of life when the risk of AD is dramatically increased, a relationship between ApoE4 and depression is observed (34).

Depression in the elderly is associated with subclinical cognitive impairment (29) and mild cognitive impairment (MCI) which is the preclinical stage of AD (25, 35). Depression has also been found to increase the risk of developing MCI (31, 36), particularly in highly educated elders (23). One study shows that in elders, cognitive impairment is associated with current depression but not a history of depression (37). Despite the majority of studies suggesting that depression increases the risk of AD, some longitudinal studies have questioned the relationship between late-onset depression and AD or cognitive decline (38, 39). We argue that depression is a heterogeneous clinical syndrome with multiple etiologies, and different depression subtypes have different prognoses due to different underlying pathologies.

Phenomenology of Geriatric Depression

Recent studies have looked at depression in younger or middle-aged adults versus the elderly. While there are many similarities, differences are emerging which may inform our understanding and approach to treatment. In the NIMH Collaborative Depression Study with 15 years of prospective data, the authors examined the initial episode of major depression and time to recurrence in four different age groups defined at intake: 17–30, 31–50, 51–64, and 65–79 years of age. Results showed similar recovery times for the four groups, but time to first recurrence was significantly shorter for the oldest group. In addition, the level of comorbid medical illness was higher in the oldest group. There was no difference in the level of pharmacotherapy dosing between the four groups. The authors conclude that elderly patients with MDD have a treatable disorder, on par with younger patients, but the risk of recurrence of depression is higher (40). This conclusion was echoed by another study, which likewise found a higher risk of recurrence in the elderly, along with medical comorbidity. It noted that medical comorbidity is a risk factor for poor treatment response and poor antidepressant tolerability (41). An Australian study found that depression is strongly linked to factors indicating increased dependency in the elderly (42). Also, comorbid medical illness has been linked to depression severity (43). In addition to differences in the course and presentation of geriatric depression, several research initiatives in geriatric depression are resulting in an understanding of the underlying biology of depression in this age group. Such research is also being conducted in younger adults as well, but the geriatric reports demonstrate the increased interest in understanding the specific biopathology in the elderly and how it may differ from other age groups. One such topic of research is in neuroimaging, looking at orbitofrontal gray matter in geriatric depression and changes in response to antidepressant treatment. There appears to be gray matter loss in depression, which can be partially reversed by antidepressant therapies (44, 45). Such findings have the potential to change our method of diagnosis, as we discover biological markers of depression (see discussion on vascular depression below). Another research initiative is looking at the role of brain-derived neurotrophic factor (BDNF) gene expression in elderly brains. BDNF has been found to have a differential blood level in depressed versus non-depressed patients, and the role of gene activity (Val66Met) with polymorphisms is being investigated as to underlying causes of variable BDNF levels (46). It may be that patients with lower activity of gene expression are more prone to depression. Other studies are looking at gene expression for serotonin (47, 48). The debate over the serotonin transporter-linked promoter region (5-HTTLPR) with its "long arm" (44-base pair inclusion) or "short arm" (44-base pair deletion) and its association with susceptibility to depression is well known in general psychiatry, and has also reached geriatric research (49). Finally, the topic of homocysteine levels and association with depression, vascular disease, and neurotransmitters is being researched, with the suggestion that high levels of homocysteine causes vascular disease, which in turn causes depression (50, 51). Such evidence is preliminary and awaits further clarification.

Diagnosis

Depressive disorders to consider in geriatrics should include not only the DSM diagnoses of major depression and dysthymia, but also *subsyndromal* depression (also called *minor* depression) characterized by depressive symptoms that do not meet criteria for other DSM diagnoses. Although not included in the DSM, some have argued that subsyndromal depression should be considered a separate entity (5). Such depressive conditions have been reported to be more common in the elderly than

Table 1 Characteristics of depressive states in the elderly (52)

Older patients report more somatic and cognitive symptoms than affective symptoms "depression without sadness" (53)
Suicide is twice as frequent as in the general population
Aging reduces suicide attempts but increases lethality
Severity of depression is strongly correlated with suicidal ideation
Depressions occurring in the context of medical illness should be treated concurrently with the medical illness
Late-onset dysthymia is not usually associated with personality disorders, but when it is, obsessive-compulsive and avoidant personality are most common
Subsyndromal or minor depressions in the elderly is associated with disability and progression to major depression in 25% of cases over 2 years; old–old patients may have longer prodromal periods (3 years) prior to onset of major depression

major depression, and may increase in prevalence with age. They should not be considered more benign forms of depression, because they are nonetheless associated with significant morbidity and disability (5). Presenting symptoms in old age may differ from those seen in younger adults, with an in increase in somatic and cognitive complaints, but with fewer affective symptoms, more specifically lacking a sad mood (52). Such complaints in an elderly person can be considered either symptoms of depression or medical illness, and can be a challenge to diagnosis (see Table 1).

Standard screening tools can be helpful in clarifying depressive states. The Mini-Mental Status Exam (MMS) is universally used as a gross assessment of cognitive functioning (54). The self-rated GDS has 30-item, 15-item, and 5-item versions, and the 5-item version has been found to have a high sensitivity (82–97%) and specificity (75–94%) (2, 55–57). The Center for Epidemiologic Studies Depression Scale is also used, but is not specifically designed for use in geriatric medically ill patients, and its many somatic questions may render false positives (10). The Hamilton Rating Scale for Depression (HAM-D) is a standard interviewer-administered instrument, as is the Cornell Scale for Depression in Dementia (CSDD) (58). Most research studies also use the Montgomery-Asberg Depression Rating Scale (MADRS). The detection of depressive symptoms is important whether or not a DSM diagnosis can be made, and screening tools can help sort out the relative severity of the symptoms, yet may fail to detect a significant portion of the depressed elderly population (59). In patients with concomitant medical illness, sorting out depression from medical symptoms presents diagnostic challenges. (See Sect. "Depression and Medical Illness" below).

Essential elements of diagnostic workup include a thorough psychiatric history and examination. Important areas of focus during such an exam are cognitive exam, neurological exam, and assessment of functioning, loss/grief, living situation, and supports in the community. Laboratory workup should include thyroid stimulating hormone, complete metabolic panel, complete blood count with differential, B12, folate, urinalysis. Computerized tomography (CT) and magnetic resonance imaging (MRI) of the head should be considered, particularly for patients without prior examination history. Chest films and EKGs may be indicated depending upon the presentation.

Depression Subtypes and Comorbidity

Vascular Depression

Vascular depression is a relatively recent concept based on the association of ischemic changes in the brain with late-life onset depression. There is a growing body of research supporting a neuropathologic basis to a form of depression characterized less by depressive ideation and more by subcortical dysfunction, apathy, and psychomotor change (60–66). Alexopoulos and associates (60) studied 33 elderly patients diagnosed with vascular depression and 32 patients with nonvascular depression based on the Cumulative Illness Rating Scale-Geriatrics. They found the symptoms of vascular depression to include cognitive dysfunction, disability, retardation, lack of insight, and limited depressive ideation. Although the underlying pathology is unknown, the resemblance of symptoms to a frontal lobe syndrome led these investigators to suggest vascular depression was related to the disruption of striato-pallido-thalamo-cortical pathways, but they also pointed out that lesions in other brain areas could produce vascular depression. More recently, Alexopoulos has proposed the term "depression-executive dysfunction syndrome." In his view, "impairment in frontolimbic and frontostriatal pathways confers vulnerability to depression and often results in impairment of executive functions" (67).

Vascular depression can be understood in the broader context of neuropsychiatry, in which lesions affecting the prefrontal-subcortical circuitry results in abnormalities of behavior, cognition, and mood. The lesions can occur in degenerative conditions such as the frontotemporal dementias, other age-related changes, or most obviously in ischemic cerebrovascular disease (68). In the Cardiovascular Health Study, 23% of 3,660 patients over age 65 with no history of stroke showed specific evidence of silent stroke by MRI (69). Post-stroke depression is a well-known phenomenon in psychiatry, but the underlying reason for depression resulting from the interruption of these circuits is poorly understood. Krishnan and colleagues (70–72) have also described subcortical white matter hyperintensities assumed to be of vascular origin in the pathogenesis of late-life depression and have proposed the term "subcortical ischemic depression" (73). Krishnan et al. note parallel prefrontal pathways originating in the frontal lobe and projecting to the ventral striatum, passing to the globus pallidus and substantia nigra and through the thalamus back to the frontal lobe. Three of these circuits exhibit behavioral correlates: executive dysfunction (dorsolateral prefrontal circuit), apathy (anterior cingulate circuit), and mood lability and disinhibition (orbitofrontal circuit). They report that subcortical ischemic disease has various clinical presentations, and that there is evidence of its contribution to the risk of late-onset depression. Subcortical lesions are more common in elderly depressed than healthy elderly control subjects, and more common in late-onset than early-onset elderly depression.

As mentioned above, several other investigators have identified the medial orbital frontal cortex (OFC) in late-life depression and smaller OFC volumes are associated with late-life depression (5, 74–78). In a postmortem study, inflammatory changes consistent with cerebral ischemia were found in the dorsal lateral prefrontal cortex in tissue from elderly depressed compared to control subjects (79). A study by Tupler and associates (80) suggested that left-sided white matter lesions were associated with older age of onset of depression, whereas right anterior white matter and left subcortical lesions were associated with melancholia. MRI imaging revealed deep white matter hyperintensities—markers of ischemic change—particularly in the dorsolateral prefrontal cortex.

While we are still characterizing vascular depression and even what to call it, treatment of this new phenomenon presents unique challenges. It has been noted that vascular depression is less responsive to conventional therapies, although relatively few studies have yet been done. There is suggestion that overall hyperintensity burden, in particular brain structures, is associated with poorer antidepressant treatment outcome, but not all studies have supported such association. Alexopoulos et al. have postulated that disrupted prefrontal-subcortical pathways in turn disrupt neural pathways necessary for antidepressant response. In a recent study, they found that deficits in one of the executive functions—response inhibition—predicted poor response to citalopram in the very old (81). The efficacy of drug therapy in late-onset depression remains controversial. There are some indications that sertraline may be effective (82). Another study found an absence of any association between the severity of subcortical hyperintensities and sertraline response (83). Microstructural white matter abnormalities 15 and 10 mm above the anterior commissure–posterior commissure (AC–PC) plane, which is located laterally to the anterior cingulate, were associated with poor response to citalopram treatment (84). These investigators hypothesized that such abnormalities interfere "with the reciprocal regulation of dorsal neocortical-ventral limbic structures and lead to a "disconnection syndrome" with poor antidepressant response."

These findings raise the possibility of more heterogeneous treatment approaches, in order to find the most effective treatment. One of the most intriguing suggestions they made was for further study of nontraditional agents for the treatment of vascular depression. Specifically, these included "anticholisterinemic and antiplatelet agents, free radical scavengers, calcium-channel blockers, glutamate *N*-methyl-D-aspartic acid receptor antagonists, gangliosides, aminosteroids, and amphetamine" (60). They also stressed that antidepressants may differ in their ability to promote neurological recovery after ischemic lesions. Another group has looked at augmentation of SSRI with nimodipine, a calcium-channel blocker, with some success (85). Another report showed efficacy of ECT in vascular depression (86). However, a clear direction, in terms of treatment, has not emerged yet.

Therefore, the concept of vascular depression challenges the ways in which we diagnose psychiatric illness. Currently, we identify symptom clusters in order to diagnose, but advances in neuroimaging and brain functioning introduce the subject of causality. Krishnan proposes a two-axial approach to diagnosis in which clinical presentation is on one axis and putative risk factors on the other (73).

Depression and Alzheimer's disease

Given that there are a large number of drugs for AD in clinical trials (87), we may have effective medications for the treatment and intervention of AD in the near future. Therefore, it is important for a clinician to diagnose and differentially diagnose a prodromal depression of AD so that the treatment can start early. Neuropathologically, history of depression is associated with increased amyloid plaques and neurofibrillary tangles, which are the neuropathological hallmarks of AD (88). Clinically, depression preceding the cognitive symptoms of AD only involves mild symptoms of depressed mood, fatigue, and indecision (25, 89). Some studies also found that recurrent major depressive disorder (MDD) in the elderly is associated with memory loss (90–92) and hippocampal atrophy (93–95), which is an important marker for the preclinical stage of AD. In addition, persistent depressive symptoms increase the risk of cognitive decline in the elderly even more than episodic depression (24).

Although depression of prodromal AD would lead to a primary memory impairment, followed by significant cognitive dysfunction across multiple cognitive domains, it is difficult to rely only on the clinical syndrome to differentially diagnose prodromal depression of AD from other depression subtypes. It is predicted that neuroimaging and biomarkers will enable a geriatric psychiatrist to make specific diagnoses of depression subtypes in late life. Qiu et al. have found that late-life depression with high plasma amyloid-β peptide40 (Aβ40) and low plasma Aβ42, important components of AD pathology, present with impairments in multiple cognitive domains, especially memory, suggesting prodromal depression of AD (96). Using PET scans with Pittsburgh Compound-B (PiB) to detect amyloid plaques of the AD brain, a study has found that the elderly with depression and MCI had higher PiB retention than those with depression and no MCI (97).

Depression can also be comorbid with dementia, including AD (98). Depression in Alzheimer's is common, with those in the mild to moderate stages more likely to have depression than those in the late stages (107–109). Some have suggested that the incidence of depression in vascular dementia or mixed vascular-Alzheimer's dementia is higher (99, 100). It is challenging to diagnose or differentially diagnose depression in dementia especially at intermediate to late stage of the disease because (1) the patients often lose the language ability needed to express their depressed mood or sadness; (2) depression often coexists with other neuropsychiatric symptoms including apathy, agitation, aggression, and psychosis. The CSDD (101) and the Neuropsychiatric Inventory (NPI), based on the information from the caregivers, are helpful to evaluate depression in dementia for both clinical practice and drug trials. The National Institute of Mental Health has devised provisional criteria for the diagnosis of depression in patients with Alzheimer's disease from the DSM-IV-TR (98). The significant differences include the requirement of fewer symptoms for the diagnosis (3 or more vs. 5 or more), less pervasiveness of symptoms, and the presence of irritability and social withdrawal or isolation. The association between depression and cognitive decline is most evident during the intermediate (limbic) stages of AD pathology.

Depression and Cognitive Decline

It is only in the past few years that we have begun looking at the interplay of depression and cognitive decline. Prior to this, studies of depression in the elderly excluded those with cognitive impairment or inadequately assessed cognitive status. At the same time, studies on cognitive impairment in the elderly excluded or failed to adequately assess those with depression. But current research is being driven by the fact that both cognitive and affective symptoms commonly occur in the elderly. A number of published studies are beginning to open our understanding to this critically important area in geriatric psychiatry (102).

Clarifying the terms "depression" and cognitive impairment" is a matter of debate. For example, major depression, as defined in the DSM as a symptom cluster, may miss subtypes of depression quite commonly noted in geriatric psychiatry—depression which is subsyndromal or in which the patient denies sadness. There is even more lack of clarity around the issue of cognitive impairment, and how to define the gray zone between normal cognitive function and dementia. Most researchers now refer to this as MCI, although other terms are also used. There is no precise definition of MCI as yet or standardized assessment. MCI is used to refer to a primarily amnestic disorder, with or without other cognitive domain impairment—presumably a precursor to Alzheimer's—as well as to a non-amnestic disorder characterized by other cognitive domain deficits (language, executive function, visuo-spatial skill), which may progress to non-Alzheimer's types of dementias (102).

Much of the current research revolves around the association of depression with MCI, and to what extent this level of cognitive impairment is predictive of further decline. The Cardiovascular Health Study reported a cumulative prevalence of 26% for depression among individuals with MCI (35) and it has been found that the combination of depression and impaired cognition doubles every 5 years (103). Much evidence suggests that late-onset depression can be a prodrome of cognitive decline (22, 26, 104–107) but other studies dispute this (39). Another study looking at the Cardiovascular Health Study results found that depression symptoms were associated with increased risk of MCI, but this association was independent of underlying vascular disease (108).

Treatment of depression in the setting of MCI or dementia is still under investigation. Most studies show that patients with executive dysfunction are particularly difficult to treat. In particular, poor scores on neuropsychological testing with Trails B, card-sorting perseveration, and errors in the Controlled Oral Work Association Test and Animal Naming predicted a poor outcome on treatment of depression (109, 110). In another study, abnormal initiation/perseveration scores and abnormal Stroop Color-Word scores predicted an unfavorable response in elderly to citalopram treatment (111). Other studies have shown that in elderly with depression and MCI, the cognitive deficits persist even if the depression is successfully treated (112, 113). As yet, there is no consensus as to what antidepressants are preferable in patients with depression and cognitive impairment.

Grief with Depression and Complicated Grief in the Elderly

There are approximately 2.4 million deaths in the United States each year, and the large majority of the deceased are older persons suffering from chronic diseases. As a result, a typical death is preceded by an extended period of time during which one or more family members, most often their spouses, provide health and support services to their disabled relative (114). Additionally, old people often lose their friends and/or neighbors, who are also old, resulting in deteriorating social support. Despite the generally positive prognosis for most bereaved, old caregivers after the death of a loved one, approximately 10–15% of people experience chronic depression (115). Another study has found that 30% of caregivers of people with dementia are at risk for clinical depression 1 year post-death, and 20% experience complicated grief (116, 117). Complicated grief is defined by (1) an intense longing and yearning for the person who died; (2) recurrent intrusive and distressing thoughts about the absence of the deceased; (3) making it difficult to concentrate and move beyond an acute state of mourning; (4) making it difficult to form other interpersonal relationships, and engage in potentially rewarding activities for 6 months or longer. Complicated grief is distinct from both depression and normal grief reactions (118), but often occurs along with other disorders such as major depression and post-traumatic stress disorder (PTSD) and is associated with suicidality and self-destructive behaviors (119).

Psychotic Depression

Psychotic depression is a variant of major depression, characterized by paranoia, delusions, or hallucinations in addition to meeting criteria for major depression. Diagnosis can be difficult as it is often challenging to distinguish between dementia with depression and psychosis. Fortunately, the treatment is often the same for both conditions, using an antidepressant concurrently with an antipsychotic medication. Electroconvulsive therapy (ECT) is an alternative effective treatment (see also Chap. 4 for a discussion on the pharmacotherapy of psychotic depression).

Suicidality

Suicidality is of particular concern in the elderly, who have the highest risk of any population group. The rate is almost twice that of the general population, and even higher in white males over 65. In the elderly, suicidal ideation is almost always associated with depression. Over 75% of those who committed suicide saw a primary care physician within a month of their death, demonstrating the need for better diagnosis and aggressive treatment (120). A widely used screening tool for assessing suicidal ideation is Beck's Scale for Suicide Ideation (SSI) (121). A more recent tool, the Geriatric Suicide Ideation Scale (GSIS), also appears to be a useful indicator of late-life suicide risk (122). There are four subscales: suicide ideation, death ideation, loss of personal and social worth, and perceived meaning in life. Each subscale can be used in a stand-alone assessment, whether for evaluation of suicidality or psychological resilience.

Much has been heard in the media about studies suggesting that antidepressant therapy is associated with an increase in suicide attempts, particularly in the child/adolescent and young adult populations. Two recent large studies of adult population suggest otherwise. In one, 131,788 patients were evaluated for suicide attempts 90 days before and 180 days after starting antidepressant treatment, in primary care, psychiatric care, or psychotherapeutic care. The pattern of suicide attempts was the same in all three treatment groups: the highest rate of attempts was in the month before starting treatment, the next highest in the month after starting treatment, and the rate declining thereafter (123). It is interesting to note that the treatment group with the highest numbers of suicide attempts was in the psychiatric treatment group, raising the question of whether that group represented a higher level of psychopathology. In another study in the Veteran's Administration system, data on 226,866 veterans were analyzed, all of whom had received a diagnosis of depression in 2003 or 2004, who had received at least a 6-month follow-up, and none who had no history of depression from 2000 to 2002. Results showed that suicide attempts declined among all patients treated with antidepressants, with the best results for patients on SSRIs. In the age group >65 years old, the rate of suicide attempts was 66/100,000 for those not on antidepressant and 25/100,000 for those on antidepressant (124). However, the question as to the role of antidepressants in suicidal patients is not resolved, as a study in 2006 looking at the risk of suicide using SSRIs in the elderly concludes that "suicides of a violent nature were distinctly more common during SSRI therapy" (125). The study included 1.2 million Ontario residents with 1,329 suicides from 1992 to 2000. They conclude a fivefold higher risk during the first month on antidepressant treatment. Because the absolute risk is low, they postulate an idiosyncratic response in a vulnerable subgroup of patients.

Depression with Concurrent Substance Abuse

Depression with concurrent substance abuse is a complicated comorbid condition ("dual diagnosis"). Substance abuse by itself can cause depression and, conversely, depression can lead to substance abuse. It is this bidirectional relationship that can make diagnosis and treatment difficult. Community-based surveys indicate that the prevalence of alcohol use disorders in the elderly depressed population is 3–4 times greater than in the nondepressed elderly. In the National Comorbidity Study, the most common concurrent psychiatric conditions for major depression included alcohol dependence and anxiety disorders (126). A past history of major depressive disorder in individuals 65 years or older is associated with a prevalence of alcohol use disorder of 13.3% compared with 4.5 % in the elderly without a past history of major depressive disorder (127). In clinically depressed samples, the comorbidity is even higher with 15–30% of depressed patients also having an alcohol use disorder (128, 129). Typically, there is a less family history density of alcoholism in elderly patients with late-onset than in patients with early onset of substance abuse. Some but not all studies show a worse prognosis for elderly depressed patients who are also diagnosed with an alcohol use disorder (129, 130). An intriguing study by Oslin looked at treating older outpatients with alcohol dependence and depression with simultaneous naltrexone and sertraline, plus weekly psychosocial support. All patients received 100 mg sertraline/day, and either naltrexone or placebo for 12 weeks. Results showed that 42% of the subjects had a remission of their depression with no drinking relapse during the trial. There was no evidence for benefit of naltrexone, but there was a significant association between relapse of drinking and poor response to depression treatment (131).

As a society we tend to not suspect our elderly of substance abuse or dependence excuse them for "nipping at the bottle" or needing a benzodiazepine to "steady their nerves". This may lead us to miss an underlying cause for a patient's mood disorder. Therefore, substance abuse screening should be a routine part of any depression workup. The usual screening tools such as the CAGE questions can be applied, and information from family members or caretakers can also be invaluable.

Depression with Anxiety

In a sample of psychiatric and primary care elderly, 23% of patients with major depression were diagnosed with an anxiety disorder at the time of interview and 35% met criteria for lifetime anxiety disorder (132). Using less rigorous criteria, 50% of 336 elderly patients with major depression had symptoms of anxiety based on rating scales; however, only 2.5% met DSM-III-R criteria for any anxiety disorder (133). The latter study has been criticized for excluding generalized anxiety disorder, which is believed to have a high prevalence in the geriatric population (134); however, other evidence supports low rates of anxiety disorders in elderly depressed patients (135–137). Comorbid anxiety disorders do not seem to diminish treatment response to antidepressants in the elderly (138), although there are few studies examining this issue. One study assessing comorbidity of lifetime anxiety and depression in elderly patients found that each disorder followed its own course, and often occurred at different times. Generalized anxiety disorder tended to be chronic (years to decades long) and typically preceded major depressive disorder in this elderly population. The authors concluded that GAD is a disorder distinct from MDD (139).

Comorbidity Depression and Personality Disorders

Kunik and associates (140) reported that 24% of a series of elderly depressed inpatients had comorbid personality disorders, mainly in the Cluster C category (avoidant, dependent, obsessive-compulsive, passive-aggressive). Devanand and associates (141) reported on a series of 76 elderly patients and found that 31.2% had concurrent personality disorders (obsessive-compulsive, 17.1%; avoidant, 11.8%;

borderline, 5.3%; narcissistic, 2.6%; and schizoid, 2.6%, and no antisocial or histrionic personality disorders). Personality disorders are associated with an earlier age of onset of depression (127) and a history of recurrent depressive episodes (142). Some studies suggest a poorer prognosis for patients with major depression and personality disorders compared to major depression alone (143, 144). Regarding the treatment of Cluster C comorbidity with depression in the elderly, Morse et al. found that such patients had a slower response to antidepressant therapy in the acute phase, and non-response to treatment in the continuation or maintenance phase (145). In addition, there was noted an inclination towards a decline in instrumental activities of daily living (IADL) in patients in maintenance therapy. Others have found a poor response to psychotherapy (146), but a recent study using dialectical behavioral therapy (DBT) in elders shows some positive effect (147).

Depression and Medical Illness

Comorbidity of depression and medical illness likewise presents a diagnostic challenge, because the criteria used in psychiatry for diagnosing depression rely on physical symptoms common to both depression and feeling ill. For example, even though the DSM-IV specifies not including "symptoms that are clearly due to a medical condition", criteria for major depression include significant weight loss and fatigue or loss of energy. There have been four major approaches proposed to differentiate psychiatric from medical symptoms (52, 148, 149):

1. Inclusive approach: Consider all depressive symptoms, somatic or psychological, as evidence of a mood disorder. For example: in a patient with anemia, a complaint of "poor energy" would be considered a depressive symptom. If there are enough symptoms to meet criteria for depression, the diagnosis is made. The problem with this approach is its over-inclusiveness that can result in poor specificity.
2. Exclusive approach: Physical or medical symptoms are not considered symptoms of a depressive disorder. In the same patient as above, "poor energy" would not contribute to a diagnosis of depression. The problem with this approach is its over-exclusiveness, leading to poor sensitivity.
3. Substitutive approach: Physical symptoms are "translated" into psychological symptoms. For example, back pain is equivalent to hopelessness. If there are enough resulting psychiatric equivalents, a diagnosis of depression can be made. The problem with this approach is that there is no evidence to establish the validity of the concept of "psychological equivalents."
4. Etiological approach: The clinician evaluates each symptom independently and makes a subjective determination whether it is related to depression or medical illness. The problem with this approach is that it relies on decisions that are not evidence based and has poor inter-rater reliability.

Other approaches to sorting out depression from medical illness have included combinations of the above approaches, use of the Hospital Anxiety and Depression Scale, use of the shortened version of the GDS, and even one study which concluded that a one-item question ("are you depressed?") was the most sensitive and specific tool. The conundrum in finding the best diagnostic method is that there is no gold standard by which to compare results, and further epidemiological research is needed. Given the tolerability and safety profile of today's antidepressants, it may be best to initiate pharmacotherapy when depression is suspected. Fortunately, a recent study suggests that elderly with comorbid medical illness are responsive to antidepressant therapy. 195 patients 70 years or older with depression were treated with proxetine and weekly interpersonal psychotherapy. Those who did not achieve sustained recovery were augmented with buproprion, nortriptyline, or lithium. Those with a high medical burden (as measured by the Cumulative Illness Rating Scale) showed a slower treatment response, but the final results were similar to the augmentation phase of the STAR*D in younger adults. It also demonstrated the value of augmentation in the elderly in that they were able to tolerate the addition of medication (150).

The issue of pain is important, as this is an issue endemic to the elderly with depression and medical illness. Pain can complicate the treatment of depression, but study results do not agree as to whether pain interferes with successful treatment of depression. One study by Karp et al. used paroxetine and interpersonal psychotherapy in patients over 68 with depression ($n=187$) and pain, measured with the Bodily Pain Index. Overall response rate was 75% in terms of depression, with non-responders reporting more pain at baseline. Body pain remained stable, independent of lessened depression (151). However, in another study by the same author looking at younger adults aged 21–65, the conclusion was that pain predicted a longer time to remission and may be a marker of a more difficult-to-treat depression (152). A larger VA study ($n=524$) looking at depressed patients aged 60 and older investigated (1) pain severity and (2) the degree to which pain interfered with work inside and outside of the home. They found that both pain and pain's interference with functioning have an impact on recovery from depression, with pain interference having a larger effect (153). Treatment of pain and depression have traditionally been treated with tricyclic medication, but with the arrival of SNRIs (duloxetine and venlafaxine) there has been renewed interest in the subject. Some studies have found favorable results for both (154–157).

Treatment of Geriatric Depression

Pharmacological Treatment Issues

The elderly face barriers in obtaining effective pharmacological treatment for depression. Most clinical trials of antidepressants are conducted in younger patients, and clinicians must therefore extrapolate results in order to treat the elderly. The aged often have serious comorbid medical conditions, which can complicate the treatment, and they are already on polypharmacy, in many cases. Older adults metabolize medications more slowly and are more susceptible to side effects.

However, as a group, they experience both low rates and low intensity of treatment. Antidepressants are often prescribed in subtherapeutic doses, and many geriatric patients simply stop taking their medications (16, 158). One study looked at what predicted adherence among the elderly to taking antidepressant medication. They noted that perceived social support had been positively linked to medication adherence in several non-psychiatric conditions; in prior studies of depression, social support had been associated with less time to remission and reduced risk of institutionalization. They noted that adherence may also be associated with beliefs about the controllability of health, and that meta-analysis has linked perceptions of lack of control over health to depression. They found that elderly who believe they have control over their health also benefited from social and non-family support, and predicted greater adherence to medication 1 year later (159). Another study looked at caretaker attitudes toward their elderly patients. If the caretaker attributed depression in the patient to cognitive or attitude problems, it predicted decreased adherence in the patient; conversely, caretakers who attributed the depression to medical or biological causes predicted increased adherence to antidepressant medication in the patient. This reveals the importance of the social environment of the patient in treatment outcome, and also the need to educate and involve caretakers in treatment planning (160).

Despite these challenges, the elderly have been prescribed antidepressants in greatly increased numbers in the last 10 years, particularly the SSRIs (161, 162). Reasons for geriatric patients being prescribed antidepressants has shifted somewhat, with antidepressant use predicted strongly by low positive affect scores, poor health status, and somatic complaints, as well as by prior antidepressant use and white race (162). Antidepressant products are being formulated to make adherence easier among the elderly. Now, there are extended release versions for once-daily and once-weekly administration, orally disintegrating tablets, and transdermal systems (163). These difficulties may be related to a relative lack of clear guidance in what the most effective treatments are for this population; the studies are relatively few, and there are many problems in conducting such studies as well as problems associated with measuring the outcome of interventions. Despite this, it is clear that treatment of depression is effective for the majority of patients.

When elderly patients present with persistent sad moods, diagnosis is rarely difficult; however, mood disorders also present solely with anxiety, impaired cognitive function, medical symptoms, decreased activity, social isolation, or reduced motivation. Overemphasis on depressed mood results in a failure to recognize treatable depression in the elderly (84).

Relatively few large efficacy studies have been done on elderly patients, but one looked at patients from 18 primary care clinics with DSM-IV diagnosable major depression and their response to usual treatment. 40% of patients showed significant symptom resolution over the 12- to 24-month observation period, and higher initial severity was predictive of improvement (164). Although there was apparently no augmentation or further treatment phases, these results are similar to STAR*D results in the citalopram (first) phase, and suggest that the treatability of geriatric depression is on a par with younger adults. A study by Reynolds' group looked at the response rate in treatment-resistant elderly patients—those with at least one adequate antidepressant trial—and found a 67% response rate using paroxetine, with augmentation by other medication if needed, and interpersonal therapy. They noted that the treatment-resistant group may require a longer period of treatment (165). A Cochrane meta-analysis of overall efficacy of antidepressants in the elderly versus placebo led to the conclusion that "TCAs, SSRIs, and MAOIs are effective in the treatment of older community patients and inpatients and at least 6 weeks of antidepressant treatment is recommended to achieve optimal therapeutic effect" (166).

There also may be clinical relevance to subtyping late-life depression. An interesting study done in a group of oldest-old nursing home patients (50 patients with mean age of 89) compared antidepressant response to fluoxetine, sertraline, and paroxetine. At 12 weeks, there was a significant overall decline in HAM-D scores and 42% had at least a 50% decline in their scores. There was no difference in efficacy between the three medications. However, it was noted that among the 50 patients, there were four kinds of depression (major depression, Alzheimer's plus depression, vascular depression, and CNS-related disorders with depression) that responded quite differently. The drop in response rate between those with "simple" major depression versus those with cognitive impairments with perhaps an underlying vascular etiology has been shown in other studies as well. The challenge clearly is to find effective treatments for diagnostic subgroups (167).

Physiology of Aging

The physiology of aging is an important consideration in prescribing psychotropic medications. There are a number of well-documented changes and potential changes involving three interrelated areas of physiologic function: homeostasis, pharmacokinetics, and pharmacodynamics (168–171).

Human beings have a reserve physiological capacity to deal with stress or acute events; this reserve capacity diminishes with age. If an individual is faced with a physiological stress that is beyond reserve capacity, there is a decompensation of the involved organ system(s). Therefore, even a minor stressor can result in the downward cascade of events referred to earlier in this chapter. Particularly, vulnerable organ systems in the elderly involve cardiovascular, central nervous system, and musculoskeletal systems. Examples of homeostatic impairments include orthostatic hypotension and other autonomic nervous system dysregulation (e.g., temperature regulation), cognitive decompensation (e.g., confusion, disorientation), bowel and bladder function, and ambulatory stability (172).

Pharmacokinetics

Pharmacokinetics, the action of a drug in the body over time, changes with age (173, 174). Specifically, the subcategories of absorption, distribution, metabolism, and excretion each have well-known age-associated changes. Individuals, however, age differently and so do organ systems in a given individual. In addition, normal aging and "pathological aging" may be difficult to distinguish.

Absorption is the pharmacokinetic function, which seems least affected by age. Despite increased gastric pH, decreased gastrointestinal blood flow, and decreased gastric motility, it appears that the bioavailability of most antidepressants does not meaningfully change (175). Medications that require active transport may be more poorly absorbed. Also, first-pass metabolism is decreased in aging, causing overall higher serum levels for drugs such as morphine and propranolol (176).

Distribution of medication in the body depends on body composition. In the elderly, there is an increase in body fat and a relative decline in lean body mass and total body water. This means that water-soluble drugs such as lithium may have a decreased volume of distribution with an increase in plasma concentration. Lipophilic drugs such as benzodiazepines may have an increase in volume of distribution but also have a longer elimination half-life (177). Distribution is also a function of plasma protein binding, particularly albumin and α_1-acid glycoprotein (178). Serum concentrations of the drug can be altered by changes in the level of these proteins, thereby altering the bound/free ratio. The clinical relevance of increased free nortriptyline in the elderly is unknown (179). Plasma protein binding alterations in aging are not thought to be as clinically important as declining hepatic or renal function or decreased cardiac output (180).

Hepatic metabolism of antidepressants may be decreased in the elderly as a consequence of reduced liver blood flow and decreased activity of the cytochrome P450 oxidative enzymes. CYP2D6 appears to be less affected by aging than CYP2C19 and CYP3A4 (181). Antipyrine clearance, a general marker of oxidative metabolism, declines with age. Cytochrome P450 content from biopsied livers showed decreased content in samples from patients 40–49 years old, compared to those 20–39 years old, but was similar to those from subjects 50–69; only in samples from subjects over 70 years old was the cytochrome P450 content lowered further (182).

With respect to specific isoenzymes, there are few data comparing in vitro models and human pharmacokinetics using known substrates. Probes for 1A2 and 3A4 indicate impaired function in aging (183, 184). Substrate challenges of 1A2 using caffeine and theophylline have demonstrated decreased clearance in the elderly (168). Metabolism of debrisoquine, a 2D6 substrate, was not altered by aging, in other studies (185, 186). Both age- and gender-related differences have been found with CYP3A4 substrates. Aging reduces clearance of erythromycin (187), nifedipine (188), and nefazodone (189).

Excretion by the kidneys is the primary site of elimination for many drugs. The glomerular filtration rate is thought to decline with age, although many elderly do not show such a decline. Medications such as lithium are dependent upon renal function, and serum levels—critical in lithium—can be affected by it (190). Alterations in renal function may lead to higher levels of hydroxy metabolites of nortriptyline, desipramine, and imipramine, which are potentially cardiotoxic (191, 192).

Determination of age-related changes in the pharmacokinetics of antidepressants relies on animal experiments, in vitro modeling, and direct drug administration to humans. von Moltke and colleagues (169) have reviewed the data for older antidepressants, emphasizing a lack of consistency in the data, most likely the result of large interindividual variation in TCA metabolism, study designs that did not use appropriate control groups, and a failure to distinguish clinical importance from statistical significance. Despite these shortcomings, they concluded that there was evidence to support reduced clearance of amitriptyline and imipramine in the elderly, but desipramine clearance was not significantly affected (175). Nortriptyline clearance does not seem to be altered, except in the presence of medical illness. TCA hydroxy metabolites are likely to accumulate in elderly patients who have reduced renal function. Trazodone clearance may also be decreased in the elderly (175).

Several pharmacokinetic studies of SSRIs in the elderly have been published. Clearance of citalopram is reduced in subjects over the age of 60 years, resulting in higher steady-state concentrations and prolonged elimination half-life (193, 194). Initial doses of citalopram in elderly are half those of younger individuals. Escitalopram area-under-the-curve and elimination half-life are increased by approximately 50% of patients 65 years or older; the initial dose should be reduced to 10 mg in these patients. In a study of 22 healthy volunteers, sertraline and desmethylsertraline plasma levels were similar in elderly men and both elderly and young women, all groups having mean concentrations about 25% higher than young men (195). These differences are unlikely to be clinically meaningful.

Studies of paroxetine have examined doses ranging from 20 to 40 mg in elderly and non-elderly patients (196–199). The two clinically important findings from these studies are that the elderly have 40% higher mean steady-state plasma concentrations than younger patients, and older patients may be more sensitive to the nonlinear kinetics of paroxetine resulting in disproportionate plasma level increases in response to dose escalation. Many clinicians begin paroxetine at doses of 10 mg daily in the elderly, rather than the usual initial dose of 20 mg.

Data on fluvoxamine are contradictory: one study showed only an insignificant increase in elimination half-life in the elderly (mean 25 vs. 22 h in young adults) (200). When the drug was still under its patent in the U.S., Solvay Pharmaceuticals reported in its product information (2002) that single dose studies of 50 mg and 100 mg in elderly (66–73 years old) and young subjects (19–35 years old) showed C_{max} values 50% higher in the elderly. Multiple dose elimination half-life was 17.4 and 25.9 h in the elderly compared to 13.6 and 15.6 h in young adults at steady state for the 50 and 100 mg dose, respectively. Clearance may be reduced by 50% in the elderly.

In a study of fluoxetine, a single 40 mg dose given to patients between 65 and 77 years old found no clinically significant differences in pharmacokinetics compared to younger patients (181). A study of adults 60 years old or greater found that 20 mg of fluoxetine for 6 weeks produced steady-state levels of fluoxetine and norfluoxetine of 209.3 ng/ml, which is comparable to the levels produced in younger adults and adolescents (201).

In a comparison of a single 50 mg dose of venlafaxine followed by 5 days of 50 mg every 8 h in elderly (60–80 years old) and young (21–44 years old), pharmacokinetic differences were not found after the single dose and only modest increases in steady-state concentrations after chronic dosing were found in the elderly, making it unlikely that dosage reduction based on pharmacokinetic factors alone would be necessary for most elderly depressed patients (202).

A small study of bupropion suggests that dosage reductions should be made in the elderly (203). Elevated plasma levels of bupropion and its metabolites suggest dosage reductions of 25–50% may be necessary. Even more significant pharmacokinetic changes in the elderly have been reported for nefazodone (189) and most clinicians begin treatment with half or less of the usual starting dose for younger adults. Mirtazapine clearance was reduced by 40% in elderly men compared to younger men after 20 mg daily doses for 7 days, but was reduced by only 10% when elderly and young women were compared.

Pharmacodynamics

Pharmacodynamics–the response of the body to a drug acting at a particular site–is altered in the elderly where there can be a heightened response or "sensitivity" to a given drug (173). Benzodiazepines are a good example of this, and there is evidence that the elderly are sensitive to the central nervous system effect of this class of drugs (177, 204–206) as well as to opiates (207). Conversely, the elderly exhibit a reduced response to other medications used in psychiatry such as β-adrenergic antagonists (190).

Altered sensitivity can lead to adverse effects, independent of increased plasma levels. Several reviews have summarized the common adverse effects of antidepressants, which may be the consequence of altered metabolism, receptor function, or signal transduction mechanisms (16, 172, 208–210).

Anticholinergic Adverse Effects

Elderly patients often take other prescribed and over-the-counter medications that have anticholinergic activity; clinicians should be aware of potential drug–drug interactions. Older individuals are more sensitive to the anticholinergic effects of TCAs, and even low doses may produce urinary retention, severe constipation, xerostomia, glaucoma, and tachycardia. More severe anticholinergic effects can include mild confusion, memory impairment, worsening of depression, and delirium. The lack of muscarinic effects makes SSRIs and some of the newer mixed action agents more appropriate as first-line agents in depressed elderly individuals. Among the SSRIs, only paroxetine has substantial anticholinergic activity; however, in vitro studies suggest a greater effect than is seen clinically. Using sera from patients (60–95 years old) treated with either nortriptyline (plasma level 100 ng/ml) or paroxetine (20–30 mg daily), the latter drug had only one-fifth the anticholinergic activity of nortriptyline (211). Also, a study by Salzman and colleagues in patients 80 years or older found no adverse effects with paroxetine (16). On the other hand, their more recent 8-week double-blind placebo-controlled study of nursing home patients, which compared paroxetine and placebo (212), found that of the study's 24 patients (mean age of 87.9 years), two subjects in the paroxetine group experienced delirium, and the paroxetine subjects also had lower MMS scores. Subjects with higher HAM-D-17 and CSDD scores of the paroxetine group experienced greater improvement than placebo subjects on the Clinical Global Impression of Change (CGI-C) scale, an interview-based outcome measure. In contrast to other studies, they found no clinically significant differences in serum anticholinergic activity between the paroxetine and placebo groups. Therefore, if cognitive impairment does occur in elderly patients treated with paroxetine, a relationship to anticholinergic effect has not been unequivocally established.

Cardiovascular Effects

As discussed in Chap. 2, cardiovascular mortality is increased in depression (213–215). There are few studies specifically addressing the association in the elderly. The relationship of depression and heart failure was studied in 2,501 individuals 65 years or older living in the community and free of heart failure at baseline (216). During a 14-year follow-up, depression in women, but not men, was associated with a greater risk of heart failure. Between 11 and 19% of the elderly living in the community reported depressive symptoms above the cutoff on the Center for Epidemiological Studies Depression Scale (217–220). In a cohort study of antihypertensive treatment, increases in depression over time, but not baseline depression scores, were predictive of stroke and myocardial infarction (MI) in the individuals 60 years old or greater (221). The Cardiovascular Health Study prospectively examined the relationship between depressive symptoms and coronary heart disease in 4,493 Americans 65 years of age or older who were free of cardiovascular disease at baseline (222). Depression was an independent risk factor for cardiovascular disease and mortality, with the more severe the depressive symptoms, the greater the risk. Similar findings were reported by Pratt and associates (215) for the general population over 18 years old—the odds ratio for MI associated with dysphoria was 2.07 (CI, 1.16–3.71) and 4.54 (95 CI, 1.65–12.44) with major depression. Given these findings, the role of antidepressant pharmacotherapy in older patients has substantial public health implications.

We are unaware of strong evidence to suggest that intervention with antidepressants or psychological treatments reduces coronary risk in the elderly with depression; however, there is a growing body of literature that supports their safety, even in patients with cardiovascular disease. In the general population, mortality rates are lower in depressed individuals who have adequate treatment of depression (223). Furthermore, preliminary data in adult smokers 30–65 years old who were hospitalized with a first MI found a lower recurrence of MI in patients treated with SSRIs than those who did not receive an SSRI (224); however, SSRIs may not confer the same benefit on individuals without a prior MI (225). In a study of the effects of treating depression after a recent MI in 2,481 patients (mean age 61 years old), antidepressant treatment was associated with a lower risk for death or nonfatal MI compared to those subjects who did not receive antidepressant treatment, although differences in depression scores were small and of questionable clinical significance (226). Potential cardioprotective biological effects of SSRIs, such as blockade of platelet serotonin receptors, complicate interpretation of these findings.

Early concerns about the cardiac effects of TCAs were raised in a report by Rodstein and Oei (227), who described 32 geriatric patients, 10 of whom received amitriptyline (20–75 mg daily for a mean 53 weeks), and 21 of whom received imipramine (20–100 mg for a mean 40 weeks), and 1 of whom received two 10 mg doses of nortriptyline. Inversion of T waves and "evidence of acute coronary insufficiency" were noted in two patients on amitriptyline. With imipramine, intermittent left bundle branch block, acute coronary insufficiency with node dysfunction, T wave inversion, and tachycardia were reported. The single patient taking nortriptyline had an acute MI after two 10 mg doses. Current opinion is that the TCAs present the greatest risk in patients with an ischemic myocardium, a conclusion inferred from the Cardiac Arrhythmia Suppression Trials discussed in Chap. 2. In the presence of myocardial ischemia, the TCAs and other Class 1A antiarrhythmics have pro-arrhythmic properties. Several studies now confirm that SSRIs, including fluoxetine (228, 229), sertraline (230), paroxetine (16, 149, 231–233), and citalopram (234) have greater cardiac safety than TCAs. Similarly, cardiac profiles of bupropion, venlafaxine, and mirtazapine are superior to TCAs, although venlafaxine is associated with hypertension in a dose-related fashion. Autonomic dysfunction, evidenced by decreased heart rate variability, may be greater in depression (235) and anticholinergic antidepressants (such as TCAs) may present greater risk of adverse cardiac events (236). Venlafaxine has undergone more scrutiny recently for its possible cardiac effects. It has been known that venlafaxine can increase blood pressure, but a recent study raises further concerns about its potential cardiac effects. In a study of 62 depressed elderly started on venlafaxine, 24% of initially normotensive patients and 54% of those with pre-existing hypertension experienced an increase in blood pressure. 29% developed orthostatic hypertension, and others developed an increase in QTc interval, dizziness, new-onset tachycardia, or palpitations. The study concluded that, overall, venlafaxine XR was well tolerated, but was associated with cardiovascular side effects in some patients, recommending systematic monitoring of patients on this medication (237).

Orthostatic Hypotension and Falls

Experienced clinicians have long been aware of the risks of orthostatic hypotension with TCAs and MAOIs. As described in Chap. 2, this is most likely a consequence of α-adrenergic blocking activity. Among the TCAs, nortritpyline is least likely to produce this adverse effect. One of the most surprising findings from SSRI research in the elderly is that SSRI are also associated with falls and fractures. In one study of 8,127 elderly women living in the community followed for an average of 4.8 years, 15% experienced a nonspine fracture, including 4% with a first hip fracture (207). Women taking narcotics and antidepressants had the greatest risk of any nonspine fracture. Women taking SSRIs and TCAs had a 1.7-fold risk for hip fracture. There was not an independent association with use of a benzodiazepine or anticonvulsant and hip fracture. Other studies have also found an increased risk of falls with SSRIs, especially when therapy is initiated; some evidence suggests that tolerance to this adverse effect develops (238–240). Studies of body sway with sertraline and paroxetine do not clarify the underlying mechanism of SSRI-associated falls (241). In a study of 104 individuals 69 years or older who were given paroxetine, psychotherapy, and augmentation therapy (with bupropion, nortriptyline, or lithium), 38% of subjects fell, of whom about half fell within the first 6 weeks of treatment (242). Memory impairment and orthostatic hypotension were risk factors for falls.

Other Adverse Effects

Recent reports have highlighted the possibility of loss of bone mineral density in persons receiving SSRIs. In two separate studies, bone density loss was demonstrated in both men and women taking SSRIs, an effect not seen in patients on tricyclic antidepressants. In women, bone mineral density declined 0.82% yearly in the hips of users compared with a decline of 0.47% in non-users (243). In the study of elderly men, those taking SSRIs had, on average, 3.9% lower density at the hip and 5.9% lower density at the lumbar spine compared with men not taking antidepressant (244). Not surprisingly, there have been reports of older patients on SSRIs with a twofold increased risk of incident clinical fracture (245). While these are relatively new reports, and it is unclear how this might influence prescribing, it may be that the SSRIs are not quite as benign as previously thought. Certainly, thought should be given to prescribing a patient an SSRI who already has bone density issues (246).

There are other adverse effects that have been reported as single cases or case series. Although the frequency of these adverse effects cannot be determined from available studies, it is our experience that they do appear more commonly, albeit still infrequently, in the elderly. Extrapyramidal symptoms associated with the SSRI have been reported, and appear to be related to reduced dopaminergic tone in aging and the effects of serotonin on dopamine activity. We believe that all SSRI can produce EPS in susceptible individuals, and that the increased number of reports with fluoxetine is related to greater clinical experience. To put this risk in perspective, Coulter and Pillans (247) reviewed 5,555 patients treated with fluoxetine, and found 15 cases of EPS, only 7 of which involved fluoxetine as the sole psychotropic. Some have suggested lower incidence of EPS with sertraline, citing its weak dopamine reuptake inhibiting activity; however, there have been reports of EPS with that drug as well (248–250).

The syndrome of inappropriate antidiuretic hormone secretion (SIADH) is an infrequent but serious adverse effect of antidepressant therapy that is more common in the elderly. Liu and colleagues (251) reviewed the published and unpublished data (1980–1995) on SIADH with fluoxetine, fluvoxamine, paroxetine, and sertraline.

They found a total of 736 cases, 75.3% with fluoxetine, 12.4% with paroxetine, 11.7% with sertraline, and 1.5% with fluvoxamine. Although most reports involved fluoxetine, this finding is most likely an artifact of its greater clinical use. The median time to onset of hyponatremia was 13 days (range 3–120 days). There are reports of SIADH with citalopram (252, 253), fluvoxamine (254–256), paroxetine (256–259), sertraline (260–262), and venlafaxine (257, 263), as well as TCAs (264–271) and MAOIs (272). Although the exact mechanism of this adverse effect is unknown, clinicians should be vigilant for sodium changes, especially early in treatment. Lethargy, disorientation, and muscle cramps are early signs of hyponatremia, with delirium and coma possible in late stages (172). Management involves discontinuation of the offending agent, fluid restriction, and in severe cases administration of hypertonic saline. When the condition has cleared, an alternative antidepressant may be started; however, there have been reports of recurrences. In severe depressions, clinicians should consider ECT.

The elderly may be more sensitive to other adverse effects that younger people are able to tolerate. Bupropion, for example, may be more likely to cause agitation in the elderly, and lower than usual doses of venlafaxine may cause blood pressure elevations. Sedative effects of antidepressants are also enhanced in the elderly. The serotonin syndrome has also been reported in elderly on monotherapy with mirtazapine (273, 274) and in combination with fluoxetine (275), as well as with the combination of paroxetine and risperidone (276).

Treatment of Major Depression

Several reviews have now reached the conclusion that first-line antidepressant agents for geriatric major depression are the SSRIs (208, 277, 278). A 2006 Cochrane Database meta-review of 32 clinical trials looked at the efficacy of antidepressant classes. The review was unable to find any differences in efficacy when comparing classes of antidepressants, but it was noted that TCAs compared less favorably with SSRIs in terms of numbers of patients withdrawn from the trials due to side effects (279).

Virtually all available SSRIs have been compared to TCAs or mixed action agents and most have found equivalent efficacy, with fewer adverse effects than tertiary amine TCAs (280).

Very little has been specifically researched about augmentation of antidepressant in the elderly, while recently there have been some significant studies of younger adult depression treatment strategies, for example the augmentation strategies in the STAR*D trials. One study targeted this issue in the aged (70 or older, $n = 195$) and found that augmentation was required for 105 patients (53%) because of inadequate initial treatment (paroxetine, 10–40 mg) response or relapse. Of those who went on augmentation therapy (sustained release buproprion, nortriptyline, or lithium), the response rate was 50%, and the response time was slower, with modestly more side effects; greater medical burden and anxiety predicted slower recovery (150).

SSRIs

All SSRIs are effective for treating late-life depression. There are minor variations in side effects which may recommend one medication over another (e.g., paroxetine is more sedating and fluoxetine is more stimulating) which may influence choice of medication. At times, these side effects may be significant. For example, elderly depressed patients who were also medically ill lost more than 5% of body weight when treated with fluoxetine (as compared with tricyclic treatment in which no weight was lost) (281). Some SSRIs also strongly inhibit hepatic-metabolizing enzymes which may affect blood levels of other medications. Since elderly individuals are likely to be taking several drugs concurrently, an SSRI such as citalopram which does not influence hepatic enzymes can be selected for treatment. A large study looking at sleep effects of SSRIs in women over 70 years old found that those on SSRI medication had a greater likelihood of sleep disturbances, including poorer sleep efficiency, longer sleep latency, and sleep fragmentation (282). Another study looked at the phenomenon of apathy among 384 elderly taking SSRI medication. They found that although depression was improved in these patients, apathy appeared to be greater in those treated with SSRI than in those not treated (283).

One study in elderly patients with depression compared citalopram (20–40 mg daily) to amitriptyline (50–100 mg daily) and found equivalent efficacy on MADRS, HAM-D, and CGI, with more adverse effects and discontinuation in the amitriptyline group (284). In a study of patients 60 years or over with unipolar major depression who were randomized to flexible dose nortriptyline or citalopram, a better response was seen in the nortriptyline group, especially in endogenous or psychotic patients (285). Although discontinuation rates due to adverse effects were similar between groups, autonomic effects were more common in the nortriptyline group. Citalopram was superior to placebo in prophylaxis of recurrent depression in a 48-week trial of maintenance therapy in outpatients 65 years or older (286). Keller (234) reported the pooled data from eight double-blind placebo-controlled studies to assess tolerability of citalopram in patients younger and older than 60 years old. In this analysis, of the 1,891 patients treated with citalopram (10–80 mg daily) or placebo, 265 were over 60 years old. The only adverse effect more common in the elderly on active treatment compared to placebo was increased sweating (7.3 vs.1.2%). Another study in the elderly with depression and dementia that found early adverse effects associated with citalopram were fatigue and emotional indifference; although by the fourth week there were no differences in adverse effects between active drug and placebo (287). A 2007 study looked at 175 depressed patients aged 60 and older, who were all given citalopram 10 mg for 6 weeks. They were first evaluated for baseline scores of depression severity, hopelessness, anxiety, cognitive functioning, coexisting medical illness burden, social support, and disability. The results were divided into full (31%), partial (43%), and non-responder (26%) groups. Predictive of the non-responders was a higher depressive score, anxiety, and/or low self-esteem seen initially (288).

Although not limited to data from studies in the elderly, the adverse effect profile of citalopram and escitalopram makes them good candidates for treatment of depression in the older individuals. In younger patients, somnolence, dry mouth, and nausea occur at rates of 5% greater than placebo, but there is some evidence that tolerance to these effects develops. Cardiovascular risk is low with all SSRIs including citalopram, which cause small declines in heart rate (4–8 bpm), and a 1% incidence of bradycardia, even in the elderly. The issues of the cardiotoxicity of the didemethylmetabolite is relevant for humans only at very high plasma levels (greater than 1,000 nM), which would require a massive overdose. With one exception, all of the reported fatalities with overdose of citalopram involved very high doses (840–3,920 mg) in combination with alcohol or sedatives.

Another important advantage for both citalopram and escitalopram over most other SSRIs is their low incidence of pharmacokinetic interactions. In a review of in vitro models, Greenblatt and colleagues (289) have reported that citalopram produces only slight inhibition of CYP1A2, with virtually no effects at CYP2C9, CYP2C19, CYP2D6, or CYP3A4 (see also Chap. 2 for a discussion of antidepressant metabolism). With the possible exception of an interaction between citalopram and metoprolol, a 2D6 substrate, studies in humans confirm the low incidence of pharmacokinetic interactions with citalopram (234). Pharmacodynamic drug interactions of citalopram and escitalopram are probably equivalent to other SSRI, and efforts should be made to avoid concomitant administration with MAOIs, other SSRI, meperidine, tramadol, or other medications that increase serotonin activity. Two small studies looked at augmenting citalopram with methylphenidate, and both concluded that this appears to be a safe and viable strategy for enhancing antidepressant response (290, 291).

Sertraline is another SSRI that is commonly prescribed in geriatric depression (292, 293). It also has the advantage of low incidence of pharmacokinetic drug interactions (289) and good tolerability.

Bondareff and colleagues (294) compared sertraline to nortriptyline in treatment of major depression (210 outpatients, all 60 years old or older, mean duration of illness 3 years, HDRS-24 scores greater or equal to 18). In a complete analysis, efficacy was similar for both groups, with 71.6% responders to sertraline (mean dose 96 mg per day at 12 weeks) versus 61.4% responders to nortriptyline (mean dose 78 mg per day at 12 weeks). Using Intent-to-Treat analysis and last observation carried forward response rates (greater or equal to 50% reduction in HAM-D scores), were not as robust but were still similar in both drug groups. Time to response was also similar for both groups, with 75% of improvement occurring by week 6. Patients who were 70 years old or over taking nortriptyline did not do as well as younger patients on nortriptyline; however, age did not appear to influence treatment response to sertraline. An additional finding of the study was a beneficial effect of sertraline on cognitive functioning (assessed by the Profile of Moods State (POMS) confusion factor, MMS, the Wechsler Adult Intelligence Scale (WAIS), and Shopping List Task (SLT)). The finding of improved cognitive function is supported by another study that found small improvements in cognitive function with sertraline but not paroxetine in normal elderly volunteers (295).

Another study found only modest improvement in cognitive function in response to sertraline treatment (296). Thirty-nine patients 50 years or older with depression (major depressive disorder, dysthymic disorder or depression NOS, HAM-D-17 ≥8) and cognitive impairment without dementia (the presence of intellectual impairment for ≥6 months and ≤10 years, and impaired neuropsychological test performance (≥1 SD below standardized norms) on at least one test from a brief neuropsychological battery) participated in an open sertraline trial of up to 200 mg per day for 12 weeks. Antidepressant response was defined as a 50% or greater decline in HAM-D scores from baseline and improvement on the CGI. Of 26 completers, 17 patients were responders and 9 were non-responders. Responders were younger, with a mean age of 66.8 years, compared to 82.3 years in non-responders. The only cognitive measures to show a significant difference between responders and non-responders was a slight but statistically significant difference in the WAIS-R digit symbol substitute test, a measure of attention and executive function. However, another test of attention, the WAIS-R digit span, did not show group differences.

The findings of another study also suggest some cognitive improvement in elderly patients treated with sertraline (297). Two hundred and thirty-six outpatients aged 60 years or older, with major depression, were assigned to a 1-week placebo wash-in followed by 12 weeks of double-blind treatment with sertraline (50–100 mg daily) or fluoxetine (20–40 mg daily). Response, defined as ≥50% reduction in HAM-D from baseline, was comparable in both groups (73% sertraline, 71% fluoxetine), with high severity depression responding more quickly in the sertraline-treated group. Equivalent responses were also seen on the CGI, MADRS, and the Hamilton Rating Scale for Anxiety (HAM-A). The sertraline group had greater improvement in verbal learning and recall as measured by the SLT as well as the WAIS-R digital symbol substitution test. Improvement in cognitive functioning did not appear to be correlated with improvement in depression. A 12-week clinical trial of patients over the age of 70 with a diagnosis of major depressive disorder by Finkel and colleagues found no statistically significant difference in the adverse effects of sertraline or fluoxetine (298).

Inconsistent data on cognitive improvement with antidepressant treatment are not limited to sertraline. Citalopram and moclobemide have been associated with cognitive improvement, while findings with tricyclic antidepressants and paroxetine have been mixed (7, 212, 287, 297, 299–301).

Despite controversies surrounding the clinical significance of cognitive changes seen with sertraline, evidence for its antidepressant efficacy and tolerability in elderly patients is consistent, although equivalency to TCAs remains unresolved. In a study of depressed patients over 60 years of age treated with sertraline (50 mg per day) or imipramine (150 mg per day), response to treatment (defined as a 50% decrease in the MADRS scale) was similar between groups. Although the completer group and the ITT group had lower MADRS scores with imipramine treatment, these differences did not reach statistical significance. Also of interest is that the dropout rate in the imipramine group was 44.4 and 28.6% in the sertraline group. Although this is not statistically significant, it does suggest better tolerability for sertraline (302, 303). Montgomery and associates (304) have suggested that improved tolerability of SSRIs compared to TCAs is most evident when the comparator drug is amitriptyline or imipramine. This would seem to be supported by an open label study of sertraline in doses up to 100 mg a day in nursing home residents in whom no differences in tolerability of sertraline and nortriptyline were found, but sertraline was less effective for the treatment of depression (305), although the dose used may have been too low.

Many of the efficacy trials of sertraline suffer from inadequate dosage and duration of treatment. In a study of elderly nursing home residents, with significant residual depression after treatment with sertraline at 100 mg per day, an increase in daily dosage to 200 mg improved response and was well tolerated (306). Efficacy studies that use nortriptyline for a comparator drug are complicated by the interaction of plasma levels, depression, and cognitive function observed with this drug. For example, a double-blind, 10-week clinical trial of regular (60–80 mg per day) versus low (10–13 mg per day) of nortriptyline found greater improvements in depression in cognitively intact patients taking the regular dose and greater improvement with low doses in those with dementia (307). In depressed patients without cognitive impairment, a curvilinear plasma response relationship was demonstrated; however, the therapeutic window may be somewhat lower (i.e., shifted to the left) compared to that seen in younger adults. Sertraline is effective in depression associated with dementia; a double-blind, placebo-controlled efficacy and safety study of sertraline in 22 Alzheimer's patients found that sertraline was superior to placebo in reducing the depression in Alzheimer's patients (308). The sertraline group also experienced significantly greater declines in the CSDD scores.

Paroxetine has been widely used in geriatric depression. An acute, 6-week, study comparing the efficacy of nortriptyline and paroxetine in 80 elderly patients (mean age 75.0 years) with a major depressive episode found neither significant differences in dropout rates nor any in relative decreases in HAM-D scores (149).

An 18-month continuation/maintenance open trial compared the efficacy of paroxetine (24.5 mg/day) and nortriptyline (51.3 mg/day; mean blood level 85.5 ng/mL) in 40 patients, 70 years or older, with major depression, no or some MCIs, and mild-to-moderate chronic medical illnesses (309). Paroxetine was found to be comparable to nortriptyline in delaying relapse and recurrence of major depression and may be better tolerated by patients in continuation/maintenance treatment than nortriptyline.

Bump and associates (310) compared the effects of paroxetine and nortriptyline in a larger, two phase continuation/maintenance open trial, beginning with a 12-week acute treatment period. Elderly patients ($n=116$) with major depression were treated with either paroxetine or nortriptyline and were openly switched to the comparator if they were not responding (defined as not achieving a HAM-D-17 score of 10 or less for 3 weeks). Patients whose depression remitted were given the opportunity to enter the second phase of the study, an 18-month follow-up trial continuing the medication to which they responded. During the follow-up, the paroxetine-treated group ($n=83$) and the nortriptyline-treated group ($n=21$) had similar relapse rates and similar time to relapse. The nortriptyline group subjects experienced both lower residual depressive symptoms and adverse effects than the paroxetine group subjects during the second phase. The study found that in elderly, paroxetine and nortriptyline have similar efficacy in depression relapse and recurrence.

A more recent double-blind study (311) in 255 elderly patients (at least 65 years old) with major depression, but without dementia, examined the efficacy and tolerability of mirtazapine and paroxetine. The study involved an 8-week acute phase followed by a 16-week extension phase. Mirtazapine exhibited more notable antidepressant effects, with greater mean changes from baseline in the HAM-D-17 scores, as well as greater score reductions in HAM-D Factor I (Anxiety/Somatization) and Factor VI (Sleep Disturbance). The mirtazapine group also experienced better drug tolerability during the acute phase and a more rapid onset of action, with a median time of 26 days compared to 40 days in the paroxetine group.

Cassano and associates (312) performed a 1-year, double-blind, parallel group study of the treatment of depression with paroxetine (20–40 mg daily) or fluoxetine (20–60 mg daily) in 242 nondemented elderly patients (mean age 75.4 years) without dementia. Subjects were assessed for cognitive performance (Buschke Selective Reminding Test, Blessed Information and Memory Test, Clifton Assessment Schedule, Cancellation Task Test, and Wechsler Paired Word T Test) and for mood functions (HAM-D and Clinical Anxiety Scale). Both paroxetine and fluoxetine were well tolerated. Most subjects in both groups experienced improved cognitive function. Based on the percentage of responders, both drug groups also exhibited good antidepressant efficacy. A 2006 study in the *New England Journal of Medicine* looked at the efficacy of paroxetine and interpersonal psychotherapy in a 2-year maintenance study. One hundred and sixteen patients were assigned to one of four maintenance programs (either paroxetine or placebo combined with either monthly psychotherapy or clinical management programs) after having demonstrated response in the lead-in phase. They found a recurrence of major depression within 2 years in 35% of patients receiving paroxetine and psychotherapy, in 37% of those receiving paroxetine and clinical management sessions, in 68% of those receiving placebo and psychotherapy, and in 58% of those receiving placebo and clinical management sessions (313).

An acute, 12-week, double-blind study (314) of nortriptyline and paroxetine in 116 elderly in- and outpatients (mean age of 72 years) with either major depression or melancholic depression found both drugs efficacious. Although paroxetine did show greater tolerability, with significantly lower discontinuation rates due to adverse effects, there were no significant differences between the response rates in the Intent-to-Treat analysis of either drug group.

A double-blind French study (315) compared the efficacy, safety, and tolerability of paroxetine (20 mg daily) and mianserin (30 mg daily) in the treatment of major depressive disorder in 116 elderly, hospitalized patients, 60 years or older. After 6 weeks, there was a marked improvement in both treatment group subjects for all assessment criteria expect the MMS. The paroxetine group patients exhibited significantly greater improvement in the COVI anxiety scale. This study supports paroxetine's therapeutic value and efficacy as a treatment for geriatric depression, especially when comorbid with anxiety.

The efficacy of reboxetine and imipramine was assessed in subjects 65 years or older with a diagnosis of depression or dysthymia in an 8-week double-blind multicenter trial (10). One hundred and seventy-six subjects were assigned to reboxetine (4–6 mg) and 171 subjects received imipramine (50–100 mg per day). The reduction in HAM-D was similar between the treatment groups with a modest, but clinically significant difference favoring imipramine in both the HAM-D and CGI. Tolerability was comparable between the two groups with 68% and 71% of the patients experiencing adverse effects in the reboxetine and imipramine groups, respectively. Hypotension and cardiovascular effects were lower with reboxetine, whereas insomnia was less common with imipramine (10).

A comparison study (316) between mirtazapine (15–45 mg/day) and amitriptyiline (30–90 mg/day) in 115 elderly depressed patients (60–85 years old) found similar reductions in total HAM-D and MADRS scores over a 6-week treatment period. Analysis of HAM-D factors revealed a statistically significant advantage for amitriptyline on the cognitive disturbance factor for weeks 2, 4, 6, and endpoint and for the retardation depression factor at week 6. Both drugs were well tolerated.

A double-blind study (317) compared buproprion sustained release to paroxetine in 100 elderly outpatients. Both medications resulted in similar improvement on the HAM-D and CGI, but the side effect profile was more favorable for buproprion. Significantly, more patients in the paroxetine group reported somnolence and gastrointestinal disturbances than the subjects taking buproprion SR. Both groups reported dry mouth, nausea, and agitation in rates from 12 to 15%. Headache occurred in 35% of patients treated with buproprion and 19% of patients treated with paroxetine. In a naturalistic study of buproprion SR, elderly patients with major depression and medical comorbidity responded well to bupriopion alone or in combination with other medications (318).

The serotonin-norepinephrine reuptake inhibitor (SNRI) antidepressants venlafaxine and duloxetine have been gaining ground in geriatric use, despite a paucity of placebo-controlled studies in this population. In one study, 300 patients were randomly assigned to venlafaxine, fluoxetine, or placebo and followed for efficacy and emergent side effects for 8 weeks. They found no significant difference in efficacy among placebo, venlafaxine, and fluoxetine. However, side effects occurred in 27% of the venlafaxine group (immediate-release formulation), 19% of the fluoxetine group, and 9% of the placebo group (319).

Another study comparing duloxetine to placebo in 90 elderly patients resulted in a remission rate of 44% in the duloxetine group versus 16% in the placebo group. The discontinuation rate was high (21%) in this study. It was also noted that there were significant reductions in overall pain, back pain, and pain while awake compared with placebo (320). A second duloxetine study compared the effects on depression, cognition, and pain in 207 patients with 104 placebo-treated patients. A standard dose of 60 mg was given for 8 weeks to this group with a median age of 72. Significant reductions were seen on the Hamilton and GDSs, while Visual Analogue Scale scores for back pain and pain while awake, and cognitive scores both showed significant improvement. The study was sponsored by Eli Lilly Co (155).

TCAs

Although TCAs are no longer the first-line pharmacologic choice for the treatment of depression, they are the most extensively studied class of antidepressant medications for the elderly. Numerous published reports indicate the efficacy of these medications for treating these depressions (278, 321). TCAs are subdivided into two groups (the pharmacology of TCAs is described in detail in Chap. 2). The tertiary amines, including amitriptyline, clomipramine, doxepin, imipramine, and trimipramine, are not recommended for elderly patients because of the frequency and intensity of their side effects. Secondary amines, especially desipramine and nortriptyline, are still widely used for treating depressed elderly patients, although usually as a second-line medication for those who have not adequately responded to a nontricyclic antidepressant.

Most recent studies of TCAs in geriatric patients have examined nortriptyline. Nortriptyline is often a comparator drug in late-life depression treatment studies (149, 227, 285, 294, 305, 307, 309, 310, 314) and has been assessed for both acute and maintenance treatment independently. A double-blind, placebo-controlled maintenance study examined the efficacy of nortriptyline (80–120 ng/mL) and interpersonal therapy (IPT) in 187 elderly patients (mean age 67.6 years) with recurrent major depression (HAM-D-17 score ≥17 and MMS score ≥27) over a 7-year period (322). All active treatment groups experienced significantly lower recurrence rates than the placebo group; 20% in the nortriptyline and IPT group, 43% in the nortriptyline and medication clinic visit group, 64% in the IPT and placebo group, and 90% in the placebo and medication clinic visit group. The combination treatment of nortriptyline and IPT had a clinically significant effect in deterring recurrence; the effect was most pronounced in the first year of maintenance in patients over 70 years.

In a 3-year double-blind study, Reynolds and associates (323) compared the efficacy of two fixed plasma levels of nortriptyline (80–120 ng/mL and 40–60 ng/mL) in the treatment of depression among 41 elderly patients with recurrent major depression histories. The rate of recurrence among the 80–120 ng/mL group (mean age 67.7 years) and the 40–60 ng/mL group (mean age 66.3 years) did not differ significantly. Compared to the 40–60 ng/mL group, the 80–120 ng/mL group had significantly fewer subsyndromal range HAM-D scores (6 vs. 25%), but experienced constipation more frequently (33 vs. 5%). With proper management of the side effects, the researchers found the 80–120 ng/mL treatment condition more efficacious.

A more recent, 1-year maintenance trial of nortriptyline and IPT assessed the social adjustment of participants (n=49; mean age 66.8 years; HAM-D score ≥17 or MMS score ≥27) during the treatment of major depression (324). The Social Adjustment Scale (comprised of performance, interpersonal behavior, friction, and satisfaction domains) was administered every 3 months until the depression recurred. The study found that the subjects in the nortriptyline and IPT group "maintained treatment-attributable improvements" in Social Adjustment Scale scores while those subjects in either monotherapy group exhibited declining scores. According to Lenze and associates, the combination therapy improved "not only the length but the quality of recovery."

Side effect severity of nortriptyline was examined in a double-blind, placebo-controlled maintenance study of recurrent major depression treatment in 37 elderly subjects (mean age 67.9 years) over 2–3 years (325). Of the 10 side effect variables monitored, treatment-by-time analysis identified only dry mouth and elevated heart rate of 6–8 bpm as more consistently exhibited in the nortriptyline group. Other complaints, such as total Asberg Rating Scale for Side Effects, physical tiredness, daytime sleepiness, and night-time sleep disturbance were found to be related to residual depression as opposed to the nortriptyline use. This trial did not support reports of nortriptyline use being associated with constipation, weight change, and orthostatic symptoms. The study suggests that nortriptyline is a safe and well-tolerated treatment option for late-life major depression.

Dew and associates (326) examined initial recovery patterns as potential predictors of maintenance treatment success in a 3-year study of nortriptyline and IPT in 140 elderly subjects (≥60 years) with recurrent, unipolar major depression. After 16 weeks of combined nortriptyline and IPT, participants were classified as "rapid, sustained responders," "delayed, sustained responders," "mixed responders without sustained improvement," or "prolonged non-responders" and were then randomized into either combined therapy (IPT and nortriptyline), monotherapy (IPT or nortriptyline), or medication clinic visits with placebo. Relative to the placebo group, "rapid responders" assigned to combined therapy or monotherapy experienced lower recurrence rates. In the "rapid responders" group, both monotherapies were equally effective in decreasing recurrence rates. The "mixed responders" group only exhibited better depression recurrence prevention compared to the placebo group when assigned to combined therapy, and was only moderately superior to the placebo group when assigned to monotherapy. The "delayed responders" receiving combined therapy experienced lower recurrence rates than the placebo group, but those receiving either of the monotherapies did not differ from the placebo group. The "prolonged non-responders" group did not experience any beneficial effects from any of the treatment conditions. This study suggests that identification of a patient's initial response to depression treatment may be a predictor of their recovery success with certain maintenance therapies.

An acute, 6-week, double-blind study focused on the sex-related differences in side effects of nortriptyline (60–120 ng/mL) in 78 subjects, age 18–85 (mean age approximately 50 in both the male and female groups), with a major depressive episode diagnosis, a HAM-D-21 score of 18 or greater, and definite, primary, unipolar depression (327). A significant increase in supine heart rate from baseline was exhibited in both the male and female nortriptyline-treated groups. Men experienced a significantly higher supine heart rate between weeks 4 and 6 compared to the women; the increased supine heart rate adverse effect had no significant group differences in age. Throughout the 6 weeks of the trial, a significantly higher percentage of females reported dry mouth/lip, while the males only reported significantly greater occurrence of dry mouth during weeks 3 and 5.

An acute, 6-month, single-blind study compared the efficacy and safety of venlafaxine (225–300 mg/day) and nortriptyline (50–100 mg/day) in treating late-life major depression (328). Sixty-eight in- and outpatients (aged 65 or over) with current major depression (HAM-D-17 score ≥21), who had been symptomatic for at least 1 month, participated in the trial. The recurrence rates and dropout percentages for both the nortriptyline and venlafaxine groups exhibited no significant differences. The venlafaxine group tolerated the medication slightly better. Those in the nortriptyline group reported significantly more episodes of orthostatic vertigo, dry mouth, and impaired accommodation, as assessed using the Udvalg for Kliniske Undersogelser (USK) Side Effect Rating Scale. The study suggests similar efficacy in venlafaxine and nortriptyline treatment of moderate to severe major late-life depression, with venlafaxine exhibiting slightly better side- effect tolerance.

Several other TCAs have also been assessed for efficacy in the treatment of late-life depression. Two acute double-blind, placebo-controlled studies compared the efficacy of nomifensine and imipramine in the treatment of late-life depression (329, 330). Both studies found that nomifensine and imipramine were comparable in their antidepressant effect and were both superior to placebo. Nomifensine and imipramine were well tolerated in both studies, with the imipramine-treated groups experiencing more uncomfortable side effects. One of the studies found imipramine to have more incidences of anticholinergic effects. The other study found no statistical differences between the two medications, but that imipramine-treated groups tended to experience more drowsiness, nervousness/restlessness, and blurred vision, while the nomifensine-treated groups tended to experience constipation more often. An earlier, 4-week, double-blind, placebo-controlled study of trazodone and imipramine in the treatment of 60 subjects (mean age 68.4 years) with unipolar depression found that both drugs were superior to placebo and had similar therapeutic effects (331). This comparison found that the imipramine-treated group reported a larger side-effect profile, including cardiovascular and anticholinergic side effects. An 8-week comparison study of buspirone and imipramine in the treatment of 177 subjects (mean age 72 years; HAM-D score ≥18) with major depression found that the imipramine-treated group experienced clinically significant reductions in total HAM-D scores, clinically significant improvement in CGI-Improvement scores, and earlier onset of improvement compared to placebo (332). Imipramine elicited a more robust therapeutic effect than buspirone, with greater changes in HAM-D scores and a significant improvement over placebo beginning at week 2 versus week 8. An acute, 8-week, double-blind trial of imipramine in the treatment of 61 elderly Alzheimer's subjects (mean age 72 years) with and without depression assessed rate of improvement with HAM-D and MMS (299). Depressed patients treated with imipramine and placebo exhibited similar rates of improvement as assessed by the HAM-D. All subjects improved over time on the MMS; there were no differences between subjects on imipramine or placebo, and subjects with depression improved significantly more than those without depression.

A comparison study of trazodone (150 mg t.i.d.), mianserin (60 mg t.i.d.), and amitriptyline (75 mg t.i.d.) assessed their efficacy and tolerability among 106 subjects (mean age 65.8 years) with major depression over 5 weeks. All three medications exhibited comparable efficacy as assessed by the HAM-D and GDS, but the trazodone-treated group experienced fewer side effects. Amitriptyline was also compared to mianserin in a placebo-controlled, depression treatment study of 75 subjects, aged 60 years or older (333). This trial found that amitriptyline and mianserin had comparable antidepressant effects, while mianserin exhibited a more tolerable side-effect profile. A more recent, 8-week, double-blind study compared the efficacy and tolerability paroxetine (20–40 mg/day) and amitriptyline (75–150 mg/day) in 191 subjects (mean age approximately 55 years) with rheumatoid arthritis and depression (334). Both medications resulted in similar improvements in MADRS and CGI scores. Paroxetine tended to be better tolerated than amitriptyline, in particular with fewer anticholinergic effects (18.1 vs. 43.8%, respectively) and fewer sedative effects (9.6 vs. 25.0%, respectively).

A 4-month study compared the efficacy of desipramine and cognitive/behavioral therapy (CBT) in the treatment of late-life depression (335). One hundred and two elderly subjects, aged 60 years or over, with major depressive disorder received either monotherapy (desipramine or CBT) or combined therapy. With respect to the per-session rate of change, significant improvements in the HAM-D scores were achieved by the combined therapy subjects compared to the desipramine-alone treated subjects. Significantly greater per-session rates of change were also exhibited by both the combined therapy and CBT-alone groups compared to the desipramine-alone group, as assessed by the Beck Depression Inventory-Short Form (BDI-SF). Intent-to-Treat analyses suggested that the combined therapy group experienced significantly greater improvement than desipramine-alone and different measures yielded conflicting results as to CBT-alone superiority over desipramine-alone.

Clinical Use of TCAs

Before treatment with a tricyclic is initiated, the elderly patient should be evaluated for cardiac disease, cerebrovascular or degenerative brain disease, glaucoma, and protastic hypertrophy, each potentially worsened by tricyclic administration. The most common side effects are orthostatic hypotension, sedation, and anticholinergic effects: dry mouth, constipation, blurred vision, urinary hesitancy, and cognitive impairment. Tricyclics also have quinidine-like properties, so that high blood levels may produce cardiac arrhythmias. For this reason, it is strongly recommended that an elderly depressed patient have a baseline EKG before tricyclic treatment is initiated. Widening of the QTc indicates approaching cardiac toxicity from the tricyclic (see also Chap. 2).

Most older patients respond to tricyclic antidepressants in approximately 6–8 weeks, the same as young and middle-aged adults. However, the quality of response is less complete in the elderly, so 12 or more weeks may be necessary for remission of the depressive symptoms. Once an older patient has responded, maintenance treatment should continue for at least 1 year (or longer) depending on the number of prior depressive episodes and the severity of the most recent depressive episode. Those elderly individuals who have been extremely ill or repeatedly ill should remain on their tricyclic antidepressant as long as possible.

Summary of Antidepressants in Geriatric Major Depression

Based on available studies, antidepressants have equivalent efficacy in geriatric major depression. SSRIs are considered first-line agents because of their safety profile, simplicity of dosing, and the lack of drug–drug interactions for citalopram and escitalopram. Other drugs that are also effective and well tolerated include sertraline, nortriptyline, venlafaxine, mirtazapine, and buproprion. Other studies indicate that TCAs can be used safely provided adequate medical monitoring occurs. ECT should always be considered in geriatric major depression (278).

Antidepressant Response in non-MDD Subtypes of Geriatric Depression

Treatment of Dysthymia and Subsyndromal Depression

Dysthymic disorder in the elderly appears to be different from dysthymia seen in younger patients and as described in the DSM. Late age of onset with limited comorbid psychiatric pathology characterizes this group of patients and is found to be similar to late-onset major depression. Contrast this with younger adults who qualify for dysthymic diagnosis with early onset and, commonly, comorbid psychiatric pathology (141, 336). Perhaps a better term is subsyndromal depression of the elderly, which underlines its probable closer association with late-onset major depression. A placebo-controlled study using fluoxetine in 71 patients with dysthymia showed a very mild efficacy favoring fluoxetine over placebo, with 37% response rate on fluoxetine versus 23% response rate on placebo (337).

The approach to treatment of subsyndromal depression (minor depression) depends on the length and relative severity of symptoms. For recent (few weeks) onset of symptoms, the best initial course is to carefully follow patients and treat with psychotherapy. If this fails after a reasonable period, addition of an antidepressant is warranted. No specific antidepressant has demonstrated superior efficacy. It should be noted that published trials are not equivalent, having used different doses of the same antidepressant, different medications, and variable durations of treatment and follow-up. Many of the clinical trials discussed above have included subjects with both major depression and dysthymia. Very few antidepressant studies have limited subjects only to those with dysthymia or minor depression.

A notable exception is a study of 415 primary care patients (mean age 71 years) with minor depression ($n=204$) or dysthymia ($n=211$) and a HAM-D of 10 or greater who were randomized to receive paroxetine (beginning at 10 mg per day and titrated to a maximum of 40 mg per day) or a behaviorally based psychotherapy designed specifically for primary care, Problem-Solving Treatment-Primary Care (PST-PC) (338). Paroxetine-treated patients showed greater declines in the Hopkins

Symptom Check List-Depression (HSCL-D) scale compared to both PST-PC and placebo groups. Improvement in depression was greater and more rapid with paroxetine; however, the change would be considered moderate by clinical standards. Both dysthymia and minor depression responded to drug treatment similarly.

Two small open trials suggest that sertraline and citalopram are effective in minor depression in the elderly. An open label trial of sertraline among nursing home residents with dysthymia ($n=12$) for 6 weeks showed no significant side effects, and 75% met criteria for remission (339). In a study of ten geriatric patients with minor depression who were given 20 mg of citalopram for 12 weeks, the medication was well tolerated and there was a marked decrease in depressive symptoms (340). Prolonged bereavement has been shown to respond to antidepressant treatment in a small number of studies (208).

Treatment of Depression with Insomnia

While aging is a risk factor for insomnia, insomnia is a clinical symptom with multiple etiologies, including late-life depression, medical disorders, pain, and side effects of some medications (341). Therefore, consideration of a treatment for insomnia must be preceded by the clinician's differential diagnosis (342). Generally, if insomnia is caused by depression or anxiety, sleep will be improved after depression or anxiety is treated and remitted. Some antidepressants have been shown to be superior to others in treating depression with insomnia. For example, mirtazapine and trazodone have been found to significantly improve insomnia among the depressed elderly (311). Additionally, paroxetine is found to be beneficial in initiating sleep onset (343, 344). Given the adverse effects in the elderly, TCA and benzodiazepine should not be considered as the first-line agents to treat late-life depression with insomnia.

Treatment of Depression Comorbid with Dementia

Depression in AD has higher rates of spontaneous resolution than vascular dementia (VaD) and MCI, and depression accompanying VaD or MCI is more resistant to antidepressant treatment than depression in AD (345). Generally, all the antidepressants used for major depression disorder (MDD) are effective for depression or dysphoria in dementia. However, the use of selective serotonin reuptake inhibitors (SSRI) is recommended given their demonstrated efficacy and safety in patients with AD (346). Lyketsos et al. conducted a randomized, placebo-controlled, double-blind clinical trial of sertraline in the treatment of depression complicating AD by starting with sertraline 25 mg and titrated to 150 mg in 6 weeks (308, 347). It was found that after 12 weeks, patients given sertraline had significantly greater mean declines from baseline in CSDD scores; the bulk of antidepressant response occurred by the third week of treatment. Another study found that both fluoxetine and placebo are equally effective in improving the depressive symptoms in AD patients (348). The TCA antidepressant, clomipramine, is found to worsen the confusion although it improves the depressive symptoms of AD patients (300). Two studies found that a placebo improves depressive symptoms in AD which suggests that some non-pharmacological treatment such as social interaction may also be helpful.

Psychosis and agitation are common among dementia patients, especially in the late stage. Although antipsychotics are shown to increase the risk, 1.6–1.7 times, of mortality among these patients, clinicians are left with limited choices, other than using atypical antipsychotics for treating demented patients with psychosis and severe agitation (342). Unlike atypical antipsychotics which are D2 receptor antagonists, aripiprazole is a D2 partial agonist with interaction with 5HT receptors. Interestingly, a randomized, double-blind, placebo-controlled study found that aripiprazole is not effective for treating psychotic symptoms in AD patients; but their symptoms of agitation, anxiety, and depression are improved by aripiprazole with a low risk of adverse events (349). Another randomized, double-blind, parallel trial shows that depressive symptoms and agitated behavior are improved by trazodone, but not by haloperidol in dementia patients (350). Although there is no double-blind, placebo-control trial yet, an open label study shows that mirtazapine may be helpful in improving depression with weight loss and anxiety in AD patients (351). Another open label study shows that mirtazapine improves depressive symptoms among the nursing home elderly with MMSE >10 (352).

While it is still unclear whether antidepressants are helpful as a cognitive enhancer, several studies suggest that classical drugs for AD might be helpful in improving patients' mood symptoms. Double-blind placebo-controlled studies show that donepezil, a cholinesterase inhibitor, improves neuropsychiatric symptoms including depression/dysphoria (353) and delays progression to AD among depressed subjects with amnestic MCI (354). Memantine is a specific, moderate affinity, uncompetitive *N*-methyl-D-aspartate (NMDA) receptor antagonist. While it slows down the cognitive decline in AD (355), memantine 20 mg/day also reduces severity of depression and dysphoria in AD patients based on the NPI scale (356).

Treatment of Complicated Grief

There are no randomized controlled trials of pharmacotherapy for complicated grief although some open-label trials show that buproprion, but not nortripline, might be helpful (357, 358). Given the lack of response to standard depression treatments for complicated grief (359, 360), Shear et al. developed a psychotherapy, complicated grief treatment (CGT) (361), which combined IPT and CBT. A randomized control trial shows that CGT has higher response rates and faster time to response than IPT among patients who have complicated grief aged 18–85 (361). However, complicated grief patients who are on an antidepressant medication are more likely to complete a full course of CGT (91 vs. 58% completed) than those who did not use antidepressants (362). In one study, in which patients with complicated grief were assigned randomly to psychotherapy exclusively by e-mail between therapists and patients or a waiting list, the results show a large treatment effect maintaining for 3 months to 1.5 years (363, 364).

Antidepressants, especially SSRIs, are effective in treating grief with MDD. One open label study shows that escitalopram improves depressive, anxiety, and grief symptoms in individuals experiencing a major depressive episode related to the loss of a loved one (365). A double-blind trial shows that nortriptyline is superior to a placebo in achieving remission of bereavement-related major depressive episodes (366). Psychotherapy, such as CBT and IPT, should be effective in treating grief with MDD in conjunction with antidepressants, as described in the treatment of MDD in the elderly.

Treatment of Post-Stroke Depression

The concept of post-stroke depression may seem unnecessary in this new age of vascular depression. Post-stroke depression assumes a vascular event large enough to be clinically detected, whereas the concept of vascular depression encompasses all infarcts, large or small, immediately detectable or with insidious onset and hyperintensities of white matter seen on MRI as evidence of an ongoing, and perhaps initially undetected, process. Therefore, the assumption may be made that post-stroke depression may be on the same continuum with vascular depression, and theoretically, the effective treatments may be the same. However, as of this writing, there exists a literature and ongoing research on post-stroke depression. The two literatures are just beginning to inform each other, even though they have to date focused on different phenomena (367), and eventually there may be a joining of effort by both camps. What follows is a review of the literature on treatment of post-stroke depression.

Depression is a risk factor for the development of stroke. The rates of stroke are 2.3–2.7 times greater in persons over the age of 65 with high versus low levels of depressive symptoms (368). Approximately 30% of patients after stroke are depressed (369). Research surrounding the biological treatment of post-stroke depression has focused on the use of antidepressant medications, psychostimulants, and ECT. Confirmation of psychostimulant and ECT efficacy requires more randomized, controlled studies although both treatments appear to be safe and well tolerated (370). Post-stroke depression responds well to antidepressant treatment. Tricyclics, especially nortriptyline, have been found particularly effective as have most SSRI antidepressants (371, 372). Most recent evidence, however, strongly favors the use of SSRIs over TCAs (373).

The efficacy and tolerability of fluoxetine (20 mg/day) in the treatment of post-stroke depression was examined in a double-blind, placebo-controlled, 6-week study of 31 post-stroke patients (374). All subjects recently experienced a stroke (<3 months) and were diagnosed with major depression (as determined by the International Classification of Diseases, 10th revision and a MADRS score >19). The fluoxetine group exhibited clinically significant improvement in mean MADRS scores than the placebo group at week 6 (11.8 vs. 18.7, respectively). The fluoxetine group also experienced significantly greater mean changes in MADRS scores than the placebo group (1.6 vs. 8.4, respectively). Fluoxetine was well tolerated, with no significant adverse effects noted.

Fluoxetine efficacy and safety was also assessed in a 3-month, double-blind, placebo-controlled study, with an 18-month, open-label follow-up (375). Subjects ($n=54$) had experienced a stroke within 2 weeks and were diagnosed with moderate to severe depression (assessed by BDI, CGI, and a HAM-D score >15). Both groups exhibited significant improvements in HAM-D scores and were not significantly different at the 3-month assessment, but at the 18-month follow-up, fluoxetine-treated subjects were significantly less depressed than subjects in the placebo group. No adverse effects to the fluoxetine treatment were exhibited. An 8-week trial of fluoxetine (20–40 mg/day) and sertraline (50–100 mg/day) in the treatment of 45 post-stroke subjects with major depression found that both SSRIs could be efficacious (376).

A 12-week, double-blind, placebo-controlled comparison study of nortriptyline (25–100 mg/day) and fluoxetine (10–40 mg/day) assessed their efficacy in the treatment of post-stroke depression in 56 patients (372). The findings of this study indicated that nortriptyline was superior to fluoxetine in treating post-stroke depression, eliciting a significantly higher response rate (77% for nortriptyline, 14% for fluoxetine, and 31% for placebo). These results appear to contradict other studies that suggest that SSRIs are superior to TCAS in post-stroke depression treatment; however, this study suffers from a higher dropout rate in the fluoxetine group and a mid-study alteration in design due to a high placebo response rate. The fluoxetine-treated group was comprised of significantly more subjects who failed to respond to placebo than the nortriptyline-treated group, which may suggest that the fluoxetine-treated subjects were more difficult to treat (370).

A 12-week, double-blind, placebo-controlled comparison study of nortriptyline (25–100 mg/day) and fluoxetine (10–40 mg/day), and examined their efficacy in the prevention of post-stroke depression in nondepressed patients ($n=48$) (377). Among study completers during the 12-week treatment period, there were significantly higher rates of depression in the placebo group than the active treatments combined. The nortriptyline-treated group was significantly more vulnerable to developing depression for over 6 months after the treatment period ended, indicating that fluoxetine may have a prophylactic effect.

Research indicates that post-stroke depression can be effectively treated by antidepressants. Both TCAs and SSRIs are well tolerated and effective; however, research supports the use of SSRIs as first-line agents in the treatment of post-stroke depression.

Electroconvulsive Therapy

Although the primary purpose of this chapter is to review the pharmacotherapy of geriatric depression, ECT is also an effective and safe treatment. In a review of treatment of depression in the elderly, Salzman and associates (278) reported on 12 publications examining the efficacy of ECT (378–389). They concluded that ECT was efficacious and well tolerated even in those patients over 80 years old. Antidepressants play an important role in ECT treatment and are often used as adjunctive therapy during a course of ECT. Because the rate of relapse after ECT treatment is high, antidepressant therapy is essential for patients "graduating" from a series of ECT treatments. In cases where antidepressant therapy cannot maintain the patient following ECT, maintenance ECT treatments are a possibility (390).

Despite ECT's well-established efficacy and safety record, ECT can have side effects of post-treatment and inter-treatment delirium, headache, muscle ache, and nausea. More rarely, longer term cognitive deficits can be seen and are often associated with the total number of treatments in a given period of time, as well as practice methods such as electrode placement. The relative risk of ECT is, however, roughly equivalent to the risk of the anesthesia itself (143, 391).

The mechanism of action of ECT has remained unknown, but a recent report has found an increase in plasma BDNF concentration in patients receiving ECT, and offers an intriguing possible neurotrophic mechanism for this treatment (392).

Psychosocial Treatments

There are a number of psychotherapies or psychosocial interventions that have proven helpful in treating geriatric depression. Briefly, there are individual, group, and family therapy approaches used with or without concurrent antidepressant medication. A large meta-analysis in 1994 showed the efficacy of various individual therapies which included cognitive, behavioral, interpersonal, supportive, reminiscence, and "eclectic" approaches. Both brief and longer psychodynamic therapies show good results in the elderly. For those patients with both dementia and depression, cognitive-behavioral therapy is a recognized treatment. Interpersonal therapy is effective, particularly so with bereavement issues.

Group treatment includes cognitive-focused work, psycho-educational, reminiscence, problem solving, and goal-focused group psychotherapies. These are conducted in inpatient settings, partial hospital programs, and day programs with good effect; but some studies have shown that patient selection is important since various disabilities need to be taken into account. If a given patient has difficulty engaging in group therapy, it may negatively influence the group process.

Family therapy is of importance, since patients are often first seen after the family has become involved and overwhelmed in trying to take care of its loved one. Family involvement in therapy offers the opportunity to gather an accurate history of the patient in order to better understand the current situation, educate the family as primary managers with regard to behaviors and medicines, and gather information about family dynamics, which may help or hinder the situation (393).

Conclusions

Depression is a significant cause of morbidity and mortality among the elderly, at enormous cost to society, and having a devastating impact on patients. It is intriguing to think not only about more effective detection and treatment of such depression but also about prevention as an attractive option (394).

The evidence for efficacy of antidepressants is strongest in major depression but somewhat weaker for minor depression or dysthymia. Although the safety and efficacy of antidepressants in the medically depressed elderly is established, the effect sizes are modest. Antidepressant augmentation strategies have not been adequately studied in the elderly, and therefore information must be extrapolated from the adult literature. However, the pharmacokinetics and pharmacodynamics of antidepressants in the elderly are altered, leading to the maxim, "start low, go slow." Older patients take longer to respond and are more likely than younger patients to experience side effects. Once treated, the elderly, as a group, are prone to relapse sooner than younger adults.

The field of geriatric psychiatry continues to grow, and research is revealing that there may be geriatric disorders separate from those seen in younger adults. Vascular depression is a prime example, and is challenging our traditional approaches to treatment. More research is needed in all forms of geriatric depression so as to determine the most effective agents to use; clearly, there is much left to achieve pharmacologically, to decrease suffering in this vulnerable, and increasingly distinct, population.

References

1. Nelson JC, Epstein LJ. Depression and Anxiety in the Old-Old. Honolulu: AAGP Annual Meeting, 2003.
2. Blazer DG. Psychiatry and the oldest old. Am J Psychiatry. 2000;157(12):1915–24.
3. Gallo JJ, Coyne JC. The challenge of depression in late life: bridging science and service in primary care. JAMA. 2000;284(12):1570–2.
4. Harman JS, Reynolds CF, III. Removing the barriers to effective depression treatment in old age. J Am Geriatr Soc. 2000;48(8):1012–3.
5. Lai T, Payne ME, Byrum CE, Steffens DC, Krishnan KR. Reduction of orbital frontal cortex volume in geriatric depression. Biol Psychiatry. 2000;48(10):971–5.
6. Behavioral Manifestations of Dementia and Depression in the Older Adult. . Honolulu: AAGP Annual Meeting, 2003.
7. Katona C, Livingston G. Impact of screening old people with physical illness for depression? Lancet. 2000;356(9224):91–2.
8. McDougall FA, Kvaal K, Matthews FE, Paykel E, Jones PB, Dewey ME, et al. Prevalence of depression in older people in England and Wales: the MRC CFA Study. Psychol Med. 2007;37(12):1787–95.
9. Niti M, Ng TP, Kua EH, Ho RC, Tan CH. Depression and chronic medical illnesses in Asian older adults: the role of subjective health and functional status. Int J Geriatr Psychiatry. 2007;22(11):1087–94.
10. Katona C, Bercoff E, Chiu E, Tack P, Versiani M, Woelk H. Reboxetine versus imipramine in the treatment of elderly patients with depressive disorders: a double-blind randomised trial. J Affect Disord. 1999;55(2–3):203–13.

11. Smalbrugge M, Jongenelis L, Pot AM, Eefsting JA, Ribbe MW, Beekman AT. Incidence and outcome of depressive symptoms in nursing home patients in the Netherlands. Am J Geriatr Psychiatry. 2006;14(12):1069–76.
12. Wilson K, Mottram P, Sixsmith A. Depressive symptoms in the very old living alone: prevalence, incidence and risk factors. Int J Geriatr Psychiatry. 2007;22(4):361–6.
13. Charney DS, Reynolds CF, III, Lewis L, Lebowitz BD, Sunderland T, Alexopoulos GS, et al. Depression and Bipolar Support Alliance consensus statement on the unmet needs in diagnosis and treatment of mood disorders in late life. Arch Gen Psychiatry. 2003;60(7):664–72.
14. Salzman C. Pharmacological treatment of depression in elderly patients. In: Schneider LS, Reynolds CF, Lebowitz BD, editors. Diagnosis and Treatment of Depression in Late Life:Results of the NIH Consensus Development Conference. Washington, D.C.: American Psychiatric Press; 1994. p. 65–9.
15. Lebowitz BD, Pearson JL, Schneider LS, Reynolds CF, III, Alexopoulos GS, Bruce ML, et al. Diagnosis and treatment of depression in late life. Consensus statement update. JAMA. 1997;278(14):1186–90.
16. Salzman C. Practical considerations for the treatment of depression in elderly and very elderly long-term care patients. J Clin Psychiatry. 1999;60 Suppl 20:30–3.
17. Patrick DL, Erickson P. Health status and health policy : quality of life in health care evaluation and resource allocation. New York: Oxford University Press; 1993.
18. Samuelsson SM, Alfredson BB, Hagberg B, Samuelsson G, Nordbeck B, Brun A, et al. The Swedish Centenarian Study: a multidisciplinary study of five consecutive cohorts at the age of 100. Int J Aging Hum Dev. 1997;45(3):223–53.
19. Larkin M. Centenarians point the way to healthy ageing. Lancet. 1999;353(9158):1074.
20. Geerlings SW, Beekman AT, Deeg DJ, Twisk JW, Van Tilburg W. The longitudinal effect of depression on functional limitations and disability in older adults: an eight-wave prospective community-based study. Psychol Med. 2001;31(8):1361–71.
21. Sutcliffe C, Burns A, Challis D, Mozley CG, Cordingley L, Bagley H, et al. Depressed mood, cognitive impairment, and survival in older people admitted to care homes in England. Am J Geriatr Psychiatry. 2007;15(8):708–15.
22. Devanand DP, Sano M, Tang MX, Taylor S, Gurland BJ, Wilder D, et al. Depressed mood and the incidence of Alzheimer's disease in the elderly living in the community. Arch Gen Psychiatry. 1996;53(2):175–82.
23. Geerlings MI, Schoevers RA, Beekman AT, Jonker C, Deeg DJ, Schmand B, et al. Depression and risk of cognitive decline and Alzheimer's disease. Results of two prospective community-based studies in The Netherlands. Br J Psychiatry. 2000;176:568–75.
24. Paterniti S, Verdier-Taillefer MH, Dufouil C, Alperovitch A. Depressive symptoms and cognitive decline in elderly people. Longitudinal study. Br J Psychiatry. 2002;181:406–10.
25. Kumar R, Parslow RA, Jorm AF, Rosenman SJ, Maller J, Meslin C, et al. Clinical and neuroimaging correlates of mild cognitive impairment in a middle-aged community sample: the personality and total health through life 60+ study. Dement Geriatr Cogn Disord. 2006;21(1):44–50.
26. Ownby RL, Crocco E, Acevedo A, John V, Loewenstein D. Depression and risk for Alzheimer disease: systematic review, meta-analysis, and metaregression analysis. Arch Gen Psychiatry. 2006;63(5):530–8.
27. Berger AK, Fratiglioni L, Forsell Y, Winblad B, Backman L. The occurrence of depressive symptoms in the preclinical phase of AD: a population-based study. Neurology. 1999;53(9):1998–2002.
28. Cervilla JA, Prince M, Joels S, Mann A. Does depression predict cognitive outcome 9 to 12 years later? Evidence from a prospective study of elderly hypertensives. Psychol Med. 2000;30(5):1017–23.
29. Ritchie K, Ledesert B, Touchon J. Subclinical cognitive impairment: epidemiology and clinical characteristics. Compr Psychiatry. 2000;41(2 Suppl 1):61–5.
30. Wilson RS, Barnes LL, Mendes de Leon CF, Aggarwal NT, Schneider JS, Bach J, et al. Depressive symptoms, cognitive decline, and risk of AD in older persons. Neurology. 2002;59(3):364–70.

31. Lopez OL, Becker JT, Sweet RA, Klunk W, Kaufer DI, Saxton J, et al. Psychiatric symptoms vary with the severity of dementia in probable Alzheimer's disease. J Neuropsychiatry Clin Neurosci. 2003;15(3):346–53.
32. Dal Forno G, Palermo MT, Donohue JE, Karagiozis H, Zonderman AB, Kawas CH. Depressive symptoms, sex, and risk for Alzheimer's disease. Ann Neurol. 2005;57(3):381–7.
33. Mauricio M, O'Hara R, Yesavage JA, Friedman L, Kraemer HC, Van De Water M, et al. A longitudinal study of apolipoprotein-E genotype and depressive symptoms in community-dwelling older adults. Am J Geriatr Psychiatry. 2000;8(3):196–200.
34. Steffens DC, Trost WT, Payne ME, Hybels CF, MacFall JR. Apolipoprotein E genotype and subcortical vascular lesions in older depressed patients and control subjects. Biol Psychiatry. 2003;54(7):674–81.
35. Lyketsos CG, Lopez O, Jones B, Fitzpatrick AL, Breitner J, DeKosky S. Prevalence of neuropsychiatric symptoms in dementia and mild cognitive impairment: results from the cardiovascular health study. JAMA. 2002;288(12):1475–83.
36. Geda YE, Knopman DS, Mrazek DA, Jicha GA, Smith GE, Negash S, et al. Depression, apolipoprotein E genotype, and the incidence of mild cognitive impairment: a prospective cohort study. Arch Neurol. 2006;63(3):435–40.
37. Palsson S, Larsson L, Tengelin E, Waern M, Samuelsson S, Hallstro T, et al. The prevalence of depression in relation to cerebral atrophy and cognitive performance in 70- and 74-year-old women in Gothenburg. The Women's Health Study. Psychol Med. 2001;31(1):39–49.
38. Jones S, Small BJ, Fratiglioni L, Backman L. Predictors of cognitive change from preclinical to clinical Alzheimer's disease. Brain Cogn. 2002;49(2):210–3.
39. Ganguli M, Du Y, Dodge HH, Ratcliff GG, Chang CC. Depressive symptoms and cognitive decline in late life: a prospective epidemiological study. Arch Gen Psychiatry. 2006;63(2):153–60.
40. Mueller TI, Kohn R, Leventhal N, Leon AC, Solomon D, Coryell W, et al. The course of depression in elderly patients. Am J Geriatr Psychiatry. 2004;12(1):22–9.
41. Mitchell AJ, Subramaniam H. Prognosis of depression in old age compared to middle age: a systematic review of comparative studies. Am J Psychiatry. 2005;162(9):1588–601.
42. Anstey KJ, von Sanden C, Sargent-Cox K, Luszcz MA. Prevalence and risk factors for depression in a longitudinal, population-based study including individuals in the community and residential care. Am J Geriatr Psychiatry. 2007;15(6):497–505.
43. Kohn R, Epstein-Lubow G. Course and outcomes of depression in the elderly. Curr Psychiatry Rep. 2006;8(1):34–40.
44. Lavretsky H, Ballmaier M, Pham D, Toga A, Kumar A. Neuroanatomical characteristics of geriatric apathy and depression: a magnetic resonance imaging study. Am J Geriatr Psychiatry. 2007;15(5):386–94.
45. Lavretsky H, Roybal DJ, Ballmaier M, Toga AW, Kumar A. Antidepressant exposure may protect against decrement in frontal gray matter volumes in geriatric depression. J Clin Psychiatry. 2005;66(8):964–7.
46. Hwang JP, Tsai SJ, Hong CJ, Yang CH, Lirng JF, Yang YM. The Val66Met polymorphism of the brain-derived neurotrophic-factor gene is associated with geriatric depression. Neurobiol Aging. 2006;27(12):1834–7.
47. Kim H, Lim SW, Kim S, Kim JW, Chang YH, Carroll BJ, et al. Monoamine transporter gene polymorphisms and antidepressant response in koreans with late-life depression. JAMA. 2006;296(13):1609–18.
48. Grunblatt E, Loffler C, Zehetmayer S, Jungwirth S, Tragl KH, Riederer P, et al. Association study of the 5-HTTLPR polymorphism and depression in 75-Year-Old nondemented subjects from the Vienna Transdanube Aging (VITA) study. J Clin Psychiatry. 2006;67(9):1373–8.
49. Taylor WD, Steffens DC, Payne ME, MacFall JR, Marchuk DA, Svenson IK, et al. Influence of serotonin transporter promoter region polymorphisms on hippocampal volumes in late-life depression. Arch Gen Psychiatry. 2005;62(5):537–44.
50. Folstein M, Liu T, Peter I, Buell J, Arsenault L, Scott T, et al. The homocysteine hypothesis of depression. Am J Psychiatry. 2007;164(6):861–7.

51. Almeida OP, Flicker L, Norman P, Hankey GJ, Vasikaran S, van Bockxmeer FM, et al. Association of cardiovascular risk factors and disease with depression in later life. Am J Geriatr Psychiatry. 2007;15(6):506–13.
52. Alexopoulos GS, Borson S, Cuthbert BN, Devanand DP, Mulsant BH, Olin JT, et al. Assessment of late life depression. Biol Psychiatry. 2002;52(3):164–74.
53. Gallo JJ, Rabins PV. Depression without sadness: alternative presentations of depression in late life. Am Fam Physician. 1999;60(3):820–6.
54. Folstein MF, Folstein SE, McHugh PR. "Mini-mental state". A practical method for grading the cognitive state of patients for the clinician. J Psychiatr Res. 1975;12(3):189–98.
55. Hoyl MT, Alessi CA, Harker JO, Josephson KR, Pietruszka FM, Koelfgen M, et al. Development and testing of a five-item version of the Geriatric Depression Scale. J Am Geriatr Soc. 1999;47(7):873–8.
56. Yesavage JA, Brink TL, Rose TL, Lum O, Huang V, Adey M, et al. Development and validation of a geriatric depression screening scale: a preliminary report. J Psychiatr Res. 1982;17(1):37–49.
57. Korner A, Lauritzen L, Abelskov K, Gulmann N, Marie Brodersen A, Wedervang-Jensen T, et al. The Geriatric Depression Scale and the Cornell Scale for Depression in Dementia. A validity study. Nord J Psychiatry. 2006;60(5):360–4.
58. Wancata J, Alexandrowicz R, Marquart B, Weiss M, Friedrich F. The criterion validity of the Geriatric Depression Scale: a systematic review. Acta Psychiatr Scand. 2006;114(6):398–410.
59. Korner A, Lauritzen L, Abelskov K, Gulmann NC, Brodersen AM, Wedervang-Jensen T, et al. Rating scales for depression in the elderly: external and internal validity. J Clin Psychiatry. 2007;68(3):384–9.
60. Alexopoulos GS, Meyers BS, Young RC, Kakuma T, Silbersweig D, Charlson M. Clinically defined vascular depression. Am J Psychiatry. 1997;154(4):562–5.
61. Alexopoulos GS, Meyers BS, Young RC, Campbell S, Silbersweig D, Charlson M. 'Vascular depression' hypothesis. Arch Gen Psychiatry. 1997;54(10):915–22.
62. Krishnan KR, Hays JC, Blazer DG. MRI-defined vascular depression. Am J Psychiatry. 1997;154(4):497–501.
63. Baldwin RC, O'Brien J. Vascular basis of late-onset depressive disorder. Br J Psychiatry. 2002;180:157–60.
64. Thomas AJ, O'Brien JT, Davis S, Ballard C, Barber R, Kalaria RN, et al. Ischemic basis for deep white matter hyperintensities in major depression: a neuropathological study. Arch Gen Psychiatry. 2002;59(9):785–92.
65. Tiemeier H, Bakker SL, Hofman A, Koudstaal PJ, Breteler MM. Cerebral haemodynamics and depression in the elderly. J Neurol Neurosurg Psychiatry. 2002;73(1):34–9.
66. Davies J, Lloyd KR, Jones IK, Barnes A, Pilowsky LS. Changes in regional cerebral blood flow with venlafaxine in the treatment of major depression. Am J Psychiatry. 2003;160(2):374–6.
67. Alexopoulos GS. The vascular depression hypothesis: 10 years later. Biol Psychiatry. 2006;60(12):1304–5.
68. Roman GC. Vascular depression: an archetypal neuropsychiatric disorder. Biol Psychiatry. 2006;60(12):1306–8.
69. Longstreth WT, Jr., Bernick C, Manolio TA, Bryan N, Jungreis CA, Price TR. Lacunar infarcts defined by magnetic resonance imaging of 3660 elderly people: the Cardiovascular Health Study. Arch Neurol. 1998;55(9):1217–25.
70. Krishnan KR, Goli V, Ellinwood EH, France RD, Blazer DG, Nemeroff CB. Leukoencephalopathy in patients diagnosed as major depressive. Biol Psychiatry. 1988;23(5):519–22.
71. Krishnan KR, Hays JC, George LK, Blazer DG. Six-month outcomes for MRI-related vascular depression. Depress Anxiety. 1998;8(4):142–6.
72. Krishnan KR. Biological risk factors in late life depression. Biol Psychiatry. 2002;52(3):185–92.

73. Taylor WD, Steffens DC, Krishnan KR. Psychiatric disease in the twenty-first century: the case for subcortical ischemic depression. Biol Psychiatry. 2006;60(12):1299–303.
74. Ebert D, Ebmeier KP. The role of the cingulate gyrus in depression: from functional anatomy to neurochemistry. Biol Psychiatry. 1996;39(12):1044–50.
75. Rajkowska G, Miguel-Hidalgo JJ, Wei J, Dilley G, Pittman SD, Meltzer HY, et al. Morphometric evidence for neuronal and glial prefrontal cell pathology in major depression. Biol Psychiatry. 1999;45(9):1085–98.
76. MacFall JR, Payne ME, Provenzale JE, Krishnan KR. Medial orbital frontal lesions in late-onset depression. Biol Psychiatry. 2001;49(9):803–6.
77. Bremner JD, Vythilingam M, Vermetten E, Nazeer A, Adil J, Khan S, et al. Reduced volume of orbitofrontal cortex in major depression. Biol Psychiatry. 2002;51(4):273–9.
78. Taylor WD, Steffens DC, McQuoid DR, Payne ME, Lee SH, Lai TJ, et al. Smaller orbital frontal cortex volumes associated with functional disability in depressed elders. Biol Psychiatry. 2003;53(2):144–9.
79. Thomas AJ, Perry R, Kalaria RN, Oakley A, McMeekin W, O'Brien JT. Neuropathological evidence for ischemia in the white matter of the dorsolateral prefrontal cortex in late-life depression. Int J Geriatr Psychiatry. 2003;18(1):7–13.
80. Tupler LA, Krishnan KR, McDonald WM, Dombeck CB, D'Souza S, Steffens DC. Anatomic location and laterality of MRI signal hyperintensities in late-life depression. J Psychosom Res. 2002;53(2):665–76.
81. Sneed JR, Roose SP, Keilp JG, Krishnan KR, Alexopoulos GS, Sackeim HA. Response inhibition predicts poor antidepressant treatment response in very old depressed patients. Am J Geriatr Psychiatry. 2007;15(7):553–63.
82. Krishnan KR, Doraiswamy PM, Clary CM. Clinical and treatment response characteristics of late-life depression associated with vascular disease: a pooled analysis of two multicenter trials with sertraline. Prog Neuropsychopharmacol Biol Psychiatry. 2001;25(2):347–61.
83. Salloway S, Correia S, Boyle P, Malloy P, Schneider L, Lavretsky H, et al. MRI subcortical hyperintensities in old and very old depressed outpatients: the important role of age in late-life depression. J Neurol Sci. 2002;203–204:227–33.
84. Alexopoulos GS, Kiosses DN, Choi SJ, Murphy CF, Lim KO. Frontal white matter microstructure and treatment response of late-life depression: a preliminary study. Am J Psychiatry. 2002;159(11):1929–32.
85. Taragano FE, Bagnatti P, Allegri RF. A double-blind, randomized clinical trial to assess the augmentation with nimodipine of antidepressant therapy in the treatment of "vascular depression". Int Psychogeriatr. 2005;17(3):487–98.
86. Ramos-Rios R, Berdullas Barreiro J, Varela-Casal P, Arauxo Vilar A. Vascular depression with melancholic symptoms: response to electroconvulsive therapy. Actas Esp Psiquiatr. 2007;35(6):403–5.
87. Roses AD. The medical and economic roles of pipeline pharmacogenetics: Alzheimer's disease as a model of efficacy and HLA-B(*)5701 as a model of safety. Neuropsychopharmacology. 2009;34(1):6–17.
88. Rapp MA, Schnaider-Beeri M, Grossman HT, Sano M, Perl DP, Purohit DP, et al. Increased hippocampal plaques and tangles in patients with Alzheimer disease with a lifetime history of major depression. Arch Gen Psychiatry. 2006;63(2):161–7.
89. Rubin EH, Veiel LL, Kinscherf DA, Morris JC, Storandt M. Clinically significant depressive symptoms and very mild to mild dementia of the Alzheimer type. Int J Geriatr Psychiatry. 2001;16(7):694–701.
90. Basso MR, Bornstein RA. Relative memory deficits in recurrent versus first-episode major depression on a word-list learning task. Neuropsychology. 1999;13(4):557–63.
91. MacQueen GM, Galway TM, Hay J, Young LT, Joffe RT. Recollection memory deficits in patients with major depressive disorder predicted by past depressions but not current mood state or treatment status. Psychol Med. 2002;32(2):251–8.

92. Rapp MA, Dahlman K, Sano M, Grossman HT, Haroutunian V, Gorman JM. Neuropsychological differences between late-onset and recurrent geriatric major depression. Am J Psychiatry. 2005;162(4):691–8.
93. Steffens DC, Byrum CE, McQuoid DR, Greenberg DL, Payne ME, Blitchington TF, et al. Hippocampal volume in geriatric depression. Biol Psychiatry. 2000;48(4):301–9.
94. Bell-McGinty S, Butters MA, Meltzer CC, Greer PJ, Reynolds CF, III, Becker JT. Brain morphometric abnormalities in geriatric depression: long-term neurobiological effects of illness duration. Am J Psychiatry. 2002;159(8):1424–7.
95. Sheline YI, Sanghavi M, Mintun MA, Gado MH. Depression duration but not age predicts hippocampal volume loss in medically healthy women with recurrent major depression. J Neurosci. 1999;19(12):5034–43.
96. Sun X, Steffens DC, Au R, Folstein M, Summergrad P, Yee J, et al. Amyloid-associated depression: a prodromal depression of Alzheimer disease? Arch Gen Psychiatry. 2008;65(5):542–50.
97. Butters MA, Klunk WE, Mathis CA, Price JC, Ziolko SK, Hoge JA, et al. Imaging Alzheimer pathology in late-life depression with PET and Pittsburgh Compound-B. Alzheimer Dis Assoc Disord. 2008;22(3):261–8.
98. Olin JT, Schneider LS, Katz IR, Meyers BS, Alexopoulos GS, Breitner JC, et al. Provisional diagnostic criteria for depression of Alzheimer disease. Am J Geriatr Psychiatry. 2002;10(2):125–8.
99. Sultzer DL, Levin HS, Mahler ME, High WM, Cummings JL. A comparison of psychiatric symptoms in vascular dementia and Alzheimer's disease. Am J Psychiatry. 1993;150(12):1806–12.
100. Naarding P, de Koning I, dan Kooten F, Dippel DW, Janzing JG, van der Mast RC, et al. Depression in vascular dementia. Int J Geriatr Psychiatry. 2003;18(4):325–30.
101. Alexopoulos GS, Abrams RC, Young RC, Shamoian CA. Cornell Scale for Depression in Dementia. Biol Psychiatry. 1988;23(3):271–84.
102. Steffens DC, Otey E, Alexopoulos GS, Butters MA, Cuthbert B, Ganguli M, et al. Perspectives on depression, mild cognitive impairment, and cognitive decline. Arch Gen Psychiatry. 2006;63(2):130–8.
103. Arve S, Tilvis RS, Lehtonen A, Valvanne J, Sairanen S. Coexistence of lowered mood and cognitive impairment of elderly people in five birth cohorts. Aging (Milano). 1999;11(2):90–5.
104. Yaffe K, Blackwell T, Gore R, Sands L, Reus V, Browner WS. Depressive symptoms and cognitive decline in nondemented elderly women: a prospective study. Arch Gen Psychiatry. 1999;56(5):425–30.
105. Bassuk SS, Berkman LF, Wypij D. Depressive symptomatology and incident cognitive decline in an elderly community sample. Arch Gen Psychiatry. 1998;55(12):1073–81.
106. Ritchie K, Gilham C, Ledesert B, Touchon J, Kotzki PO. Depressive illness, depressive symptomatology and regional cerebral blood flow in elderly people with sub-clinical cognitive impairment. Age Ageing. 1999;28(4):385–91.
107. Chen P, Ganguli M, Mulsant BH, DeKosky ST. The temporal relationship between depressive symptoms and dementia: a community-based prospective study. Arch Gen Psychiatry. 1999;56(3):261–6.
108. Barnes DE, Alexopoulos GS, Lopez OL, Williamson JD, Yaffe K. Depressive symptoms, vascular disease, and mild cognitive impairment: findings from the Cardiovascular Health Study. Arch Gen Psychiatry. 2006;63(3):273–9.
109. Simpson S, Baldwin RC, Jackson A, Burns AS. Is subcortical disease associated with a poor response to antidepressants? Neurological, neuropsychological and neuroradiological findings in late-life depression. Psychol Med. 1998;28(5):1015–26.
110. Potter GG, Kittinger JD, Wagner HR, Steffens DC, Krishnan KR. Prefrontal neuropsychological predictors of treatment remission in late-life depression. Neuropsychopharmacology. 2004;29(12):2266–71.

111. Alexopoulos GS, Kiosses DN, Heo M, Murphy CF, Shanmugham B, Gunning-Dixon F. Executive dysfunction and the course of geriatric depression. Biol Psychiatry. 2005;58(3):204–10.
112. Murphy CF, Alexopoulos GS. Longitudinal association of initiation/perseveration and severity of geriatric depression. Am J Geriatr Psychiatry. 2004;12(1):50–6.
113. Nebes RD, Pollock BG, Houck PR, Butters MA, Mulsant BH, Zmuda MD, et al. Persistence of cognitive impairment in geriatric patients following antidepressant treatment: a randomized, double-blind clinical trial with nortriptyline and paroxetine. J Psychiatr Res. 2003;37(2):99–108.
114. Emanuel EJ, Fairclough DL, Slutsman J, Alpert H, Baldwin D, Emanuel LL. Assistance from family members, friends, paid care givers, and volunteers in the care of terminally ill patients. N Engl J Med. 1999;341(13):956–63.
115. Hensley PL. Treatment of bereavement-related depression and traumatic grief. J Affect Disord. 2006;92(1):117–24.
116. Schulz R, Mendelsohn AB, Haley WE, Mahoney D, Allen RS, Zhang S, et al. End-of-life care and the effects of bereavement on family caregivers of persons with dementia. N Engl J Med. 2003;349(20):1936–42.
117. Schulz R, Boerner K, Shear K, Zhang S, Gitlin LN. Predictors of complicated grief among dementia caregivers: a prospective study of bereavement. Am J Geriatr Psychiatry. 2006;14(8):650–8.
118. Schulz R, Hebert R, Boerner K. Bereavement after caregiving. Geriatrics. 2008;63(1):20–2.
119. Latham AE, Prigerson HG. Suicidality and bereavement: complicated grief as psychiatric disorder presenting greatest risk for suicidality. Suicide Life Threat Behav. 2004;34(4):350–62.
120. Alexopoulos GS, Katz IR, Reynolds CF, III, Carpenter D, Docherty JP. The expert consensus guideline series. Pharmacotherapy of depressive disorders in older patients. Postgrad Med. 2001;Spec No Pharmacotherapy:1–86.
121. Beck AT, Kovacs M, Weissman A. Assessment of suicidal intention: the Scale for Suicide Ideation. J Consult Clin Psychol. 1979;47(2):343–52.
122. Heisel MJ, Flett GL. The development and initial validation of the geriatric suicide ideation scale. Am J Geriatr Psychiatry. 2006;14(9):742–51.
123. Simon GE, Savarino J. Suicide attempts among patients starting depression treatment with medications or psychotherapy. Am J Psychiatry. 2007;164(7):1029–34.
124. Gibbons RD, Brown CH, Hur K, Marcus SM, Bhaumik DK, Mann JJ. Relationship between antidepressants and suicide attempts: an analysis of the Veterans Health Administration data sets. Am J Psychiatry. 2007;164(7):1044–9.
125. Juurlink DN, Mamdani MM, Kopp A, Redelmeier DA. The risk of suicide with selective serotonin reuptake inhibitors in the elderly. Am J Psychiatry. 2006;163(5):813–21.
126. Kessler RC, Nelson CB, McGonagle KA, Liu J, Swartz M, Blazer DG. Comorbidity of DSM-III-R major depressive disorder in the general population: results from the US National Comorbidity Survey. Br J Psychiatry Suppl. 1996(30):17–30.
127. Devanand DP. Comorbid psychiatric disorders in late life depression. Biol Psychiatry. 2002;52(3):236–42.
128. Blixen CE, McDougall GJ, Suen LJ. Dual diagnosis in elders discharged from a psychiatric hospital. Int J Geriatr Psychiatry. 1997;12(3):307–13.
129. Oslin DW, Katz IR, Edell WS, Ten Have TR. Effects of alcohol consumption on the treatment of depression among elderly patients. Am J Geriatr Psychiatry. 2000;8(3):215–20.
130. Cook BL, Winokur G, Garvey MJ, Beach V. Depression and previous alcoholism in the elderly. Br J Psychiatry. 1991;158:72–5.
131. Oslin DW. Treatment of late-life depression complicated by alcohol dependence. Am J Geriatr Psychiatry. 2005;13(6):491–500.
132. Lenze EJ, Mulsant BH, Shear MK, Schulberg HC, Dew MA, Begley AE, et al. Comorbid anxiety disorders in depressed elderly patients. Am J Psychiatry. 2000;157(5):722–8.
133. Mulsant BH, Reynolds CF, III, Shear MK, Sweet RA, Miller M. Comorbid anxiety disorders in late-life depression. Anxiety. 1996;2(5):242–7.

134. Ben-Arie O, Swartz L, Dickman BJ. Depression in the elderly living in the community. Its presentation and features. Br J Psychiatry. 1987;150:169–74.
135. Alexopoulos GS. Anxiety-depression syndromes in old age. Int J Geriatr Psychiatry. 1990(5):351–3.
136. Parmelee PA, Katz IR, Lawton MP. Anxiety and its association with depression among institutionalized elderly. Am J Geriatr Psychiatry. 1993;46:46–58.
137. Henderson AS, Jorm AF, Korten AE, Jacomb P, Christensen H, Rodgers B. Symptoms of depression and anxiety during adult life: evidence for a decline in prevalence with age. Psychol Med. 1998;28(6):1321–8.
138. Lenze EJ, Mulsant BH, Shear MK, Alexopoulos GS, Frank E, Reynolds CF, III. Comorbidity of depression and anxiety disorders in later life. Depress Anxiety. 2001;14(2):86–93.
139. Lenze EJ, Mulsant BH, Mohlman J, Shear MK, Dew MA, Schulz R, et al. Generalized anxiety disorder in late life: lifetime course and comorbidity with major depressive disorder. Am J Geriatr Psychiatry. 2005;13(1):77–80.
140. Kunik ME, Mulsant BH, Rifai AH, Sweet RA, Pasternak R, Zubenko GS. Diagnostic rate of comorbid personality disorder in elderly psychiatric inpatients. Am J Psychiatry. 1994;151(4):603–5.
141. Devanand DP, Turret N, Moody BJ, Fitzsimons L, Peyser S, Mickle K, et al. Personality disorders in elderly patients with dysthymic disorder. Am J Geriatr Psychiatry. 2000;8(3):188–95.
142. Kunik ME, Mulsant BH, Rifai AH, Sweet RA, Pasternak R, Rosen J. Personality Disorders in Elderly Inpatients with Major Depression. Am J Geriatr Psychiatry. 1993;1:38–45.
143. Abrams RC, Alexopoulos GS, Spielman LA, Klausner E, Kakuma T. Personality disorder symptoms predict declines in global functioning and quality of life in elderly depressed patients. Am J Geriatr Psychiatry. 2001;9(1):67–71.
144. Salzman C. A 60-year-old woman who has felt sad for much of her life. JAMA. 2006;295(3):318–23.
145. Morse JQ, Pilkonis PA, Houck PR, Frank E, Reynolds CF, III. Impact of cluster C personality disorders on outcomes of acute and maintenance treatment in late-life depression. Am J Geriatr Psychiatry. 2005;13(9):808–14.
146. Thompson LW, Gallagher D, Czirr R. Personality disorder and outcome in the treatment of late-life depression. J Geriatr Psychiatry. 1988;21(2):133–53.
147. Lynch TR, Cheavens JS, Cukrowicz KC, Thorp SR, Bronner L, Beyer J. Treatment of older adults with co-morbid personality disorder and depression: a dialectical behavior therapy approach. Int J Geriatr Psychiatry. 2007;22(2):131–43.
148. Rapp SR, Vrana S. Substituting nonsomatic for somatic symptoms in the diagnosis of depression in elderly male medical patients. Am J Psychiatry. 1989;146(9):1197–200.
149. Mulsant BH, Pollock BG, Nebes RD, Miller MD, Little JT, Stack J, et al. A double-blind randomized comparison of nortriptyline and paroxetine in the treatment of late-life depression: 6-week outcome. J Clin Psychiatry. 1999;60 Suppl 20:16–20.
150. Dew MA, Whyte EM, Lenze EJ, Houck PR, Mulsant BH, Pollock BG, et al. Recovery from major depression in older adults receiving augmentation of antidepressant pharmacotherapy. Am J Psychiatry. 2007;164(6):892–9.
151. Karp JF, Weiner D, Seligman K, Butters M, Miller M, Frank E, et al. Body pain and treatment response in late-life depression. Am J Geriatr Psychiatry. 2005;13(3):188–94.
152. Karp JF, Scott J, Houck P, Reynolds CF, III, Kupfer DJ, Frank E. Pain predicts longer time to remission during treatment of recurrent depression. J Clin Psychiatry. 2005;66(5):591–7.
153. Mavandadi S, Ten Have TR, Katz IR, Durai UN, Krahn DD, Llorente MD, et al. Effect of depression treatment on depressive symptoms in older adulthood: the moderating role of pain. J Am Geriatr Soc. 2007;55(2):202–11.
154. Wise TN, Wiltse CG, Iosifescu DV, Sheridan M, Xu JY, Raskin J. The safety and tolerability of duloxetine in depressed elderly patients with and without medical comorbidity. Int J Clin Pract. 2007;61(8):1283–93.

155. Raskin J, Wiltse CG, Siegal A, Sheikh J, Xu J, Dinkel JJ, et al. Efficacy of duloxetine on cognition, depression, and pain in elderly patients with major depressive disorder: an 8-week, double-blind, placebo-controlled trial. Am J Psychiatry. 2007;164(6):900–9.
156. Ibor JJ, Carrasco JL, Prieto R, Garcia-Calvo C. Effectiveness and safety of venlafaxine extended release in elderly depressed patients. Arch Gerontol Geriatr. 2008;46(3):317–26.
157. Staab JP, Evans DL. Efficacy of venlafaxine in geriatric depression. Depress Anxiety. 2000;12 Suppl 1:63–8.
158. Kivela S. Treatment of depressive disorders in old age. Curr Opin Psychiatry. 2001;14:387–93.
159. Voils CI, Steffens DC, Flint EP, Bosworth HB. Social support and locus of control as predictors of adherence to antidepressant medication in an elderly population. Am J Geriatr Psychiatry. 2005;13(2):157–65.
160. Sher I, McGinn L, Sirey JA, Meyers B. Effects of caregivers' perceived stigma and causal beliefs on patients' adherence to antidepressant treatment. Psychiatr Serv. 2005;56(5):564–9.
161. Raymond CB, Morgan SG, Caetano PA. Antidepressant utilization in British Columbia from 1996 to 2004: increasing prevalence but not incidence. Psychiatr Serv. 2007;58(1):79–84.
162. Blazer DG, Hybels CF, Fillenbaum GG, Pieper CF. Predictors of antidepressant use among older adults: have they changed over time? Am J Psychiatry. 2005;162(4):705–10.
163. Keith S. Advances in psychotropic formulations. Prog Neuropsychopharmacol Biol Psychiatry. 2006;30(6):996–1008.
164. Katon WJ, Fan MY, Lin EH, Unutzer J. Depressive symptom deterioration in a large primary care-based elderly cohort. Am J Geriatr Psychiatry. 2006;14(3):246–54.
165. Tew JD, Jr., Mulsant BH, Houck PR, Lenze EJ, Whyte EM, Miller MD, et al. Impact of prior treatment exposure on response to antidepressant treatment in late life. Am J Geriatr Psychiatry. 2006;14(11):957–65.
166. Wilson K, Mottram P, Sivanranthan A, Nightingale A. Antidepressant versus placebo for depressed elderly. Cochrane Database Syst Rev. 2001(2):CD000561.
167. Trappler B, Cohen CI. Use of SSRIs in "very old" depressed nursing home residents. Am J Geriatr Psychiatry. 1998;6(1):83–9.
168. Loi CM, Vestal RE. Drug metabolism in the elderly. Pharmacol Ther. 1988;36(1):131–49.
169. von Moltke LL, Greenblatt DJ, Shader RI. Clinical pharmacokinetics of antidepressants in the elderly. Therapeutic implications. Clin Pharmacokinet. 1993;24(2):141–60.
170. O'Mahony MS, Woodhouse KW. Age, environmental factors and drug metabolism. Pharmacol Ther. 1994;61(1–2):279–87.
171. Zubenko GS, Sunderland T. Geriatric psychopharmacology: why does age matter? Harv Rev Psychiatry. 2000;7(6):311–33.
172. Pollock BG. Adverse reactions of antidepressants in elderly patients. J Clin Psychiatry. 1999;60 Suppl 20:4–8.
173. Salzman C. Key concepts in geriatric psychopharmacology. Altered pharmacokinetics and polypharmacy. Psychiatr Clin North Am. 1982;5(1):181–90.
174. von Moltke LL, Greenblatt DJ, Hartmatz JS, Shader RI. Psychotropic drug metabolism in old age: principles and problems of assessment. In: Bloom FE, Kupfer DJ, editors. Psychopharmacology: The fourth generation of progress. New York: Raven; 1995. p. 1461–9.
175. Abernethy DR, Greenblatt DJ, Shader RI. Imipramine and desipramine disposition in the elderly. J Pharmacol Exp Ther. 1985;232(1):183–8.
176. Iber FL, Murphy PA, Connor ES. Age-related changes in the gastrointestinal system. Effects on drug therapy. Drugs Aging. 1994;5(1):34–48.
177. Greenblatt DJ, Harmatz JS, Shader RI. Clinical pharmacokinetics of anxiolytics and hypnotics in the elderly. Therapeutic considerations (Part I). Clin Pharmacokinet. 1991;21(3):165–77.
178. Verbeeck RK, Cardinal JA, Wallace SM. Effect of age and sex on the plasma binding of acidic and basic drugs. Eur J Clin Pharmacol. 1984;27(1):91–7.
179. Young RC, Dhar AK, Hull J, Kakuma T, Alexopoulos GS. Age and nortriptyline concentrations in plasma ultrafiltrate. Int J Geriatr Psychiatry. 2000;15(11):1009–12.
180. Grandison MK, Boudinot FD. Age-related changes in protein binding of drugs: implications for therapy. Clin Pharmacokinet. 2000;38(3):271–90.

181. DeVane CL, Pollock BG. Pharmacokinetic considerations of antidepressant use in the elderly. J Clin Psychiatry. 1999;60 Suppl 20:38–44.
182. Sotaniemi EA, Arranto AJ, Pelkonen O, Pasanen M. Age and cytochrome P450-linked drug metabolism in humans: an analysis of 226 subjects with equal histopathologic conditions. Clin Pharmacol Ther. 1997;61(3):331–9.
183. Schmucker DL, Woodhouse KW, Wang RK, Wynne H, James OF, McManus M, et al. Effects of age and gender on in vitro properties of human liver microsomal monooxygenases. Clin Pharmacol Ther. 1990;48(4):365–74.
184. Loi CM, Parker BM, Cusack BJ, Vestal RE. Aging and drug interactions. III. Individual and combined effects of cimetidine and cimetidine and ciprofloxacin on theophylline metabolism in healthy male and female nonsmokers. J Pharmacol Exp Ther. 1997;280(2):627–37.
185. Pollock BG, Perel JM, Altieri LP, Kirshner M, Fasiczka AL, Houck PR, et al. Debrisoquine hydroxylation phenotyping in geriatric psychopharmacology. Psychopharmacol Bull. 1992;28(2):163–8.
186. May DG, Porter J, Wilkinson GR, Branch RA. Frequency distribution of dapsone N-hydroxylase, a putative probe for P4503A4 activity, in a white population. Clin Pharmacol Ther. 1994;55(5):492–500.
187. Miglioli PA, Pivetta P, Strazzabosco M, Orlando R, Okolicsanyi L, Palatini P. Effect of age on single- and multiple-dose pharmacokinetics of erythromycin. Eur J Clin Pharmacol. 1990;39(2):161–4.
188. Robertson DR, Waller DG, Renwick AG, George CF. Age-related changes in the pharmacokinetics and pharmacodynamics of nifedipine. Br J Clin Pharmacol. 1988;25(3):297–305.
189. Barbhaiya RH, Shukla UA, Greene DS. Single-dose pharmacokinetics of nefazodone in healthy young and elderly subjects and in subjects with renal or hepatic impairment. Eur J Clin Pharmacol. 1995;49(3):221–8.
190. Beyth RJ, Shorr RI. Medication Use. In: Duthie EH, editor. Practice of Geriatrics. Philadelphia: Saunders; 1998.
191. Young RC, Alexopoulos GS, Dhar AK, Kutt H. Plasma 10-hydroxynortriptyline and renal function in elderly depressives. Biol Psychiatry. 1987;22(10):1283–7.
192. Rudorfer MV, Potter WZ. Metabolism of tricyclic antidepressants. Cell Mol Neurobiol. 1999;19(3):373–409.
193. Foglia JP, Pollock BG, Kirshner MA, Rosen J, Sweet R, Mulsant B. Plasma levels of citalopram enantiomers and metabolites in elderly patients. Psychopharmacol Bull. 1997;33(1):109–12.
194. Fredericson Overo K, Toft B, Christophersen L, Gylding-Sabroe JP. Kinetics of citalopram in elderly patients. Psychopharmacology (Berl). 1985;86(3):253–7.
195. Ronfeld RA, Tremaine LM, Wilner KD. Pharmacokinetics of sertraline and its N-demethyl metabolite in elderly and young male and female volunteers. Clin Pharmacokinet. 1997;32 Suppl 1:22–30.
196. Bayer AJ, Roberts NA, Allen EA, Horan M, Routledge PA, Swift CG, et al. The pharmacokinetics of paroxetine in the elderly. Acta Psychiatr Scand Suppl. 1989;350:85–6.
197. Ghose K. The pharmacokinetics of paroxetine in elderly depressed patients. Acta Psychiatr Scand Suppl. 1989;350:87–8.
198. Kaye CM, Haddock RE, Langley PF, Mellows G, Tasker TC, Zussman BD, et al. A review of the metabolism and pharmacokinetics of paroxetine in man. Acta Psychiatr Scand Suppl. 1989;350:60–75.
199. Lundmark J, Scheel Thomsen I, Fjord-Larsen T, Manniche PM, Mengel H, Moller-Nielsen EM, et al. Paroxetine: pharmacokinetic and antidepressant effect in the elderly. Acta Psychiatr Scand Suppl. 1989;350:76–80.
200. De Vries MH, Van Harten J, Van Bemmel P, Raghoebar M. Pharmacokinetics of fluvoxamine maleate after increasing single oral doses in healthy subjects. Biopharm Drug Dispos. 1993;14(4):291–6.
201. Wilens TE, Cohen L, Biederman J, Abrams A, Neft D, Faird N, et al. Fluoxetine pharmacokinetics in pediatric patients. J Clin Psychopharmacol. 2002;22(6):568–75.

202. Klamerus KJ, Maloney K, Rudolph RL, Sisenwine SF, Jusko WJ, Chiang ST. Introduction of a composite parameter to the pharmacokinetics of venlafaxine and its active O-desmethyl metabolite. J Clin Pharmacol. 1992;32(8):716–24.
203. Sweet RA, Pollock BG, Kirshner M, Wright B, Altieri LP, DeVane CL. Pharmacokinetics of single- and multiple-dose bupropion in elderly patients with depression. J Clin Pharmacol. 1995;35(9):876–84.
204. Salzman C, Shader RI, Harmatz J, Robertson L. Psychopharmacologic investigations in elderly volunteers: effect of diazepam in males. J Am Geriatr Soc. 1975;23(10):451–7.
205. Shader RI, Greenblatt DJ, Salzman C, Kochansky GE, Harmatz JS. Benzodiazepines: safety and toxicity. Dis Nerv Syst. 1975;36(5 Pt. 2):23–6.
206. Salzman C, Shader RI, Greenblatt DJ, Harmatz JS. Long v short half-life benzodiazepines in the elderly. Kinetics and clinical effects of diazepam and oxazepam. Arch Gen Psychiatry. 1983;40(3):293–7.
207. Ensrud KE, Blackwell T, Mangione CM, Bowman PJ, Bauer DC, Schwartz A, et al. Central nervous system active medications and risk for fractures in older women. Arch Intern Med. 2003;163(8):949–57.
208. Montgomery SA. Late-life depression: rationalizing pharmacological treatment options. Gerontology. 2002;48(6):392–400.
209. Skerritt U, Evans R, Montgomery SA. Selective serotonin reuptake inhibitors in older patients. A tolerability perspective. Drugs Aging. 1997;10(3):209–18.
210. Mulchahey JJ, Malik MS, Sabai M, Kasckow JW. Serotonin-selective reuptake inhibitors in the treatment of geriatric depression and related disorders. Int J Neuropsychopharmacol. 1999;2(2):121–7.
211. Pollock BG, Mulsant BH, Nebes R, Kirshner MA, Begley AE, Mazumdar S, et al. Serum anticholinergicity in elderly depressed patients treated with paroxetine or nortriptyline. Am J Psychiatry. 1998;155(8):1110–2.
212. Burrows AB, Salzman C, Satlin A, Noble K, Pollock BG, Gersh T. A randomized, placebo-controlled trial of paroxetine in nursing home residents with non-major depression. Depress Anxiety. 2002;15(3):102–10.
213. Malzberg B. Mortality Among Patients with Involutional Melancholia. Am J Psychiatry. 1937;93:1231–8.
214. Dreyfuss F, Dasberg H, Assael MI. The relationship of myocardial infarction to depressive illness. Psychother Psychosom. 1969;17(2):73–81.
215. Pratt LA, Ford DE, Crum RM, Armenian HK, Gallo JJ, Eaton WW. Depression, psychotropic medication, and risk of myocardial infarction. Prospective data from the Baltimore ECA follow-up. Circulation. 1996;94(12):3123–9.
216. Williams SA, Kasl SV, Heiat A, Abramson JL, Krumholz HM, Vaccarino V. Depression and risk of heart failure among the elderly: a prospective community-based study. Psychosom Med. 2002;64(1):6–12.
217. Berkman LF, Berkman CS, Kasl S, Freeman DH, Jr., Leo L, Ostfeld AM, et al. Depressive symptoms in relation to physical health and functioning in the elderly. Am J Epidemiol. 1986;124(3):372–88.
218. Kaplan GA, Roberts RE, Camacho TC, Coyne JC. Psychosocial predictors of depression. Prospective evidence from the human population laboratory studies. Am J Epidemiol. 1987;125(2):206–20.
219. Gatz M, Hurwicz ML. Are old people more depressed? Cross-sectional data on Center for Epidemiological Studies Depression Scale factors. Psychol Aging. 1990;5(2):284–90.
220. Blazer D, Burchett B, Service C, George LK. The association of age and depression among the elderly: an epidemiologic exploration. J Gerontol. 1991;46(6):M210–5.
221. Wassertheil-Smoller S, Applegate WB, Berge K, Chang CJ, Davis BR, Grimm R, Jr., et al. Change in depression as a precursor of cardiovascular events. SHEP Cooperative Research Group (Systoloc Hypertension in the elderly). Arch Intern Med. 1996;156(5):553–61.

222. Ariyo AA, Haan M, Tangen CM, Rutledge JC, Cushman M, Dobs A, et al. Depressive symptoms and risks of coronary heart disease and mortality in elderly Americans. Cardiovascular Health Study Collaborative Research Group. Circulation. 2000;102(15):1773–9.
223. Avery D, Winokur G. Mortality in depressed patients treated with electroconvulsive therapy and antidepressants. Arch Gen Psychiatry. 1976;33(9):1029–37.
224. Sauer WH, Berlin JA, Kimmel SE. Selective serotonin reuptake inhibitors and myocardial infarction. Circulation. 2001;104(16):1894–8.
225. Meier CR, Schlienger RG, Jick H. Use of selective serotonin reuptake inhibitors and risk of developing first-time acute myocardial infarction. Br J Clin Pharmacol. 2001;52(2):179–84.
226. Berkman LF, Blumenthal J, Burg M, Carney RM, Catellier D, Cowan MJ, et al. Effects of treating depression and low perceived social support on clinical events after myocardial infarction: the Enhancing Recovery in Coronary Heart Disease Patients (ENRICHD) Randomized Trial. JAMA. 2003;289(23):3106–16.
227. Rodstein M, Oei LS. Cardiovascular side effects of long-term therapy with tricyclic antidepressants in the aged. J Am Geriatr Soc. 1979;27(5):231–4.
228. Roose SP, Glassman AH, Attia E, Woodring S, Giardina EG, Bigger JT, Jr. Cardiovascular effects of fluoxetine in depressed patients with heart disease. Am J Psychiatry. 1998;155(5):660–5.
229. Strik JJ, Honig A, Lousberg R, Lousberg AH, Cheriex EC, Tuynman-Qua HG, et al. Efficacy and safety of fluoxetine in the treatment of patients with major depression after first myocardial infarction: findings from a double-blind, placebo-controlled trial. Psychosom Med. 2000;62(6):783–9.
230. Shapiro PA, Lesperance F, Frasure-Smith N, O'Connor CM, Baker B, Jiang JW, et al. An open-label preliminary trial of sertraline for treatment of major depression after acute myocardial infarction (the SADHAT Trial). Sertraline Anti-Depressant Heart Attack Trial. Am Heart J. 1999;137(6):1100–6.
231. Boyer WF, Blumhardt CL. The safety profile of paroxetine. J Clin Psychiatry. 1992;53 Suppl:61–6.
232. Dunner DL, Dunbar GC. Optimal dose regimen for paroxetine. J Clin Psychiatry. 1992;53 Suppl:21–6.
233. Hutchinson DR, Tong S, Moon CA, Vince M, Clarke A. Paroxetine in the treatment of elderly depressed patients in general practice: a double-blind comparison with amitriptyline. Int Clin Psychopharmacol. 1992;6 Suppl 4:43–51.
234. Keller MB. Citalopram therapy for depression: a review of 10 years of European experience and data from U.S. clinical trials. J Clin Psychiatry. 2000;61(12):896–908.
235. Carney RM, Blumenthal JA, Stein PK, Watkins L, Catellier D, Berkman LF, et al. Depression, heart rate variability, and acute myocardial infarction. Circulation. 2001;104(17):2024–8.
236. Yeragani VK, Roose S, Mallavarapu M, Radhakrishna RK, Pesce V. Major depression with ischemic heart disease: effects of paroxetine and nortriptyline on measures of nonlinearity and chaos of heart rate. Neuropsychobiology. 2002;46(3):125–35.
237. Johnson EM, Whyte E, Mulsant BH, Pollock BG, Weber E, Begley AE, et al. Cardiovascular changes associated with venlafaxine in the treatment of late-life depression. Am J Geriatr Psychiatry. 2006;14(9):796–802.
238. Ray WA, Griffin MR, Schaffner W, Baugh DK, Melton LJ, III. Psychotropic drug use and the risk of hip fracture. N Engl J Med. 1987;316(7):363–9.
239. Ruthazer R, Lipsitz LA. Antidepressants and falls among elderly people in long-term care. Am J Public Health. 1993;83(5):746–9.
240. Liu B, Anderson G, Mittmann N, To T, Axcell T, Shear N. Use of selective serotonin-reuptake inhibitors or tricyclic antidepressants and risk of hip fractures in elderly people. Lancet. 1998;351(9112):1303–7.
241. Laghrissi-Thode F, Pollock BG, Miller MC, Mulsant BH, Altieri L, Finkel MS. Double-blind comparison of paroxetine and nortriptyline on the postural stability of late-life depressed patients. Psychopharmacol Bull. 1995;31(4):659–63.

242. Joo JH, Lenze EJ, Mulsant BH, Begley AE, Weber EM, Stack JA, et al. Risk factors for falls during treatment of late-life depression. J Clin Psychiatry. 2002;63(10):936–41.
243. Diem SJ, Blackwell TL, Stone KL, Yaffe K, Haney EM, Bliziotes MM, et al. Use of antidepressants and rates of hip bone loss in older women: the study of osteoporotic fractures. Arch Intern Med. 2007;167(12):1240–5.
244. Haney EM, Chan BK, Diem SJ, Ensrud KE, Cauley JA, Barrett-Connor E, et al. Association of low bone mineral density with selective serotonin reuptake inhibitor use by older men. Arch Intern Med. 2007;167(12):1246–51.
245. Richards JB, Papaioannou A, Adachi JD, Joseph L, Whitson HE, Prior JC, et al. Effect of selective serotonin reuptake inhibitors on the risk of fracture. Arch Intern Med. 2007;167(2):188–94.
246. Editorial. Mend the mind, but mind the bones! Balancing benefits and potential skeletal risks of serotonin reuptake inhibitors. Arch Intern Med. 2007;167:1231–2.
247. Coulter DM, Pillans PI. Fluoxetine and extrapyramidal side effects. Am J Psychiatry. 1995;152(1):122–5.
248. Settle EC, Jr. Akathisia and sertraline. J Clin Psychiatry. 1993;54(8):321.
249. Shihabuddin L, Rapport D. Sertraline and extrapyramidal side effects. Am J Psychiatry. 1994;151(2):288.
250. Leo RJ. Movement disorders associated with the serotonin selective reuptake inhibitors. J Clin Psychiatry. 1996;57(10):449–54.
251. Liu BA, Mittmann N, Knowles SR, Shear NH. Hyponatremia and the syndrome of inappropriate secretion of antidiuretic hormone associated with the use of selective serotonin reuptake inhibitors: a review of spontaneous reports. CMAJ. 1996;155(5):519–27.
252. Barclay TS, Lee AJ. Citalopram-associated SIADH. Ann Pharmacother. 2002;36(10):1558–63.
253. Zullino D, Brauchli S, Horvath A, Baumann P. Inappropriate antidiuretic hormone secretion and rhabdomyolysis associated with citalopram. Therapie. 2000;55(5):651–2.
254. Baliga RR, McHardy KC. Syndrome of inappropriate antidiuretic hormone secretion due to fluvoxamine therapy. Br J Clin Pract. 1993;47(2):62–3.
255. Inaguma D, Kitagawa W, Hayashi H, Kanoh T, Kurata K, Kumon S. [Three cases of severe hyponatremia under taking selective serotonin reuptake inhibitor (SSRI)]. Nippon Jinzo Gakkai Shi. 2000;42(8):644–8.
256. Arinzon ZH, Lehman YA, Fidelman ZG, Krasnyansky, II. Delayed recurrent SIADH associated with SSRIs. Ann Pharmacother. 2002;36(7–8):1175–7.
257. Meynaar IA, Peeters AJ, Mulder AH, Ottervanger JP. Syndrome of inappropriate ADH secretion attributed to the serotonin re-uptake inhibitors, venlafaxine and paroxetine. Neth J Med. 1997;50(6):243–5.
258. van der Klooster JM, Peters R, Ashruf RZ, Grootendorst AF. Hyponatraemia and the syndrome of inappropriate antidiuretic hormone secretion with convulsions, coma and pulmonary oedema in a patient using paroxetine. Neth J Med. 1997;51(6):237–9.
259. Monmany J, Vazquez G, Rodriguez J, Domingo P. Syndrome of inappropriate secretion of antidiuretic hormone induced by paroxetine. Arch Intern Med. 1999;159(17):2089–90.
260. Llorente MD, Gorelick M, Silverman MA. Sertraline as the cause of inappropriate antidiuretic hormone secretion. J Clin Psychiatry. 1994;55(12):543–4.
261. Bradley ME, Foote EF, Lee EN, Merkle L. Sertraline-associated syndrome of inappropriate antidiuretic hormone: case report and review of the literature. Pharmacotherapy. 1996;16(4):680–3.
262. Raphael K, Tokeshi J. Hyponatremia associated with sertraline and fluoxetine: a case report. Hawaii Med J. 2002;61(3):46–7.
263. Masood GR, Karki SD, Patterson WR. Hyponatremia with venlafaxine. Ann Pharmacother. 1998;32(1):49–51.
264. Luzecky MH, Burman KD, Schultz ER. The syndrome of inappropriate secretion of antidiuretic hormone associated with amitriptyline administration. South Med J. 1974;67(4):495–7.
265. Beckstrom D, Reding R, Cerletty J. Syndrome of inappropriate antidiuretic hormone secretion associated with amitriptyline administration. JAMA. 1979;241(2):133.

266. Lydiard RB. Desipramine-associated SIADH in an elderly woman: case report. J Clin Psychiatry. 1983;44(4):153–4.
267. Liskin B, Walsh BT, Roose SP, Jackson W. Imipramine-induced inappropriate ADH secretion. J Clin Psychopharmacol. 1984;4(3):146–7.
268. Mitsch RA, Lee AK. Syndrome of inappropriate antidiuretic hormone with imipramine. Drug Intell Clin Pharm. 1986;20(10):787–9.
269. Adlakha A, Manocha AP, Bechard DL. Imipramine-induced syndrome of inappropriate antidiuretic hormone secretion. South Med J. 1991;84(12):1507–9.
270. Colgate R. Hyponatraemia and inappropriate secretion of antidiuretic hormone associated with the use of imipramine. Br J Psychiatry. 1993;163:819–22.
271. Sommer BR. Syndrome of inappropriate antidiuretic hormone (SIADH) in an 80-year-old woman given clomipramine. Am J Geriatr Psychiatry. 1997;5(3):268–9.
272. Peterson JC, Pollack RW, Mahoney JJ, Fuller TJ. Inappropriate antidiuretic hormone secondary to a monamine oxidase inhibitor. JAMA. 1978;239(14):1422–3.
273. Hernandez JL, Ramos FJ, Infante J, Rebollo M, Gonzalez-Macias J. Severe serotonin syndrome induced by mirtazapine monotherapy. Ann Pharmacother. 2002;36(4):641–3.
274. Ubogu EE, Katirji B. Mirtazapine-induced serotonin syndrome. Clin Neuropharmacol. 2003;26(2):54–7.
275. Benazzi F. Serotonin syndrome with mirtazapine-fluoxetine combination. Int J Geriatr Psychiatry. 1998;13(7):495–6.
276. Karki SD, Masood GR. Combination risperidone and SSRI-induced serotonin syndrome. Ann Pharmacother. 2003;37(3):388–91.
277. Solai LK, Mulsant BH, Pollock BG. Selective serotonin reuptake inhibitors for late-life depression: a comparative review. Drugs Aging. 2001;18(5):355–68.
278. Salzman C, Wong E, Wright BC. Drug and ECT treatment of depression in the elderly, 1996–2001: a literature review. Biol Psychiatry. 2002;52(3):265–84.
279. Mottram P, Wilson K, Strobl J. Antidepressants for depressed elderly. Cochrane Database Syst Rev. 2006(1):CD003491.
280. Mittmann N, Herrmann N, Einarson TR, Busto UE, Lanctot KL, Liu BA, et al. The efficacy, safety and tolerability of antidepressants in late life depression: a meta-analysis. J Affect Disord. 1997;46(3):191–217.
281. Brymer C, Winograd CH. Fluoxetine in elderly patients: is there cause for concern? J Am Geriatr Soc. 1992;40(9):902–5.
282. Ensrud KE, Blackwell TL, Ancoli-Israel S, Redline S, Yaffe K, Diem S, et al. Use of selective serotonin reuptake inhibitors and sleep disturbances in community-dwelling older women. J Am Geriatr Soc. 2006;54(10):1508–15.
283. Wongpakaran N, van Reekum R, Wongpakaran T, Clarke D. Selective serotonin reuptake inhibitor use associates with apathy among depressed elderly: a case-control study. Ann Gen Psychiatry. 2007;6:7.
284. Kyle CJ, Petersen HE, Overo KF. Comparison of the tolerability and efficacy of citalopram and amitriptyline in elderly depressed patients treated in general practice. Depress Anxiety. 1998;8(4):147–53.
285. Navarro V, Gasto C, Torres X, Marcos T, Pintor L. Citalopram versus nortriptyline in late-life depression: a 12-week randomized single-blind study. Acta Psychiatr Scand. 2001; 103(6):435–40.
286. Klysner R, Bent-Hansen J, Hansen HL, Lunde M, Pleidrup E, Poulsen DL, et al. Efficacy of citalopram in the prevention of recurrent depression in elderly patients: placebo-controlled study of maintenance therapy. Br J Psychiatry. 2002;181:29–35.
287. Nyth AL, Gottfries CG, Lyby K, Smedegaard-Andersen L, Gylding-Sabroe J, Kristensen M, et al. A controlled multicenter clinical study of citalopram and placebo in elderly depressed patients with and without concomitant dementia. Acta Psychiatr Scand. 1992;86(2):138–45.
288. Saghafi R, Brown C, Butters MA, Cyranowski J, Dew MA, Frank E, et al. Predicting 6-week treatment response to escitalopram pharmacotherapy in late-life major depressive disorder. Int J Geriatr Psychiatry. 2007;22(11):1141–6.

289. Greenblatt DJ, von Moltke LL, Harmatz JS, Shader RI. Drug interactions with newer antidepressants: role of human cytochromes P450. J Clin Psychiatry. 1998;59 Suppl 15:19–27.
290. Lavretsky H, Kim MD, Kumar A, Reynolds CF, III. Combined treatment with methylphenidate and citalopram for accelerated response in the elderly: an open trial. J Clin Psychiatry. 2003;64(12):1410–4.
291. Lavretsky H, Park S, Siddarth P, Kumar A, Reynolds CF, III. Methylphenidate-enhanced antidepressant response to citalopram in the elderly: a double-blind, placebo-controlled pilot trial. Am J Geriatr Psychiatry. 2006;14(2):181–5.
292. Muijsers RB, Plosker GL, Noble S. Sertraline: a review of its use in the management of major depressive disorder in elderly patients. Drugs Aging. 2002;19(5):377–92.
293. Muijsers RB, Plosker GL, Noble S. Spotlight on sertraline in the management of major depressive disorder in elderly patients. CNS Drugs. 2002;16(11):789–94.
294. Bondareff W, Alpert M, Friedhoff AJ, Richter EM, Clary CM, Batzar E. Comparison of sertraline and nortriptyline in the treatment of major depressive disorder in late life. Am J Psychiatry. 2000;157(5):729–36.
295. Furlan PM, Kallan MJ, Ten Have T, Pollock BG, Katz I, Lucki I. Cognitive and psychomotor effects of paroxetine and sertraline on healthy elderly volunteers. Am J Geriatr Psychiatry. 2001;9(4):429–38.
296. Devanand DP, Pelton GH, Marston K, Camacho Y, Roose SP, Stern Y, et al. Sertraline treatment of elderly patients with depression and cognitive impairment. Int J Geriatr Psychiatry. 2003;18(2):123–30.
297. Newhouse PA, Krishnan KR, Doraiswamy PM, Richter EM, Batzar ED, Clary CM. A double-blind comparison of sertraline and fluoxetine in depressed elderly outpatients. J Clin Psychiatry. 2000;61(8):559–68.
298. Finkel SI, Richter EM, Clary CM, Batzar E. Comparative efficacy of sertraline vs. fluoxetine in patients age 70 or over with major depression. Am J Geriatr Psychiatry. 1999;7(3):221–7.
299. Reifler BV, Teri L, Raskind M, Veith R, Barnes R, White E, et al. Double-blind trial of imipramine in Alzheimer's disease patients with and without depression. Am J Psychiatry. 1989;146(1):45–9.
300. Petracca G, Teson A, Chemerinski E, Leiguarda R, Starkstein SE. A double-blind placebo-controlled study of clomipramine in depressed patients with Alzheimer's disease. J Neuropsychiatry Clin Neurosci. 1996;8(3):270–5.
301. Kindermann SS, Brown GG. Depression and memory in the elderly: a meta-analysis. J Clin Exp Neuropsychol. 1997;19(5):625–42.
302. Forlenza OV, Stoppe Junior A, Hirata ES, Ferreira RC. Antidepressant efficacy of sertraline and imipramine for the treatment of major depression in elderly outpatients. Sao Paulo Med J. 2000;118(4):99–104.
303. Forlenza OV, Almeida OP, Stoppe A, Jr., Hirata ES, Ferreira RCR. Antidepressant efficacy and safety of low-dose sertraline and standard-dose imipramine for the treatment of depression in older adults: results from a double-blind, randomized, controlled clinical trial. Int Psychogeriatr. 2001;13(1):75–84.
304. Montgomery SA, Kasper S. Comparison of compliance between serotonin reuptake inhibitors and tricyclic antidepressants: a meta-analysis. Int Clin Psychopharmacol. 1995;9 Suppl 4:33–40.
305. Oslin DW, Streim JE, Katz IR, Smith BD, DiFilippo SD, Ten Have TR, et al. Heuristic comparison of sertraline with nortriptyline for the treatment of depression in frail elderly patients. Am J Geriatr Psychiatry. 2000;8(2):141–9.
306. Weintraub D, Streim JE, Datto CJ, Katz IR, DiFilippo SD, Oslin DW. Effect of increasing the dose and duration of sertraline trial in the treatment of depressed nursing home residents. J Geriatr Psychiatry Neurol. 2003;16(2):109–11.
307. Streim JE, Oslin DW, Katz IR, Smith BD, DiFilippo S, Cooper TB, et al. Drug treatment of depression in frail elderly nursing home residents. Am J Geriatr Psychiatry. 2000;8(2):150–9.
308. Lyketsos CG, Sheppard JM, Steele CD, Kopunek S, Steinberg M, Baker AS, et al. Randomized, placebo-controlled, double-blind clinical trial of sertraline in the treatment of

depression complicating Alzheimer's disease: initial results from the Depression in Alzheimer's Disease study. Am J Psychiatry. 2000;157(10):1686–9.
309. Walters G, Reynolds CF, III, Mulsant BH, Pollock BG. Continuation and maintenance pharmacotherapy in geriatric depression: an open-trial comparison of paroxetine and nortriptyline in patients older than 70 years. J Clin Psychiatry. 1999;60 Suppl 20:21–5.
310. Bump GM, Mulsant BH, Pollock BG, Mazumdar S, Begley AE, Dew MA, et al. Paroxetine versus nortriptyline in the continuation and maintenance treatment of depression in the elderly. Depress Anxiety. 2001;13(1):38–44.
311. Schatzberg AF, Kremer C, Rodrigues HE, Murphy GM, Jr. Double-blind, randomized comparison of mirtazapine and paroxetine in elderly depressed patients. Am J Geriatr Psychiatry. 2002;10(5):541–50.
312. Cassano GB, Puca F, Scapicchio PL, Trabucchi M. Paroxetine and fluoxetine effects on mood and cognitive functions in depressed nondemented elderly patients. J Clin Psychiatry. 2002;63(5):396–402.
313. Reynolds CF, III, Dew MA, Pollock BG, Mulsant BH, Frank E, Miller MD, et al. Maintenance treatment of major depression in old age. N Engl J Med. 2006;354(11):1130–8.
314. Mulsant BH, Pollock BG, Nebes R, Miller MD, Sweet RA, Stack J, et al. A twelve-week, double-blind, randomized comparison of nortriptyline and paroxetine in older depressed inpatients and outpatients. Am J Geriatr Psychiatry. 2001;9(4):406–14.
315. Dalery J, Aubin V. [Comparative study of paroxetine and mianserin in depression in elderly patients: efficacy, tolerance, serotonin dependence]. Encephale. 2001;27(1):71–81.
316. Hoyberg OJ, Maragakis B, Mullin J, Norum D, Stordall E, Ekdahl P, et al. A double-blind multicentre comparison of mirtazapine and amitriptyline in elderly depressed patients. Acta Psychiatr Scand. 1996;93(3):184–90.
317. Weihs KL, Settle EC, Jr., Batey SR, Houser TL, Donahue RM, Ascher JA. Bupropion sustained release versus paroxetine for the treatment of depression in the elderly. J Clin Psychiatry. 2000;61(3):196–202.
318. Steffens DC, Doraiswamy PM, McQuoid DR. Bupropion SR in the naturalistic treatment of elderly patients with major depression. Int J Geriatr Psychiatry. 2001;16(9):862–5.
319. Schatzberg A, Roose S. A double-blind, placebo-controlled study of venlafaxine and fluoxetine in geriatric outpatients with major depression. Am J Geriatr Psychiatry. 2006;14(4):361–70.
320. Nelson JC, Wohlreich MM, Mallinckrodt CH, Detke MJ, Watkin JG, Kennedy JS. Duloxetine for the treatment of major depressive disorder in older patients. Am J Geriatr Psychiatry. 2005;13(3):227–35.
321. Alexopoulos GS, Salzman C. Treatment of depression with heterocyclic antidepressants, monoamine oxidase inhibitors, and psychomotor stimulants. In: Salzman C, editor. Clinical Geriatric Pharmacology. Baltimore: Williams & Wilkins; 1998. p. 184–244.
322. Reynolds CF, III, Frank E, Perel JM, Imber SD, Cornes C, Miller MD, et al. Nortriptyline and interpersonal psychotherapy as maintenance therapies for recurrent major depression: a randomized controlled trial in patients older than 59 years. JAMA. 1999;281(1):39–45.
323. Reynolds CF, III, Perel JM, Frank E, Cornes C, Miller MD, Houck PR, et al. Three-year outcomes of maintenance nortriptyline treatment in late-life depression: a study of two fixed plasma levels. Am J Psychiatry. 1999;156(8):1177–81.
324. Lenze EJ, Dew MA, Mazumdar S, Begley AE, Cornes C, Miller MD, et al. Combined pharmacotherapy and psychotherapy as maintenance treatment for late-life depression: effects on social adjustment. Am J Psychiatry. 2002;159(3):466–8.
325. Marraccini RL, Reynolds CF, III, Houck PR, Miller MD, Frank E, Perel JM, et al. A double-blind, placebo-controlled assessment of nortriptyline's side-effects during 3-year maintenance treatment in elderly patients with recurrent major depression. Int J Geriatr Psychiatry. 1999;14(12):1014–8.
326. Dew MA, Reynolds CF, III, Mulsant B, Frank E, Houck PR, Mazumdar S, et al. Initial recovery patterns may predict which maintenance therapies for depression will keep older adults well. J Affect Disord. 2001;65(2):155–66.

327. Pomara N, Shao B, Choi SJ, Tun H, Suckow RF. Sex-related differences in nortriptyline-induced side-effects among depressed patients. Prog Neuropsychopharmacol Biol Psychiatry. 2001;25(5):1035–48.
328. Gasto C, Navarro V, Marcos T, Portella MJ, Torra M, Rodamilans M. Single-blind comparison of venlafaxine and nortriptyline in elderly major depression. J Clin Psychopharmacol. 2003;23(1):21–6.
329. Cohn JB, Varga L, Lyford A. A two-center double-blind study of nomifensine, imipramine, and placebo in depressed geriatric outpatients. J Clin Psychiatry. 1984;45(4 Pt 2):68–72.
330. Merideth CH, Feighner JP, Hendrickson G. A double-blind comparative evaluation of the efficacy and safety of nomifensine, imipramine, and placebo in depressed geriatric outpatients. J Clin Psychiatry. 1984;45(4 Pt 2):73–7.
331. Gerner R, Estabrook W, Steuer J, Jarvik L. Treatment of geriatric depression with trazodone, imipramine, and placebo: a double-blind study. J Clin Psychiatry. 1980;41(6):216–20.
332. Schweizer E, Rickels K, Hassman H, Garcia-Espana F. Buspirone and imipramine for the treatment of major depression in the elderly. J Clin Psychiatry. 1998;59(4):175–83.
333. Branconnier RJ, Cole JO, Ghazvinian S, Rosenthal S. Treating the depressed elderly patient: the comparative behavioral pharmacology of mianserin and amitriptyline. Adv Biochem Psychopharmacol. 1982;32:195–212.
334. Bird H, Broggini M. Paroxetine versus amitriptyline for treatment of depression associated with rheumatoid arthritis: a randomized, double blind, parallel group study. J Rheumatol. 2000;27(12):2791–7.
335. Thompson LW, Coon DW, Gallagher-Thompson D, Sommer BR, Koin D. Comparison of desipramine and cognitive/behavioral therapy in the treatment of elderly outpatients with mild-to-moderate depression. Am J Geriatr Psychiatry. 2001;9(3):225–40.
336. Devanand DP, Nobler MS, Singer T, Kiersky JE, Turret N, Roose SP, et al. Is dysthymia a different disorder in the elderly? Am J Psychiatry. 1994;151(11):1592–9.
337. Devanand DP, Nobler MS, Cheng J, Turret N, Pelton GH, Roose SP, et al. Randomized, double-blind, placebo-controlled trial of fluoxetine treatment for elderly patients with dysthymic disorder. Am J Geriatr Psychiatry. 2005;13(1):59–68.
338. Williams JW, Jr., Barrett J, Oxman T, Frank E, Katon W, Sullivan M, et al. Treatment of dysthymia and minor depression in primary care: a randomized controlled trial in older adults. JAMA. 2000;284(12):1519–26.
339. Rosen J, Mulsant BH, Pollock BG. Sertraline in the treatment of minor depression in nursing home residents: a pilot study. Int J Geriatr Psychiatry. 2000;15(2):177–80.
340. Thompson TL, 2nd, Moran MG, Nies AS. Drug therapy: psychotropic drug use in the elderly (first of two parts). N Engl J Med. 1983;308(3):134–8.
341. Ancoli-Israel S. Sleep and its disorders in aging populations. Sleep Med. 2009;10 Suppl 1:S7–11.
342. Salzman C. Pharmacologic treatment of disturbed sleep in the elderly. Harv Rev Psychiatry. 2008;16(5):271–8.
343. Ancoli-Israel S, Ayalon L, Salzman C. Sleep in the elderly: normal variations and common sleep disorders. Harv Rev Psychiatry. 2008;16(5):279–86.
344. Salzman C, Jeste DV, Meyer RE, Cohen-Mansfield J, Cummings J, Grossberg GT, et al. Elderly patients with dementia-related symptoms of severe agitation and aggression: consensus statement on treatment options, clinical trials methodology, and policy. J Clin Psychiatry. 2008;69(6):889–98.
345. Li YS, Meyer JS, Thornby J. Longitudinal follow-up of depressive symptoms among normal versus cognitively impaired elderly. Int J Geriatr Psychiatry. 2001;16(7):718–27.
346. Thompson S, Herrmann N, Rapoport MJ, Lanctot KL. Efficacy and safety of antidepressants for treatment of depression in Alzheimer's disease: a metaanalysis. Can J Psychiatry. 2007;52(4):248–55.
347. Lyketsos CG, DelCampo L, Steinberg M, Miles Q, Steele CD, Munro C, et al. Treating depression in Alzheimer disease: efficacy and safety of sertraline therapy, and the benefits of depression reduction: the DIADS. Arch Gen Psychiatry. 2003;60(7):737–46.

348. Petracca GM, Chemerinski E, Starkstein SE. A double-blind, placebo-controlled study of fluoxetine in depressed patients with Alzheimer's disease. Int Psychogeriatr. 2001;13(2):233–40.
349. Streim JE, Porsteinsson AP, Breder CD, Swanink R, Marcus R, McQuade R, et al. A randomized, double-blind, placebo-controlled study of aripiprazole for the treatment of psychosis in nursing home patients with Alzheimer disease. Am J Geriatr Psychiatry. 2008;16(7):537–50.
350. Sultzer DL, Gray KF, Gunay I, Wheatley MV, Mahler ME. Does behavioral improvement with haloperidol or trazodone treatment depend on psychosis or mood symptoms in patients with dementia? J Am Geriatr Soc. 2001;49(10):1294–300.
351. Raji MA, Brady SR. Mirtazapine for treatment of depression and comorbidities in Alzheimer disease. Ann Pharmacother. 2001;35(9):1024–7.
352. Nelson JC, Holden K, Roose S, Salzman C, Hollander SB, Betzel JV. Are there predictors of outcome in depressed elderly nursing home residents during treatment with mirtazapine orally disintegrating tablets? Int J Geriatr Psychiatry. 2007;22(10):999–1003.
353. Gauthier S, Feldman H, Hecker J, Vellas B, Ames D, Subbiah P, et al. Efficacy of donepezil on behavioral symptoms in patients with moderate to severe Alzheimer's disease. Int Psychogeriatr. 2002;14(4):389–404.
354. Lu PH, Edland SD, Teng E, Tingus K, Petersen RC, Cummings JL. Donepezil delays progression to AD in MCI subjects with depressive symptoms. Neurology. 2009;72(24):2115–21.
355. Reisberg B, Doody R, Stoffler A, Schmitt F, Ferris S, Mobius HJ. Memantine in moderate-to-severe Alzheimer's disease. N Engl J Med. 2003;348(14):1333–41.
356. Gauthier S, Wirth Y, Mobius HJ. Effects of memantine on behavioural symptoms in Alzheimer's disease patients: an analysis of the Neuropsychiatric Inventory (NPI) data of two randomised, controlled studies. Int J Geriatr Psychiatry. 2005;20(5):459–64.
357. Pasternak RE, Reynolds CF, III, Schlernitzauer M, Hoch CC, Buysse DJ, Houck PR, et al. Acute open-trial nortriptyline therapy of bereavement-related depression in late life. J Clin Psychiatry. 1991;52(7):307–10.
358. Zisook S, Shuchter SR, Pedrelli P, Sable J, Deaciuc SC. Bupropion sustained release for bereavement: results of an open trial. J Clin Psychiatry. 2001;62(4):227–30.
359. Zygmont M, Prigerson HG, Houck PR, Miller MD, Shear MK, Jacobs S, et al. A post hoc comparison of paroxetine and nortriptyline for symptoms of traumatic grief. J Clin Psychiatry. 1998;59(5):241–5.
360. Shear MK, Zuckoff A, Frank E. The syndrome of traumatic grief. CNS Spectr. 2001;6(4):339–46.
361. Shear MK, Frank E, Foa E, Cherry C, Reynolds CF, III, Vander Bilt J, et al. Traumatic grief treatment: a pilot study. Am J Psychiatry. 2001;158(9):1506–8.
362. Simon NM, Shear MK, Fagiolini A, Frank E, Zalta A, Thompson EH, et al. Impact of concurrent naturalistic pharmacotherapy on psychotherapy of complicated grief. Psychiatry Res. 2008;159(1–2):31–6.
363. Wagner B, Knaevelsrud C, Maercker A. Internet-based cognitive-behavioral therapy for complicated grief: a randomized controlled trial. Death Stud. 2006;30(5):429–53.
364. Wagner B, Maercker A. A 1.5-year follow-up of an Internet-based intervention for complicated grief. J Trauma Stress. 2007;20(4):625–9.
365. Hensley PL, Slonimski CK, Uhlenhuth EH, Clayton PJ. Escitalopram: an open-label study of bereavement-related depression and grief. J Affect Disord. 2009;113(1–2):142–9.
366. Reynolds CF, III, Miller MD, Pasternak RE, Frank E, Perel JM, Cornes C, et al. Treatment of bereavement-related major depressive episodes in later life: a controlled study of acute and continuation treatment with nortriptyline and interpersonal psychotherapy. Am J Psychiatry. 1999;156(2):202–8.
367. Robinson RG. Vascular depression and poststroke depression: where do we go from here? Am J Geriatr Psychiatry. 2005;13(2):85–7.
368. Simonsick EM, Wallace RB, Blazer DG, Berkman LF. Depressive symptomatology and hypertension-associated morbidity and mortality in older adults. Psychosom Med. 1995;57(5):427–35.

369. Roose SP, Glassman AH, Seidman SN. Relationship between depression and other medical illnesses. JAMA. 2001;286(14):1687–90.
370. Whyte EM, Mulsant BH. Post stroke depression: epidemiology, pathophysiology, and biological treatment. Biol Psychiatry. 2002;52(3):253–64.
371. Robinson RG, Schultz SK, Paradiso S. Treatment of Poststroke psychiatric disorders. In: Nelson JC, editor. Geriatric Psychopharmacology. New York: Marcel Deckker; 1998. p. 161–85.
372. Robinson RG, Schultz SK, Castillo C, Kopel T, Kosier JT, Newman RM, et al. Nortriptyline versus fluoxetine in the treatment of depression and in short-term recovery after stroke: a placebo-controlled, double-blind study. Am J Psychiatry. 2000;157(3):351–9.
373. Cole MG, Elie LM, McCusker J, Bellavance F, Mansour A. Feasibility and effectiveness of treatments for post-stroke depression in elderly inpatients: systematic review. J Geriatr Psychiatry Neurol. 2001;14(1):37–41.
374. Wiart L, Petit H, Joseph PA, Mazaux JM, Barat M. Fluoxetine in early poststroke depression: a double-blind placebo-controlled study. Stroke. 2000;31(8):1829–32.
375. Fruehwald S, Gatterbauer E, Rehak P, Baumhackl U. Early fluoxetine treatment of post-stroke depression--a three-month double-blind placebo-controlled study with an open-label long-term follow up. J Neurol. 2003;250(3):347–51.
376. Spalletta G, Guida G, Caltagirone C. Is left stroke a risk-factor for selective serotonin reuptake inhibitor antidepressant treatment resistance? J Neurol. 2003;250(4):449–55.
377. Narushima K, Kosier JT, Robinson RG. Preventing poststroke depression: a 12-week double-blind randomized treatment trial and 21-month follow-up. J Nerv Ment Dis. 2002;190(5):296–303.
378. Philibert RA, Richards L, Lynch CF, Winokur G. Effect of ECT on mortality and clinical outcome in geriatric unipolar depression. J Clin Psychiatry. 1995;56(9):390–4.
379. Tomac TA, Rummans TA, Pileggi TS, Li H. Safety and efficacy of electroconvulsive therapy in patients over age 85. Am J Geriatr Psychiatry. 1997;5(2):126–30.
380. Flint AJ, Rifat SL. Two-year outcome of psychotic depression in late life. Am J Psychiatry. 1998;155(2):178–83.
381. Flint AJ, Rifat SL. The treatment of psychotic depression in later life: a comparison of pharmacotherapy and ECT. Int J Geriatr Psychiatry. 1998;13(1):23–8.
382. Gormley N, Cullen C, Walters L, Philpot M, Lawlor B. The safety and efficacy of electroconvulsive therapy in patients over age 75. Int J Geriatr Psychiatry. 1998;13(12):871–4.
383. Stoudemire A, Hill CD, Marquardt M, Dalton S, Lewison BJ. Recovery and relapse in geriatric depression after treatment with antidepressants and ECT in a medical-psychiatric population. Gen Hosp Psychiatry. 1998;20(3):170–4.
384. Tew JD, Jr., Mulsant BH, Haskett RF, Prudic J, Thase ME, Crowe RR, et al. Acute efficacy of ECT in the treatment of major depression in the old-old. Am J Psychiatry. 1999;156(12):1865–70.
385. Brodaty H, Hickie I, Mason C, Prenter L. A prospective follow-up study of ECT outcome in older depressed patients. J Affect Disord. 2000;60(2):101–11.
386. de Carle AJ, Kohn R. Electroconvulsive therapy and falls in the elderly. J ECT. 2000;16(3):252–7.
387. Manly DT, Oakley SP, Jr., Bloch RM. Electroconvulsive therapy in old-old patients. Am J Geriatr Psychiatry. 2000;8(3):232–6.
388. Rao V, Lyketsos CG. The benefits and risks of ECT for patients with primary dementia who also suffer from depression. Int J Geriatr Psychiatry. 2000;15(8):729–35.
389. O'Connor MK, Knapp R, Husain M, Rummans TA, Petrides G, Smith G, et al. The influence of age on the response of major depression to electroconvulsive therapy: a C.O.R.E. Report. Am J Geriatr Psychiatry. 2001;9(4):382–90.
390. Gagne GG, Jr., Furman MJ, Carpenter LL, Price LH. Efficacy of continuation ECT and antidepressant drugs compared to long-term antidepressants alone in depressed patients. Am J Psychiatry. 2000;157(12):1960–5.

391. APA. A Task Force Report of the American Psychiatric Association. Washington, D.C.: American Psychiatric Association, 2001.
392. Marano CM, Phatak P, Vemulapalli UR, Sasan A, Nalbandyan MR, Ramanujam S, et al. Increased plasma concentration of brain-derived neurotrophic factor with electroconvulsive therapy: a pilot study in patients with major depression. J Clin Psychiatry. 2007;68(4):512–7.
393. Spar JE, LaRue A. Concise Guide to Geriatric Psychiatry. Washington, D.C.: American Psychiatric Publishing; 2002.
394. Whyte EM, Rovner B. Depression in late-life: shifting the paradigm from treatment to prevention. Int J Geriatr Psychiatry. 2006;21(8):746–51.

Treatment of Psychotic Disorders

Oliver Freudenreich and Donald C. Goff

Introduction

Depression is common among patients with schizophrenia and is associated with a wide range of poor outcomes, including psychotic relapse and suicide. Although some dysphoria may be an adverse medication effect from conventional neuroleptics and some depressive reactions may follow resolution of a psychotic episode or represent demoralization, often depression appears to be a chronic, comorbid condition that can be present throughout the entire course of the illness, from prodromal schizophrenia to aging schizophrenia patients.

In this chapter, the epidemiology and clinical characteristics of depression in schizophrenia are briefly reviewed, including differential diagnosis of depressive symptoms and dysphoria. The older literature describing augmentation of conventional neuroleptics is also reviewed, along with the studies of electroconvulsive therapy. Evidence suggesting that the newer atypical antipsychotics possess antidepressant efficacy is presented. Unfortunately, very little data are available regarding augmentation of atypical agents when depressive symptoms persist, although addition of antidepressants is a common practice. For this reason, potential pharmacokinetic interactions between atypical antipsychotics and selective serotonin reuptake inhibitors will be outlined.

Prevalence and Course of Depression in Schizophrenia

Depression is common in schizophrenia and may represent a core symptom cluster of the illness. Factor analyses of individual items of the Positive and Negative Syndrome Scale (PANSS) in large samples of patients with schizophrenia have

O. Freudenreich (✉)
Schizophrenia Program, Massachusetts General Hospital, Freedom Trail Clinic, 25 Staniford Street, Boston, MA 02114, USA
and
Harvard Medical School, Boston, MA, USA
e-mail: ofreudenreich@partners.org

D.A. Ciraulo and R.I. Shader (eds.), *Pharmacotherapy of Depression*,
DOI 10.1007/978-1-60327-435-7_4, © Springer Science+Business Media, LLC 2011

identified a symptom cluster representing depression and anxiety, which remains consistent even after treatment with an atypical antipsychotic (1, 2). Rates of depressive episodes have varied from 20 to 80% between schizophrenia patient samples, reflecting in part differing definitions of depression and assessment methods (3, 4). Most studies have identified dysphoric mood only or threshold scores on depression rating scales rather than establishing a diagnosis of major depression. Siris (5) calculated a modal depression rate of 25% derived from over three dozen published studies in schizophrenia patients. Although subsyndromal depressive symptoms are consistently found in the majority of patients, the prevalence of full major depression is quite variable between studies (6, 7).

Depressive symptoms can occur at any time period during the course of schizophrenia (8). The schizophrenia prodrome is frequently associated with depression, which often becomes the initial target of treatment until psychotic symptoms emerge and the diagnosis of schizophrenia is established (7). In a prospective study of 29 prodromal patients, 28% were diagnosed with a current DSM-IV depressive disorder, and 59% had a life-time diagnosis for a DSM-IV depressive disorder (9). Clinically-significant depressive symptoms have been reported in as many as 75% of first episode patients (10). A significant minority of first-episode patients fulfill syndromal severity criteria for major depression in their first psychotic episode. For example, 23% of patients who were part of a large, epidemiologically defined first-episode sample fulfilled the ICD-10 criteria for a current depressive episode when they were evaluated at first admission (11). Once treatment for the first psychotic episode is initiated and psychosis during this acute illness phase resolves, the high rate of clinically-relevant comorbid depressive syndromes characteristic of first-episode cohorts decreases, for example, from a point prevalence of 62.8% during the first episode to 33.3% 6 months after hospital admission in the aforementioned epidemiological cohort study. However, depression remains a clinical problem beyond the prodrome and first episode of psychosis. Data again from the longitudinal cohort study of first-episode schizophrenia showed that 106 out of 107 patients experienced at least one depressive syndrome during a 12-year follow-up period (12). In any given month, 30–35% of patients experienced at least one of the core symptoms of the depressive syndrome. Depression is also common among older schizophrenia patients. Jin et al. (13) reported that 66% of elderly schizophrenia outpatients scored in the moderate-to-severe range on the Hamilton Depression Rating Scale. Hogarty et al. (14) found that most "distressed" schizophrenia patients experience chronic depression, often accompanied by anxiety, rather than discrete, time-limited episodes of depression.

Although certain features of depression, such as anergia, psychomotor retardation, and anhedonia, overlap with the negative symptoms of schizophrenia, usually the two syndromes can be differentiated based on the presence or absence of dysphoric mood (15). The Calgary Depression Scale for Schizophrenia (CDSS) was developed specifically to distinguish depressive symptoms from the deficit syndrome by identifying depressive symptoms that do not overlap with negative symptoms (16). Despite the partial phenomenological overlap with negative symptoms, in several studies the severity of depression correlated positively with the severity of psychotic symptoms rather than negative symptoms (6, 17, 18).

Functional Consequences of Depression in Schizophrenia

The presence of depression at the onset of schizophrenia has been associated with a favorable outcome in some studies (19). However, comorbid depressive symptoms generally carry a high illness burden since they are associated with increased risk for suicide and relapse, involvement with law enforcement agencies as well as poorer quality of life (20). In a survey of older schizophrenia outpatients, depressive symptoms were significantly associated with worse everyday functioning (13). In a large prospective clinical trial, improvement of mood with risperidone or olanzapine significantly correlated with improved quality of life scores (21). Improved interpersonal relationships represented the factor most strongly correlated with reductions in depression. Furthermore, worsening of depressive symptoms also significantly predicted a relapse over a 4-week period (22). Several other studies have also linked depressive symptoms to relapse in schizophrenia patients (23, 24). In addition, comorbid depression has been identified as a significant risk factor contributing to the high incidence of suicide in schizophrenia patients (23, 25–27). Depression correlates with the degree of illness insight in first-episode patients (28), a correlation that appears to have clinical significance: Crumlish et al. (29) found that good insight 6 months after presentation with a first-episode of psychosis predicted depression and attempted suicide at 4 years.

Differential Diagnosis of Depression in Schizophrenia

The first step in treating depression in a schizophrenia patient should involve a careful diagnostic assessment (3). Depressive symptoms may reflect conditions other than comorbid endogenous depression. Negative symptoms, including anhedonia, social isolation, constricted affect, and apathy, may mimic depression, although as discussed previously, the absence of depressed mood usually distinguishes negative symptoms, or the deficit syndrome, from depression. Antipsychotics, in particular the conventional neuroleptics, can produce side effects that also may be mistaken for depression. The mask-like facies, psychomotor retardation, and dysphoria of neuroleptic-induced parkinsonism may resemble depression, but can be distinguished on the basis of tremor, increased muscle tone, and impaired gait. Neuroleptics may also produce dysphoria as an isolated side effect, which presents with a sense of physical discomfort and anxiety (30); neuroleptic-induced dysphoria may be accompanied by akinesia, or agitation, but is not accompanied by neurovegetative symptoms of depression (31, 32). In theory, neuroleptic dose reduction or addition of an anticholinergic agent should improve neuroleptic-induced dysphoria, although Hogarty et al. (14) found no improvement in dysphoria with increasing doses of anticholinergic medication and only modest improvements 6 weeks after fluphenazine dose reduction. Switching a patient to an atypical antipsychotic represents a more compelling strategy for eliminating neuroleptic-induced dysphoria (33).

Substance abuse also may contribute to dysphoric mood in schizophrenia patients. Almost half of schizophrenia patients surveyed in the Epidemiologic Catchment Area

Study (34) reported abusing drugs, with alcohol and stimulants being the most frequently abused substances. Self-reporting of substance abuse is notoriously unreliable among schizophrenia patients (35), making assessment of the contribution of alcohol and stimulants to dysphoric mood quite difficult. Studies of schizophrenia patients who use cocaine have consistently reported elevated levels of depression and anxiety associated with cocaine use; dramatic increases in hospitalization rates during periods of cocaine ingestion have also been observed (36, 37). Alcohol can cause depression, as can a host of medications such as antihypertensives, steroids, or interferon.

After other medical etiologies of dysphoria have been ruled-out, the clinician should assess whether the patient has affective symptoms complicating schizophrenia, versus a primary affective disorder with psychotic features, such as bipolar disorder or psychotic depression. The distinction between schizoaffective disorder, depressed type, and schizophrenia with superimposed depression is of unclear clinical or theoretical significance, not to mention of uncertain diagnostic reliability (38).

When affective symptoms complicate schizophrenia, they can do so concurrent with or without acute psychosis (39). Depressive symptoms in conjunction with acute psychotic exacerbations frequently recede as psychosis recedes (10), although persistent depression can develop in the post-psychotic period (40). However, most recent studies of "post-psychotic depression" have indicated that depression usually is present at the earliest stages of the illness and becomes more prominent as the florid psychotic symptoms resolve with treatment (41, 42). Any stipulated temporal relationship in post-psychotic depressions with the acute psychotic episode has been further called into question by the finding of similar incident rates of depressive episode within 12 months following a psychotic episode (i.e., the ICD-10 "post-schizophrenic depression" time cut-off) and outside this time period (43). Depression in remitted schizophrenia patients (i.e., without active psychosis) can develop acutely and can herald an impending psychotic relapse (44). Dysphoria can also indicate psychosocial stress that could lead to an adjustment disorder with depression and anxiety. In this case, environmental and interpersonal stressors should be identified and remedied if possible. Some patients with schizophrenia experience chronic depression. Depression and dysphoria experienced by individuals with schizophrenia may in some cases reflect demoralization, especially early in the course of the illness as patients first come to terms with the devastating effects of schizophrenia upon their lives. Psychoeducational interventions and supportive counseling for patients and family members are crucial to assist this coping process, but depressed mood in most cases should not be viewed solely as an appropriate psychological reaction to losses associated with the illness.

Treatment

Atypical Antipsychotics

In the landmark Clozapine Collaborative Study, Kane et al. (45) demonstrated a significant reduction in a broad range of symptoms with clozapine compared with chlorpromazine in refractory schizophrenia patients. Depressive symptoms and anxiety were among the symptom clusters that displayed a preferential response to clozapine. Subsequent trials with other atypical antipsychotic agents have found superior efficacy against depressive symptoms, best demonstrated with olanzapine, risperidone, and ziprasidone (2, 33, 46, 47). Although the atypical antipsychotics appear to possess greater antidepressant efficacy than the conventional agents, it is unclear whether significant differences in antidepressant efficacy exist between atypical antipsychotics (48). Comparisons between risperidone and olanzapine have found inconsistent differences (22, 49, 50). A meta-analysis of the North American trials of risperidone found that risperidone 6 mg daily produced a larger antidepressant effect compared with haloperidol 20 mg daily, with a between-treatment group effect size of 0.30, which was larger than effect sizes for other symptom domains (2). However, risperidone monotherapy was less effective than the combination of haloperidol and amitriptyline in a 6-week trial involving 123 patients with psychosis and depression. The superior efficacy of haloperidol and amitriptyline was most apparent in patients with psychotic depression; no significant difference was found between the two treatments in depressed schizophrenia patients and patients with schizoaffective disorder, depressed type. Of note, olanzapine was found to enhance antidepressant efficacy when added to fluoxetine in patients with treatment-resistant unipolar depression, but produced only modest antidepressant effects when administered as monotherapy (51).

Electroconvulsive Therapy

A largely uncontrolled literature supports the use of electroconvulsive therapy (ECT) in treatment-refractory schizophrenia (52, 53). In general, treatment has been found most effective when administered early in the course of the illness; the presence of affective symptoms has predicted a positive outcome in some studies, but not all. ECT has not been studied in schizophrenia patients with comorbid major depression, but has shown efficacy for depressive and anxiety symptoms in samples of treatment-resistant and first-episode patients (52, 54). The effect on depressive symptoms has been of a smaller magnitude than the effect on positive symptoms, although this could reflect the absence of major depression and possibly a confusion between negative and depressive symptoms on the rating scales employed.

Augmentation of Antipsychotics

Efficacy

In 1989, Kramer et al. (55) published results from a 4-week, placebo-controlled trial of desipramine and amitriptyline in 58 acutely decompensated schizophrenia patients who remained depressed after 5 weeks of haloperidol monotherapy. The tricyclic antidepressants did not enhance resolution of depressive symptoms compared with placebo and appeared to retard the response of psychotic symptoms. This rigorous study was a major factor in subsequent recommendations that antidepressants not be prescribed in acutely psychotic depressed schizophrenia patients (56). In contrast, studies conducted in patients whose psychosis had been fully stabilized with conventional neuroleptics tended to find more positive results. Singh et al. (57) added trazodone 150–300 mg daily to phenothiazines in a 6-week placebo-controlled trial involving 60 chronic schizophrenia patients with "marked depressive symptoms." Trazodone was associated with significant reduction in Hamilton Depression Scale scores compared with placebo, without worsening of psychosis. In a series of studies culminating in a placebo-controlled trial, Siris et al. (58) similarly demonstrated that imipramine 200 mg daily significantly improved depressive symptoms when added to depot fluphenazine for 6 weeks in 33 schizophrenia patients with major or minor depression who were not actively psychotic. All subjects were treated with benztropine to minimize neuroleptic-induced akinesia. Imipramine was not associated with worsening of psychosis, but did improve measures of negative symptoms (59). Siris et al. (60) subsequently demonstrated that maintenance treatment with imipramine can prevent relapse of depression in patients who responded to an initial course of treatment. Hogarty et al. (14) randomly assigned 57 persistently depressed or anxious schizophrenia patients to augmentation of low-dose fluphenazine decanoate with either desipramine, lithium, or placebo. At 6 weeks, desipramine augmentation did not differ from placebo, but at the end of the 12-week study significant reductions in depression, anxiety, and psychosis were observed in the desipramine group compared with that of placebo. Response to desipramine was most evident among female subjects and did not correlate with serum desipramine blood levels. There was no evidence of psychotic exacerbation or relapse in patients treated with desipramine. Similarly, lithium 900–1,200 mg/day was associated with significant improvement in anxiety and depression compared with placebo at week 12. Unlike desipramine, the lithium-treated group exhibited an increase in ratings of akinesia and akathisia.

Results from other placebo-controlled trials of antidepressants added to conventional neuroleptics in schizophrenia have been less positive. Prusoff et al. (61) randomized 40 schizophrenia patients with elevated depression scores to amitriptyline 100–200 mg/day or placebo added to perphenazine for 1–6 months. Hamilton Depression Scale scores were significantly reduced in the amitriptyline group; however, ratings of thought disorder and agitation showed significant worsening with amitriptyline when compared with placebo and the drop-out rate was 47% at 4 months. Waehrens and Gerlach (62) found no effect with maprotiline 50–200 mg/day added to neuroleptics in 20 schizophrenia patients in a 6-week, placebo controlled cross-over trial. Subjects had been stabilized for at least 2 months on neuroleptics and were selected for study on the basis of elevated anergia ratings on the BPRS, rather than meeting formal criteria for depression. Finally, no effect was found by Johnson (63) when nortriptyline 75–150 mg/day was added for 5 weeks to low-dose fluphenazine or flupenthixol decanoate in 50 schizophrenia patients with elevated scores on the Beck Depression Inventory. Blood levels of nortriptyline were not obtained – in light of the reported "therapeutic window" for nortriptyline and the possible elevation of tricyclic antidepressant blood levels by phenothiazines – it is possible that subjects in this study did not receive optimal nortriptyline dosing (64). It is an interesting observation that antidepressants added to conventional antipsychotics to treat pronounced negative symptoms rather than depression seem to show some efficacy (65).

Surprisingly, only two placebo-controlled trials of augmentation with a selective serotonin reuptake inhibitor (SSRI) in depressed schizophrenia patients have been reported. Mullholland et al. (66) reported a trend toward improvement in depressive symptoms compared with placebo with sertraline 50 mg daily added to conventional and atypical antipsychotics for 6 weeks in 26 schizophrenia patients in a preliminary report. Addington et al. (67) conducted a multi-center placebo-controlled trial of sertraline in 48 chronic schizophrenia patients meeting criteria for major depression. Twenty-eight of the 48 subjects were receiving atypical antipsychotics; the remainders were treated with conventional neuroleptics. All subjects were first treated with an anticholinergic for 1 week to exclude neuroleptic-induced akinesia, and then were randomized to placebo or sertraline at a dose of 50 mg daily for 4 weeks. Sertraline could be increased to 100 mg daily during the final 2 weeks of the 6-week trial. Less than 5% of patients dropped out from either treatment group. Significant improvements in depression were recorded in both placebo and sertraline groups, with no evidence of superiority with sertraline. The response rates, defined by a 50% or greater improvement in the Calgary Depression Scale for Schizophrenia, were 48% with placebo and 43% with sertraline. Levels of psychosis did not differ between treatment groups. In the only other controlled study of an SSRI, Kirli and Caliskan (68) randomized 40 depressed schizophrenia patients to sertraline and imipramine and found no significant difference between treatment groups.

Safety

Similar to lack of efficacy data for combining antidepressants and antipsychotics for depression in schizophrenia patients, the safety of this combination has not been well defined. Studies combining conventional neuroleptics with tricyclic antidepressants and SSRIs have been generally reported good tolerability, although the goal of most of these studies has been the amelioration of negative symptoms (69), a strategy that has even some evidence for efficacy according to a recent meta-analysis (65). Additive side effects represent a potential problem; particularly anticholinergic side effects arising from the combination of a highly anticholinergic tricyclic antidepressant and a low-potency neuroleptic or clozapine. Other potential additive side effects from drug combinations include sedation and dizziness. Clinicians must also be aware of potential pharmacokinetic interactions between antidepressants and antipsychotics. Phenothiazines are reported to elevate blood levels of tricyclic antidepressants, potentially resulting in serum concentrations high enough to produce serious toxicity (64, 70). Most conventional antipsychotics are primarily metabolized by the hepatic cytochrome 2D6; metabolism of these drugs may be significantly inhibited by certain selective serotonin reuptake inhibitors. For example, fluoxetine 20 mg daily increased haloperidol serum concentrations by 20% and fluphenazine serum concentrations by 65% in one placebo-controlled augmentation trial for negative symptoms (71). However, measures of extrapyramidal symptoms did not change significantly. Addington et al. (72) measured antipsychotic drug levels in the aforementioned double-blind sertraline add-on trial (67). At the maximum dose of sertraline used in this trial, 100 mg/day, antipsychotic drug levels showed only minor fluctuations. Spina et al. (73) studied drug levels in 11 patients who received sertraline added onto risperidone and found that the dose of sertraline did have an effect on risperidone levels: 50 mg/day of sertraline did not change risperidone levels, 100 mg/day increased risperidone insignificantly by a mean of 15%, but a dose of 150 mg/day increased risperidone by up to 52%. Perhaps of most clinical concern is the inhibition of clozapine metabolism by fluvoxamine on the basis of cytochrome 1A2 inhibition. In one well-controlled trial, fluvoxamine coadministration raised serum clozapine levels by more than threefold (74). In contrast, sertraline produced no effect on clozapine in one study, and paroxetine produces a small effect (75). Buchanan et al. (76) found that fluoxetine up to 40 mg daily was well tolerated when added to clozapine in a placebo-controlled parallel group trial in 33 treatment-resistant schizophrenia patients, although depressive symptoms did not improve. Pharmacokinetic studies have found only modest interactions between fluoxetine and olanzapine (77).

Conclusion

Depressed affect is common in schizophrenia and often is chronic. The illness burden from depressive symptoms is high: the presence of depression predicts a worse outcome, including quality of life measures, psychotic relapse, and heightened risk of suicide. The conventional neuroleptics may produce or exacerbate dysphoria in schizophrenia patients, whereas atypical antipsychotics appear to possess substantial antidepressant activity. The clinician should first carefully evaluate a depressed patient for medical etiologies, including substance abuse and neuroleptic-induced dysphoria. Differentiating comorbid depression from negative symptoms and from primary affective psychoses is also crucial. Switching dysphoric patients from conventional neuroleptics to atypical agents is probably the most sensible first step. Augmentation of atypical antipsychotics with antidepressants has not been adequately studied – there is no compelling evidence for efficacy either in acutely depressed schizophrenia patients or in chronically dysphoric patients. A systematic meta-analytic review of antidepressants for depression in schizophrenia found only weak evidence for the effectiveness of antidepressants that could be explained by publication bias (78). In addition, high rates of placebo response have been reported in several studies, suggesting that major depressive episodes may resolve spontaneously, whereas chronic dysphoria is less likely to resolve. The addition of SSRIs to atypical antipsychotics does not seem to hinder antipsychotic response, a concern raised with older antidepressants added to conventional antipsychotics. Any combination of antidepressants with antipsychotics should be guided by an understanding of potential pharmacokinetic interactions – the combination that is potentially most dangerous is the addition of fluvoxamine to clozapine. Although similarly not well-studied, psychosocial interventions should also be made available to dysphoric patients and their families.

References

1. Lindenmayer J-P, Grochowski S, Hyman RB. Five factor model of schizophrenia: replication across samples. Schizophr Res. 1995;14:229–34.
2. Marder SR, Davis JM, Chouinard G. The effects of risperidone on the five dimensions of schizophrenia derived by factor analysis: combined results of the North American trials. J Clin Psychiatry. 1997;58:538–46.
3. Bartels SJ, Drake RE. Depressive symptoms in schizophrenia: comprehensive differential diagnosis. Compr Psychiatry. 1988;29:467–83.
4. DeLisi LE. Depression in Schizophrenia. Washington: American Psychiatric Press; 1990.
5. Siris SG. Depression in schizophrenia: perspective in the era of "atypical" antipsychotic agents. Am J Psychiatry. 2000;157:1379–89.
6. Zisook S, McAdams LA, Kuck J, Harris MJ, Bailey A, Patterson TL, et al. Depressive symptoms in schizophrenia. Am J Psychiatry. 1999;156:1736–43.
7. Wassink TH, Flaum M, Nopoulos P, Andreasen NC. Prevalence of depressive symptoms early in the course of schizophrenia. Am J Psychiatry. 1999;156:315–6.
8. Sands JR, Harrow M. Depression during the longitudinal course of schizophrenia. Schizophr Bull. 1999;25:157–71.
9. Rosen JL, Miller TJ, D'Andrea JT, McGlashan TH, Woods SW. Comorbid diagnoses in patients meeting criteria for the schizophrenia prodrome. Schizophr Res. 2006;85:124–31.
10. Koreen AR, Siris SG, Chakos M, Alvir J, Mayerhoff D, Lieberman J. Depression in first-episode schizophrenia. Am J Psychiatry. 1993;150:1643–8.
11. Hafner H, Maurer K, Trendler G, an der Heiden W, Schmidt M, Konnecke R. Schizophrenia and depression: challenging the paradigm of two separate diseases – a controlled study of schizophrenia, depression and healthy controls. Schiz Res. 2005;77:11–24.
12. an der Heiden W, Konnecke R, Maurer K, Ropeter D, Hafner H. Depression in the long-term course of schizophrenia. Eur Arch Psychiatry Clin Neurosci. 2005;255:174–84.
13. Jin H, Zisook S, Palmer BW, Patterson TL, Heaton RK, Jeste DV. Association of depressive symptoms with worse functioning in schizophrenia: a study in older outpatients. J Clin Psychiatry. 2001;62:797–803.
14. Hogarty GE, McEvoy JP, Ulrich RF, DiBarry AL, Bartone P, Cooley S, et al. Pharmacotherapy of impaired affect in recovering schizophrenic patients. Arch Gen Psychiatry. 1995;52:29–41.
15. Newcomer JW, Faustman WO, Yeh W, Csernansky JG. Distinguishing depression and negative symptoms in unmedicated patients with schizophrenia. Psychiatry Res. 1989;31: 243–50.
16. Addington D, Addington T, Maticka-Tyndale E. Reliability and validity of a depression rating scale for schizophrenics. Schizophr Res. 1992;6:201–8.
17. Norman RMG, Malla AK. Dysphoric mood and symptomatology in schizophrenia. Psychol Med. 1991;21:897–903.

18. Sax KW, Strakowski SM, Keck PEJ, Upadhyaya VH, West SA, McElroy SL. Relationships among negative, positive, and depressive symptoms in schizophrenia and psychotic depression. Br J Psychiatry. 1996;168:68–71.
19. Vaillant GE. Prospective prediction of schizophrenic remission. Arch Gen Psychiatry. 1964;11:509–18.
20. Conley RR, Ascher-Svanum H, Zhu B, Faries DE, Kinon BJ. The burden of depressive symptoms in the long-term treatment of patients with schizophrenia. Schizophr Res. 2007;90:186–97.
21. Tollefson GD, Andersen SW. Should we consider mood disturbance in schizophenia as an important determinant of quality of life? J Clin Psychiatry. 1999;60 (suppl 5):23–9.
22. Tollefson GD, Andersen SW, Tran PV. The course of depressive symptoms in predicting relapse in schizophrenia: a double-blind, randomized comparison of olanzapine and risperidone. Biol Psychiatry. 1999;46:365–73.
23. Johnson DAW. The significance of depression in the prediction of relapse in chronic schizophrenia. Br J Psychiatry. 1988;152:320–3.
24. Mandel MR, Severe JB, Schooler NR, Gelenberg AJ, Mieske M. Development and prediction of postpsychotic depression in neuroleptic-treated schizophrenics. Arch Gen Psychiatry. 1982;39:197–203.
25. Roy A, Thompson R, Kennedy S. Depression in chronic schizophrenia. Br J Psychiatry. 1983;142:465–70.
26. Caldwell CB, Gottesman II. Schizophrenics kill themselves too: a review of risk factors for suicide. Schizophr Bull. 1990;16:571–89.
27. Palmer BA, Pankratz VS, Bostwick JM. The lifetime risk of suicide in schizophrenia: a reexamination. Arch Gen Psychiatry. 2005;62:247–53.
28. Saeedi H, Addington J, Addington D. The association of insight with psychotic symptoms, depression, and cognition in early psychosis: a 3-year follow-up. Schizophr Res. 2007;89:123–8.
29. Crumlish N, Whitty P, Kamali M, Clarke M, Browne S, McTigue O, et al. Early insight predicts depression and attempted suicide after 4 years in first-episode schizophrenia and schizophreniform disorder. Acta Psychiatr Scand. 2005;112:449–55.
30. Voruganti LP, Awad AG. Is neuroleptic dysphoria a variant of drug-induced extrapyramidal side effects? Can J Psychiatry. 2004;49:285–9.
31. Van Putten T, May PRA. ‘Akinetic depression’ in schizophrenia. Arch Gen Psychiatry. 1978;35:1101–7.
32. Van Putten T, May PRA. Subjective response as a predictor of outcome in pharmacotherapy. Arch Gen Psychiatry. 1978;35:477–80.
33. Tollefson GD, Sanger TM, Lu Y, Thieme ME. Depressive signs and symptoms in schizophrenia: A prospective blinded trial of olanzapine and haloperidol. Arch Gen Psychiatry. 1998;55:250–8.
34. Regier DA, Farmer ME, Rae DS, Locke BZ, Keith SJ, Judd LL, et al. Comorbidity of mental disorders with alcohol and other drug abuse. Results from the Epidemiological Catchment Area (ECA) Study. JAMA. 1990;264:2511–8.
35. Wilkins JN, Shaner AL, Patterson CM, Setoda D, Gorelick D. Discrepancies between patient report, clinical assessment, and urine analysis in psychiatric patients during inpatient admission. Psychopharmacol Bull. 1991;27:149–54.
36. Shaner A, Eckman TA, Roberts LJ, Wilkins JN, Tucker DE, Tsuang JW, et al. Disability income, cocaine use, and repeated hospitalization among schizophrenic cocaine abusers. N Engl J Med. 1995;333:777–83.
37. Serper MR, Alpert M, Richardson NA, Dickson S, Allen MH, Werner A. Clinical effects of recent cocaine use on patients with acute schizophrenia. Am J Psychiatry. 1995;152:1464–9.
38. Vollmer-Larsen A, Jacobsen TB, Hemmingsen R, Parnas J. Schizoaffective disorder – the reliability of its clinical diagnostic use. Acta Psychiatr Scand. 2006;113:402–7.
39. Hausmann A, Fleischhacker WW. Differential diagnosis of depressed mood in patients with schizophrenia: a diagnostic algorithm based on a review. Acta Psychiatr Scand. 2002;106:83–96.

40. Siris SG, Rifkin A, Reardon GT, Doddi SR, Strahan A, Hall KS. Stability of the postpsychotic depression syndrome. J Clin Psychiatry. 1986;47:86–8.
41. Knights A, Hirsch SR. "Revealed" depression and drug treatment for schizophrenia. Arch Gen Psychiatry. 1981;38:806–11.
42. Green MF, Nuechterlein KH, Ventura J, Mintz J. The temporal relationship between depressive and psychotic symptoms in recent-onset schizophrenia. Am J Psychiatry. 1990;147:179–82.
43. Bressan RA, Chaves AC, Pilowsky LS, Shirakawa I, Mari JJ. Depressive episodes in stable schizophrenia: critical evaluation of the DSM-IV and ICD-10 diagnostic criteria. Psychiatry Res. 2003;117:47–56.
44. Herz M. Prodromal symptoms and prevention of relapse in schizophrenia. J Clin Psychiatry. 1985;46:22–5.
45. Kane J, Honigfeld G, Singer J, Meltzer H. Clozapine for the treatment-resistant schizophrenic. A double-blind comparison with chlorpromazine. Arch Gen Psychiatry. 1988;45:789–96.
46. Davis JM, Chen N. The effects of olanzapine on the 5 dimensions of schizophrenia derived by factor analysis: combined results of the North American and international trials. J Clin Psychiatry. 2001;62:757–71.
47. Keck Jr. P, Buffenstein A, Ferguson J, Feighner J, Jaffe W, Harrigan EP, et al. Ziprasidone 40 and 120 mg/day in the acute exacerbation of schizophrenia and schizoaffective disorder: a 4-week placebo-controlled trial. Psychopharmacology. 1998;140:173–84.
48. Moeller HJ. Occurrence and treatment of depressive comborbidity/cosyndromality in schizophrenic psychoses: conceptual and treatment issues. World J Biol Psychiatry. 2005;6:247–63.
49. Tran P, Hamilton S, Kuntz A, Potvin J, Andersen S, Beasley C, et al. Double-blind comparison of olanzapine versus risperidone in the treatment of schizophrenia and other psychotic disorders. J Clin Psychopharmacology. 1997;17:407–18.
50. Conley RR, Mahmoud R. A randomized double-blind study of risperidone and olanzapine in the treatment of schizophrenia or schizoaffective disorder. Am J Psychiatry. 2001;158:765–74.
51. Shelton RC, Tollefson GD, Tohen M, Stahl S, Gannon KS, Jacobs TG, et al. A novel augmentation strategy for treating resistant major depression. Am J Psychiatry. 2001;158:131–4.
52. Brandon S, Cowley P, McDonald C. Leicester ECT trial: results in schizophrenia. Br J Psychiatry. 1985;146:177–83.
53. Fink M, Sackeim HA. Convulsive therapy in schizophrenia? Schizophr Bull. 1996;22:27–39.
54. Taylor P, Fleminger JJ. ECT for schizophrenia. Lancet. 1980;1:1380–3.
55. Kramer M, Vogel W, DiJohnson C, Dewey D, Sheves P, Cavicchia S, et al. Antidepressants in 'depressed' schizophrenic inpatients: a controlled trial. Arch Gen Psychiatry. 1989;46:922–8.
56. Plasky P. Antidepressant usage in schizophrenia. Schizophr Bull. 1991;17:649–57.
57. Singh AN, Saxena B, Nelson HL. A controlled clinical study of trazodone in chronic schizophrenic patients with pronounced depressive symptomatology. Curr Ther Res. 1978;23:485–501.
58. Siris SG, Morgan V, Fagerstrom R, Rifkin A, Cooper TB. Adjunctive imipramine in the treatment of postpsychotic depression. Arch Gen Psychiatry. 1987;44:533–9.
59. Siris SG, Bermanzohn PC, Gonzalez A, Mason SE, White CV, Shuwall MA. The use of antidepressants for negative symptoms in a subset of schizophrenic patients. Psychopharmacol Bull. 1991;27:331–5.
60. Siris S, Bermazohn P, Mason S, Shuwall M. Maintenance imipramine therapy for secondary depression in schizophrenia. Arch Gen Psychiatry. 1994;51:109–15.
61. Prusoff VA, Williams DH, Weissman MM, Astrachan BM. Treatment of secondary depression in schizophrenia. Arch Gen Psychiatry. 1979;36:569–75.
62. Waehrens J, Gerlach J. Antidepressant drugs in anergic schizophrenia. Acta Psychiatr Scand. 1980;61:438–44.
63. Johnson D. Studies of depressive symptoms in schizophrenia. Br J Psychiatry. 1981;139:89–101.

64. Freudenreich O, Goff DC. Antipsychotics. In: Ciraulo DA, Shader RI, Greenblatt D, Creelman W, editors. Drug interactions in psychiatry. 3rd ed. Philadelphia, PA: Lippincott Williams & Wilkins. 2005.
65. Rummel C, Kissling W, Leucht S. Antidepressants as add-on treatment to antipsychotics for people with schizophrenia and pronounced negative symptoms: a systematic review of randomized trials. Schizophr Res. 2005;80:85–97.
66. Mulholland C, Lynch G, Cooper SI. A double-blind, placebo-controlled trial of sertraline for depressive symptoms in stable chronic schizophrenia. Biol Psychiatry. 1997;42:188S.
67. Addington D, Addington J, Patten S, Remington G, Moamai J, Labelle A, et al. Double-blind, placebo-controlled comparison of the efficacy of sertraline as treatment for a major depressive episode in patients with remitted schizophrenia. J Clin Psychopharmacol. 2002;22:20–5.
68. Kirli S, Caliskan M. A comparative study of sertraline versus imipramine in postpsychotic depressive disorder of schizophrenia. Schizophr Res. 1998;33:103–11.
69. Evins A, Goff D. Adjunctive antidepressant drug therapies in the treatment of negative symptoms of schizophrenia. CNS Drugs. 1996;6:130–47.
70. Siris SG, Cooper TB, Rifkin AE, Brenner R, Lieberman JA. Plasma imipramine concentrations in patients receiving concomitant fluphenazine decanoate. Am J Psychiatry. 1982;139:104–6.
71. Goff D, Midha K, Sarid-Segal O, Hubbard J, Amico E. A placebo-controlled trial of fluoxetine added to neuroleptic in patients with schizophrenia. Psychopharmacology. 1995;117:417–23.
72. Pierson K, Addington D, Addington J, Patten S. Serum monitoring of antipsychotic drug levels during concomitant administration of sertraline and antipsychotic medication. Can J Psychiatry. 2006;51:715–8.
73. Spina E, D'Arrigo C, Migliardi G, Morgante L, Zoccali R, Ancione M, et al. Plasma risperidone concentrations during combined treatment with sertraline. Ther Drug Monit. 2004;26:386–90.
74. Wetzel H, Anghelescu I, Szegedi A, Wiesner J, Weigmann H, Hartter S, et al. Pharmacokinetic interactions of clozapine with selective serotonin reuptake inhibitors: differential effects of fluvoxamine and paroxetine in a prospective study. J Clin Psychopharmacol. 1998;18:2–9.
75. Spina E, Avenoso A, Salemi M, Facciola G, Scordo MG, Ancione M. Plasma concentrations of clozapine and its major metabolites during combined treatment with paroxetine or sertraline. Pharmacopsychiatry. 2000;33:213–7.
76. Buchanan RW, Kirkpatrick B, Bryant N, Ball P, Breier A. Fluoxetine augmentation of clozapine treatment in patients with schizophrenia. Am J Psychiatry. 1996;153:1625–7.
77. Gossen D, De Suray J, Vandenhende F, Onkelinx C, Gangji D. Influence of fluoxetine on olanzapine pharmacokinetics. AAPS Pharmsci. 2002;4:E11.
78. Whitehead C, Moss S, Cardno A, Lewis G. Antidepressants for the treatment of depression in people with schizophrenia: a systematic review. Psychol Med. 2003;330:589–99.

Treatment of Bipolar Depression

Robert M. Post

Introduction

Scope of Depression in Bipolar Illness

The challenge of treating depression in patients with bipolar illness has been both underestimated and understudied for a variety of reasons. The role of traditional unimodal antidepressants in bipolar illness had been highly controversial, and now with the publication of the results of a clinical trial addressing the issue (1) in the *NEJM*, the entire area needs to be reevaluated. They found that augmentation of mood stabilizers (MSs) with antidepressants was no more effective in bipolar depression than with placebo. Treatment of the depressed phase is also complicated by the fact that three of the major MSs, lithium, carbamazepine, and valproate, are each better antimanic agents than they are antidepressants.

Perhaps not surprisingly, when a large group of intensively treated outpatients was prospectively assessed on a daily basis, it was found that they had three times as many days of depression as they did days of mania, even though bipolar I disorder (BD I) was the predominant diagnosis in this group (2–5). Among these patients, group I or about 25% remained ill for more than three-fourths of the year, with the majority of these having ultra-rapid cycling frequencies and 7% having chronic depression. In group II comprising 40% of the patients, they continued to show intermittent patterns of illness despite the intensive therapy; the majority of these had intermittent major depressions either with full-blown mania intervening in 9.7%, hypomania in 19%, or no mania in 5.8%; another 5.8% had mostly intermittent manic episodes. Disappointingly, in group III, only one third were minimally impacted by their affective illness over the prospective year, and only 11.2% were judged symptom-free.

Although bipolar illness begins in half of all patients with episodes of depression rather than mania, these patients contribute disproportionally to the population of

R.M. Post (✉)
Bipolar Collaborative Network, 5415 W. Cedar Lane, Suite 201-B, Bethesda, MD 20814, USA
e-mail: robert.post@speakeasy.net

D.A. Ciraulo and R.I. Shader (eds.), *Pharmacotherapy of Depression*,
DOI 10.1007/978-1-60327-435-7_5, © Springer Science+Business Media, LLC 2011

those with more episodes and more rapid cycling patterns over the course of their illness. These patients with BD whose illness begins with depression, and the 20–40% of bipolar patients in these academic cohorts who actually have bipolar II disorder (BD II) or BD not otherwise specified (BD-NOS), undergo extremely long delays before they are properly treated (6, 7).

Although it is estimated that roughly 1% of the US population will have a diagnosis of BD I over their lifetime, current estimates suggest that an additional 2–4% will have bipolar spectrum disorder. Epidemiological studies indicate that 40% of patients with BD meeting the criteria for BD I are not receiving treatment at the time of the diagnostic interview. In a survey of more than 80,000 US households, using the self-rated mood disorder questionnaire – which has been validated as a screening instrument to detect bipolar illness (8) – investigators determined that only 20% were diagnosed bipolar in the community, and the majority of these were not receiving appropriate treatment. In most cases treatment involved the use of antidepressants without concomitant MSs.

Traditional antidepressants (9) have not been widely systematically studied even as adjuncts to MSs in bipolar depression, and existing studies even prior to the Sachs et al. (1) findings suggested less than robust long-term efficacy of these compounds.

Evidence that the depressive components of bipolar illness remain a major contributor to morbidity (10) and that the illness is markedly under diagnosed and undertreated in the community has important ramifications for mortality associated with the illness. It has been estimated that about 10–20% of patients with this diagnosis will die by suicide (11). The major phases of the illness that drive suicide attempts are the depressive ones, along with dysphoric mania (12, 13). We have ascertained that patients who have made serious suicide attempts (which require medical treatment) have a history of more prior depressive episodes, and demonstrate prospectively on follow-up that they experience more severe depression and are many more times depressed (14).

Therefore, there is a great need for a better approach to depression in bipolar illness to prevent both depressive morbidity and mortality by suicide. Additionally, depression is a risk factor for premature death from a variety of other medical illnesses, such as heart attack and stroke. It is estimated that inadequately treated patients with recurrent unipolar and bipolar depression have an average of a 7-year reduction in life expectancy compared with the general population. As discussed later, long-term therapy with lithium reduces the risk of suicide dramatically (15, 16) and normalizes the excess medical mortality that is associated with recurrent affective illness. Patients with four or more episodes of depression are at a twofold higher risk of late life dementia than those with two or fewer depressive episodes (17). These and a variety of other data suggest that inadequately treated bipolar illness can be progressive, with faster recurrences, greater disability, and increased treatment resistance.

Each episode of depression (and mania) is associated with decrements in serum brain-derived neurotrophic factor (BDNF) in proportion to the severity of the episode (18, 19). This is also accompanied by increases in oxidative stress measured in blood cell elements (20). Together the BDNF decreases and increases in free radical toxins provide a highly plausible mechanism for episode sensitization and illness progression. The clinical data above supplemented by this conception of the underlying neurobiology provide a strong rationale for attempting to intervene earlier and with more consistent long-term prophylaxis to prevent recurrence of depressions and their multiple untoward consequences for the individuals and their brains.

Potential Reasons for Understudy of This Phase of the Illness

Despite the association of BD with a considerable depressive illness burden and high rate of suicide, the illness in general and depression in particular has been disappointingly understudied for a number of reasons. These include the following:

1. The initial perception is that lithium was adequate treatment for the vast majority of patients. It is now recognized that only a minority of patients with BD respond well to lithium, whether it is administered as monotherapy or in combination therapy with an antidepressant, antimanic, benzodiazepine, or other type of adjunctive agent.
2. Patients with bipolar depression have traditionally been excluded from trials of antidepressants for fear of their switching into a manic episode and confounding interpretation of antidepressant responsivity. Thus, there is little information about the efficacy in bipolar illness of the antidepressants despite their wide use. Only recently this need has been recognized by the pharmaceutical industry and they have targeted this population for study.
3. Moreover, almost all drugs now being used in BD were initially studied in mania, i.e., the antipsychotic agents for schizophrenia or the anticonvulsants. Rarely has a drug been studied initially or at all for its potential efficacy in the acute treatment of bipolar depression, with the recent exceptions of the anticonvulsant lamotrigine and the secondary exploration of the antidepressant effects of the atypical antipsychotics olanzapine and quetiapine.
4. Perhaps the most important issue responsible for the lack of research in bipolar illness is the complexity of its presentation and course, which often confounds the most highly respected investigators in the field and prevents them from reaching agreement on appropriate study methodology and appropriate grant funding. Disagreements about optimal research methodology, design, and outcome measures have markedly reduced the number of studies funded. Currently, few studies on the efficacy of pharmacological agents in bipolar illness are even submitted for consideration for funding to the extramural program of the National Institute of Mental Health because of this controversial history (21).

Implications for Treatment Recommendations

The limited amount of research into BD therapy has had a considerable effect in the field of clinical therapeutics. In this chapter, we review the open and systematic literature that exists on the treatment of depression in bipolar illness, but acknowledge from the outset that there is a paucity of information in this regard, and that a very large part of clinical practice and treatment of bipolar depression is currently based on uncontrolled clinical observations and clinical wisdom and intuition. As such, much of what we discuss and present in this chapter remains highly provisional and subject to revision as more systematic data become available from controlled clinical trials.

Conventional wisdom had suggested that therapy for bipolar depression should begin with combination therapy using an antidepressant and a MS, but this remained highly controversial even prior to the study of Sachs et al. (1), indicating lack of benefit of two of the most widely used agents, bupropion and paroxetine. Another well recognized option is lamotrigine monotherapy, particularly for bipolar II depression, for which it is not yet FDA-approved. Many authorities have recommended the avoidance of antidepressants in patients with rapid cycling, continuous cycling, and/or polyphasic episodes, favoring the use of one or more MSs or atypical antipsychotics instead to control the rate of occurrence and reduce mood instability. A considerable diversity of opinion exists regarding the next step when these initial options fail, particularly because of the multiple agents available in each drug class and the wide variety of potential augmentation strategies that can be used.

As the search for agents moves from first-line to second- or third-line options for patients with BD, guidance from controlled clinical trials drops from minimal to virtually nonexistent. A number of possible options and strategies for patients with substantial residual depressive morbidity – which comprise a large percentage of this patient population – are described later in this chapter.

Second Generation Antidepressants: Their Limitations Despite Preference Over TCAs

Antidepressants that are widely used in the treatment of bipolar depression are bupropion, the serotonin selective reuptake inhibitors (SSRIs), and the serotonin norepinephrine reuptake inhibitors (SNRIs), venlafaxine, and duloxetine. For several reasons, these agents had generally supplanted the first-generation antidepressants – the tricyclic antidepressants (TCAs) and monoamine oxidase inhibitors (MAOIs). Although the efficacy is approximately the same, the second-generation antidepressants are much better tolerated. In particular, they have fewer anticholinergic adverse effects and are less likely to induce orthostatic hypotension, both of which can be particularly problematic in older individuals and at higher doses. Second-generation antidepressants are also generally safer than the TCAs in terms of the risk of lethality from overdose.

There is also some evidence that first-generation drugs compared with second generation antidepressants are more likely to induce a switch to mania or promote rapid cycling (22). For these reasons, the first-generation agents are largely to be avoided, except for MAOIs in patients with refractory bipolar depression and anergic or atypical depressive syndromes (23–25). The efficacy of MAOIs is likely better than that of TCAs in bipolar depression (23). Additionally, anergic or atypical depressive syndromes are more common in bipolar than unipolar patients (26).

Evidence of the risk for mania induction by antidepressants varies widely across several studies. Mania induction rates of 25–50% have been reported for TCAs and MAOIs (27–29). Considerably lower rates (range 2.5–12%) have been reported in studies of acute treatment with second-generation antidepressants (22, 30) vs. placebo (4.2% switch rate) (30). The reversible MAOI moclobemide is effective in bipolar depression and appears to have lower switch rates than TCAs (31, 32).

Variables contributing to the wide range of switch rates appear to be the duration of observation (acute vs. prophylactic studies), as well as patient population characteristics. Regarding the latter, in studies including patients with rapid cycling or with a greater number of manic episodes (28, 33, 34), switch rates are usually higher than studies that exclude patients with these disorders. In one meta-analysis by Rouillon et al. (27), switch rates for placebo as well as combination therapy using an antidepressant (usually a TCA) and a MS was approximately 25%. The switch rate rose to about 50% for antidepressant monotherapy, suggesting that concomitant use of a MS can help limit antidepressant-induced switch rates.

A number of studies have examined factors associated with an increased rate of switching into mania, even when antidepressants are used as adjuncts to MSs. These include the following:

1. Younger age of diagnosed patients (35)
2. BP-I vs. BP-II subtype (34, 36)
3. Counting recurrent brief hypomanias, as well as more sustained hypomania and mania (37)
4. TCAs vs. second-generation antidepressants (22)
5. Rapid cycling in the previous year
6. History of substance abuse (38)
7. Increased relative norepinephrine (NE) activity as with DMI vs. bupropion (39) or with venlafaxine vs. sertraline (33) or venlafaxine vs. paroxetine (40)
8. Mixed depression (i.e., increased rate of speech or thoughts) (41)

All of these attributes and characteristics are relatively common in bipolar depression, making a switch into hypomania much more likely than was previously appreciated. While many would consider this a clinically benign occurrence, in the patient with recurrent depressions and/or rapid cycling, these "overswings" may propel cycle acceleration and faster recurrence of the next depression, or a pattern of continuous cycling.

The risks of switching taken with the evidence (discussed below) of less than robust acute or longer-term antidepressant effectiveness has led to the view that antidepressant augmentation should not be the first choice in treatment of bipolar depression.

In patients with new-onset bipolar depression, the antidepressant agents discussed below are sometimes started as monotherapy for the first day or two, to determine their side-effects profiles, and thereafter are administered as combination therapy with a MS. Starting both the antidepressant and MS concomitantly is also a common approach.

A variety of soft clinical predictors of individual response to MSs are described later; these may be of assistance to the clinician in choosing initial and secondary treatment options because they remain the core treatment of bipolar depression.

Bupropion

Bupropion was reported effective for bipolar depression in two small controlled studies (39, 42). Yet, the recent large study of Sachs et al. (1) indicated a lack of efficacy of bupropion in doses up to 575 mg/day compared with placebo. Although the SSRIs are most widely used to treat unipolar depression, bupropion is often recommended for patients with BD because of its general tolerability and side-effects profile, which is well attuned to patients with BD, who often have atypical depression with reverse vegetative symptoms. This drug can be slightly excitatory for the anergic patient and may help delay sleep onset for the hypersomnic patient. It is also weight neutral and few individuals experience sexual dysfunction with this antidepressant compared with SSRIs. In a randomized comparison of three adjunctive antidepressants, bupropion had the lowest rate of switch into mania/hypomania, with the SSRI sertraline intermediate between bupropion and venlafaxine (33, 34).

Open clinical trial literature supports the use of combination therapy using bupropion with lithium carbonate even for those with rapid cycling presentations. It can also be used effectively with valproate or carbamazepine, although carbamazepine induces bupropion to be metabolized to form an active hydroxymetabolite.

The drug is said to carry approximately 0.1% seizure liability, particularly at doses of 450 mg or more. Although divided and spaced doses are necessary with the bupropion immediate-release preparation, this is less of a concern with the available extended-release preparations, and seizure risk may be even lower when the drug is used in combination with anticonvulsants. Individual case reports indicate that unexpected switches into hypomania and mania can still occur with this drug, despite use in conjunction with MSs (43). However, low switch rates on this drug were observed even in rapid cyclers (33, 34).

SSRIs

The SSRIs have been thought to be effective for bipolar depression, with small controlled studies providing some support for the use of fluoxetine (44, 45), paroxetine (40, 46, 47), and citalopram (48). The study of Sachs et al. (1) now raises grave doubts about the effectiveness of paroxetine in doses up to 40 mg/day. SSRIs are well tolerated as a class, although headache, insomnia, GI upset, and sexual dysfunction can sometimes limit their use. Recent controlled studies of SSRIs as adjuncts to MSs suggest a switch rate typically in the range of 5–10% and in several instances significantly less than the rates for older TCAs. Of note, patients receiving concomitant paroxetine and lithium may develop a serotonin syndrome (49). The switch rates on sertraline were intermediate between those of bupropion and venlafaxine (33, 34).

Nefazodone is essentially an SSRI with the additional mechanism of blocking 5-HT_2 receptors, an action associated with an increase in slow-wave sleep. This agent has not been studied systematically in bipolar patients, but has been reported particularly effective for sleep disturbance in patients with post-traumatic stress disorder, and may therefore be useful for patients with BD and this comorbidity. Nefazodone has not been associated with the same degree of sexual dysfunction as pure SSRIs, likely because of the 5-HT_2 receptor antagonist properties of this agent.

SNRIs

Venlafaxine was reported effective for bipolar depression in small trials (40, 50). Because it inhibits the reuptake of both serotonin (5-HT) and NE, it is thought to have a potency exceeding that of the SSRIs and definitely superior antinociceptive effects (as does duloxetine). Two recent meta-analyses support the contention of an increased rate or magnitude of response in patients with unipolar depression, although this is unlikely to occur in patients with bipolar depression.

Venlafaxine was not more acutely effective in bipolar depression than bupropion or sertraline, but did show an increased rate of switch into mania compared with sertraline or bupropion (33, 34). Those with a history of rapid cycling in the prior year were at particular risk for switching into mania on venlafaxine. Vieta et al. (40) also found higher switch rates on venlafaxine than the SSRI paroxetine.

For some individuals gastrointestinal adverse effects are problematic, particularly during the first week of treatment, but these are usually time-limited. Venlafaxine has been associated with a small increase in blood pressure, which may be problematic for patients with borderline or frank hypertension.

Mirtazapine

Mirtazapine exerts actions on both the serotonergic and noradrenergic systems through its blockade of inhibitory noradrenergic alpha_2-autoreceptors. However, it has substantial sedating properties and is often associated with considerable weight gain, which can limit its utility to patients with BD who often present with reverse vegetative symptoms such as psychomotor retardation, hypersomnia, and increased appetite.

Pramipexole

Pramipexole is a dopamine (DA) agonist with high intrinsic activity and modest selectivity for D_3 or D_2 receptors and, therefore, perhaps for mesolimbic dopaminergic systems. Goldberg et al. (51) found pramipexole to be superior to placebo in

24 patients with bipolar depression, as did Zarate et al. (52). This is consistent with previous case series (53, 54), and a large controlled study in 174 patients found pramipexole equal to fluoxetine in unipolar depression (55). It is likely that pramipexole is a unimodal antidepressant, because there have been reports of mania induction. The DA D_2 and D_3 agonist ropinirole may have similar activity (56).

Use of Antidepressant in Depression Breaking Through Ongoing Treatment with a Mood Stabilizer: Duration of Treatment

The most typical presentation of depression in bipolar illness is that of breakthrough depression during ongoing treatment with a MS that was initiated for the treatment of one or more manic episodes. This not only involves many of the issues discussed earlier, but also introduces the controversial issue of optimal duration of prophylactic antidepressant augmentation therapy in the face of the need to simultaneously limit the risk for mania induction.

Because of the perceived risk of switching patients into a manic episode, inducing cycle acceleration or continuous mood cycling with the unimodal antidepressants, circumscribed use of antidepressants in bipolar illness has generally been recommended. Some authorities recommend discontinuation of antidepressants as soon as possible after the depressive episode ends, to limit the risk for switching. The findings of Frankle et al. (57) were consistent with this approach. However, Sachs et al. (1) found no excess of switching on bupropion or paroxetine augmentation compared with placebo – about 10% switch rate in both randomized arms.

In a retrospective chart review, these investigators found no difference in the length of depressive episodes among 50 patients with BD, whether they received antidepressants ($n=33$) or not ($n=17$) (57). One way to limit unimodal antidepressants is to use combination MS therapy; this approach is supported indirectly by data showing that prophylaxis is enhanced with various combinations of MSs (58–61).

In new short-term and longer-term studies, questions have been raised about this strategy. In a 6-week study, Young et al. (62) observed superior antidepressant effects and no differences in switch rates in patients with BD when paroxetine was added to a MS vs. the addition of a second MS.

In two studies of patients who remained stable for 2 months while taking adjunctive antidepressants – a retrospective chart review (58) and a prospective study (63) – the outcomes for patients who continued antidepressants vs. those who discontinued were compared. In both studies, antidepressant continuation was associated with a lower risk of depressive relapse over 1 year (30–40%) with antidepressant continuation, vs. 65–70% with antidepressant discontinuation. Strikingly, the lower relapse rate into depression in those who continued on antidepressants was achieved without an increased risk for switching to mania. Joffe et al. (64) also reported similar findings. However, these three studies were naturalistic, and the initial randomized open data of Ghaemi et al. (65) suggest few differences in antidepressant continuation vs. discontinuation. However, antidepressant continuation in rapid cyclers resulted in increased depressive morbidity and cycling.

Another caveat in the interpretation of the studies of Altshuler et al. (58, 63) is that they included only a highly selective subgroup of about 15% of all those treated with antidepressants who, in fact, remained well for 2 months. Eighty-five percent of antidepressant-exposed patients did not achieve this initial degree of stabilization, suggesting that the majority of bipolar depressed patients do not fare well in the long-term upon antidepressant augmentation of a MS. Consistent with these observations are the finding that only 17% of the antidepressant trials and 25% of the patients remained well acutely and through their continuation phase without relapsing or switching into a hypomanic episode (34). Those data suggesting the lack of effectiveness of antidepressant augmentation are also consistent with those of the STEP-BD Network (1), and indicate the need to explore other agents that have more acute and sustained efficacy.

However, these data of Altshuler et al. (58, 63) and Joffe et al. (64) appear consistent with the general proposition that if the illness is stable, a conservative approach should be taken and pharmacological regimens should not be revised. In the case of continued mood instability, however, a more aggressive approach may be necessary, using a revised pharmacological intervention.

Our personal algorithm involves considering antidepressant augmentation of MSs or atypicals after other options have been tried. When depressions emerge within the context of rapid or continuous cycling, we recommend the use of a second or perhaps a third mood stabilizing agent or an atypical before adding a unimodal antidepressant. In this fashion, the primary problem of the combination of mood instability and cycling would be addressed before an antidepressant is used, and hopefully, the combination of several MSs would be sufficient and preclude the need for unimodal antidepressant therapy, or prevent a switch into mania if one is used. In cases of rapid or continuous cycling, we strongly endorse the use of lamotrigine or lithium augmentation, if these agents are not already part of the therapeutic regimen.

Mood Stabilizers in the Treatment of Bipolar Depression

Lithium, carbamazepine, and valproate all demonstrate some efficacy in the acute treatment of bipolar depression, but this effect is less well documented and apparently less impressive than their rapid onset of efficacy in mania. However, effectiveness of long-term prophylaxis against depressive episodes with each of these agents may be roughly equivalent to that of their ability to prevent manic relapses. Lamotrigine is a clear exception in this regard because it is clearly a superior antidepressant than antimanic both acutely and also prophylactically (for which it is FDA-approved).

Lithium

A substantial number of studies in the literature – including the off-on-off studies of Goodwin et al. (66) and other groups, as well as a number of placebo-controlled, parallel group studies – suggests that lithium has both acute (immediate) and prophylactic antidepressant efficacy in its own right; however, the acute antidepressant effects of lithium remain controversial (11, 67). The weight of evidence suggests that lithium is more effective in patients with bipolar vs. unipolar depression. Lithium was judged effective as short-term therapy for bipolar depression in 79% of 164 patients in seven controlled studies. Additionally, lithium was found equal to a TCA in 4 of 5 studies, but had a slower onset of action – about 3–4 weeks before first changes in the depressive syndrome were seen.

Lithium has been widely used in the prophylaxis of recurrent unipolar illness in Europe; in patients with BD it appears to prevent depressive as well as manic episodes. Lithium was reported effective for the prophylaxis of depression and mania in 63% of 739 patients in ten controlled studies. Newer studies show prophylaxis of depression was better in BP-II than BP-I patients (68). Lithium has been associated with an eightfold lower rate of hospitalization and a sevenfold lower rate of suicide (69–71). Lithium may even have antisuicide effects when poorly effective for mood (69). Unfortunately, long-term studies indicate good outcome in less than 40% of patients (68, 72). Additionally, newer studies show that lithium prophylaxis of mania or hypomania is better than for depression, and that efficacy in rapid cycling patients was only about 30% (61, 73, 74).

Less controversially, lithium can augment the antidepressant effects of almost any unimodal antidepressant used to treat unipolar depression (75). Improvement rates of 50–65% are typically reported when lithium is used as an adjunct to an antidepressant.

Unfortunately, few studies have specifically examined lithium augmentation of antidepressant response in patients with BD. Traditionally, lithium is already in the regimen; therefore, the antidepressant is added to lithium rather than the reverse, as in patients with unipolar depression.

Clinical predictors of lower rates of response to lithium during short-term therapy and pharmacoprophylaxis of bipolar illness in general (if not in depression per se) include presentations with dysphoric mania; rapid cycling; comorbid anxiety disorder; comorbid substance abuse, and personality disorder; negative family history of unipolar or bipolar illness in first degree relatives; continuous cycling patterns; more episodes prior to instituting lithium prophylaxis; and the pattern of depressions (D)-mania (M) and then a well interval (I) (the D-M-I pattern), rather than the converse pattern of M-D-I.

In the German collaborative studies of Greil et al., lithium (in contrast to carbamazepine) worked best in those with classical BD-I presentations without psychotic elements and without substance abuse comorbidity. One study suggested that while high doses/blood levels were better for preventing mania, lower levels were better for preventing depression (76). It is important to note that these are only relative correlates of responsivity and many exceptions can occur; certainly, lithium may be efficacious in particular patients, despite negative predictors (and vice versa).

Carbamazepine (Tegretol, Equetro)

The acute effects of carbamazepine as an acute treatment for bipolar depression have been less well studied than its acute antimanic efficacy. Its overall efficacy in depression was observed to be 44% of 108 patients in six controlled studies (77). Carbamazepine's acute antidepressant response appears to take several times longer than its antimanic effects (78). The efficacy of carbamazepine in the prophylaxis of depression and mania was reported to be 63% of 191 patients in 14 controlled studies (77, 79). Efficacy in rapid cycling was about 50% better than for lithium (30%) (74), although even lower than lithium in another study (61). Two long-term studies found carbamazepine equal to lithium (80), but lithium has been found more effective in "classic" BPI presentations (81). In a series using an off-on-off design, 17 of 54 patients with refractory affective disorders had at least a moderate response to the drug (21, 60). Those with more severe cases of depression and increased acuity were among those who responded best. The possibility of a placebo response was mitigated by the observation that a second course of blind carbamazepine therapy was again effective in a subgroup of ten initially responsive patients. Thus, in at least a small subgroup of initially responsive patients, the efficacy of carbamazepine as an acute treatment for bipolar depression was unequivocally confirmed. Their response during the second carbamazepine exposure indicates that their initial response to carbamazepine was not a placebo response.

Using the more conventional placebo parallel group design, Zhang et al. (82) recently found evidence of acute antidepressant effects of carbamazepine with response rates of 64% vs. 35% on placebo. Interestingly, when a Chinese herbal root preparation called FEW-P was included, response was even higher (85%) despite this preparation's markedly lowering blood levels of carbamazepine. These data, in conjunction with the on-off-on-off data noted above, support the view that a subgroup of bipolar depressed patients may be acutely responsive to this drug, and that the effects may be sustained in long-term prophylaxis in the majority, even though there is evidence of the development of loss of effectiveness (i.e., treatment resistance via a tolerance mechanism) in 25–40% of responsive patients observed on regimens including carbamazepine after several years (60).

A key clinical issue has been determining which patients respond to carbamazepine as opposed to other MSs. Additionally, despite structural similarity to TCAs, carbamazepine exerts numerous opposite biochemical effects. For example, rather than decreasing beta adrenergic receptors in the frontal cortex, an action of most traditional antidepressant modalities, chronic carbamazepine treatment increases them. Instead of upregulating glucocorticoid receptors and decreasing cortisol secretion like many antidepressants, upon chronic administration carbamazepine increases cortisol as revealed by increased secretion of 24-h urinary free cortisol in patients and normal volunteers. On the basis of these and other mechanistic dissimilarities from traditional antidepressant modalities, the carbamazepine responsive subgroup may be different from that responsive to more traditional antidepressant modalities.

Consistent with this suggestion, Ketter et al. (83) found that carbamazepine exerted antidepressant effects in a subgroup of patients who had an atypical pattern of frontal and paralimbic hypermetabolism on their PET scans, rather than the more classic pattern of frontal hypometabolism associated with the depressive syndrome. In particular, the degree of hypermetabolism in the left insular cortex was correlated with the degree of response to carbamazepine; interestingly, the opposite relationship was observed for response to nimodipine. For this dihydropyridine L-type calcium blocker with some antidepressant efficacy, the degree of left insular hypometabolism was associated with the degree of response. In general, relative hypometabolism at baseline appears to be a marker of response to a variety of other antidepressant modalities including lamotrigine, while baseline limbic hyperactivity appears to be a correlate of a positive response to carbamazepine, sleep deprivation, and low (as opposed to high) frequency repeated transcranial magnetic stimulation (rTMS).

Studies have indicated that carbamazepine is effective in alcohol withdrawal syndromes, both in preclinical laboratory studies and in clinical populations. Carbamazepine is used for this indication in a number of Scandinavian countries, and improvement in alcohol-related dysphoria has been observed during maintenance therapy. Several studies suggest that carbamazepine is an effective treatment for BP depression in patients with a history of prior alcoholism (in contrast, this appears to be a relative correlate of lithium nonresponse).

In a German collaborative study, Greil et al. (81) assessed differential correlates of prophylactic response to carbamazepine vs. lithium in a randomized study discussed earlier. They found that lithium was more effective in patients with classical bipolar I illness who did not have mood-incongruent delusions or any comorbidities. In contrast, carbamazepine showed a tendency to be more effective than lithium in patients with bipolar II and bipolar NOS presentations, recurrent mood incongruent delusions, and comorbid substance abuse. Patients with schizoaffective depressive presentations appeared to be particularly responsive to carbamazepine in long-term prophylaxis.

Valproate (VPA, Divalproex Sodium, or Depakote)

Valproate is FDA approved for the treatment of acute mania. Several studies do suggest antidepressant properties for valproate (84), although more systematic studies remain to be performed and the potential clinical and biological predictors of response examined. Earlier review of its overall efficacy in depression was 32% of 170 patients in seven uncontrolled studies (77), including an 8 week open study with 66% response rate in 33 unipolar depressed patients (85). In a recent 12-week open study, Ketter et al. (86) found valproate highly effective as monotherapy for bipolar II depression.

In the prophylaxis of depression and mania, a recent 12-month controlled study found valproate superior to placebo or lithium for depression, but not mania (87, 88). Prior to this study, valproate's overall efficacy in prophylaxis was 64% of 496 patients in 11 uncontrolled studies (77). Valproate has been found to have approximately equal efficacy in rapid cyclers, in contrast to lithium (74). There are few controlled studies regarding the efficacy of valproate in depression. Sachs and Collins (89) in a recent double-blind, randomized study vs. placebo, found valproate nonsignificantly superior to placebo on most measures but at several time points during the study (weeks 3, 4, and 6) the differences were significant. Davis et al. (84) reported that monotherapy compared with placebo showed highly significant positive effects on depression and even stronger antianxiety effects in acute bipolar depression. These data, taken with open observations of the effectiveness of valproate in several primary anxiety disorders, suggest the utility of valproate in patients with characteristics of bipolar depression likely to be associated with antidepressant-nonresponse or with antidepressant-related switching, as noted above.

In open trials of adjunctive therapy and monotherapy studies in patients with rapid cycling bipolar depression, a slightly different picture emerged, one that is more consistent with conventional wisdom about valproate's psychotrophic profile (90–92). In a study of more than 100 treatment-resistant patients with rapid cycling bipolar depression, Calabrese et al. found excellent efficacy for valproate in manic and mixed states, with a substantially lesser degree of efficacy during the depressive phase of the illness. Correlates of valproate efficacy in that study included a patient history of a stable (nonaccelerating) course of illness, lack of psychosis or personality disorder, and less severe depression; additionally, the more severe the mania over the course of illness, the better the antidepressant outcome.

In a series of patients studied at the NIMH using double-blind nurses' ratings, we observed very different individual responsiveness to the group of anticonvulsants, with some patients responding well to carbamazepine and not valproate or phenytoin, and other patients revealing the opposite pattern by failing to respond to carbamazepine (even with adjunctive lithium), and showing a complete response to valproate (93–95). Thus, response to anticonvulsant therapy in bipolar illness cannot be considered a class effect, which makes it increasingly important to identify potential clinical and biological predictors of such differential responsivity. Because of the high incidence of comorbid migraine in bipolar disorder, valproate would have appeal as a possible medication yielding a "two for one" response given its FDA approval for primary migraine prophylaxis. Since valproate increases homocysteine levels, concurrent treatment with folic acid (which decreases homocysteine) would appear indicated.

Lamotrigine (Lamictal)

As noted in the introduction, lamotrigine appears to be an exception to the other three widely used MSs, lithium, carbamazepine, and valproate, which all appear to show a better antimanic than antidepressant efficacy. Lamotrigine is more effective in the treatment of depression than mania, probably both for acute treatment and prophylaxis. A randomized double-blind, placebo-controlled trial in patients with acute depression by Calabrese et al. (96) found the efficacy of both lamotrigine 50 and 200 mg/day dosages to be significantly superior to that of placebo ($p<0.05$), based on the Montgomery-Asberg depression rating scale (MADRS) score while 50 mg/day had a trend for superior efficacy vs. placebo ($p=0.058$).

Interestingly, such a statistical difference was not seen using the Hamilton depression rating scale (HAM-D), which many investigators have found less sensitive to antidepressant effects in bipolar illness. Lamotrigine has not been found to be efficacious in the treatment of patients with acute mania, but the need for slow dose titration may compromise the ability to see such an effect.

In a 6-week double-blind study of lamotrigine vs. gabapentin vs. placebo (which was followed by two 6-week crossover phases designed to expose each patient to all three treatment arms) in 31 highly treatment-refractory patients, most of whom had bipolar depression, Frye et al. (97) found superior overall efficacy and antidepressant efficacy for lamotrigine compared with both placebo and gabapentin. In both the Calabrese et al. (96) and Frye et al. (97) studies, the switch rate into mania on lamotrigine did not exceed that of placebo (also see (98, 99)).

However, the four industry-sponsored studies of lamotrigine in acute bipolar depression following the Calabrese et al. (31) study did not show statistical significance, although the meta-analysis of these studies (whether or not the initial study of Calabrese et al. was included) did show significance. Nierenberg et al. (100) found a 23% response rate to lamotrigine vs. 17% to inositol and 5% to risperidone. This suggestive difference was not significant, possibly because the study was underpowered and terminated prematurely by the data safety monitoring board because of the low overall response rate. More recently, Van der Loos (101) found that lamotrigine was highly significantly more effective than placebo for acute bipolar depression when either was added to ongoing lithium therapy.

The prophylactic antidepressant effects for lamotrigine were seen in two 76-week, double-blind, randomized, placebo-controlled studies of lamotrigine vs. lithium, which led to FDA approval of lamotrigine for prevention of depressed, manic, and mixed episodes. Interestingly, lithium had a superior prophylactic effect for mania in these studies, compared with lamotrigine and placebo. In contrast, lamotrigine was more effective than lithium or placebo on the primary outcome measure of time-to-intervention for a "depressive episode." Taken together with the findings of a substantial number of open trials (102) and recent randomized, placebo-controlled studies, evidence clearly supports lamotrigine for prophylaxis, but remains more ambiguous for acute short-term therapy in patients with bipolar depression.

Given this view, it would appear most efficient to start lamotrigine as early in an acute episode as possible because of the necessity of the very slow dose titration (to prevent rash), so that adequate doses may be achieved with the goal of prevention of the next episode. Using this strategy, lamotrigine might even contribute to the acute antidepressant effects of the other agents in the regimen.

Such a view is mirrored by the revised American Psychiatric Association (APA) guidelines for treatment of bipolar depression, which place lamotrigine in a first- or second-line position among treatment approaches to bipolar depression. Lamotrigine also appears to benefit affective lability, demonstrating good responses in patients with rapid cycling bipolar depression (96, 99), and showing benefits for patients with borderline personality disorder (103).

Lamotrigine carries the risk for inducing rash and severe and potentially life-threatening dermatologic reactions including Stevens–Johnson syndrome (SJS) and toxic epidermal necrolysis (TEN). When lamotrigine was rapidly titrated in early studies in seizure patients, the incidence of SJS/TEN was approximately 1 in 1,000. With more conservative dosing strategies and a much slower dose escalation, the incidence is now reported to be 1 in 5,000 patients in adults and 1/2,500 children.

Calabrese et al. (104) recently reported the findings of a retrospective analysis of lamotrigine rash in 12 multicenter mood disorder studies. In the 1,198 patients who received lamotrigine and the 1,056 patients who received placebo, the rash rates were 8.3 and 6.4%, respectively; no cases of SJS were observed with lamotrigine. In open-label settings, 1,955 patients taking lamotrigine exhibited a rash rate of 13.1%, including two cases of serious rash, and one (mild) case of SJS apparently not requiring hospitalization. TEN was not observed in any of these settings.

There are other risk factors for rash, SJS, and TEN (105). If a patient had any prior drug allergy, the risk of rash increases two to threefold, and if the patient had a prior anticonvulsant allergy, the rash risk increases three to fourfold. Rash risk increases two to threefold in children. For 57 cases of Stevens–Johnson syndrome ($n=43$) and TEN ($n=14$), the median time to onset was 17 days and the median dosages 50 and 87.5 mg/day, respectively. In 74% of Stevens–Johnson syndrome cases and 64% of TEN cases, concomitant valproate had been used. The Stevens–Johnson syndrome group was younger than the TEN group (21 vs. 31 years). The risk of SJS TEN in children is fivefold higher than in adults (105). Cyclosporin, IgG, and plasmaphoresis have been used to treat SJS/TEN associated with lamotrigine.

Valproate essentially doubles the blood levels of lamotrigine, necessitating reducing the starting and target doses by one-half, and slowing the rate of titration compared with the schedule used in patients treated with lamotrigine alone. The conventional rate of upward titration is 25 mg/day during the first 2 weeks and 50 mg/day for the next 2 weeks, with subsequent increases not exceeding 50 mg/week, but a limit of 25 mg/week increments is more conservative. In contrast, carbamazepine induces the metabolism of lamotrigine and reduces lamotrigine levels approximately by half; this results in the ability to more rapidly titrate to achieve the same blood level of lamotrigine as is seen in monotherapy.

Lamotrigine has an advantage over several other anticonvulsants, such as carbamazepine and valproate in not being sedating. Some patients find it slightly activating or even generating some degree of insomnia. This latter effect may actually be helpful for some bipolar patients experiencing reverse vegetative symptoms, including hypersomnia rather than the more classic insomnia, which often accompanies unipolar depression. Lamotrigine also is weight neutral and does not appear to cause sexual dysfunction, as is often problematic for the serotonin selective antidepressants.

Recent reports have suggested differential predictors of positive response to lamotrigine vs. gabapentin (106) and vs. lithium (107). Lamotrigine response was correlated with male gender, fewer hospitalizations, and fewer medication trials, while gabapentin response correlated with younger age and lower baseline body weight (106). Lamotrigine appeared more effective in those with a personal and family history of anxiety disorders and substance abuse disorders, while lithium appeared more effective in those with a positive family history of affective illness, including unipolar depression in first degree relatives (107–109).

Gabapentin and Pregabalin

The role of gabapentin in the treatment of patients with bipolar depression is not clear. In a placebo-controlled short-term trial of gabapentin to augment neuroleptic therapy in patients with mania, Pande et al. (110) found a lack of efficacy for gabapentin compared with placebo (111). Similarly, in the study of Frye et al. (97), gabapentin and placebo were inferior to lamotrigine in highly treatment-refractory patients.

These controlled data stand in sharp contrast to those produced by open trials and case-series literature, which suggested the usefulness of gabapentin as augmentation therapy in patients inadequately responsive to a range of current pharmacotherapies (98, 112, 113). One possible interpretation of this discordance is that gabapentin may have a number of therapeutic properties of particular use to patients with bipolar illness that are not primarily antimanic or mood stabilizing. Considerable evidence from controlled studies indicates that gabapentin is effective in patients with anxiety disorders, including social phobia, as well as in patients with somatic complaints (which are common in patients with BD) or headache or a variety of other pain syndromes. Gabapentin has also been reported helpful as adjunctive therapy in patients with restless leg syndrome, insomnia, and alcohol withdrawal, all of which are often comorbid with bipolar illness.

It is also possible that gabapentin is more effective as an adjunct than in monotherapy. Consistent with this view are the data of Vieta et al. (114) that gabapentin compared with placebo was a more effective adjunct in long-term prophylaxis.

Thus, more definitive evidence is required before it can be determined whether gabapentin has primary antidepressant effects in patients with bipolar depression or is merely a useful adjunct that targets a variety of comorbidities, especially anxiety disorders. In the studies of Frye et al. (97) and Obrocea et al. (106), patients who had the best responses to gabapentin were relatively younger and had a relatively shorter duration of illness and relatively lower weight at baseline. Since the role of GABA in the central nervous system changes from excitatory early in development to inhibitory, perhaps an examination of potential efficacy in younger individuals is indicated.

Pregabalin (Lyrica) has not been widely studied in bipolar depression and until such data become available, one must assume that many of its effects will be similar to that of its close congener gabapentin. The $alpha_2$ delta subunit of the

L-type calcium channel is where gabapentin is thought to bind selectively and account for its antinociceptive and anti anxiety properties. Pregabalin compared with gabapentin is even more potent in binding to this subunit, so one might presume (without direct evidence) that pregabalin might be a more potent antinociceptive agent than gabapentin. How the rest of its positive profile in anxiety disorders fit with the treatment of bipolar depression remains to be determined.

Topiramate (Topamax)

Topiramate studies have had discrepant results in the clinical literature on bipolar disorder. A large series of open studies suggested that topiramate may be useful as an adjunct in treatment of mania and cycling (115, 116). However, the findings of a recent series of three large multi-center randomized, double-blind, placebo-controlled studies indicate that topiramate monotherapy is not effective in acute mania. In contrast, lithium – the comparator drug in two of these studies – did show the expected positive efficacy profile compared with placebo.

The role of topiramate in bipolar depression is even less clear. During an open label study in 56 bipolar outpatients, McElroy et al. (116) found that the response to adjunctive topiramate was much lower in patients with acute-onset depression (27%) than in those with mania and cycling (i.e., 50–60%). However, in a single-blind, randomized study of topiramate compared with bupropion as add-on therapy for breakthrough bipolar depression, a response rate of about 55% was seen for both drugs (117), suggesting the need to further explore the potential antidepressant effects of topiramate. A role for adjunctive topiramate therapy for prophylaxis in patients with depression and mania is suggested by a 6-month study in 34 bipolar patients, in which investigators found that 55% of depressed patients and 59% of manic patients were considered as responders (116). Several open trials have produced results suggesting that topiramate may play a role in the treatment of PTSD. This efficacy may be due to topiramate's unique mechanism of action in blocking glutamate receptors of the AMPA-kainate subtype, which are involved in the maintenance of long-term memory, as revealed in the hippocampal slice model of long-term potentiation (LTP).

The findings of a placebo-controlled study have also suggested utility for topiramate in primary alcohol abuse (118), and these results have recently been replicated. A placebo-controlled study in primary cocaine abuse was also positive (118). PTSD and alcohol abuse are not uncommon in patients with bipolar illness; thus, topiramate could play a therapeutic role despite its lack of intrinsic antimanic effects.

Topiramate also has carbonic anhydrase inhibiting properties, resulting in about 1% incidence of renal calculi and a higher rate of parathesias. In an open trial of the carbonic anhydrase inhibitor acetazolamide, investigators found improvement in 7 of 16 treatment-refractory patients with BD, with all responders having depressed or rapid cycling (119).

In studies of patients with epilepsy and with affective disorder, topiramate has the effect of producing mild to more substantial weight loss. This may be a positive side effect in bipolar illness in those 50% of women and two-thirds of men who are overweight (120). Topiramate can be used concurrently with weight-gain prone drugs to prevent weight gain, or later to facilitate weight loss.

The magnitude of weight loss on topiramate parallels that of the FDA-approved weight loss drug sibutramine. However, in this randomized open study, many patients dropped out early on topiramate and later on sibutramine for intolerance or ineffectiveness (121). Topiramate is also effective in bulimia, reducing the number and quantity of binges.

Some 5% or more of epileptic and affectively ill patients may have mild to severe cognition impairment (word finding difficulties) on topiramate, such that starting with a dose of 25 mg/day and slowly increasing it as tolerated may be prudent.

Other Anticonvulsants

Oxcarbazepine (Trileptal)

Oxcarbazepine is the keto-congener of carbamazepine. In controlled studies of oxcarbazepine in patients with trigeminal neuralgia and epilepsy, it demonstrated clinical effectiveness similar to that of carbamazepine (77). Two randomized studies suggested comparable efficacy to lithium and haloperidol, with better tolerability of oxcarbazepine compared with the latter drug. The findings of two small retrospective studies (122, 123) in patients with mania (124) and in treatment-refractory patients, most of whom had bipolar depression (125), suggested mild-to-moderate mood stabilizing benefits with oxcarbazepine. In contrast to these suggestions of possible equivalency to carbamazepine, Wagner et al. (126) reported that oxcarbazepine was similar to placebo in the treatment of child and adolescent onset mania, although it was superior to placebo in the youngest children.

The epilepsy literature indicates that oxcarbazepine has a wider therapeutic window than carbamazepine, and fewer adverse effects (111, 127) with the exception of more frequent hyponatremia induction (128, 129). Oxcarbazepine has less cytochrome P450 enzyme system auto- and heteroinduction than carbamazepine (119, 120), but still requires use of higher dosage forms of estrogen in birth control pills. Changing from carbamazepine to oxcarbazepine can result in large increases in neuroleptic plasma levels and extrapyramidal symptoms due to enzyme de-induction (130).

Levetiracetam (Keppra)

The potential antidepressant effects of levetiracetam and zonisamide have not yet been adequately delineated. Levetiracetam is noteworthy for its unique profile of action, given that it is not effective against maximum electroconvulsive seizures (MES) or (PTZ), but is effective in both the development and completed phases of amygdala kindling. It appears to act, in part, by blocking inhibitory modulators (i.e., zinc and beta-carboline) of the GABA-A-benzodiazepine-chloride-ionophore, thus indirectly enhancing the efficacy of GABA. It also has a stereospecific binding site in the brain, the SV-40 binding site involved with neurotransmitter release. Interestingly, levetiracetam had recently been reported to have additive or potentiating effects in an animal model of mania when used in combination with valproate, but comparable data in the clinic have not been forthcoming.

In an open add-on study, we observed inconsistent antimanic and antidepressant effects of levetiracetam, but the results were confounded by the high drop-out rate for sedation because dose escalation toward 2,000–3,000 mg/day may have proceeded too rapidly (37). Although many mildly depressed patients appeared to respond to levetiracetam, none of the severely depressed patients responded. Lower starting doses (250–500 mg/day H.S.) may be useful to reevaluate. However, other studies have suggested more positive effects in bipolar depressed patients.

Zonisamide (Zonegran)

Zonisamide is not only a sodium channel blocker, but also has complex effects on DA and serotonin metabolism, raising the possibility that these actions may contribute to its positive effects in affective disorders, although this remains to be demonstrated. One small open study reported positive antimanic effects for zonisamide (131). McElroy et al. (132) replicated and extended these observations in an open add-on study. She found positive acute antimanic effects in the first week in about three-quarters of patients and milder and delayed antidepressant effects in about one-third of patients.

However, as others have observed (133), weight loss was a significant side effect with a magnitude approximately similar to topiramate. Zonisamide is also positive for use in bulimia, reducing number and amount of binges. Thus, zonisamide would appear to be a useful alternative to topiramate in those unable to tolerate its side effects when patients are seeking assistance with weight loss or bulimia, or as a recent report suggests in alcohol abuse.

Tiagabine (Gabitril)

The utility of the GABAergic agent valproate in mania apparently does not extend to other GABAergic anticonvulsants such as tiagabine, vigabatrin, or gabapentin, and these appear to be poor choices for the primary mood disorders. Open reports do not indicate efficacy of tiagabine in mania or depression. Grunze et al. (134) found that tiagabine was not an effective antimanic agent, as none of their first eight patients showed good response. Similarly, Suppes et al. (135) reported clinically relevant effects in only 3 of 17 treatment-refractory bipolar patients exposed to adjunctive tiagabine. At least one patient in each of the above studies had a seizure while taking tiagabine; none of these individuals had a history of seizure disorders.

Schaffer et al. (136) had 8 of 22 bipolar outpatients benefit from add-on tiagabine therapy, but 14 patients could not tolerate it. Vigabatrin also is not promising, possibly owing to its reported ability to induce depression and affective psychosis (137, 138) as well as cause visual field defects.

Second Generation Atypical Antipsychotic Agents

All of the conventional first generation antipsychotic (or neuroleptic) agents also have antimanic properties. This principal now seems to extend to the atypical antipsychotic agents as well. What was more problematic was the lack of adequate acute or prophylactic antidepressant properties of these first generation antipsychotic agents. Is an open question whether the antidepressant therapeutic spectrum will be better achieved with the atypical as a class; however, the initial data with several agents are supportive of this possibility (139, 140).

From a mechanistic perspective, considerable theoretical reasons exist for assuming that the atypicals will have a better antidepressant profile. As a group, the atypicals have a wider range of receptor effects, which are thought to be related to potential antidepressant mechanisms, such as the blockade of 5-HT_2 receptors as well as 5-HT_{1A} and DA receptors beyond the D_2 subtype, which are potentially involved in the effects of the typical antipsychotics.

Clozapine is paradigmatic of this shift, with studies of *c-fos* induction indicating that the neuroanatomical distribution of its actions are much more mesolimbic and mesocortical, compared with the more exclusively striatal mechanisms of the typical antipsychotic agent haloperidol. In addition to this distribution of effects rendering this atypical less likely to cause extrapyramidal side effects and the long-term liabilities of tardive dyskinesia, this redistribution of activity may be more relevant to antidepressant properties as well.

With the availability of six atypical antipsychotic agents beginning with clozapine in 1990, risperidone in 1994, olanzapine in 1996, quetiapine in 1997, ziprasidone in 2001, and aripiprazole in 2002, the crucial question has switched from their antimanic to their long-term tolerability and antidepressive efficacy.

The issues of weight gain, diabetes mellitus, and the metabolic syndrome now require careful monitoring and selectivity. In this regard, clozapine and olanzapine appear most problematic, risperidone and quetiapine less so, and ziprasidone and aripiprazole relatively weight neutral, at least in adults.

Clozapine

A series of open studies have suggested that clozapine is more effective in bipolar disorder than in schizoaffective disorder and least effective in schizophrenia, despite it being recognized as a drug of choice for treatment-resistant schizophrenia (141, 142).

Clozapine is particularly effective in treatment-refractory rapid cycling patients or those with dysphoric components of mania. Its antidepressant efficacy is less well delineated. Utility for acute treatment and prophylaxis of depression has been suggested by open studies (143). However, Barbini et al. (144) found that although 19 bipolar and schizoaffective patients receiving add-on clozapine had less mania and psychosis at 12 months, there was no difference in depression for these patients vs. 19 other bipolar and schizoaffective patients not receiving add-on clozapine.

Risperidone

Vieta et al. (145) studied 299 patients with BDI and 183 with bipolar-type schizoaffective disorder treated with risperidone (4.0 mg/day) for 6 months. While the minority of patients presented with psychotic depressive episodes, the mean Hamilton (HAM-D) score declined highly significantly from 12.8 ± 7.9 at baseline to 4.1 ± 4.8 at 6 months, suggesting antidepressant effects in this open study. In a controlled study, Janicak et al. (146) found that risperidone decreased HAM-D scores more than haloperidol in 62 schizoaffective patients: 33 bipolar subtypes and 29 depressed subtype. Additional suggestions of utility in depression comes efficacy as an adjunct to prophylaxis of depression and mania as an adjunct (147), and from risperidone augmentation of SSRIs (148, 149). However, Mullen et al. (150), in a randomized study in patients with diverse psychotic disorders, found an equivalent efficacy on PANSS scores, but quetiapine showed a greater reduction in the HAM-D score (5.4 ± 0.38; $n = 491$) than risperidone (4.0 ± 0.59, $n = 150$, $p < 0.028$). Tolerability was equivalent based on drop-out rates, while quetiapine showed greater somnolence, dry mouth, and dizziness than risperidone, and risperidone showed a greater incidence of extrapyramidal side effects (mean daily dose 3.17 mg for quetiapine, 4.7 mg for risperidone).

Olanzapine

Similarly, olanzapine's antidepressant effects are suggested by effectiveness in a chart review finding improvement with olanzapine in 67% of 15 patients with psychotic depression (151), in 60% of patients in a chart review of Ghaemi et al. (152), and with superior depressive symptom improvement vs. haloperidol in schizoaffective bipolar subtype (70). Recent double-blind studies in unipolar and bipolar depressed patients provide some support for this perspective. Olanzapine showed some efficacy in bipolar depression compared with placebo, while in combination with the SSRI fluoxetine, it had much more dramatic antidepressant effects (153). Similar results were observed in patients with unipolar depression (154). This led to the FDA approval of the olanzapine/fluoxetine combination for the treatment of bipolar depression. A randomized, 1-year study showed that olanzapine has superior prophylactic antimanic effects to lithium and equal antidepressant effects (155).

Quetiapine

In an open study examining the add-on quetiapine, risperidone, or clozapine presented by Keck et al. at the APA 2001 (156), preliminary analysis revealed improved depression ratings on the inventory of depressive symptoms (IDS) for quetiapine. Improvement with quetiapine therapy was detectable within the first month of treatment and was maintained through the second to fourth month. In contrast, there were no significant decrements in IDS ratings when risperidone or clozapine were used as open add-ons and assessed in the same fashion. These preliminary observations lead to the conduct of more formal RCTs of quetiapine monotherapy in bipolar depression.

The studies of Calabrese et al. (140) and Thase et al. (139) led to FDA approval of the first monotherapy for bipolar depression. Quetiapine 300 or 600 mg H.S. showed rapid onset (in week 1) of antidepressant, antianxiety, and anti-insomnia effects compared with placebo ($p<0.001$). The effects were robust for both bipolar I and bipolar II depressed patients, and the 300 and 600 mg doses yielded similar degrees of effectiveness, suggesting the ideal antidepressant dose might be 300 mg/day or below. The effective size for quetiapine monotherapy was of a similar magnitude to that of the olanzapine/fluoxetine combination.

New data suggest that quetiapine may have potent effects on NE reuptake and $5HT_{1A}$ partial agonism (157), in addition to its effects in preventing stress-induced decreases in BDNF (158) as potential mechanisms of quetiapine's antidepressant effects.

Sedation was the major side effect and some investigators have recommended test doses of quetiapine 25 mg H.S. (on a Friday or Saturday night) to see who might be particularly sensitive to carry-over A.M. lethargy and sedation that might interfere with usual weekday functioning. Quetiapine was also recently FDA approved for long term prophylaxis of depression and mania when used as an adjunct to either lithium or valproate

Ziprasidone and Aripiprazole

The potential antidepressant effects of the two latest atypicals ziprasidone and aripiprazole remain to be systematically assessed, but have the advantage of being relatively weight neutral, at least in adults. Ziprasidone blocks $5\text{-}HT_2$ and D2 receptors as other atypical antipsychotic agents, but it also has some 5-HT and NE reuptake inhibition and $5\text{-}HT_1$ receptor agonist activity. Ziprasidone's pharmacological profile in inhibiting stress-induced decrements in BDNF (159) also suggests it may have some antidepressant activity. Recent RCT of ziprasidone in bipolar depression was not positive, however.

Aripiprazole is a partial dopaminergic agonist with intermediate intrinsic activity, acting at D1, D2, D3; it also is a partial agonist at 5-HT_{1A} receptors and blocks 5-HT_2 receptors. It is a mechanistically promising agent, perhaps conveying some of the properties of Carlsson's long sought after "DA buffer." A large controlled study in schizophrenia and schizoaffective disorder found aripiprazole equal to haloperidol by PANSS and CGI, but better tolerated (160).

McElroy et al. (161) reported suggestive antidepressant effects of aripiprazole in bipolar depression. Large positive placebo-controlled trials in unipolar depression were positive (162), but in bipolar depression, higher doses were used and had a higher dropout rate, and were not significant (163). In patients with borderline personality disorder, Nickel et al. (164) reported highly significant effects of aripiprazole over placebo on measures of both depression and anxiety.

Affectively ill depressed patients may be particularly sensitive to the activating or akathesia-inducing effects of aripiprazole, and it may be helpful to start these individuals on "baby" doses of drug, i.e., 1 to 2 mg/day and then titrate slowly according to efficacy and side effects toward a presumptive range of 5 to 10 mg/day.

Superior Effectiveness of Atypical vs. Typical Antipsychotics in Bipolar Depression

Thus, in contrast to the typical antipsychotics where several studies have suggested possible increases in severity of depression or duration of depressive episodes from long-term maintenance treatment, the initial studies reviewed above suggest that the atypicals, in accord with their different mechanisms of action and fewer extrapyramidal side-effects, are more promising in the treatment of bipolar depressive phases of the illness. Given the incidence of extrapyramidal side effects of the conventional antipsychotic agents and the associated 20–40% risk of tardive dyskinesia in BD patients, use of the atypicals in bipolar illness in general, and in bipolar depression in particular, appears to be indicated in preference to the first-generation antipsychotic agents.

Thus, while some have argued that the CATIE trial in schizophrenia demonstrated equal effectiveness of the typical fluphenazine compared with several atypicals, Helena Cramer highlighted that the study was not randomized (because those with extrapyramidal side effects were not given fluphenazine) and that few conclusions could be derived from the study. Despite the selection for no extrapyramidal effects, more patients dropped out on this drug because of extrapyramidal side effects. Bipolar patients, especially those in depressed phases (165), are highly prone to the development of tardive dyskinesia, and for this reason and poor performance of the typicals in bipolar depression, the atypicals are highly preferred for this diagnostic group of patients, even though equivalency is claimed for those with schizophrenia. While the potential mood stabilizing properties of several of the atypicals appear highly promising, the ability of other agents beside quetiapine to prevent depressive recurrences in long-term prophylaxis remains to be further studied.

Sequential Treatment Approaches

Acute Episode

Given the very substantial residual depressive morbidity typically observed following conventional treatment for BD noted in the introduction, how should this problem be addressed, particularly given the wide range of treatment options available? Again, we begin this section with the caveat that most of the following recommendations are not based on evidence from systematic, controlled clinical trials. As such they should be considered very preliminary and should be changed as warranted by new data. We focused mainly on the issue of therapeutic approaches to breakthrough depression occurring during ongoing treatment with one or more MSs.

As noted previously, in the face of an isolated bipolar depressive episode breaking through a MS, the addition of unimodal antidepressant to the MS regimen had often been recommended as first-line treatment, but their liability of potentially switching patients into hypomania or mania has been reviewed above, as well as their less than optimal effects in acute depression long-term prophylaxis. If there had been a prior pattern of manic and depressive recurrences, particularly if they have rapid or ultra-rapid cycling, lamotrigine or an alternate MS or atypical antipsychotic should be considered for adjunctive therapy instead of an antidepressant, especially given the findings of Sachs et al. (1).

If depressions persisted or recurred in spite of the use of two MSs, or a MS and an atypical, the addition of a unimodal antidepressant might then be considered. If this antidepressant is not effective in relieving chronic depression, another antidepressant – one with an alternative mechanism of action – may be indicated. If an SSRI was utilized, the clinician might consider the addition of bupropion or as switch to venlafazine or duloxetine.

If the depression persists, one might also want to consider one or more additional augmentation strategies, including the utilization of folate (1 mg/day for women and 2 mg/day for men), ascorbate (3,000 mg/day), and T_3 (25–37.5 mg/day). This approach is suggested as it would appear to be a low risk proposition in each instance, with each of these agents having a modicum of data to support their potential utility in unipolar, if not bipolar illness. For example, Coppen et al. (166) reported folate potentiation of antidepressant effects of the SSRIs in unipolar patients and folate potentiation of lithium prophylaxis in bipolar illness. Recent studies indicate that higher homocysteine levels are a risk factor for cognitive dysfunction (167) and lack of achievement of "well intervals" (168), further enhancing the rationale for using folate, since it helps lower homocysteine levels.

If lithium were not already in the therapeutic regimen, it would be useful to consider it as an option for adjunctive therapy. A lower serum free T_4 level, even in the normal range, has been associated with greater mood instability in-patient with BD being maintained with lithium (169). Thyroid augmentation may thus be more routinely useful. Kocsis et al. found that T_3 augmentation of lithium improves cognitive functioning even when baseline thyroid values were normal (170, 171).

Similarly, in the face of inadequate response, major revisions of the basic MS regimen and the antidepressant regimen may be in order as well. This is in light of the substantial evidence that individual patients may be responsive to lithium, valproate, or carbamazepine, even when they have failed to respond to the other two agents. In patients with a rapid cycling course, Denicoff et al. (61) found a much better response rate for the combination of lithium and carbamazepine compared with a year of either drug as monotherapy.

Obviously, if the depression included psychotic symptoms, earlier use of atypical antipsychotic agents would be indicated. Use of atypicals after one or more revisions of MSs and antidepressant modalities would also appear particularly worthwhile given the new evidence of the antidepressant effects of olanzapine and quetiapine, especially when olanzapine is used in combination with fluoxetine. Insomnic vs. hypersomnic depressive presentations would differentially suggest the initial use of sedating vs. activating atypicals respectively, whose side effects profile is most in accord with these differences.

In those who are overweight, considering the less well-studied and more difficult to titrate agents ziprasidone and aripiprazole in preference to other atypical might even be considered.

As one moves toward the use of complex combination therapy by necessity (because the patient has not responded adequately to various simplified regimens), it becomes increasingly important to titrate doses of each added agent against the side effects incurred, as a primary concern is for the tolerability of the entire drug regimen. Another augmenting strategy has considerable merit. Michael Berk and colleagues from Australia found benefit over placebo at 3 and 6 months of treatment with N-acetyl cysteine (NAC) 1,000mg B.I.D. Of great interest are also reports that NAC has positive effects in placebo controlled trials in cocaine, heroin, and gambling addiction, as well as in trichotillomania. As addiction comorbidities are common in bipolar disorder, the potential for positive affects on mood and substance abuse is particularly intriguing. A recent double blind randomized trial of T4 (the 4 should be little; I couldn't format it here) slowly titrated to 300 ug/day showed noteable significant effects over placebo in females, but not in males (Michael Bauer, 2009, unpublished observations).

Supraphysiologic Thyroid Hormone Augmentation

Use of supraphysiologic or hypermetabolic doses of levothyroxine (T_4) is another augmentation strategy in bipolar illness (172, 173). Following slow increases in the dose of T_4 into the range of 200–400 μg/day (which usually produces free thyroxine index 150% of normal), a substantial response rate (>50%) has been observed, with relatively good tolerability. The most frequent adverse effects indicate a mild hyperthyroidism, for example, tachycardia, sweating at night, and increased tremulousness.

Bauer and Whybrow (173) have found that this approach is not only helpful in patients with treatment-refractory rapid cycling, but also in those with persistent treatment-refractory depression. It might be useful to attempt this approach (in the absence of medical contraindications) prior to considering more aggressive and invasive approaches, such as maintenance electroconvulsive therapy (ECT) or a vagal nerve stimulator (VNS) implant.

Omega-3-Fatty Acids (OFAs)

The status of augmentation therapy using omega-3-fatty acids (OFAs) remains somewhat ambiguous (174). Stoll et al. (174) originally reported success in bipolar depression with 9 grams of a preparation containing the mixture of docosahexaenoic acid (DHA) and eicosapentaenoic acid (EPA). Peet and Horrobin (175) reported antidepressant effects for 2 g/day of EPA in patients with unipolar depression, as did Nemets et al. (176). Several other investigators have found positive effects of low-dose EPA or DHA, most recently Frangou et al. (177).

Negative reports include Marangell et al. (12) with 4–6 g/DHA and Keck et al. (178) using 6 g pure EPA.

Keck et al. (178) found EPA no more effective than placebo in a 4-month randomized, double-blind, controlled trial in patients experiencing either a refractory depressive episode or cycling. However, in post hoc analysis, younger patients exceeded placebo, but older patients worsened on active drug. Failure to see superior effects vs. placebo may be associated with a variety of factors, one of which is based on the findings by Horrobin et al. (179) of an inverted U-shaped dose-response curve for EPA on arachidonic acid levels in schizophrenia (arachidonic acid is thought to be important for its antidepressant and mood stabilizing effects). They observed that lower doses of EPA increased arachidonic acid levels as expected, but the highest dose actually caused arachidonic acid levels to decrease compared with baseline. These changes corresponded with better antipsychotic effects at 2 g/day than those observed at the higher doses of EPA.

Another alternative explanation was offered by Hibbeln and Salem (180), also from their experience with EPA in the treatment of schizophrenia. In their study, they found no overall positive effect of EPA compared with placebo. However, for those patients who received low doses of EPA and demonstrated the expected increase in cell membrane DHA levels, a significant improvement in schizophrenia was seen. However, in patients in whom a decrease in membrane DHA levels was seen, symptoms worsened compared with placebo.

Thus, other doses and preparations of this drug in specific patient subgroups should be studied before the negative findings from the study of Keck et al. (178) using 6 g of EPA can be generalized to augmentation strategies in all patients with treatment-refractory depression.

Inositol

An interesting pilot study suggested that inositol may be a useful adjunctive treatment for bipolar depression (181). In a randomized, placebo-controlled trial of inositol, 12 g/day or D-glucose added to stable mood-stabilizer regimens (n=24), 67% of inositol-treated patients improved vs. 33% of placebo patients, based on MADRS scores; however, no difference in CGI scores was detected. Recent observations are less positive.

The STEP-BD program compared the addition of lamotrigine, inositol, and risperidone for persisting bipolar depression (89, 100). Not many patients responded; 24% on lamotrigine, but only about 15% inositol, and 4.6% on risperidone.

Focus on Long-Term Prevention

If an effective antidepressive response from short-term therapy is achieved without adverse effects, the same regimen should be considered for continuation and long-term prophylaxis. This recommendation is based on the observation that a moderate depressive relapse rate occurs, even in patients who responded and are continued on their regimens. Moreover, an even higher rate of relapse into depression has been observed when patients who were maintained well for 2 months discontinue their antidepressant drugs (58, 63, 64). Filkowski et al. (182) in their randomized open study found a longer time to relapse into depression in those who continued on antidepressants, but no overall difference in morbidity.

Evidence is weaker for the need to continue other adjunctive elements for long term; however, in light of the generally high relapse rates into depression, it is suggested that full doses of these agents generally be maintained as well. One caveat would be that in the face of at least a moderate increase in the incidence of adverse effects, clinicians should attempt to reduce the dose of the agent most likely to be responsible in order to achieve better tolerability and avoid jeopardizing a sustained antidepressant response because of noncompliance.

Another reason for continuing short-term therapy as long-term prophylaxis is that when a good response is achieved during the first year or two of therapy, there is still a moderate risk for an eventual loss of efficacy by means of a pharmacodynamic tolerance (i.e., gradual loss of effect despite maintenance of good blood levels). Development tolerance that results in treatment resistance has been observed to some extent with essentially all of the MSs. One of the factors thought to be relevant to the development of tolerance is use of minimally effective doses, so that dose reduction or drug regimen simplification (in the absence of the need to do this to prevent adverse effects) may put the patient at increased risk for breakthrough episodes.

Other Therapies Including ECT, rTMS, and VNS

ECT has been used effectively in patients with bipolar depression (183). There is some evidence that bipolar patients respond more rapidly than patients with unipolar depression (183). A number of investigative groups have anecdotally noted some success with prophylactic ECT, although large, even semisystematic case series have not yet been reported to our knowledge. One group suggested using prophylactic ECT with the atypical antipsychotic clozapine because this agent lowers the seizure threshold and does not interfere with the induction or duration of the ECT seizures, as do some mood-stabilizing anticonvulsants. Moreover, there is the theoretical possibility that prophylactic ECT would exert protective anticonvulsant effects against the risk for clozapine-induced seizures; thus, patients for whom high-dose clozapine therapy was prescribed might not also need an anticonvulsant drug. This possibility is based on the original observations that ECT was an effective anticonvulsant modality in patients with epilepsy prior to the advent of more widespread use of pharmacological anticonvulsant compounds.

However, in bipolar patients with rapid recurrences, this author would recommend that a course of ECT be delayed until other options are explored, unless it was a life-threatening situation. As reported by Prudic et al. (184), there is an extraordinarily high relapse rate as a function of the increasing number of weeks following the last treatment. Responsive patients relapse at a rate of 4% per week, such that by 10 weeks, 40% have already relapsed, and the sustained response and remission rates at 6 months are 20% or less. Thus, after a good acute response, one would still be left without good data about what might be the best long-term prophylactic approach. Kellner et al. (185) also reported in unipolar patients the lack of superiority of continuation ECT compared with treatment with lithium plus nortriptyline. This author has seen about ten individuals with no particular risk factors emerge from their series of ECT with profound degrees of retrograde amnesia, and a few of those had anterograde problems as well. These anecdotal observations now converge with the report of Sackeim et al. (186) that the severity of retrograde amnesia measured on tests of autobiographical memory at 6 months is directly proportional to the number of bilateral ECTs received. Given the high rates of relapse, even after good acute response to ECT, and the risks of considerable degrees of memory loss, it would appear that trying to use pharmacological treatment of the acute episode with approaches that then may inform longer-term prophylaxis has much with which to recommend itself. If ECT is used, recent findings suggest the benefits of right unilateral ultra-brief pulse treatment to minimize cognitive impairment.

Meta-analyses have suggested that there is a significant effect of moderate to high frequency (5–20 Hz) rTMS over stimulation of the left prefrontal cortex in the treatment of unipolar or bipolar depression compared with sham stimulation (187, 188). The overall effect sizes are moderate; a number of studies have not shown positive results, and the field has not yet agreed on optimal treatment parameters. The best results do appear to be obtained with the most intense treatment parameters, i.e., 110–120% motor threshold (MT) instead of 80–90% MT at 10 Hz, and longer periods of treatment beyond the usual 2-week clinical trial (189–191). Cognitive side effects with rTMS are negligible and substantially less than with ECT.

VNS is available in many European countries and Canada, and recently was approved by the FDA in the United States. Initial open studies suggested that approximately 30% to 50% of patients with treatment-refractory depression respond to this unique type of augmentation treatment (12, 192, 193), which was originally FDA-approved for refractory epileptic seizures. The procedure used in patients with either an affective illness or epilepsy appears to be well tolerated and apparently triggers a gradually increasing response in affectively ill patients. Although most long-term pharmacological treatments show some loss of efficacy over time, the effects of the

VNS appear to increase both in magnitude and in the number of responders over 6–12 months of treatment. This suggests that a placebo effect is unlikely. However, a recent comparison had equivocal results for active VNS vs. sham stimulation.

Furthermore, the availability of third-party reimbursement for VNS treatment for patients with treatment-refractory unipolar and bipolar depression in the United States is currently uncertain. Several groups have begun to explore the use of VNS in bipolar patients with more cyclic presentations, with preliminary reports of success (193). More formal assessment of VNS for this subgroup of patients is eagerly awaited. A majority of bipolar patients apparently would choose a course of rTMS or even VNS implantation (if they were available) over the option of prophylactic ECT for a variety of reasons including expense, inconvenience, inadequate documentation of long-term efficacy in controlled trials, requirement for anesthesia, the need to induce a seizure, and concerns about effects of ECT on memory.

A night of total sleep deprivation (TSD) has been found to improve bipolar depression, albeit temporarily until the patient sleeps again, in about 50% of patients (144). Treatments that may enhance and extend the improvement afforded by TSD include lithium, light therapy, pindolol, and circadian phase advance manipulations (194, 195, 196). Another, still experimental, approach to rapid onset antidepressant effects is that of using the NMDA receptor antagonist Ketamine (197), or even an NR2B glutamate receptor subunit antagonist (198). The antidepressant and antisuicidality effects of Ketamine are observed in 2 hours and last for about 3 days. These findings and the rapid response to both sleep deprivation and TRH suggest that the requirement of several weeks for antidepressant effects to become manifest seen with routine treatment may ultimately be circumvented.

A Critical Role for Psychoeducation and Targeted Psychotherapy

Bipolar disorder patients benefit from psychosocial treatments, and controlled trials support the efficacy of such approaches, especially for targeted educational and cognitive behavior therapy interventions compared with treatment as usual (199, 200) Strikingly, several types of therapy were more effective than treatment as usual (199) when, in the same patients, antidepressant augmentation was ineffective (1). Therapy and education should also proceed as appropriate to the stage of illness evolution (37, 201). Work on relapse prevention and maintenance of remission should increasingly be introduced and emphasized as acute episodes and symptoms are resolved.

Rationale for Early Detection and Intervention

Perhaps our strongest recommendation is for the clinician to attempt to intervene pharmacologically with primary and adjunctive agents and utilize psychotherapeutic and educational techniques as early in the development of bipolar illness as possible.

Many studies have indicated that there is an (almost incredible) average duration of some 10 years between first affective symptoms meeting diagnostic thresholds and first treatment in bipolar patients. Our group (34, 202, 203) and Kessler et al. (202) have observed that the delays to first treatment are the longest in those with the earliest onsets. During this time, repeated episodes of depression and/or mania may not only interfere with patient functioning and cause a substantial morbidity and psychosocial loss, but could also be worsening the subsequent course of illness and its responsiveness to pharmacological (3, 204, 205) and psychotherapeutic (206) intervention more difficult and problematic.

The findings of Kessing et al. (207) support one of the fundamental postulates of the sensitization hypothesis, which suggests that neurobiological vulnerabilities accrue with each successive episode. Kraepelin (208) was the first to report a tendency over the first several episodes for the interval of wellness between successive episodes to decrease (i.e., cyclic acceleration), and for stressors to be less important in the precipitation of episodes later compared with earlier in the course of illness. These findings have generally been replicated in more recent systematic studies (209).

Using the Danish case registry, Kessing et al. (207) found support for this notion with the findings that the best predictor for the rate and latency to relapse into a depressive episode in either unipolar or bipolar patients was the number of prior episodes of depression requiring hospitalizations. Although these data can be interpreted in other ways, they strongly suggest the importance of intervening early and preventing episodes in the hopes that this would reduce the risk of recurrence. The observations that serum BDNF decreases and oxidative stress increases with each episode of depression (noted in the introduction) offer a potential mechanism for episode acceleration and illness progression.

Adolescents with bipolar illness are seven- to ninefold more likely than adolescents in the general population to adopt substance abuse (210), and this risk would appear to increase in the absence of treatment. Great numbers of prior depressions are associated with neuropsychological deficits, functional impairment, and treatment resistance. Depressed patients are also at increased risk of catastrophic medical disorders such as myocardial infarction and stroke as well as more difficult courses of treatment associated with many common ailments such as diabetes.

Against this sobering picture of potential illness progression, complications, and deterioration that all too often accompanies bipolar illness as conventionally treated in the community are the new data that: the MS lithium, valproate, carbamazepine, and lamotrigine; all antidepressant treatments; and the atypicals, quetiapine and ziprasidone, either increase BDNF or prevent stress-induced BDNF decrements and thus may help protect the brain. This protection could occur directly via increases in BDNF and related factors or indirectly by preventing episodes and their associated decreases in BDNF and increases in oxidative stress. These data should be presented to patients so that they can make the best informed decision about the need for long-term sustained treatment to protect themselves and their brains based on the most accurate and complete evaluation of the risk/benefit ratios for such a therapeutic approach.

References

1. Sachs GS, Nierenberg AA, Calabrese JR, Marangell LB, Wisniewski SR, Gyulai L, et al. Effectiveness of adjunctive antidepressant treatment for bipolar depression. New Engl J Med. 2007;356(17):1711–22.
2. Post RM, Denicoff KD, Leverich GS, Altshuler LL, Frye MA, Suppes TM, et al. Morbidity in 258 bipolar outpatients followed for 1 year with daily prospective ratings on the NIMH Life Chart Method. J Clin Psychiatry. 2003;64(6):680–90.
3. Nolen WA, Luckenbaugh DA, Altshuler LL, Suppes T, McElroy SL, Frye MA, et al. Correlates of 1-year prospective outcome in bipolar disorder: results from the Stanley Foundation Bipolar Network. Am J Psychiatry. 2004;161(8):1447–54.
4. Kupka RW, Luckenbaugh DA, Post RM, Suppes T, Altshuler LL, Keck PE, Jr., et al. Comparison of rapid-cycling and non-rapid-cycling bipolar disorder based on prospective mood ratings in 539 outpatients. Am J Psychiatry. 2005;162(7):1273–80.
5. Kupka R, Altshuler L, Nolen W, Suppes T, Luckenbaugh D, Leverich G, et al. Three times more days depressed than manic or hypomanic in both bipolar I and bipolar II disorder. Bipolar Disord. 2007;9(5):531–535.
6. Akiskal HS, Bourgeois ML, Angst J, Post R, Moller H, Hirschfeld R. Re-evaluating the prevalence of and diagnostic composition within the broad clinical spectrum of bipolar disorders. J Affect Disord. 2000;59 Suppl 1:S5–30.
7. Ghaemi SN, Sachs GS, Chiou AM, Pandurangi AK, Goodwin K. Is bipolar disorder still underdiagnosed? Are antidepressants overutilized? J Affect Disord. 1999;52(1–3):135–44.
8. Hirschfeld RM, Calabrese JR, Weissman MM, Reed M, Davies MA, Frye MA, et al. Screening for bipolar disorder in the community. J Clin Psychiatry. 2003;64(1):53–9.
9. Raadsheer FC, van Heerikhuize JJ, Lucassen PJ, Hoogendijk WJ, Tilders FJ, Swaab DF. Corticotropin-releasing hormone mRNA levels in the paraventricular nucleus of patients with Alzheimer's disease and depression. Am J Psychiatry. 1995;152(9):1372–6.
10. Hlastala SA, Frank E, Mallinger AG, Thase ME, Ritenour AM, Kupfer DJ. Bipolar depression: an underestimated treatment challenge. Depress Anxiety. 1997;5(2):73–83.
11. Goodwin FK, Jamison KR. Manic-depressive illness. New York: Oxford University Press; 1990.
12. Marangell LB, Bauer M, Dennehy EB, Wisniewski SR, Allen MH, Miklowitz DJ, et al. Prospective predictors of suicide and suicide attempts in 1.556 patients with bipolar disorders followed for up to 2 years. Bipolar Disord. 2006;8(5):566–76
13. Valtonen HM, Suominen K, Mantere O, Leppamaki S, Arvilommi P, Isometsa ET. Prospective study of risk factors for attempted suicide among patients with bipolar disorder. Bipolar Disord. 2006;8(5 Pt 2):576–85.
14. Leverich GS, Altshuler LL, Frye MA, Suppes T, Keck PE, McElroy SL, et al. Factors associated with suicide attempts in 648 patients with bipolar disorder in the Stanley Foundation Bipolar Network. J Clin Psychiatry. 2003;64(5):506–15.
15. Gonzalez-Pinto A, Mosquera F, Alonso M, Lopez P, Ramirez F, Vieta E, et al. Suicidal risk in bipolar I disorder patients and adherence to long-term lithium treatment. Bipolar Disord. 2006;8(5 Pt 2):618–24.
16. Baldessarini RJ, Tondo L, Davis P, Pompili M, Goodwin FK, Hennen J. Decreased risk of suicides and attempts during long-term lithium treatment: a meta-analytic review. Bipolar Disord. 2006;8(5 Pt 2):625–39.
17. Kessing LV, Andersen PK. Does the risk of developing dementia increase with the number of episodes in patients with depressive disorder and in patients with bipolar disorder? J Neurol Neurosurg Psychiatry. 2004;75(12):1662–6.
18. Post RM. Role of BDNF in bipolar and unipolar disorder: Clinical and theoretical implications. J Psychiatr Res. 2007;41(12):979–90.
19. Duman RS, Monteggia LM. A neurotrophic model for stress-related mood disorders. Biol Psychiatry. 2006;59(12):1116–27.

20. Kapczinski F, Vieta E, Audreazza AC, Frey BN, Gomes FA, Tramontina J, Kauer-Sant'Anna M, Grassi-Olivera R, Post RM. Allostatic load in bipolar disorder: implications for pathophysiology and treatment. Neurosci Biobehav Rev 2008;32:675–692.
21. Post RM. Bipolar depression. The stepchild, preface and overview. Clin Neurosci Res. 2002;2:122–6.
22. Gijsman HJ, Geddes JR, Rendell JM, Nolen WA, Goodwin GM. Antidepressants for bipolar depression: a systematic review of randomized, controlled trials. Am J Psychiatry. 2004;161(9):1537–47.
23. Thase ME, Mallinger AG, McKnight D, Himmelhoch JM. Treatment of imipramine-resistant recurrent depression, IV: a double-blind crossover study of tranylcypromine for anergic bipolar depression. Am J Psychiatry. 1992;149(2):195–8.
24. Potter WZ, Murphy DL, Wehr TA, Linnoila M, Goodwin FK. Clorgyline. A new treatment for patients with refractory rapid-cycling disorder. Arch Gen Psychiatry. 1982;39:505–10.
25. Himmelhoch JM, Thase ME, Mallinger AG, Houck P. Tranylcypromine versus imipramine in anergic bipolar depression. Am J Psychiatry. 1991;148:910–6.
26. Benazzi F. Prevalence of bipolar II disorder in atypcal depression. Eur Arch Psychiatry Clin Neurosci. 1999;249(2):62–5.
27. Rouillon F, Lejoyeux M, Filteau MJ, Montgomery SA, Rouillon F. Unwanted effects of long-term treatment. Long-term treatment of depression. Chichester: Wiley; 1992, pp. 81–111.
28. Boerlin HL, Gitlin MJ, Zoellner LA, Hammen CL. Bipolar depression and antidepressant-induced mania: a naturalistic study. J Clin Psychiatry. 1998;59(7):374–9.
29. Bottlender R, Rudolf D, Strauss A, Moller HJ. Mood-stabilisers reduce the risk of developing antidepressant-induced maniform states in acute treatment of bipolar I depressed patients. J Affect Disord. 2001;63(1–3):79–83.
30. Peet M. Induction of mania with selective serotonin re-uptake inhibitors and tricyclic antidepressants. Br J Psychiatry. 1994;164(4):549–50.
31. Calabrese JR, Rapport DJ, Kimmel SE, Shelton MD. Controlled trials in bipolar I depression: focus on switch rates and efficacy. Eur Neuropsychopharmacol. 1999;9 Suppl 4:S109–12.
32. Silverstone T. Moclobemide vs. imipramine in bipolar depression: a multicentre double-blind clinical trial. Acta Psychiatr Scand. 2001;104(2):104–9.
33. Post RM, Altshuler LL, Leverich GS, Frye MA, Nolen WA, Kupka RW, et al. Mood switch in bipolar depression: comparison of adjunctive venlafaxine, bupropion and sertraline. Br J Psychiatry. 2006;189(2):124–31.
34. Leverich GS, Altshuler LL, Frye MA, Suppes T, McElroy SL, Keck PE, Jr., et al. Risk of switch in mood polarity to hypomania or mania in patients with bipolar depression during acute and continuation trials of venlafaxine, sertraline, and bupropion as adjuncts to mood stabilizers. Am J Psychiatry. 2006;163(2):232–9.
35. Martin A, Young C, Leckman JF, Mukonoweshuro C, Rosenheck R, Leslie D. Age effects on antidepressant-induced manic conversion. Arch Pediatr Adolesc Med. 2004;158(8): 773–80.
36. Altshuler LL, Suppes T, Black DO, Nolen WA, Leverich G, Keck PE, Jr., et al. Lower switch rate in depressed patients with bipolar II than bipolar I disorder treated adjunctively with second-generation antidepressants. Am J Psychiatry. 2006;163(2):313–5.
37. Post RM, Leverich GS. The role of psychosocial stress in the onset and progression of bipolar disorder and its comorbidities: the need for earlier and alternative modes of therapeutic intervention. Dev Psychopathol. 2006;18(4):1181–211.
38. Goldberg JF, Whiteside JE. The association between substance abuse and antidepressant-induced mania in bipolar disorder: a preliminary study. J Clin Psychiatry. 2002;63(9): 791–5.
39. Sachs GS, Lafer B, Stoll AL, Banov M, Thibault AB, Tohen M, et al. A double-blind trial of bupropion versus desipramine for bipolar depression. J Clin Psychiatry. 1994;55(9): 391–3.
40. Vieta E, Martinez-Aran A, Goikolea JM, Torrent C, Colom F, Benabarre A, et al. A randomized trial comparing paroxetine and venlafaxine in the treatment of bipolar depressed patients taking mood stabilizers. J Clin Psychiatry. 2002;63(6):508–12.

41. Frye MA, McElroy SL, Hellemann G, Nolen WA, Suppes T, Grunze HC, et al. Clinical correlates associated with antidepressant-related mania. American Psychiatric Association Annual Meeting, Toronto, Canada, May 20–25, 2006. 2006.
42. Grossman F, Potter WZ, Brown EA, Maislin G. A double-blind study comparing idazoxan and bupropion in bipolar depressed patients. J Affect Disord. 1999;56(2–3):237–43.
43. Fogelson DL, Bystritsky A, Pasnau R. Bupropion in the treatment of bipolar disorders: the same old story? J Clin Psychiatry. 1992;53:443–6.
44. Cohn JB, Collins G, Ashbrook E, Wernicke JF. A comparison of fluoxetine, imipramine and placebo in patients with bipolar depressive disorder. Int Clin Psychopharmacol. 1989;4:313–22.
45. Amsterdam JD, Garcia-Espana F, Fawcett J, Quitkin FM, Reimherr FW, Rosenbaum JF, et al. Efficacy and safety of fluoxetine in treating bipolar II major depressive episode. J Clin Psychopharmacol. 1998;18(6):435–40.
46. Ambrosio LA, Buccomino D, Filippo A, Morelli A, Musacchio R, Pupo F, et al. Efficacy and tolerability of paroxetine in the treatent of the depresive phase of bipolar disorders. Minerva Psychiatr. 1996;37(2):91–7.
47. Nemeroff CB, Evans DL, Gyulai L, Sachs GS, Bowden CL, Gergel IP, et al. Double-blind, placebo-controlled comparison of imipramine and paroxetine in the treatment of bipolar depression. Am J Psychiatry. 2001;158(6):906–12.
48. Kupfer DJ, Chengappa KN, Gelenberg AJ, Hirschfeld RM, Goldberg JF, Sachs GS, et al. Citalopram as adjunctive therapy in bipolar depression. J Clin Psychiatry. 2001;62(12):985–90.
49. Fagiolini A, Buysse DJ, Frank E, Houck PR, Luther JF, Kupfer DJ. Tolerability of combined treatment with lithium and paroxetine in patients with bipolar disorder and depression. J Clin Psychopharmacol. 2001;21(5):474–8.
50. Amsterdam J. Efficacy and safety of venlafaxine in the treatment of bipolar II major depressive episode. J Clin Psychopharmacol. 1998;18(5):414–7.
51. Goldberg JF, Burdick KE, Endick CJ. A Placebo-contolled trial of pramipexole for bipolar depression. 155th annual meeting of the American Psychiatric Association, Philadelphia, May 22, 2002.
52. Zarate CA, Jr., Payne JL, Singh J, Quiroz JA, Luckenbaugh DA, Denicoff KD, et al. Pramipexole for bipolar II depression: a placebo-controlled proof of concept study. Biol Psychiatry. 2004;56(1):54–60.
53. Goldberg JF, Frye MA, Dunn RT. Pramipexole in refractory bipolar depression [letter]. Am J Psychiatry. 1999;156(5):798.
54. Sporn J, Ghaemi SN, Sambur MR, Rankin MA, Recht J, Sachs GS, et al. Pramipexole augmentation in the treatment of unipolar and bipolar depression: a retrospective chart review. Ann Clin Psychiatry. 2000;12(3):137–40.
55. Corrigan MH, Denahan AQ, Wright CE, Ragual RJ, Evans DL. Comparison of pramipexole, fluoxetine, and placebo in patients with major depression. Depress Anxiety. 2000;11(2):58–65.
56. Perugi G, Toni C, Ruffolo G, Frare F, Akiskal H. Adjunctive dopamine agonists in treatment-resistant bipolar II depression: an open case series. Pharmacopsychiatry. 2001;34(4):137–41.
57. Frankle WG, Perlis RH, Deckersbach T, Grandin LD, Gray SM, Sachs GS, et al. Bipolar depression: relationship between episode length and antidepressant treatment. Psychol Med. 2002;32(8):1417–23.
58. Altshuler L, Kiriakos L, Calcagno J, Goodman R, Gitlin M, Frye M, et al. The impact of antidepressant discontinuation versus antidepressant continuation on 1-year risk for relapse of bipolar depression: a retrospective chart review. J Clin Psychiatry. 2001;62(8):612–6.
59. Tohen M, Chengappa KN, Suppes T, Baker RW, Zarate CA, Bowden CL, et al. Relapse prevention in bipolar I disorder: 18-month comparison of olanzapine plus mood stabiliser v. mood stabiliser alone. Br J Psychiatry. 2004;184:337–45.
60. Post RM, Speer AM, Leverich GS. Complex combination therapy: the evolution toward rational polypharmacy in lithium-resistant bipolar illness. In: Akiskal HS, Tohen M, eds. Bipolar Psychopharmacotherapy Caring for the Patient. Chichester: Wiley; 2006, pp. 135–167.

61. Denicoff KD, Smith-Jackson EE, Disney ER, Ali SO, Leverich GS, Post RM. Comparative prophylactic efficacy of lithium, carbamazepine, and the combination in bipolar disorder. J Clin Psychiatry. 1997;58(11):470–8.
62. Young LT, Joffe RT, Robb JC, MacQueen GM, Marriott M, Patelis-Siotis I. Double-blind comparison of addition of a second mood stabilizer versus an antidepressant to an initial mood stabilizer for treatment of patients with bipolar depression. Am J Psychiatry. 2000;157(1):124–6.
63. Altshuler L, Suppes T, Black D, Nolen WA, Keck PE, Jr., Frye MA, et al. Impact of antidepressant discontinuation after acute bipolar depression remission on rates of depressive relapse at 1-year follow-up. Am J Psychiatry. 2003;160(7):1252–62.
64. Joffe RT, MacQueen GM, Marriott M, Young LT. One-year outcome with antidepressant – treatment of bipolar depression. Acta Psychiatr Scand. 2005;112(2):105–9.
65. Ghaemi SN, Ostacher MM, El-Mallakh RS, Borrelli D, Baldassano CF, Kelley ME, et al. Antidepressant discontinuation in bipolar depression: a systematic treatment enhancement program for bipolar disorder (STEP-BD) randomized clinical trial of long-term effectiveness and safety. J Clin Psychiatry 2010;71(4):372–380.
66. Goodwin FK, Murphy DL, Dunner DL, Bunney WE, Jr. Lithium response in unipolar versus bipolar depression. Am J Psychiatry. 1972;129:76–9.
67. Goodwin FK, Jamison KR. Manic-depressive illness. New York: Oxford; 2007.
68. Goldberg JF, Harrow M, Leon AC. Lithium treatment of bipolar affective disorders under naturalistic followup conditions. Psychopharmacol Bull. 1996;32(1):47–54.
69. Ahrens B, Muller-Oerlinghausen B. Does lithium exert an independent antisuicidal effect? Pharmacopsychiatry. 2001;34(4):132–6.
70. Tohen M, Zhang F, Keck PE, Feldman PD, Risser RC, Tran PV, et al. Olanzapine versus haloperidol in schizoaffective disorder, bipolar type. J Affect Disord. 2001;67(1–3):133–40.
71. Baldessarini RJ, Tondo L, Hennen J. Treating the suicidal patient with bipolar disorder. Reducing suicide risk with lithium. Ann N Y Acad Sci. 2001;932:24–38.
72. Maj M, Pirozzi R, Magliano L, Bartoli L. Long-term outcome of lithium prophylaxis in bipolar disorder: a 5-year prospective study of 402 patients at a lithium clinic. Am J Psychiatry. 1998;155(1):30–5.
73. Swann AC, Bowden CL, Morris D, Calabrese JR, Petty F, Small J, et al. Depression during mania. Treatment response to lithium or divalproex. Arch Gen Psychiatry. 1997;54:37–42.
74. Okuma T. Effects of carbamazepine and lithium on affective disorders. Neuropsychobiology. 1993;27(3):138–45.
75. Bauer M, Bschor T, Kunz D, Berghofer A, Strohle A, Muller-Oerlinghausen B. Double-blind, placebo-controlled trial of the use of lithium to augment antidepressant medication in continuation treatment of unipolar major depression. Am J Psychiatry. 2000;157(9):1429–35.
76. Kleindienst N, Severus WE, Moller HJ, Greil W. Is polarity of recurrence related to serum lithium level in patients with bipolar disorder? Eur Arch Psychiatry Clin Neurosci. 2005;255(1):72–4.
77. Dunn RT, Frye MS, Kimbrell TA, Denicoff KD, Leverich GS, Post RM. The efficacy and use of anticonvulsants in mood disorders. Clin Neuropharmacol. 1998;21(4):215–35.
78. Post RM, Uhde TW, Rubinow DR, Huggins T. Differential time course of antidepressant effects after sleep deprivation, ECT, and carbamazepine: clinical and theoretical implications. Psychiatry Res. 1987;22(1):11–9.
79. Ketter TA, Wang PW, Post R. Carbamazepine and Oxcarbazepine. In: Schatzberg AF, Nemeroff CB, eds. Textbook of Psychopharmacology, Fourth Edition. Arlington: The American Psychiatric Publishing; 2007.
80. Simhandl C, Denk E, Thau K. The comparative efficacy of carbamazepine low and high serum level and lithium carbonate in the prophylaxis of affective disorders. J Affect Disord. 1993;28:221–31.
81. Greil W, Kleindienst N, Erazo N, Muller-Oerlinghausen B. Differential response to lithium and carbamazepine in the prophylaxis of bipolar disorder. J Clin Psychopharmacol. 1998;18(6):455–60.

82. Zhang ZJ, Kang WH, Tan QR, Li Q, Gao CG, Zhang FG, et al. Adjunctive herbal medicine with carbamazepine for bipolar disorders: a double-blind, randomized, placebo-controlled study. J Psychiatr Res. 2007;41(3–4):360–9.
83. Ketter TA, Kimbrell TA, George MS, Willis MW, Benson BE, Danielson A, et al. Baseline cerebral hypermetabolism associated with carbamazepine response, and hypometabolism with nimodipine response in mood disorders. Biol Psychiatry. 1999;46(10):1364–74.
84. Davis LL, Bartolucci A, Petty F. Divalproex in the treatment of bipolar depression: a placebo-controlled study. J Affect Disord. 2005;85(3):259–66.
85. Davis LL, Kabel D, Patel D, Choate AD, Foslien-Nash C, Gurguis GN, et al. Valproate as an antidepressant in major depressive disorder. Psychopharmacol Bull. 1996;32:647–52.
86. Ketter TA, Wang PW, Nowakowska C, Chandler RA, Hill SJ, Nam JY, et al. Divalproex-extended release monotherapy and adjunctive therapy in bipolar II depression. Seventh International Conference on Bipolar Disorder, Pittsburgh, PA, June 7–9, 2007.
87. Bowden CL, Calabrese JR, McElroy SL, Gyulai L, Wassef A, Petty F, et al. A randomized, placebo-controlled 12-month trial of divalproex and lithium in treatment of outpatients with bipolar I disorder. Divalproex Maintenance Study Group. Arch Gen Psychiatry. 2000;57(5):481–9.
88. Gyulai L, Bowden CL, McElroy SL, Calabrese JR, Petty F, Swann AC, et al. Maintenance efficacy of divalproex in the prevention of bipolar depression. Neuropsychopharmacology. 2003;28(7):1374–82.
89. Sachs GS, Collins G. A placebo-controlled trial of divlproex sodium in acute bipolar depression. 40th annual meeting of the American College of Neuropsychopharmacology, Waikola, Hawaii, Dec 9–13, 2001.
90. Calabrese JR, Markovitz PJ, Kimmel SE, Wagner SC. Spectrum of efficacy of valproate in 78 rapid-cycling bipolar patients. J Clin Psychopharmacol. 1992;12(1 Suppl):53S–6.
91. Calabrese JR, Delucchi GA. Spectrum of efficacy of valproate in 55 patients with rapid-cycling bipolar disorder. Am J Psychiatry. 1990;147:431–4.
92. Calabrese JR, Delucchi GA. Phenomenology of rapid cycling manic depression and its treatment with valproate. J Clin Psychiatry. 1989;50:30–4.
93. Post RM, Ketter TA, Pazzaglia PJ, Denicoff K, George MS, Callahan A, et al. Rational polypharmacy in the bipolar affective disorders. Epilepsy Res Suppl. 1996;11:153–80.
94. Post RM, Berrettini WH, Uhde TW, Kellner CH. Selective response to the anticonvulsant carbamazepine in manic-depressive illness: a case study. J Clin Psychopharmacol. 1984;4(4):178–85.
95. Post RM. Non-lithium treatment for bipolar disorder. J Clin Psychiatry. 1990;51 Suppl:9–16.
96. Calabrese JR, Suppes T, Bowden CL, Sachs GS, Swann AC, McElroy SL, et al. A double-blind, placebo-controlled, prophylaxis study of lamotrigine in rapid-cycling bipolar disorder. Lamictal 614 Study Group. J Clin Psychiatry. 2000;61(11):841–50.
97. Frye MA, Ketter TA, Kimbrell TA, Dunn RT, Speer AM, Osuch EA, et al. A placebo-controlled study of lamotrigine and gabapentin monotherapy in refractory mood disorders. J Clin Psychopharmacol. 2000;20(6):607–14.
98. Perugi G, Toni C, Ruffolo G, Sartini S, Simonini E, Akiskal H. Clinical experience using adjunctive gabapentin in treatment-resistant bipolar mixed states. Pharmacopsychiatry. 1999;32(4):136–41.
99. Bowden CL, Calabrese JR, McElroy SL, Rhodes LJ, Keck PE, Jr., Cookson J, et al. The efficacy of lamotrigine in rapid cycling and non-rapid cycling patients with bipolar disorder. Biol Psychiatry. 1999;45(8):953–8.
100. Nierenberg AA, Ostacher MJ, Calabrese JR, Ketter TA, Marangell LB, Miklowitz DJ, et al. Treatment-resistant bipolar depression: a STEP-BD equipoise randomized effectiveness trial of antidepressant augmentation with lamotrigine, inositol, or risperidone. Am J Psychiatry. 2006;163(2):210–6.
101. van der Loos M, Nolen W. Lamotrigine as add-on to lithium in bipolar depression. 160th Annual Meeting of the American Psychiatric Association, San Diego, CA, 2007.
102. Sporn J, Sachs G. The anticonvulsant lamotrigine in treatment-resistant manic-depressive illness. J Clin Psychopharmacol. 1997;17:185–9.

103. Pinto OC, Akiskal HS. Lamotrigine as a promising approach to borderline personality: an open case series without concurrent DSM-IV major mood disorder. J Affect Disord. 1998;51(3):333–43.
104. Calabrese JR, Sullivan JR, Bowden CL, Suppes T, Goldberg JF, Sachs GS, et al. Rash in multicenter trials of lamotrigine in mood disorders: clinical relevance and management. J Clin Psychiatry. 2002;63(11):1012–9.
105. Schlienger RG, Shapiro LE, Shear NH. Lamotrigine-induced severe cutaneous adverse reactions. Epilepsia. 1998;39 Suppl 7:S22–6.
106. Obrocea GV, Dunn RM, Frye MA, Ketter TA, Luckenbaugh DA, Leverich GS, et al. Clinical predictors of response to lamotrigine and gabapentin monotherapy in refractory affective disorders. Biol Psychiatry. 2002;51(3):253–60.
107. Grof P, Duffy A, Cavazzoni P, Grof E, Garnham J, MacDougall M, et al. Is response to prophylactic lithium a familial trait? J Clin Psychiatry. 2002;63(10):942–7.
108. Duffy A, Alda M, Kutcher S, Cavazzoni P, Robertson C, Grof E, et al. A prospective study of the offspring of bipolar parents responsive and nonresponsive to lithium treatment. J Clin Psychiatry. 2002;63(12):1171–8.
109. Alda M, Passmore MJ, Garnham J, Duffy A, MacDougall M, Munro M, et al. Clinical presentation of bipolar disorders responsive to lithium or lamotrigine. Int J Neuropsychopharmacol. 2002;5(Suppl 1):S58.
110. Pande AC, Crockatt JG, Janney CA, Werth JL, Tsaroucha G. Gabapentin in bipolar disorder: a placebo-controlled trial of adjunctive therapy. Gabapentin Bipolar Disorder Study Group. Bipolar Disord. 2000;2(3 Pt 2):249–55.
111. Houtkooper MA, Lammertsma A, Meyer JWA, Goedhart DM, Meinardi H, Blom GF, et al. Oxcarbazepine (GP 47.680): a possible alternative to carbamazepine? Epilepsia. 1987;28:693–8.
112. McElroy SL, Soutullo CA, Keck PE, Jr., Kmetz GF. A pilot trial of adjunctive gabapentin in the treatment of bipolar disorder. Ann Clin Psychiatry. 1997;9:99–103.
113. Cabras PL, Hardoy MJ, Hardoy MC, Carta MG. Clinical experience with gabapentin in patients with bipolar or schizoaffective disorder: results of an open-label study. J Clin Psychiatry. 1999;60(4):245–8.
114. Vieta E, Goikolea JM, Martínez-Arán A, Comes M, Verger K, Masramon X, et al. A double-blind, randomized, placebo-controlled, prophylaxis study of adjunctive gabapentin for bipolar disorder. J Clin Psychiatry. 2006;67(3):473-7
115. Marcotte D. Use of topiramate, a new anti-epileptic as a mood stabilizer. J Affect Disord. 1998;50:245–51.
116. McElroy SL, Suppes T, Keck PE, Frye MA, Denicoff KD, Altshuler LL, et al. Open-label adjunctive topiramate in the treatment of bipolar disorders. Biol Psychiatry. 2000;47(12):1025–33.
117. McIntyre RS, Mancini DA, McCann S, Srinivasan J, Sagman D, Kennedy SH. Topiramate versus bupropion SR when added to mood stabilizer therapy for the depressive phase of bipolar disorder: a preliminary single-blind study. Bipolar Disord. 2002;4(3):207–13.
118. Johnson BA, Ait-Daoud N, Bowden CL, DiClemente CC, Roache JD, Lawson K, et al. Oral topiramate for treatment of alcohol dependence: a randomised controlled trial. Lancet. 2003;361(9370):1677–85.
119. Hayes SG. Acetazolamide in bipolar affective disorders. Ann Clin Psychiatry. 1994;6(2):91–8.
120. McElroy SL, Arnold LM, Shapira NA, Keck PE, Jr., Rosenthal NR, Karim MR, et al. Topiramate in the treatment of binge eating disorder associated with obesity: a randomized, placebo-controlled trial. Am J Psychiatry. 2003;160(2):255–61.
121. McElroy SL, Frye MA, Altshuler LL, Suppes T, Hellemann G, Black D, et al. A 24-week, randomized, controlled trial of adjunctive sibutramine versus topiramate in the treatment of weight gain in overweight or obese patients with bipolar disorders. Bipolar Disord. 2007;9(4):426–34.

122. Emrich H, Schiwy W, Silverstone T. Carbamazepine and oxcarbazepine in psychiatry. London: Clinical Neuroscience Publishers; 1990.
123. Emrich HM. Studies with oxcarbazepine (Trileptal) in acute mania. Int Clin Psychopharmacol. 1990;5(Suppl 1):83–8.
124. Hummel B, Walden J, Stampfer R, Dittmann S, Amann B, Sterr A, et al. Acute antimanic efficacy and safety of oxcarbazepine in an open trial with an on-off-on design. Bipolar Disord. 2002;4(6):412–7.
125. Ghaemi SN, Ko JY, Katzow JJ. Oxcarbazepine treatment of refractory bipolar disorder: a retrospective chart review. Bipolar Disord. 2002;4:70–4.
126. Wagner KD, Kowatch RA, Emslie GJ, Findling RL, Wilens TE, McCague K, et al. A double-blind, randomized, placebo-controlled trial of oxcarbazepine in the treatment of bipolar disorder in children and adolescents. Am J Psychiatry. 2006;163(7):1179–86.
127. Dam M, Ekberg R, Lyning Y, Waltimo O, Jakobsen K. A double-blind study comparing oxcarbazepine and carbamazepine in patients with newly diagnosed, previously untreated epilepsy. Epilepsy Res. 1989;3:70–6.
128. Dickinson RG, Hooper WD, Pendlebury SC, Moses D, Eadie MJ. Further clinical and pharmacokinetic observations on the new anticonvulsant, oxcarbazepine. Clin Exp Neurol. 1988;25:127–33.
129. Pendlebury SC, Moses DK, Eadie MJ. Hyponatraemia during oxcarbazepine therapy. Hum Toxicol. 1989;8:337–44.
130. Raitasuo V, Lehtovaara R, Huttunen MO. Effect of switching carbamazepine to oxcarbazepine on the plasma levels of neuroleptics. A case report. Psychopharmacology. 1994;116(1):115–6.
131. Kanba S, Yagi G, Kamijima K, Suzuki T, Tajima O, Otaki J, et al. The first open study of zonisamide, a novel anticonvulsant, shows efficacy in mania. Prog Neuropsychopharmacol Biol Psychiatry. 1994;18(4):707–15.
132. McElroy SL, Suppes T, Keck PE, Jr., Black D, Frye MA, Altshuler LL, et al. Open-label adjunctive zonisamide in the treatment of bipolar disorders: a prospective trial. J Clin Psychiatry. 2005;66(5):617–24.
133. Yang Y, Nowakowska C, Becker OV. Weight loss during the first two months of open adjunctive zonisamide for obesity in bipolar disorder patients. 156th annual meeting of the Amareican Psychiatric Association, San Francisco, CA, May 2003.
134. Grunze H, Erfurth A, Amann B, Normann C, Walden J. Gabapentin in the treatment of mania. Fortschr Neurol Psychiatr. 1999;67(6):256–60.
135. Suppes T, Chisholm KA, Dhavale D, Frye MA, Altshuler LL, McElroy SL, et al. Tiagabine in treatment refractory bipolar disorder: a clinical case series. Bipolar Disord. 2002;4(5):283–9.
136. Schaffer LC, Schaffer CB, Howe J. An open case series on the utility of tiagabine as an augmentation in refractory bipolar outpatients. J Affect Disord. 2002;71(1–3):259–63.
137. Ring HA, Crellin R, Kirker S, Reynolds EH. Vigabatrin and depression. J Neurol Neurosurg Psychiatry. 1993;56:925–8.
138. Aldenkamp AP, Vermeulen J, Mulder OG, Overweg J, Van Parys JA, Beun AM, et al. Gamma-vinyl GABA (vigabatrin) and mood disturbances. Epilepsia. 1994;35(5):999–1004.
139. Thase ME, Macfadden W, Weisler RH, Chang W, Paulsson B, Khan A, et al. Efficacy of quetiapine monotherapy in bipolar I and II depression: a double-blind, placebo-controlled study (the BOLDER II study). J Clin Psychopharmacol. 2006;26(6):600–9.
140. Calabrese JR, Keck PE, Jr., Macfadden W, Minkwitz M, Ketter TA, Weisler RH, et al. A randomized, double-blind, placebo-controlled trial of quetiapine in the treatment of bipolar I or II depression. Am J Psychiatry. 2005;162(7):1351–60.
141. Suppes T, Webb A, Paul B, Carmody T, Kraemer H, Rush AJ. Clinical outcome in a randomized 1-year trial of clozapine versus treatment as usual for patients with treatment-resistant illness and a history of mania. Am J Psychiatry. 1999;156(8):1164–9.

142. Ciapparelli A, Dell'Osso L, Pini S, Chiavacci MC, Fenzi M, Cassano GB. Clozapine for treatment-refractory schizophrenia, schizoaffective disorder, and psychotic bipolar disorder: a 24-month naturalistic study. J Clin Psychiatry. 2000;61(5):329–34.
143. Ranjan R, Meltzer HY. Acute and long-term effectiveness of clozapine in treatment-resistant psychotic depression. Biol Psychiatry. 1996;40:253–8.
144. Barbini B, Colombo C, Benedetti F, Campori E, Bellodi L, Smeraldi E. The unipolar-bipolar dichotomy and the response to sleep deprivation. Psychiatry Res. 1998;79(1):43–50.
145. Vieta E, Goikolea JM, Corbella B, Benabarre A, Reinares M, Martinez G, et al. Risperidone safety and efficacy in the treatment of bipolar and schizoaffective disorders: results from a 6-month, multicenter, open study. J Clin Psychiatry. 2001;62(10):818–25.
146. Janicak PG, Keck PE, Jr., Davis JM, Kasckow JW, Tugrul K, Dowd SM, et al. A double-blind, randomized, prospective evaluation of the efficacy and safety of risperidone versus haloperidol in the treatment of schizoaffective disorder. J Clin Psychopharmacol. 2001;21(4):360–8.
147. Ghaemi SN, Sachs GS. Long-term risperidone treatment in bipolar disorder: 6-month follow up. Int Clin Psychopharmacol. 1997;12(6):333–8.
148. Ostroff RB, Nelson JC. Risperidone augmentation of selective serotonin reuptake inhibitors in major depression. J Clin Psychiatry. 1999;60(4):256–9.
149. Shelton RC, Stahl SM. Risperidone and paroxetine given singly and in combination for bipolar depression. J Clin Psychiatry. 2004;65(12):1715–9.
150. Mullen J, Jibson MD, Sweitzer D. A comparison of the relative safety, efficacy, and tolerability of quetiapine and risperidone in outpatients with schizophrenia and other psychotic disorders: the quetiapine experience with safety and tolerability (QUEST) study. Clin Ther. 2001;23(11):1839–54.
151. Rothschild AJ, Bates KS, Boehringer KL, Syed A. Olanzapine response in psychotic depression. J Clin Psychiatry. 1999;60(2):116–8.
152. Ghaemi SN, Cherry EL, Katzow JA, Goodwin FK. Does olanzapine have antidepressant properties? A retrospective preliminary study. Bipolar Disord. 2000;2(3):196–9.
153. Tohen M, Baker RW, Altshuler LL, Zarate CA, Suppes T, Ketter TA, et al. Olanzapine versus divalproex in the treatment of acute mania. Am J Psychiatry. 2002;159(6):1011–7.
154. Shelton RC, Tollefson GD, Tohen M, Stahl S, Gannon KS, Jacobs TG, et al. A novel augmentation strategy for treating resistant major depression. Am J Psychiatry. 2001;158(1):131–4.
155. Sanger TM, Grundy SL, Gibson PJ, Namjoshi MA, Greaney MG, Tohen MF. Long-term olanzapine therapy in the treatment of bipolar I disorder: an open-label continuation phase study. J Clin Psychiatry. 2001;62(4):273–81.
156. Keck PE. New Antiepileptics in the treatment of bipolar disorders. Symposium 34: "Clinical Issues in Bipolar Disorder," American Psychiatric Association Syllabus & Proceedings Summary, 2001.
157. Goldstein JM, Cristoph G, Grimm S, Liu JW, Widzowski D, Brecher M. Unique mechanism of acton for the antidepressant properties of the atypical antipsychotic quetiapine. 160th Annual Meeting of the American Psychiatric Association, San Diego, CA, 2007.
158. Park SW, Lee SK, Kim JM, Yoon JS, Kim YH. Effects of quetiapine on the brain-derived neurotrophic factor expression in the hippocampus and neocortex of rats. Neurosci Lett. 2006;402(1–2):25–9.
159. Kim YH, Lee JG, Lee CH, Park SW. Effects of ziprasidone on the immobiliztion stress-induced BDNF mRNA expression in rat brain. 160th Annual Meeting of the American Psychiatric Association, San Diego, CA, 2007.
160. Kane JM, Carson WH, Saha AR, McQuade RD, Ingenito GG, Zimbroff DL, et al. Efficacy and safety of aripiprazole and haloperidol versus placebo in patients with schizophrenia and schizoaffective disorder. J Clin Psychiatry. 2002;63(9):763–71.
161. McElroy SL, Suppes T, Frye MA, Altshuler LL, Stanford K, Martens B, et al. Open-label aripiprazole in the treatment of acute bipolar depression: a prospective pilot trial. J Affect Disord. 2007;101:275–81.

162. Berman RM, Marcus RM, Swanink R, McQuade RD, Kahn A. Efficacy and safety of aripiprazole as adjunctive therapy in MDD; A multicenter, randomized, double-blind, placebo-controlled study. 160th Annual Meeting of the American Psychiatric Association, San Diego, CA, 2007.
163. Marcus RN, Owen R, Swanink R, McQuade RD, Iwamoto T. Two studies to evaluate the safety and efficacy of ariiprazole monotherapy in outpatients with bipolar I disorder with a major depressive episode without psychotic features. 160th Annual Meeting of the American Psychiatric Association, San Diego, CA, 2007.
164. Nickel MK, Muehlbacher M, Nickel C, Kettler C, Pedrosa GF, Bachler E, et al. Aripiprazole in the treatment of patients with borderline personality disorder: a double-blind, placebo-controlled study. Am J Psychiatry. 2006;163(5):833–8.
165. Cutler NR, Post RM. State-related cyclical dyskinesias in manic-depressive illness. J Clin Psychopharmacol. 1982;2(5):350–4.
166. Coppen A, Chaudhry S, Swade C. Folic acid enhances lithium prophylaxis. J Affect Disord. 1986;10:9–13.
167. Dittmann S, Seemuller F, Kleindienst N, Schwarz M, Stampfer R, Zach J, et al. Association of cognitive deficits with elevated homocysteine plasma levels in euthymic bipolar patients. Bipolar Disord. 2005;7(Suppl 2):48.
168. Osher Y, Sela BA, Levine J, Belmaker RH. Elevated homocysteine levels in euthymic bipolar disorder patients showing functional deterioration. Bipolar Disord. 2004;6(1):82–6.
169. Frye MA, Denicoff KD, Bryan AL, Smith-Jackson EE, Ali SO, Luckenbaugh D, et al. Association between lower serum free T4 and greater mood instability and depression in lithium-maintained bipolar patients. Am J Psychiatry. 1999;156(12):1909–14.
170. Hatterer JA, Kocsis JH, Stokes PE. Thyroid function in patients maintained on lithium. Psychiatr Res. 1988;26:249–57.
171. Joffe RT. The use of thyroid supplements to augment antidepressant medication. J Clin Psychiatry. 1998;59 Suppl 5:26–9.
172. Baumgartner A, Bauer M, Hellweg R. Treatment of intractable non-rapid cycling bipolar afective disorder with high-dose thyroxine: an open clinical trial. Neuropsychopharmacol. 1994;10(3):183–9.
173. Bauer MS, Whybrow PC. Rapid cycling bipolar affective disorder. II. Treatment of refractory rapid cycling with high-dose levothyroxine: a preliminary study. Arch Gen Psychiatry. 1990;47:435–40.
174. Stoll AL, Severus WE, Freeman MP, Rueter S, Zboyan HA, Diamond E, et al. Omega 3 fatty acids in bipolar disorder: a preliminary double-blind, placebo-controlled trial. Arch Gen Psychiatry. 1999;56(5):407–12.
175. Peet M, Horrobin DF. A dose-ranging study of the effects of ethyl-eicosapentaenoate in patients with ongoing depression despite apparently adequate treatment with standard drugs. Arch Gen Psychiatry. 2002;59(10):913–9.
176. Nemets B, Stahl Z, Belmaker RH. Addition of omega-3 fatty acid to maintenance medication treatment for recurrent unipolar depressive disorder. Am J Psychiatry. 2002;159(3):477–9.
177. Frangou S, Lewis M, McCrone P. Efficacy of ethyl-eicosapentaenoic acid in bipolar depression: randomised double-blind placebo-controlled study. Br J Psychiatry. 2006; 188(1):46–50.
178. Keck PE, Jr., Mintz J, McElroy SL, Freeman MP, Suppes T, Frye MA, et al. Double-blind, randomized, placebo-controlled trials of ethyl-eicosapentanoate in the treatment of bipolar depression and rapid cycling bipolar disorder. Biol Psychiatry. 2006;60(9):1020–2.
179. Horrobin DF, Jenkins K, Bennett CN, Christie WW. Eicosapentaenoic acid and arachidonic acid: collaboration and not antagonism is the key to biological understanding. Prostaglandins Leukot Essent Fatty Acids. 2002;66(1):83–90.
180. Hibbeln JR, Salem N, Jr. Dietary polyunsaturated fatty acids and depression: when cholesterol does not satisfy. Am J Clin Nutr. 1995;62(1):1–9.
181. Chengappa KN, Levine J, Gershon S, Mallinger AG, Hardan A, Vagnucci A, et al. Inositol as an add-on treatment for bipolar depression. Bipolar Disord. 2000;2(1):47–55.

182. Filkowski MM, Stan VA, Borrelli DJ, Ostacher MJ, El-Mallach RS, Baldassano CF, et al. Effect of antidepressant treatment on mood epiode cycling in bipolar disorder: a randomized study. 160th Annual Meeting of the American Psychiatric Association, San Diego, CA, 2007.
183. Daly JJ, Prudic J, Devanand DP, Nobler MS, Lisanby SH, Peyser S, et al. ECT in bipolar and unipolar depression: differences in speed of response. Bipolar Disord. 2001;3(2):95–104.
184. Prudic J, Olfson M, Marcus SC, Fuller RB, Sackeim HA. Effectiveness of electroconvulsive therapy in community settings. Biol Psychiatry. 2004;55(3):301–12.
185. Kellner CH, Knapp RG, Petrides G, Rummans TA, Husain MM, Rasmussen K, et al. Continuation electroconvulsive therapy vs pharmacotherapy for relapse prevention in major depression: a multisite study from the Consortium for Research in Electroconvulsive Therapy (CORE). Arch Gen Psychiatry. 2006;63(12):1337–44.
186. Sackeim HA, Prudic J, Fuller R, Keilp J, Lavori PW, Olfson M. The cognitive effects of electroconvulsive therapy in community settings. Neuropsychopharmacology. 2007;32(1):244–54.
187. Rossini D, Lucca A, Zanardi R, Magri L, Smeraldi E. Transcranial magnetic stimulation in treatment-resistant depressed patients: a double-blind, placebo-controlled trial. Psychiatry Res. 2005;137(1–2):1–10.
188. Hausmann A, Pascual-Leone A, Kemmler G, Rupp CI, Lechner-Schoner T, Kramer-Reinstadler K, et al. No deterioration of cognitive performance in an aggressive unilateral and bilateral antidepressant rTMS add-on trial. J Clin Psychiatry. 2004;65(6):772–82.
189. Avery DH, Isenberg KE, Sampson S, Janicak PG, Lisanby SH, Maixner DF, et al. TMS in the acute treatment of major depression: clinical response in an open label extension trial. 160th Annual Meeting of the Americn Psychiatric Association, San Diego, CA, 2007.
190. Avery DH, Holtzheimeriii PE, Fawaz W, Russo J, Neumaier J, Dunner DL, et al. A controlled study of repetitive transcranial magnetic stimulation in medication-resistant major depression. Biol Psychiatry. 2006;59(2):187–94.
191. Post R, Speer AM. Repetitive transcranial magnetic therapies: prospescts for the future. In: George MS, Belmaker RH, eds. Transcranial Magnetic Stimulation in Clinical Psychiatry. Arlington: American Psychiatric Publishing; 2007, pp. 225–55.
192. Rush AJ, George MS, Sackeim HA, Marangell LB, Husain MM, Giller C, et al. Vagus nerve stimulation (VNS) for treatment-resistant depressions: a multicenter study. Biol Psychiatry. 2000;47(4):276–86.
193. George MS, Sackeim HA, Rush AJ, Marangell LB, Nahas Z, Husain MM, et al. Vagus nerve stimulation: a new tool for brain research and therapy. Biol Psychiatry. 2000;47(4):287–95.
194. Smeraldi E, Benedetti F, Barbini B, Campori E, Colombo C. Sustained antidepressant effect of sleep deprivation combined with pindolol in bipolar depression. A placebo-controlled trial. Neuropsychopharmacology. 1999;20(4):380–5.
195. Colombo C, Lucca A, Benedetti F, Barbini B, Campori E, Smeraldi E. Total sleep deprivation combined with lithium and light therapy in the treatment of bipolar depression: replication of main effects and interaction. Psychiatry Res. 2000;95(1):43–53.
196. Baxter LR, Jr., Liston EH, Schwartz JM, Altshuler LL, Wilkins JN, Richeimer S, et al. Prolongation of the antidepressant response to partial sleep deprivation by lithium. Psychiatry Res. 1986;19(1):17–23.
197. Zarate CA, Jr., Singh JB, Carlson PJ, Brutsche NE, Ameli R, Luckenbaugh DA, et al. A randomized trial of an N-methyl-D-aspartate antagonist in treatment-resistant major depression. Arch Gen Psychiatry. 2006;63(8):856–64.
198. Preskorn SD, Baker B, Omo K, Kolluri S, Menniti F, Landen J. A placebo-controlled trial of the NR2B specific NMDA antagonist CP-101, 606 plus paroxetine fo treatment resistant depression. 160th Annual Meeting of the American Psychiatric Association, San Diego, CA, 2007.
199. Miklowitz DJ, Otto MW, Frank E, Reilly-Harrington NA, Wisniewski SR, Kogan JN, et al. Psychosocial treatments for bipolar depression: a 1-year randomized trial from the Systematic Treatment Enhancement Program. Arch Gen Psychiatry. 2007;64(4):419–26.
200. Scott J, Gutierrez MJ. The current status of psychological treatments in bipolar disorders: a systematic review of relapse prevention. Bipolar Disord. 2004;6(6):498–503.

201. Post RM, Post SLW, Steiner H. Molecular and cellular developmental vulnerabilities to the onset of affective disorders in children and adolescents: some implications for therapeutics. Handbook of Mental Health Interventions in Children and Adolescents. San Francisco: Jossey-Bass; 2004, pp. 140–92.
202. Kessler RC, Berglund P, Demler O, Jin R, Merikangas KR, Walters EE. Lifetime prevalence and age-of-onset distributions of DSM-IV disorders in the National Comorbidity Survey Replication. Arch Gen Psychiatry. 2005;62(6):593–602.
203. Post RM, Kowatch RA. The heath care crisis of childhood onset bipolar illness: some recommendations for its amelioration. J Clin Psychiatry. 2006;67(1):115–25.
204. Post RM. Kindling and sensitization as models for affective episode recurrence, cyclicity, and tolerance phenomena. Neurosci Biobehav Rev. 2007;31(6):858–73.
205. Post RM, Schacter SC, Holmes GL, Trenite DG (eds). Animal models of mood disorders: kindling as a model of affective illness progression. In: Schacter SC, Holmes GL, Trenite DG eds. Behavioral Aspects of Epilepsy: Principles and Practice. New York: Demos Medical Publishing; 2008, pp. 19–27.
206. Scott J, Colom F, Vieta E. A meta-analysis of relapse rates with adjunctive psychological therapies compared to usual psychiatric treatment for bipolar disorders. Int J Neuropsychopharmacol. 2007;10(1):123–9.
207. Kessing LV, Agerbo E, Mortensen PB. Does the impact of major stressful life events on the risk of developing depression change throughout life? Psychol Med. 2003;33(7):1177–84.
208. Kraepelin E, Robertson GM, Barclay RM. Manic-depressive insanity and paranoia. Edinburgh: E.S. Livingstone; 1921.
209. Post RM. Transduction of psychosocial stress into the neurobiology of recurrent affective disorder. Am J Psychiatry. 1992;149(8):999–1010.
210. Wilens TE, Biederman J, Millstein RB, Wozniak J, Hahesy AL, Spencer TJ. Risk for substance use disorders in youths with child- and adolescent-onset bipolar disorder. J Am Acad Child Adolesc Psychiatry. 1999;38(6):680–5.

Substance Abuse and Depression

John A. Renner, Jeffrey Baxter, Joji Suzuki, and Domenic A. Ciraulo

Introduction

Depression, complicated by substance abuse, is a common clinical problem and is often associated with poor clinical outcomes. Clinicians need to understand the relationship between these two conditions and must adjust their treatment plans to address both disorders simultaneously. It is critical that the clinician not confuse a substance-induced mood disorder with an independent depressive disorder. Unfortunately, the relationship between substance abuse and depression is not well understood, and there are relatively few well controlled studies to help guide the treatment of these patients.

The nature of the relationship between substance abuse and psychopathology has long been an area of controversy. Meyer identified six paradigms to explain this relationship, including the possibility that psychiatric disorders are a consequence of substance abuse or that they are a risk factor for substance abuse (1). There is a high familial incidence of both alcoholism and depression, suggesting a common genetic vulnerability for both conditions. Genetic research suggests that alcoholism and depression are two common but independent conditions that sometimes run in the same families (2, 3). Analysis of the Mid-Atlantic Twin Registry showed that individuals with major depression were at increased risk for alcohol abuse or dependence. This study indicated that there are environmental and genetic factors that influence both disorders. While these factors overlap, they are not identical. The authors concluded that these findings do not support a model in which alcoholism causes major depression, or major depression causes alcoholism (4). To date, no single gene has been identified that links both conditions.

This chapter will review the epidemiology of major depressive disorder (MDD) complicated by substance abuse and will describe common clinical presentations. The differential diagnosis of these conditions will also be addressed. Evidence will

J.A. Renner (✉)
Department of Veterans Affairs, Boston University School of Medicine,
Boston, MA, USA
e-mail: john.renner@va.gov

D.A. Ciraulo and R.I. Shader (eds.), *Pharmacotherapy of Depression*,
DOI 10.1007/978-1-60327-435-7_6, © Springer Science+Business Media, LLC 2011

be reviewed on the efficacy of antidepressant medications in this comorbid population. The potential anti-craving effect of some of the SSRIs will also be considered. Finally, recommendations will be made for comprehensive treatment plans that address both the pharmacotherapy of the depressive disorder and management of the substance use disorder.

Prevalence and Comorbidity

Over the past 20 years, a number of studies have shown a high rate of cooccurrence, or "comorbidity" of depression and other affective disorders with substance-related disorders. In studies of psychiatric patients, the range of comorbid alcoholism has been from 10 to 30% (5, 6). Two studies used structured interviews of large samples to estimate the incidence of these disorders in the general population. They supply the highest quality information available about the rates of psychiatric disorders in the general population (7).

The Epidemiological Catchment Area (ECA) Study found increased rates of depression in alcoholic individuals. The rate in men was 5%, while for women alcoholics the rate was almost three times the national rate (19% vs. 7%) (8). Analysis of these data indicated that individuals suffering from depression or other affective disorders had increased rates of substance-related disorders, and that the reverse relationship was true as well. Selections from these data listed in Table 1 show the rates of these disorders found in the general population, as well as the increased rates of additional psychiatric diagnoses in individuals already identified as having psychiatric problems.

The analyses showed increased rates of Cooccuring affective disorders in people with substance-related problems. Individuals with alcohol or drug-related disorders were 1.9 and 4.7 times respectively,more likely to have a history of affective disorders than the general population. Individuals with depression or dysthymia were found to have increased incidence of alcohol problems (16.5–21.9% vs. 13.5%) and drug problems (18–18.9% vs. 6.1%). Interestingly, individuals with alcohol or drug problems were much more likely to have other substance-related disorders, with over seven times the risk of an additional substance-related diagnosis. The authors summarized their impressions of the impact of their findings in the following statement: "These data provide clear and persuasive evidence that mental disorders must be addressed as a central part of substance abuse prevention efforts in this country" (8).

In the National Comorbidity Survey (NCS), a representative sample of over 8,000 people was interviewed. This study found that major depression and alcohol dependence were the most commonly identified psychiatric diagnoses, with lifetime incidence rates of 17 and 14.1%, respectively; alcohol abuse without dependence had a lifetime incidence rate of 9.4%. Other drug dependence was found in 7.5% of this population. Just over half of the population surveyed had no psychiatric histories, and another fifth had only a single diagnosis. The study also identified

Table 1 Lifetime prevalence and comorbidity of substance-related and affective disorders

		Diagnosis studied					
		Any nonsubstance related psych. disorder	Any affective disorder	Unipolar major depression	Dysthymia	Alcohol abuse or dependence	Drug abuse or dependence
Population studied	General population	22.5%	8.3%	4.9%	3.3%	13.5%	6.1%
	Dependent on or abusing alcohol	36.6%RR 2.3	13.4%RR 1.9			N/A	21.5%RR 7.1
	Dependent on or abusing drugs	53.1%RR 4.5	26.4%RR 4.7			47.3%RR 7.1	N/A
	Unipolar major depression					16.5%RR 1.3	18%RR 3.8
	Dysthymia					20.9%RR 1.7	18.9%RR 3.9

Incidence: percentage (%) per 100 individuals interviewed
RR: adjusted odds ratio, or relative risk
Adapted from the ECA Study (8)

a high degree of comorbidity, with 13% reporting two diagnoses and 14% reporting three or more diagnoses. This concentration of many different psychiatric diseases in a small segment of the population suggests that comorbid depression and substance abuse are the norm in some of the most seriously impaired psychiatric patients in the United States (9). Analysis of the NCS data also focused on the temporal sequences of diagnoses. These data set indicated that anxiety disorders, and depression to a lesser degree, tended to precede the development of alcohol dependence (10).

The most recent comprehensive study on cooccurring disorders was the National Epidemiologic Survey on Alcohol and Related Conditions (NESARC), published in 2004 (11). This NIAAA sponsored study targeted 43,093 noninstitutionalized US citizens, including military living off base, and individuals in rooming houses, nontransient hotels and motels, shelters, college dormitories, and group homes. Hospitals, prisons and jails were not included. During the same 12-month period, 19.67% of the respondents with any substance use disorder had at least one independent mood disorder. Among respondents with any substance use disorder, 17.71% had at least one independent anxiety disorder; 3.30–14.50% had a specific mood disorder, and 1.46–10.54% had a specific anxiety disorder. Rates of cooccurring disorders were consistently lower for abuse than for dependence, and were highest for individuals with any drug dependence. Individuals with substance use disorders were more likely to have major depression and specific phobia than any other mood or anxiety disorder. Also, 19.97% of respondents with any 12-month mood disorder had at least one substance use disorder, and among those with any 12-month anxiety disorder, 14.96% had at least one substance use disorder (11).

Wilson compared the NESARC data from 2001 to 2002 with the NIAAA sponsored National Longitudinal Alcohol Epidemiologic Survey (NLAES), conducted in 1991–1992. This comparison showed that the prevalence of comorbid major depression and substance use disorders increased from 10.0% in 1991–1992 to 15.1% in 2001–2002 (12).

Huang reviewed the NESARC data from the perspective of race-ethnicity. In respondents with major depression, the odds ratio of having an alcohol use disorder was overall 2.6 (2.2 when adjusted for age, sex, income, marital status, education, region, urbanicity; when separated by race and ethnicity, the odds ratios were whites 2.4, blacks 3.3, Native Americans 2.8, Asians 3.7, Hispanics 2.6). In those with major depression, the odds ratios of having a drug use disorder was overall 4.9 (3.5 when adjusted; when separated by race and ethnicity, whites 4.1, blacks 7.1, Native Americans 10.0, Asians 3.2, Hispanics 5.4). The authors noted the strikingly high rates of major depression, anxiety disorders, personality disorders, and alcohol and drug use disorders in the Native American population. The analysis also showed that the rates of comorbidity were greater among blacks than whites, and the association between personality disorders and alcohol use disorders was greater in Asians. The strength of the association between drug use disorder and major depression was stronger in blacks and Native Americans than in whites (13).

One recent study compared the features of independent major depressive episodes with substance-induced major depressive episodes in individuals with cooccurring substance use disorders. Subjects with both types of depressions had more life-time depressive symptoms, more cooccurring anxiety disorders, and were more likely to have attempted suicide (14). Other studies have described high rates of depression in various populations with substance-related problems. Gold surveyed 6,355 substance abuse patients and found a lifetime incidence of major depression of 43.7% (15). Miller found a 28% prevalence of major depression in alcohol and drug users treated in a variety of clinical settings (16). Hasin and Grant (17) reported a fourfold increased risk for major depression in a community sample of individuals with a history of alcohol dependence, despite the fact that a majority of them had not used alcohol for more than 2 years. In a review of a community sample of individuals with alcohol dependence, Kirchner noted that comorbid depression was more likely in women and that they were more likely to have comorbid drug use disorders (18). Depressed elderly patients are three to four times more likely to have an alcohol use disorder when compared with the nondepressed elderly. Devanand (19) reported a prevalence of 15–30% of comorbid alcoholism in patients with late life major depression.

In a sample of drug-dependent individuals in treatment, Compton found a 24% lifetime prevalence of major depression. This sample was not specific for any one drug of abuse (20). Specific details on the comorbidity of depression in opiate and cocaine abusers will be covered later in this chapter.

Minimal information is available about the relationship between other drugs of abuse and depression. MDMA (ecstasy) has been shown to deplete serotonin in animal models. Two recent studies have shown increased levels of depressive symptoms in ecstasy users (21, 22). Increased rates of depression and suicidal ideation have also been found in individuals with methamphetamine dependence (23).

One often-overlooked issue is the cooccurrence of depression and nicotine dependence, which has been demonstrated in adolescents in a number of studies (24, 25). It is also thought that depression and substance-related disorders influence the progression of nicotine dependence in teenagers (26). Although these are important topics, the treatment of these disorders in adolescents and the treatment of comorbid depression and nicotine dependence in general fall outside the scope of this chapter.

Several studies have reported an association between marijuana use and the later development of major depression (27–30). Data from the NSC suggested a "moderate" to "modest" association (29). Research done in 44 schools in Australia showed that regular marijuana use in girls predicted later depression. Daily users were at the highest risk, with a fivefold increase in the odds of reporting later depression (30). In none of these studies was there evidence that depressive symptoms in teenagers predicted later heavy marijuana use.

Considering these high rates of cooccurrence of depression and substance-related disorders, clinicians must become skilled in the evaluation and management of these complex, dually diagnosed patients. Findings to date on the sequence of onset of these disorders have been inconsistent. With alcohol, cocaine, and opiates, depressive symptoms typically precede the development of substance abuse problems; with marijuana, the reverse seems to be true. To treat these patients effectively, clinicians need to carefully separate the symptoms of substance abuse from those of depression, and to determine which symptoms reflect an independent psychiatric disorder and which symptoms are the result of alcohol or drug use or abuse (substance-induced).

Functional Consequences of Comorbid Depression and Substance Abuse

Recognizing the high rate of cooccurrence of depression and substance-related disorders, researchers have studied the effects that the presence of one of these disorders has on the clinical course of the other disorder. A number of studies showed that the treatment of alcoholism in the presence of any comorbid psychiatric disorder was associated with a poorer prognosis (31–35). One prospective treatment outcome study compared patients with alcoholism alone to alcoholics with cooccurring psychiatric disorders. At 1-year follow-up, the alcoholics with psychiatric comorbidity had a more stressful course but not necessarily a poorer outcome (36). Among women, even moderate social drinking (up to three drinks per week) is associated with increased Beck depression (BDI) and anxiety (BAI) scores when compared with abstinent women (37).

Mueller et al. followed a group of patients who entered treatment for depression; all subjects met full Research Diagnostic Criteria for MDD. Over the course of 10 years, patients with active alcoholism were significantly less likely to recover from depression than either alcoholics in remission or people with no history of alcohol problems (38). In a 5-year study, Hasin et al. (39) demonstrated that the resolution of alcohol problems both increased the chance of recovering from depression and decreased the chance of the depression recurring.

Studies have shown that 15–25% of successful suicides involve alcohol (40, 41). Although depression and substance abuse each are associated with increased risk of suicide, the risk is increased even more when both types of disorders are present (42–44). An analysis of substance use disorder cooccurring in major depressive disorder in patients enrolled in the Sequenced Treatment Alternatives to Relieve Depression (STAR*D) study showed that subjects with these cooccurring conditions were more likely to be men, either divorced or never married, to have a younger age of onset of depression and to have a higher rate of suicide attempts (45).

Recent studies have also evaluated the effect of depression on outcomes for the treatment of substance-related disorders. In a group of male veterans followed for 12 months after alcohol detoxification, those with depressive symptoms at 3 months were significantly more likely to relapse during the study period. Furthermore, the risk of relapse increased with the severity of the depressive symptoms (46).

In another study, individuals with depression and various types of substance dependence were followed for 18 months after inpatient treatment. Patients with histories of major depression that occurred before the onset of substance dependence were less likely to achieve remission. This difference remained even after patients with active depression were factored out of the analysis. Patients with depression that occurred after the development of substance dependence and persisted during periods of sobriety were at triple the risk for relapse to substance dependence after periods of stable remission. Even patients meeting criteria for major depression that would be categorized as "substance-induced," with depressive symptoms that resolve within 2–4 weeks of detoxification, were less likely to achieve stable remission of substance dependence (47).

These poor-outcome cases may be related to impaired coping skills. Kahler reviewed a group of depressed alcohol-dependent patients and compared coping skills in individuals with independent MDD, substance-induced depressive disorder, and those who never met criteria for a depressive disorder. He noted greater cognitive vulnerabilities and defective coping skills in those with an independent MDD, suggesting that they were at higher risk for recurrent depression (48).

Overall, this evidence suggests that for patients with depression and substance-related disorders, the prognosis is worse compared to individuals with a single disorder. In addition, successful treatment of one disorder may in part depend on adequate treatment of the cooccurring disorder. Alcoholics with all types of depression (independent MDD, substance-induced depressive disorder, and dysthymia) are at increased risk for relapse, but those with independent MDD probably experience the most malignant course of illness.

Clinical Evaluation and Differential Diagnosis

The Importance of an Adequate History

Appropriate diagnosis is dependent upon an accurate history. It is critical to determine the initial, presenting condition. Which symptoms developed first, the depression or the alcohol/drug use? An accurate history of the sequence of symptoms is necessary to separate the presentation of an underlying depressive illness from those symptoms induced by specific substance abuse. Unfortunately, it is difficult for some patients to provide an adequate history. Neurological impairment may limit or distort the patient's recall. Denial and/or repression may also confound the evaluation process. Ideally, the patient's history should be confirmed with relatives or significant others. It is critical to determine whether depressive symptoms were present prior to any substance use and during any drug-free periods, and if there is a family history of depressive disorders.

MDD vs. Substance-Induced Mood Disorder

There are no specific symptoms that reliably distinguish an independent depressive disorder from a substance-induced mood disorder. DSM-IV-TR identifies a substance-induced mood disorder as a mood disturbance that develops during or within a month of substance intoxication or withdrawal and substance use is thought to be etiologically related to the mood disturbance (49). An accurate history, coupled with clinical observations following 2–4 weeks sobriety, can help clarify whether the depressive symptoms represent an independent illness or are simply secondary to alcohol or drug use. A history of depression prior to the development of a substance use disorder, or during periods of extended sobriety, along with a history of depression in biologic family members increases the likelihood that a depressed substance abuse patient has an independent affective disorder (50).

Evaluation for Suicide Risk

All substance abuse patients need to be assessed for depression and suicidal risk at the time of admission to treatment. Close observation and suicide precautions should be initiated when indicated. Intoxicated patients or those in acute withdrawal are at particular risk for acting on such suicidal ideas. Such depressive symptoms may be the result of an alcohol-induced mood disorder and neither necessarily indicate the presence of an independent depressive disorder, nor the need for ongoing pharmacotherapy for depression.

Dysthymia

Substance abuse patients may also suffer from chronic forms of dysthymia. Prolonged hypophoric states have been described in alcoholics following detoxification (51). Khantzian (52) proposed that chronic problems with affect regulation, including underlying depressive disorders, lead some individuals to self-medicate with alcohol or other drugs. Based on this theory, successful addiction treatment requires the treatment of both the addiction and the underlying psychiatric disorder.

Depression After Prolonged Sobriety

Alcoholics often describe episodes of depression occurring after extended periods of sobriety. Behar reported a 15% incidence of "disabling" depression after a mean period of 36 months sobriety (53). If there is a history of prior depressive episodes independent of drinking, this can be presumed to be the recurrence of a major depression and managed as such. If there is no prior history of depression, this may represent part of the psychological process of recovery from addiction. These patients should initially be referred for psychotherapy to help them mourn the real losses in their lives: families, health, self-respect, careers, time, opportunities, etc. Clinicians should be particularly alert to identify such depressive syndromes in alcoholic women. Some patients become very discouraged when they realize that sobriety does not resolve all of life's problems. Reliance on the disease model of alcoholism leads some recovering alcoholics to expect that sobriety will eliminate most of their problems. The realization that sobriety is not a panacea can be profoundly discouraging for many alcoholics. If significant symptoms of depression persist for more than 1 month, we recommend antidepressant pharmacotherapy for these patients.

Clinical Presentations

Alcohol Dependence

Depression and Acute Intoxication

As many as 70% of alcoholics are clinically depressed at the time of admission for detoxification. These patients often score in the severely depressed range on the Beck Depression Inventory (BDI) (54). Symptoms may include suicidal ideation or behavior, which is often the primary reason for hospitalization. Such patients are at serious risk for suicide and will require observation on a secure unit. Typically this presentation is a symptom of an alcohol-induced depressive disorder; these patients usually improve rapidly following detoxification. Within 2 weeks, the patients generally score in the mildly depressed range on the BDI. At that point, the number of clinically depressed patients has dropped to 6–7% among male alcoholics and 11–13% among women alcoholics. This pattern suggests that the majority of depressive syndromes seen in acutely intoxicated individuals are transient and do not reflect an independent psychiatric disorder (55).

Beyond necessary supervision during periods of suicidal ideation, the primary treatment needed is alcohol detoxification. There is no evidence or rationale to justify the use of antidepressant medication in this subgroup. The primary long-term management for this condition is to help the patient maintain sobriety. Those patients who remain depressed beyond this period, or develop a depression during extended periods of sobriety, most likely have an independent MDD and require therapy for this comorbid condition.

Alcohol Dependence and Depression

There is no consistent agreement on the relationship between depression and alcoholism. Jaffe and Ciraulo (51) described at least ten possible causes of depressive symptoms in alcoholics, ranging from the direct pharmacologic effect of alcohol on the brain to alcohol withdrawal and major affective disorders. Depending on the diagnostic criteria used and the point at which the diagnosis is established, the reported incidence of depression in alcoholics ranges from 8 to 70% (55–57). It is difficult to compare these studies because of a lack of consensus on diagnostic approaches and the failure to separate substance-induced disorders from independent depressive disorders. Abraham screened 375 depressed psychiatric outpatients for comorbid substance use disorders to determine the age of onset and the sequence of symptoms (58). In this outpatient clinic population, he determined that alcohol dependence followed the onset of depression on average by 4.7 years. Similarly, cocaine dependence followed the first major depressive episode by 6.8 years. In a study of inpatients admitted for alcoholism treatment, Hesselbrock documented a lifetime and current prevalence of major depression of 32% in men and 52% in women. Only 3% of men and women reported bipolar affective disorder. In 41% of the men and 65% of the women, major depression preceded the development of alcohol abuse and/or dependence (59). One study has suggested that depressed alcoholics who present with physical/neurologic complaints and little or no irritation or agitation are more likely to remain depressed after 30 days in substance abuse treatment (60).

Alcoholic Hypophoria

Substance abusers who do not meet criteria for major depression may still present with clinically significant symptoms. Jaffe and Ciraulo (51) studied male alcoholic veterans hospitalized for detoxification and observed low level symptoms of dysphoria and low self esteem that they labeled "Alcoholic Hypophoria." Using the Present Affect Rating Scale developed by Kay, the Hypophoria Scale showed persistent elevations in negative mood following detoxification (see Table 2) (61). When compared with the patients' ZUNG scores, which dropped quickly following detoxification, BDI scores did not normalize, and the Hypophoria Scale remained elevated for many weeks. Alcoholics sober for 6 months in Alcoholics Anonymous continued to demonstrate elevated hypophoria scores when compared with nonalcoholic, hospitalized medical patients. These patients' complaints can easily be missed because the patients did not meet full criteria for a diagnosis of a major depression (Table 3). TCAs were not effective in treating these low level depressive symptoms (51). Although benzodiazepines may relieve hypophoric symptoms temporarily in abstinent alcoholics (see Fig. 1), they also explain the high comorbidity of sedative abuse in alcoholics.

Pharmacotherapy of Depression in the Alcoholic

Clinical Pharmacology of Antidepressants in Alcoholism

Consideration of antidepressant interactions in patients with substance abuse is complicated not only by prescribed medications, but also by the many illicit and prescription drugs that such individuals may consume. With respect to TCAs, both pharmacokinetic and pharmacodynamic interactions may occur. Pharmacodynamic interactions are the most common, and most important clinically. In general, concurrent ingestion of ethanol and cyclic antidepressants leads to impaired psychomotor

Table 2 Alcoholic hypophoria following detoxification

Group	Mean hypophoria scores
Inpatient alcoholics	
Abstinent 1 week	38.4
Abstinent 2 weeks	35.8
Abstinent 4–6 weeks	35.9
Alcoholics anonymous group	27.3
Nonalcoholic medical patients	20.5

Adapted from Jaffe and Ciraulo (51)

The Hypophoria Scale shares many items with The Addiction Research Center Inventory – Morphine Benzedrine Group scale (189) colloquially referred to as the "euphoria" scale. Alcoholics show increases in scores on this scale after the administration of either alprazolam or diazepam whereas control subjects do not (190). These findings suggest that alcohol-dependent patients self-medicate with GABA agonists such as benzodiazepines because of a desire to enhance mood. The finding that subjects without a personal or family history of alcoholism do not experience an enhanced mood after a benzodiazepine and suggests that this is a pharmacodynamic unique to alcoholics and children of alcoholics

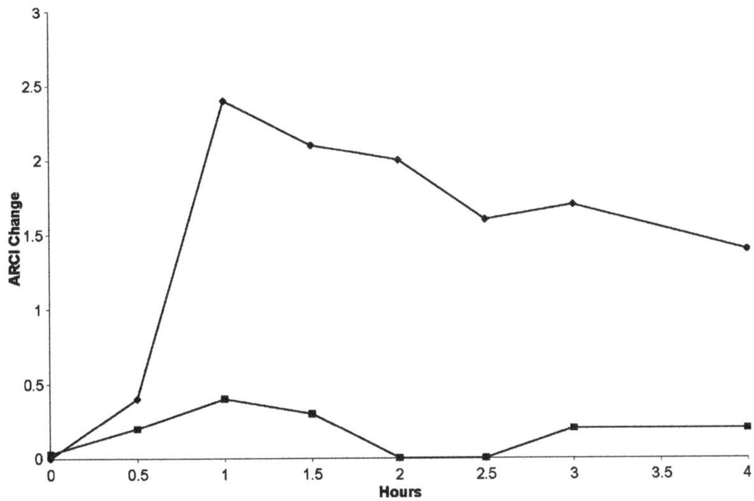

Fig. 1 The *upper line of the graph* indicates that abstinent alcoholics experienced greater euphoria (ARCI change) after a single dose of alprazolam compared with control subjects (*lower line of the graph*)

function and sedation, and the combination is particularly dangerous in overdose (62, 63). Interestingly, bupropion may antagonize the sedative effects of ethanol without affecting the perception of inebriation. Acute ingestion of ethanol and SSRIs or mixed action agents, such as venlafaxine, appear less likely to interfere with laboratory measures of psychomotor performance (64), although some patients will report that the subjective effects of an alcohol containing beverage change when they are taking SSRIs. This is consistent with the modest decreases in alcohol consumption observed in studies of heavy drinkers taking fluoxetine, zimelidine, or citalopram (64, 65). This action does not appear to generalize to all alcoholics, since the SSRIs have not proved effective therapies in alcoholism (see later).

Pharmacokinetic interactions with antidepressants differ little between classes. Acute ethanol impairs the metabolizing capacity in the liver and gut, resulting in high plasma concentrations of the antidepressant. With chronic ethanol use, hepatic enzyme capacity is usually enhanced, and tricyclic antidepressants that are hepatically metabolized will have increased clearance and lower steady state levels. Unbound fractions of imipramine, desipramine, and their hydroxy metabolites are decreased in chronic alcoholics, with corresponding increases in α_1 acid glycoproteins (64, 66).

Initiating Pharmacotherapy

Placebo-controlled trials of medication in depressed alcoholics have demonstrated significant improvement in comorbid depression (67). A diagnostic evaluation should be repeated after 2 weeks sobriety for those patients who continue to present symptoms of depression. If the depression has cleared at that time, or has significantly diminished, no antidepressant treatment is required, and alcoholism can be assumed to be the primary problem. If there is no improvement in depressive symptoms by the second week, it is likely that the patient has a comorbid depression, and it is appropriate to initiate specific pharmacotherapy. In patients with a history of depressive symptoms prior to the development of alcohol dependence, depression during extended periods of sobriety, or a strong family history of depression, there is a strong presumption that they have an independent depressive disorder. There is no reason to delay pharmacotherapy once these patients have completed detoxification. In any case, symptoms of major depression that persist longer than 2 weeks postdetoxification should always be treated.

Tricyclic Antidepressants (TCAs)

There are relatively few controlled studies of the efficacy of TCAs in depressed alcoholics. Alcoholics given 150 mg imipramine had significantly lower plasma levels compared to nonalcoholic depressed patients and BDI scores got worse, when compared with controls who are given no medication. Lower plasma levels of desipramine and imipramine, lasting at least 5 weeks, have been documented in recently detoxified alcoholics. These TCAs are primarily metabolized by the hepatic microsomal drug oxidizing system; this system is induced in chronic alcoholics without cirrhosis (68). Desipramine clearance is less affected, suggesting this is the preferred TCA for use in recently detoxified depressed alcoholics (69, 70). This enzyme induction will dissipate over time if the patient remains sober. The clinician needs to monitor plasma TCA levels and must adjust doses correspondingly to insure that plasma levels remain within the appropriate therapeutic range. In addition, recently detoxified alcoholics appear to be more sensitive to the cardiac effects of imipramine, desipramine, and their hydroxy metabolites (see Figs. 2–4) (66). The metabolism of TCAs is also inhibited in patients with cirrhosis. Lower doses may therefore be adequate in such cases, though plasma levels should always be monitored.

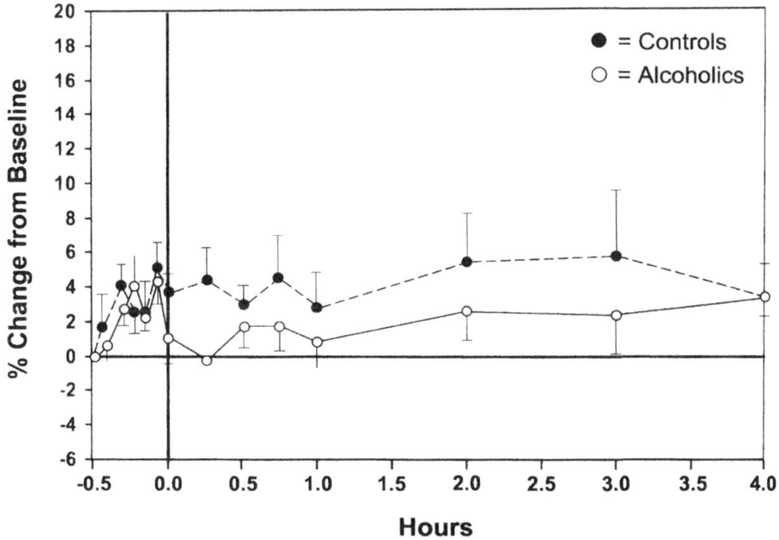

Fig. 2 Mean (± SEM) percent change from baseline in QTc interval vs. time during and following an intravenous infusion of 2-hydroxyimipramine in alcoholic and control subjects (Redrawn from data from (62))

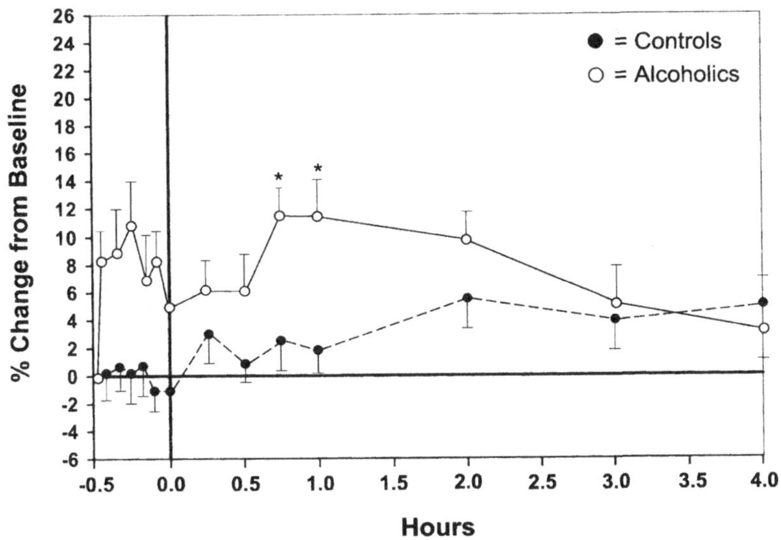

Fig. 3 Mean (± SEM) percentage change from baseline in P–R interval vs. time both during and following an intravenous infusion of 2-hydroxyimipramine in alcoholic and control subjects (*asterisks* indicates $P<0.05$) (Redrawn from data from (62))

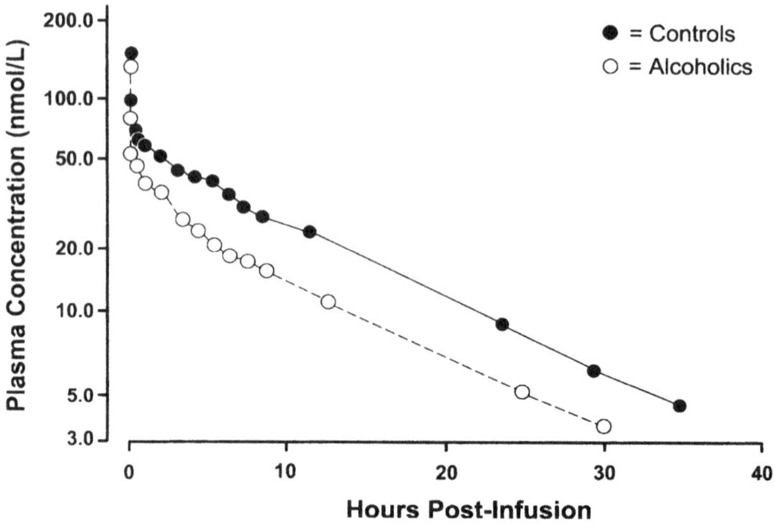

Fig. 4 Mean 2-hydroxyimipramine plasma concentration vs. time data for alcoholic and control subjects following an intravenous infusion of 2-hydroxyimipramine 10 mg (Redrawn from data from (62))

One double-blind, placebo-controlled trial of desipramine in depressed alcoholics showed that medicated subjects were significantly less depressed than controls. After 6 months treatment, there was no significant difference in the rate of sobriety between the two groups, though the desipramine treated subjects appeared to have longer periods of sobriety (71). Plasma levels were monitored in this study. This is similar to our experience with MAO inhibitors in alcoholics with atypical depression. Symptoms of depression often respond well, but there is no evidence that relapse rates are diminished in the medication-treated group; furthermore, the risks of food and drug interactions with MAOIs rarely justify their use in in-patients with substance use disorders (Ciraulo, 2003, unpublished data).

An uncontrolled, open-label study of imipramine in depressed alcoholics showed improvement in mood and drinking patterns in 45% of the patients. Addition of disulfiram to the protocol produced improvement in an additional 13% of the subjects. At the completion of this trial, the patients were randomized to either imipramine or placebo for an additional 6 months. Thirty-one percent of the patients on imipramine relapsed, when compared with a 70% relapse rate for those on placebo (72). A double-blind, placebo-controlled trial of imipramine showed efficacy in treating depression in alcoholics, but no improvement in drinking patterns (73). Another double-blind, placebo-controlled trial of desipramine showed improvement in both depression and a reduction in the rate of relapse to drinking (74).

In summary, these studies demonstrate that the TCAs are effective in treating depression in substance abuse patients. Unfortunately, the TCAs have no predictable effect on the rate of relapse to substance use. It is therefore critical that these patients participate in a comprehensive substance abuse treatment program. Although there has been an anecdotal report of the abuse of amitriptyline when used to treat depressed alcoholics (75), we do not think there is significant abuse liability for this class of drugs. A greater risk is lethality of overdose, especially when combined with alcohol or other drugs.

Serotonin Reuptake Inhibitors (SSRIs)

Animal studies have shown that serotonin systems regulate drug taking and other consummatory behavior. SSRIs have been shown to reduce drug-seeking behavior in animals. Research has also shown lower 5-HIAA in the CSF of alcoholics, suggesting an abnormality in serotonin metabolism. These findings suggest that the SSRIs may both reduce alcohol craving and treat affective symptoms in depressed alcoholics (76, 77). The side effect profile of the SSRIs makes them more acceptable to substance abuse alcoholic patients when compared with the TCAs and suggests improved compliance with treatment. There have been no reports of accelerated metabolism or altered pharmacokinetics of SSRIs in alcoholics, and there is also less risk of overdose and life-threatening side effects (78).

There have been relatively few studies on the use of the SSRIs to treat depression in alcoholics. One 4-week trial compared tianeptine (a serotonin enhancer) to amitriptyline in treating depressed alcoholics. Tianeptine was slightly more effective in this study, but there were no placebo controls (79). Cornelius et al. (80) conducted an open trial of fluoxetine in 12 seriously depressed suicidal patients who met DSM-III-R criteria for both MDD and for alcohol dependence. After 8 weeks, all subjects showed improvement in measures of both depression and postdischarge alcohol consumption. These results were not duplicated in a large randomized, placebo-controlled trial of fluoxetine in 101 alcoholics. Kranzler reported that mood improved in those alcoholics with mild depressive symptoms, but there was no difference between drug and placebo on drinking patterns (81).

In a second study of fluoxetine, Cornelius reported both reduced drinking and improved mood in a double-blind, placebo-controlled trial in 51 severely depressed alcoholics (82). In a subset of patients in this trial, there were 17 individuals who abused both alcohol and cocaine. Within that group, there was no improvement in either their depression or their alcohol or cocaine use (83). In a 1-year follow-up on the 31 patients who responded to fluoxetine in the original 1997 trial, the responders showed fewer depressive symptoms and less drinking than the placebo group (84).

There has been a single small, open label trial of fluoxetine in adolescents with comorbid major depression and an alcohol use disorder. Significant decreases were found in both depressive symptoms and drinking (85). Five year follow-up on this cohort showed decreased alcohol and marijuana use and improved academic functioning. However, the long-term clinical course for their depressive symptoms was poor (86). Riggs reported a similar reduction in depressive symptoms in an open trial of fluoxetine in abstinent adolescent delinquents with major depression and comorbid substance use disorders (87).

Roy (88) reported the successful treatment of depressive symptoms with sertraline in a double-blind, placebo-controlled trial in 36 depressed, recently abstinent alcoholics. However, Pettinati did not find a benefit for sertraline in a double-blind, placebo-controlled trial in 100 alcohol-dependent subjects. Drinking was reduced in those subjects with no history of depression. For subjects who met DSM-III-R criteria for past or current depressive disorder, sertraline was no better than placebo in reducing drinking (89). These results suggest the need to subtype alcoholics on the basis of the presence or the absence of a history of MDD.

There have been three other placebo-controlled double-blind trials of sertraline in depressed alcoholics. Moak studied 82 depressed, actively drinking alcoholics and noted lower drinks per drinking day in subjects receiving sertraline in combination with cognitive behavioral therapy, but no impact on other drinking measures. Depressive symptoms were reduced only in female alcoholics (90). Gual conducted a similar trial in 83 recently detoxified alcohol-dependent subjects with cooccurring depressive disorder. After 24 weeks, there were no significant differences between the groups, though there was a trend toward improvement in depressive symptoms in subjects on sertraline (91). Kranzler reported a 10-week trial of sertraline compared with placebo in 328 subjects with cooccurring major depression and alcohol dependence. He found that alcohol consumption and depressive symptoms decreased substantially in both groups, but there were no significant medication group differences in either depression or drinking outcomes (92).

Citalopram has been studied for its anticraving effect in alcoholics, but not in a depressed alcoholic population. This SSRI reduced alcohol craving and drinking in nondepressed alcoholics in two double-blind, placebo-controlled trails (93, 94), but only worked with less severe drinkers in a third study (95). In a related study of citalopram as an anticraving drug in nondepressed mild to moderate alcoholics, Naranjo reported a 44% reduction in drinks per day in men vs. a 27% decrease in women, suggesting that sex may be a significant variable in the response of alcoholics to pharmacotherapy (96).

Muhonen reported an open-label random assignment 26 week outpatient trial that compared the efficacy of escitalopram with memantine (a noncompetitive glutamate-*N*-methyl-D-aspartate (NMDA)-receptor blocker) in 80 alcohol-dependent subjects with cooccurring major depressive disorder. Twenty-nine subjects in both groups completed the trial. An intent-to-treat analysis showed that both medications significantly reduced baseline levels of depression and anxiety as measured by the Montgomery–Asberg Depression Rating Scale and Ham-A. There were no significant inter-group differences in these measures; however, the age of onset of the first major depressive episode significantly correlated with the treatment response in the escitalopram group. The author suggested that early age of onset of depression may predict a response to escitalopram in this study population. Alcohol consumption and craving were significantly reduced in both groups, though patients who were abstinent at baseline had higher rates of completion (97–99).

However, it is clear that the majority of trials of SSRIs have shown relatively little impact on drinking behavior despite efficacy in reducing depressive symptoms. In reviewing these findings, Pettinati (100) suggested the potential benefit of adding anticraving medications to the antidepressant treatment. Gopalakrishnan reported the natural course of 74 depressed alcoholics who were followed for 6–12 months after the completion of a 12-week trial of sertraline, naltrexone, and compliance enhancement therapy. Individuals who showed a full response to the initial 12-week combination trial sustained a better overall outcome compared with partial or non-responders (101). Pettinati recently completed a double-blind placebo-controlled trial of the combination of sertraline and naltrexone, using doses that exceed the FDA approved standard. Subjects were randomly assigned to 14 weeks treatment with either 200 mg/day sertraline alone, 100 mg/day naltrexone alone, the combination of sertraline and naltrexone, or double placebo. All 170 subjects received weekly cognitive behavioral therapy. The study found that 53% of the subjects receiving both medications remained abstinent throughout the study, compared with an abstinent rate that ranged from 21.3 to 27.5% in the other three arms of the study. The mean duration of time to relapse to heavy drinking was 63.6 days in the combination group compared with an aggregate of 42.4 days in the other three groups. Interestingly, there were also fewer adverse events reported in the medication combination group (102). These promising results require replication in additional studies, but they clearly suggest the value of SSRIs in combination with anticraving medications in depressed alcohol-dependent individuals.

Insomnia is frequently reported by depressed alcoholic patients treated with SSRIs. Supplemental trazodone, 25–75 mg hs, works well to alleviate this complaint (103). The effect of trazodone (150–200 mg) on sleep quality was compared with placebo in a small number of inpatient alcoholics (104). Sleep efficiency was significantly increased in the trazodone group, primarily because of differences in the number of awakenings, wake time after sleep onset, and non-REM sleep compared to placebo. Baseline/endpoint differences in the trazodone group included these measures as well as the apnea index and number of stage shifts. Much recent research has focused on the association of persistent sleep disturbances and relapse in alcoholism, fueling the search for nonaddictive sleep-promoting agents. Other antidepressants and some anticonvulsants (e.g., gabapentin) have been used clinically and are currently being studied. Sexual dysfunction is also a commonly reported side effect with the SSRIs. In our male patients, this has responded well to treatment with sildenafil.

The SSRIs appear to have significant efficacy in treating depression in abstinent substance abuse patients, irrespective of any effect on drinking behavior or drug use. Results are less clear in depressed individuals who actively abuse drugs or alcohol. The data regarding a specific SSRI anticraving effect are inconsistent. The recent work of Pettinati (89, 105, 106), Johnson (107), and Naranjo (96) suggests that there may be subtypes of alcoholics that obtain a specific anticraving effect from various medications. Specifically, Types A/B, early/late onset, gender, or specific genetic polymorphisms may influence SSRI response. This may explain why some depressed alcoholics actually increase drinking when treated with SSRIs. Additional research is needed to clarify these findings. When this phenomenon is better understood, it may be possible to clarify the inconsistent results seen in some of the SSRI trials.

Nefazodone

Nefazodone has been noted to be effective for depressed, anxious alcoholics and also to be helpful in normalizing sleep patterns (108). Roy-Byrne treated 64 alcohol-dependent subjects with comorbid MDD with nefazodone in a 12-week, double-blind, placebo-controlled trial. The medication group showed a significant decrease in depression scores but did not show any advantage over the placebo/psycho-education group in terms of drinking outcome. Both groups showed a similar decrease in alcohol consumption (109). Hernandez-Avila studied 41 alcoholics with cooccurring major depression in a 10-week double-blind, placebo-controlled trial of nefazodone. There were reductions in both depressive and anxiety symptoms, but the results did not reach statistical significance. However, subjects on nefazodone showed a significantly greater reduction in total drinks and in heavy drinking days, as compared to placebo (110). Because of the risk of hepatotoxicity associated with nefazodone, this drug must now be considered a second-line agent and must be used with caution in this population.

We have been unable to locate any placebo-controlled trials of bupropion, mirtazapine, or venlafaxine in the treatment of depression in substance abusing patients. Liappas reported on a 4–5 week open-label, random assignment inpatient trial comparing mirtazapine and venlafaxine in 60 recently detoxified depressed alcohol-dependent subjects. A control group received cognitive behavioral therapy alone; the two study groups received cognitive behavioral therapy plus one of the study medications. All three groups showed improvement during detoxification, but the mirtazapine group showed significantly greater improvement compared to the other groups after 4–5 weeks treatment (Hamilton Depression Rating Scale: 3.8 mirtazapine vs. 8.6 controls and 8.2 venlafaxine) (111). Altintoprak conducted a double-blind trial comparing the effectiveness of amitriptyline and mirtazapine in 44 alcoholic patients with cooccurring depressive disorder. Among the 36 patients who completed the trial, there was significant improvement in the Hamilton Depression Rating Scale and in alcohol craving scores in both study groups. There was no statistical difference in outcome between the two drugs though mirtazapine appeared to be better tolerated than amitriptyline (112). Yoon reported an 8-week open label trial of mirtazapine in alcohol-dependent subjects with cooccurring depressive disorders. He noted a "significant" reduction in both depressive symptoms and alcohol craving (113). In a similar 24-week open label trial of venlafaxine in 90 subjects, Garcia-Portilla (114) reported a decrease in Ham-D scores and some decrease in alcohol consumption.

Mood Stabilizing Antidepressants

Sixty percent of bipolar patients have a history of addiction to alcohol, drugs, or both (115). Ostacher described a prospective study of 3,750 subjects with either bipolar I or bipolar II disorder enrolled in the Systematic Treatment Enhancement Program for Bipolar Disorder (STEP-BD). Past or current substance use disorder did not predict a longer time to recovery from a depressive episode relative to individuals with no substance use comorbidity; however, it did predict a greater risk for switching from depression directly to a manic, hypomanic, or mixed state (116).

Three double-blind placebo-controlled trials have now been completed for this population. Salloum reported a 24-week trial with 150 subjects with cooccurring bipolar disorder and alcohol dependence, comparing valproate maintenance to placebo. The valproate group had significantly lower heavy drinking days, and trended toward fewer drinks per heavy drinking days. Higher serum levels of valproate were associated with better outcomes and the placebo group had higher GGT levels (117). Brown conducted a randomized, double-blind, placebo-controlled 12-week add-on trial of quetiapine in outpatients with bipolar disorder and alcohol use disorders that reported a significant decrease in depressive symptoms, but not in alcohol consumption (118).

Most studies of bipolar patients have had high dropout rates. Our clinical experience supports the value of lithium or selected anticonvulsant drug therapy for these patients. Once there is satisfactory control of mood fluctuations, alcoholic problems are generally amenable to substance abuse treatment (119). Brady reported an open-label trial of valproate in a group of nine patients with comorbid bipolar disorder and substance abuse. She believes that valproate is of particular value for bipolar II patients (120). In another open-label trial of valproate in 20 inpatients with comorbid mood disorder and substance abuse, Albanese reported valproate to be both efficacious and safe, alone and in combination with other psychiatric drugs (121). In the only reported double-blind parallel group maintenance study, Kemp compared lithium to the combination of lithium and divalproex. Of the 149 subjects with rapid-cycling bipolar disorder enrolled in the initial 6 month open-label stabilization phase, 79% discontinued prematurely. Only 21% ($N=31$) entered the randomly assigned double-blind maintenance phase. The addition of divalproex to lithium conferred no additional prophylactic benefit compared with lithium alone. The rate of relapse into a mood episode was 56% for the subjects on lithium alone and 53% for subjects on the combination therapy. Among the 19 alcohol-dependent subjects who completed the 6 month stabilization phase, 11 (58%) no longer met criteria for alcohol abuse or had entered into full remission. Among the nine subjects with cocaine use disorder, seven (78%) showed full or partial remission of their substance use disorder. Unfortunately, the small number of subjects makes it difficult to generalize from these data (122).

There has been one recent open-label trial of lamotrigine in this patient population. Rubio reported a 12-week open label trial with lamotrigine in subjects with cooccurring bipolar disorder and alcohol dependence, and found significant reductions in alcohol craving, and scores for Ham-D, Young Mania Rating Scale, and BPRS (123).

Hertzman (124) reported a retrospective chart review of patients treated with valproate for comorbid substance abuse and mood disorders. He noted diminished substance use in response to treatment. In another retrospective chart review of 204 bipolar I patients treated with anticonvulsant mood stabilizers or lithium, Goldberg reported that bipolar patients with a substance abuse history had a better response to anticonvulsant mood stabilizers than lithium (125). Despite the lack of well-controlled studies, these reports all suggest that lithium and the anticonvulsant mood stabilizers can be effective treating this population.

The most convincing evidence for efficacy of anticonvulsants is the report of Johnson et al. (126), who found that topiramate reduced ethanol consumption in individuals with alcohol abuse and dependence. These investigators proposed that a combination of enhanced GABA and decreased glutamatergic activity are likely mechanisms of action. Although not FDA approved for alcohol dependence at this time, we have found the effects dramatic in some patients, and that effective doses may be as low as 50 mg (much lower than the doses used by Johnson et al.). Cognitive impairment, especially difficulty word finding, may be associated with topiramate, especially at higher doses; therefore, we recommend trials at 25–50 mg daily for at least 2 weeks prior to increasing the dose. Monitoring of cognitive function is also recommended.

Cocaine

Depression and other affective disorders have long been recognized as complications of both intoxication and withdrawal from cocaine (127–129). A recent study reviewed the association between the severity of cocaine dependence and psychiatric and substance use disorder comorbidity. Psychiatric disorders were associated with an increased likelihood of participation in cocaine treatment or self-help groups, but not with most measures of cocaine dependence severity. Conversely, other cooccurring substance use disorders were strongly associated with more severe cocaine dependence (130). One survey of 243 cocaine-dependent adults reported that 10.3% met DSM-IV criteria for major depression (131). In cocaine users entering treatment, rates of depression as high as 47% have been identified (132), although another study has suggested that the high rate of concurrent alcohol abuse with cocaine abuse likely complicates the analysis of cocaine-associated symptoms (133). Gawin (127) reported a 30% incidence of major depression and a 15% incidence of bipolar or cyclothymic disorder in chronic cocaine abusers. Depression is also common during the withdrawal (crash) following a cocaine binge. Users may complain of suicidal ideation, insomnia, loss of energy, anhedonia, and loss of interest in sex. Once cocaine use has stopped, symptoms of severe depression will usually clear within 48 h. However, anhedonia may continue for months during early sobriety.

Chronic cocaine use will deplete CNS dopamine and norepinephrine (NE). The depletion of catecholamines is thought to explain the symptoms of depression and anhedonia that typically persist for the first 3 months of sobriety. TCA's have been suggested as treatment for the post-cocaine anhedonia and drug craving because of their ability to potentiate NE neurotransmission. Desipramine has been reported to enhance abstinence in early recovery (134), but Weiss (135) also noted that it can trigger relapse when taken by patients already abstinent. Ziedonis reported improvement in depressive symptoms and reduced cocaine usage in a randomized, double-blind trial of despiramine in depressed, cocaine-abusing, methadone maintenance patients (136). In a placebo-controlled, randomized trial of imipramine as a treatment for cocaine abuse, Nunes noted minimal effect on cocaine use, except in those individual with comorbid depression (137). In a more recent randomized placebo-controlled trial of desipramine in 111 depressed cocaine dependent subjects, McDowell reported improvement in depressive symptoms but no difference in cocaine use (138). In another study, Gonzalez reported a 12-week double blind, placebo controlled trial of desipramine in 149 cocaine-abusing subjects maintained on buprenorphine. Fifty-three subjects had a history of major depression, and 96 had no such history, and desipramine or placebo was paired with either contingency management or noncontingency management. He found that participation in contingency management increased the number of drug-free urines in patients with history of major depression, but treatment with desipramine appeared to benefit patients who never had a history of major depression (139). Brown also reported two open-label trials for lamotrigine in cocaine-dependent bipolar subjects. In the first 12-week study of 30 subjects, significant decreases were found in scores for Ham-D, Young Mania Scale, BPRS, and money spent on cocaine (140). In a later report, Brown reported a continuation of the previous study for a 36-week open-label trial with lamotrigine in 32 subjects, and found significant decreases in scores for Ham-D, Young Mania Scale, BPRS, and money spent on cocaine (141).

There have been two trials of fluoxetine in cocaine-dependent patients who were comorbid for MDD. Neither trial demonstrated a drug-related improvement in depressive symptoms or a significant reduction in cocaine use. In the previously described trial of fluoxetine in 17 depressed cocaine and alcohol-abusing patients, Cornelius noted an increase in BDI scores and worse clinical outcomes as compared to depressed alcoholics given fluoxetine (80). Schmitz reported a 12-week, placebo-controlled, double-blind study of 68 patients whose depressive symptoms decreased over time, unrelated to medication. Fluoxetine had no significant effect on their cocaine use (142).

McDowell reported a successful trial of venlafaxine in a small study of depressed cocaine abusers, all of whom had been in a larger double-blind trial of desipramine and had failed to respond to desipramine or were unable to tolerate its side effects. There were significant improvements in mood in 11 of 13 patients and all patients who completed the trial reported a greater than 75% reduction in cocaine intake (143). McDowell's report on the positive effect of venlafaxine is promising; however, in nondepressed cocaine dependent subjects, the NIDA/DVA Medication Development Research Units did not find efficacy for venlafaxine.

The National Institute on Drug Abuse and the Department of Veterans Affairs conducted a series of clinical trials searching for a "signal" of drug efficacy in cocaine dependence (144). Several antidepressants were included in these short-term trials, including paroxetine, venlafaxine, and sertraline. By most standards, these studies would be considered negative, that is, the drugs had no effect on cocaine use; however, a slight signal was seen for one study of sertraline.

There is now an encouraging trial involving bupropion for the treatment of cocaine dependence in methadone maintained patients. Poling has reported a

25-week double blind placebo controlled trial with bupropion in 106 methadone maintained cocaine users. He also paired bupropion with either contingency management or voucher control. He showed that subjects receiving bupropion and contingency management significantly decreased their cocaine use, while those on placebo and contingency management increased their cocaine use (145).

There is also some evidence that mood stabilizing anticonvulsants, such as tiagabine or topiramate, may be effective in cocaine dependence. Kampman reported a 13-week double blind placebo controlled trial of topiramate in 40 subjects, which demonstrated that topiramate treated subjects were more likely to remain abstinent (146). Gonzalez reported a 10-week double blind placebo controlled trial with tiagabine, gabapentin, and placebo in 76 cocaine-dependent subjects. He reported that the tiagabine group had significantly higher retention in treatment and drug-free urines than both gabapentin and placebo, while gabapentin did not show any improvement over placebo in retention or drug-free urines (147). Furthermore, Bisaga reported a 16-week double blind placebo controlled trial involving 128 cocaine-dependent subjects comparing gabapentin to placebo, which showed no difference in cocaine use (148). Brady reported a 12-week double blind placebo controlled trial with carbamezapine in 139 cocaine-dependent subjects with or without cooccurring affective disorder. Subjects with an affective disorder trended toward fewer cocaine positive urines and had a significantly longer time to first cocaine use. However, those without an affective disorder did not show any improvement with carbamezpaine (149).

In separate studies, early data on selegeline were encouraging, but Elkashef reported a 10-week double-blind, placebo-controlled trial in 300 cocaine-dependent subjects using transdermal selegiline, which showed no effect of selegiline over placebo as evidenced by self-report and urine BE (150). Dackis reported an 8-week double blind placebo controlled trial of modafinil in 63 cocaine-dependent subjects, which showed that modafinil treated patients had significantly more BE-negative urine samples than placebo, and were more likely to achieve abstinence of greater than 3 weeks (151). Ciraulo reported on the use of nefazodone in a double-blind placebo controlled trial of 69 cocaine-dependent subjects with cooccurring depressive symptoms. Median weekly BE levels and cocaine craving scores were significantly lower in the nefazodone treated group, compared to placebo. Both groups showed an equal improvement in mood and self-reported cocaine use (152). Lithium has been found to be effective only in those cocaine users with clear evidence of bipolar disease (153).

There is also a preliminary report of ondansetron being used for cocaine dependence. Johnson reported a 10-week double blind placebo controlled trial with ondansetron in 63 subjects, which showed that those subjects receiving 4.0 mg of ondansetron had the lowest dropout rate among all treatment groups and a greater improvement in cocaine use compared with 1.0 mg ondansetron or placebo (154). In addition, there are open label trials for risperidone (155) and vigabatrin (156, 157) showing improvement in cocaine use. Efficacy of vigabatrin was also found in a double-blind, placebo controlled study (158).

As Meyer noted in 1992 in his review of pharmacotherapies for cocaine dependence, most well designed double-blind studies failed to document the efficacy of desipramine in the long-term treatment of cocaine abuse, and did not support the optimistic results seen in early open trials (159). More recent trials with the TCAs in depressed cocaine abusers have shown improvement in depressive symptoms, but this does not consistently correlate with a decrease in cocaine use. Trials with SSRIs in this population have not demonstrated a beneficial effect on either the depression or the cocaine use. In a review of 18 trials of antidepressants for the treatment of cocaine dependence, Lima found no evidence to support the clinical use of antidepressants in the treatment of cocaine dependence (160). On the other hand depressed cocaine addicts demonstrated decreased use when measured by urine BE but not by self report (152). It should be pointed out that studies using quantitative urine BE as an outcome measure sometimes find positive results whereas studies using self report do not (161).

Opiates

In opiate addicts, symptoms of depression and anxiety are usually overshadowed by withdrawal symptoms and by the patient's characterological features. Once detoxified, or stabilized on methadone maintenance, they should be carefully evaluated for evidence of comorbid psychopathology. The lifetime incidence of any affective disease in this population is 74% (162). Brooner et al. conducted diagnostic interviews with 716 opiate-dependent patients who had been admitted to and stabilized on methadone maintenance therapy. Almost half of these patients had another nonsubstance related psychiatric disorder in their lifetimes, with over one-third of them meeting criteria for two or more other diagnoses. They found a 15.8% lifetime incidence of major depression, which is almost three times the rate found in the general population in the ECA study. They also found a strong correlation between the severity of the substance abuse disorder and the degree of psychiatric comorbidity in these patients (163). Despite the frequency of depression in opiate addicts, significant improvement is commonly seen following primary treatment for opiate dependence with either methadone, buprenorphine, or residential treatment (164). Trials of antidepressant medications have produced mixed results and provide little guidance to the clinician (165). Major depression is particularly common in women seeking treatment for opiate dependence and typically precedes the development of opiate dependence. These patients should also be carefully evaluated for PTSD and early childhood trauma.

Woody studied a group of depressed methadone maintenance patients and compared standard drug counseling to either supportive-expressive or cognitive behavioral therapy and showed measurable improvements with psychotherapy (166).

Woody also reported that doxepin was more effective than placebo in reducing depressive symptoms in a double-blind study of 35 depressed methadone maintenance patients (167). Titievsky reported similar results with doxepin in a study of 46 depressed methadone maintenance patients (168).

Other trials using other TCAs in this population were not promising. In a trial of 46 depressed methadone maintenance patients, Kleber found that imipramine was no more effective than placebo for treating depression. He noted that both placebo and imipramine groups showed similar levels of improvement. Kleber suspected this was caused by the intensive nonpharmacologic treatment provided to both groups by the methadone maintenance clinic (169). However, in a more recent large double-blind, placebo-controlled trial of methadone maintenance patients with evidence of a primary MDD, Nunes reported a 57% positive response rate to imipramine in those 84 patients judged to have received "adequate" treatment compared with a 7% response rate in the placebo group (170). These results may be explained by improved TCA dosing techniques. Since methadone has been reported to induce higher serum desipramine levels, it is now clear that TCA levels must be monitored when prescribed to methadone patients (171).

SSRIs are attractive options for treating depression in methadone maintenance patients because of their low toxicity and their minimal abuse potential. While there is evidence that some SSRIs may inhibit the metabolism of methadone, in most circumstances this does not have clinical significance. However, caution should be exercised when SSRIs are prescribed in conjunction with methadone doses over 100 mg and/or with other medications known to prolong the QTc interval (172, 173). Unfortunately, there is minimal research to support the use of SSRIs in depressed methadone maintenance patients. Fluoxetine has not been found to be effective in treating depressed opiate addicts in methadone maintenance. In a double-blind, placebo controlled trial, depressive symptoms decreased over the 12-week trial. However, there was no medication effect, even in those subjects with the most severe depression (174). Dean reported similar results in 49 depressed methadone maintenance patients randomized to either fluoxetine or placebo for 12 weeks. Depression and functioning improved in both groups, but there was no medication effect observed (175). Hamilton described a 12-week, placebo-controlled trial of sertraline in this population, but did not report any outcome data. He did note that sertraline may produce a modest increase in serum methadone levels during the first 6 weeks of therapy (176). Carpenter reported on a 12-week double-blind placebo-controlled trial of sertraline in 95 depressed methadone maintenance patients. There were no medication effects on either depression or illicit drug use, though patients living in less stressful environments had a better outcome (177). We have not been able to locate reports describing the use of paroxetine, citalopram, or any of the newer antidepressants in methadone maintenance patients.

There has been one randomized open label trial of antidepressants in 53 depressed injection drug users. Subjects were randomly assigned to either a "treatment-as-usual" control group that received a single session of post-HIV testing counseling or to the study group that received individual cognitive behavioral

Table 3 Five common patient profiles

PRIMARY AFFECTIVE DISORDER and SECONDARY ALCOHOLISM
2–5% of all alcoholics: (2% of male and 13% of female alcoholics)
Depressive symptoms clearly antedate the alcoholism
Depression continues after detoxification; symptoms are likely to be severe
Requires treatment for BOTH depression and alcoholism; suggest use of an antidepressant medication in therapeutic doses
PRIMARY ALCOHOLISM and SECONDARY ALCOHOLIC HYPOPHORIA
Occurs in 30–50% of all alcoholics
Symptoms similar to primary depression, but less severe
Symptoms are only present during drinking bouts and gradually diminish after detoxification
Requires no specific treatment for depression
May have greater tendency to use other drugs (marijuana and LSD, compared with alcoholics with no symptoms of depression)
Look for symptoms of persistent HYPOPHORIA in this group (51)
PRIMARY ALCOHOLISM and PRIMARY AFFECTIVE DISORDER
Occurs in 3–7% of all alcoholics
Depressive symptoms are severe and do not moderate with sobriety
Symptoms may be present during and between episodes of drinking
Requires treatment for both depression and alcoholism
BIPOLAR AFFECTIVE DISEASE and SECONDARY ALCOHOLISM
Drinking usually begins AFTER the onset of manic-depressive cycles
These patients rarely drink while depressed or in normal phases
Drinking is evident mainly in manic phase
Primary treatment is a mood stabilizer; these patients may not require specific treatment for alcoholism (119)
SUB-SYNDROMAL MANIC DEPRESSIVE ILLNESS and ALCOHOLISM
Patients often present with personality maladjustments (borderline, antisocial, alcohol and drug abuse, emotional liability)
May complain of "RACING THOUGHTS"
Complaints of depression are rare, or may not be obvious
These patients benefit from a mood stabilizer
Alcoholism treatment is also REQUIRED (191)

therapy plus citalopram. If the subjects did not respond to citalopram, the study physician could prescribe either venlafaxine, bupropion, or sertraline. Among the study group, 43.3% were fully adherent to treatment (attended 75% or more of counseling sessions and 75% adherence to pharmacotherapy). The frequency of ongoing heroin use was inversely associated with adherence to treatment (178).

To date, only doxepin and imipramine have been clearly demonstrated to be effective for treating depressed opiate addicts. However, we had positive clinical experience using other agents, especially citalopram, in this patient group, similar to that seen in the Stein study. The presence of severe comorbid psychopathology clearly determines the outcome of opiate addiction treatment (33, 179). Patients with minimal psychopathology do well with standard drug abuse counseling. Patients with severe psychopathology usually get worse in a therapeutic community. They generally do better on methadone maintenance, but require skilled psychotherapists and long-term treatment (180), and access to skilled psychopharmacologic therapy. Traditional psychotherapy does not help antisocial personality disorders; they will do better in a therapeutic community. Unfortunately, this form of treatment is expensive and is of limited availability in many areas. Addiction treatment increases the likelihood of addicts remaining abstinent, but major depression and life crisis increase the risk for relapse (181).

Depression and Opiate Detoxification

Depression has a significant impact on the success of detoxification from methadone maintenance. The development of depressive symptoms in maintenance patients undergoing slow detoxification was associated with a failure to successfully complete detoxification treatment (182). These finding demonstrate the importance of careful screening for depression before and during methadone detoxification. If depressed, detoxification patients should be treated with an antidepressant to maximize their potential for successful treatment outcome. Methadone itself has been thought to have some primary antidepressant effects and to be beneficial in treating comorbid depression (169). Once such patients are detoxified from methadone, it may be impossible for them to avoid relapse unless they are aggressively treated for depression.

Treatment Failures

1. *Check plasma drug levels* in alcoholics and other drug abusers who have not responded to TCAs. If plasma levels are below the therapeutic range, increase the dose. If the depression does not improve, despite adequate serum levels, consider switching to a different TCA, or to an SSRI. If that fails, try one of the newer antidepressants; if there is no response, try lithium.
2. Patients who fail to respond to antidepressant therapy *may be drinking or using drugs again*. No treatment is likely to succeed if the patient does not maintain sobriety. Depressed patients whose symptoms are secondary to a nonaffective psychiatric condition (such as alcoholism, drug use, or an anxiety disorder) are much more likely to fail to respond to antidepressant therapy and to develop chronic symptoms (183).
3. If there are repeated alcohol or drug abuse relapses consider *enforced treatment* utilizing disulfiram, mandatory 12-step groups, and random breathalyzer tests or drug screens, in addition to treatment with antidepressants (184).
4. In alcoholics who continue to drink, consider adding an *anticraving medication*. Naltrexone may be helpful in patients with less severe alcoholism, if they struggle with significant carving (185, 186). Ondansetron has also been reported to reduce drinking in early onset alcoholics (107). Topiramate (126) and acamprosate should also be considered as adjunctive anticraving medications (187).

Conclusion

Depression is one of the most common problems seen in substance abuse patients. Dysphoria and more serious forms of depression may persist for months or years after detoxification. Unfortunately, difficulty in the management of such "dual diagnosis" problems has discouraged many clinicians from working with these patients. Matching these patients to appropriate types of psychiatric treatment has clearly improved treatment outcome. This requires that all substance abuse patients be carefully screened for other psychiatric disorders and that psychiatric treatment be provided, when needed, as a part of the routine treatment for addictive disorders (188).

Clinicians need to distinguish carefully between substance-induced mood disorders and independent depressive disorders, and must become expert in the evaluation and management of these patients. When symptoms of depression have not cleared following detoxification, it is important to initiate antidepressant treatment, including both psychotherapy and pharmacotherapy. Major depression seen in substance abuse patients will usually respond to standard antidepressant pharmacotherapy, as long as the patient is able to achieve sobriety. Except in alcoholics with bipolar affective disease, it is not clear that treating dysphoria or depression will alter drinking. In most patients, antidepressant pharmacotherapy alone is unlikely to reduce the use of alcohol or other drugs. Research has shown that matching such patients to both addiction treatment and appropriate psychiatric treatment will improve the outcome for both conditions. No specific antidepressant is superior in the treatment of substance-induced mood disorders. Clinical practitioners will typically begin with an SSRI, aware of some evidence that early onset heavy drinkers may not respond. Evidence for efficacy of TCA's is strong for improving mood in these patients but drinking reductions do not always follow improvement in depressed mood. Furthermore, TCA's produce risk of lethal overdose. Clinical experience suggests that depressed mood in these patients responds to most of the standard antidepressants, as long as medications are prescribed in adequate doses and the treatment is integrated into a comprehensive substance abuse treatment program.

References

1. Meyer RE. How to understand the relationship between psychopathology and addictive disorders: another example of the chicken and the egg. In: Meyer RE, ed. Psychopathology and Addictive Disorders. New York: Guilford, 1986.
2. Merikangas KR, Leckman JF, Prusoff BA, et al. Familial transmission of depression and alcoholism. Arch Gen Psychiatry 1985;42:367–372.
3. Grove WM, Andreasen NC, Winokur G. Primary and secondary affective disorders: unipolar patients compared on family aggregation. Compr Psychiatry 1987;28:113–126.
4. Prescott CA, Aggen SH, Kendler KS. Sex-specific genetic influences on the comorbidity of alcoholism and major depression in a population-based sample of US twins. Arch Gen Psychiatry 2000;57:803–811.
5. Moore RD, Bone LR, Geller G, Mamon JA, Stokes EJ, Levine DM. Prevalence, detection, and treatment of alcoholism in hospitalized patients. JAMA 1989;261:403–407.

6. Glass IB, Jackson P. Maudsley Hospital Survey: prevalence of alcohol problems and other psychiatric disorders in a hospital population. Br J Addict 1988;83:1105–1111.
7. Narrow WE, Rae DS, Robins LN, Regier DA. Revised prevalence estimates of mental disorders in the United States: using a clinical significance criterion to reconcile 2 surveys' estimates. Arch Gen Psychiatry 2002;59:115–123.
8. Regier DA, Farmer ME, Rae DS, et al. Comorbidity of mental disorders with alcohol and other drug abuse: results from the epidemiological catchment area (ECA) study. JAMA 1990;264:2511–2518.
9. Kessler RC. Lifetime and 12-month prevalence of DSM-III-R psychiatric disorders in the United States. Results from the National Comorbidity Study. Arch Gen Psychiatry 1994;51:8–19.
10. Bucholz KK. Nosology and epidemiology of addictive disorders and their comorbidity. Psychiatr Clin North Am 1999;22:221–240.
11. Grant BF, Stinson FS, Dawson DA, et al. Prevalence and co-occurrence of substance use disorders and independent mood and anxiety disorders: results from the National Epidemiologic Survey on Alcohol and Related Conditions. Arch Gen Psychiatry 2004;61:807–816.
12. Wilson MC, Kevin PC, Frederick SS, Bridget FG. Changes in the prevalence of major depression and comorbid substance use disorders in the United States between 1991–1992 and 2001–2002. Am J Psychiatry 2006;163:2141–2147.
13. Huang B, Grant BF, Dawson DA, et al. Race-ethnicity and the prevalence and co-occurrence of Diagnostic and Statistical Manual of Mental Disorders, Fourth Edition, alcohol and drug use disorders and Axis I and II disorders: United States, 2001 to 2002. Compr Psychiatry 2006;47(4):252–257.
14. Niciu MJ, Chan G, Gelernter J, et al. Subtypes of major depression in substance dependence. Addiction 2009;104:1700–1709.
15. Gold MS, Miller NS, Hoffmann NG. Depression in drug dependency (abstract). American Psychiatric Association Annual Meeting, May 25, 1994.
16. Miller NS, Ninonuevo F, Hoffmann NG, Astrachan BM. Predictors of treatment outcome: lifetime depression versus continuum of care. Am J Addict 1999;8:243–253.
17. Hasin DS, Grant BF. Major depression in 6050 former drinkers: association with past alcohol dependence. Arch Gen Psychiatry 2002;59:794–800.
18. Kirchner JE, Curran GM, Thrush CR, et al. Depressive disorders and alcohol dependence in a community population. Community Ment Health J 2002;38:361–373.
19. Devanand DP. Comorbid psychiatric disorders in late life depression. Biol Psychiatry 2002;52:236–242.
20. Compton WM, Cottler LB, Ben Abdallah A, et al. Substance dependence and other psychiatric disorders among drug dependent subjects: race and gender correlates. Am J Addict 2000;9:113–125.
21. Gamma A, Buck A, Berthold T, Vollenweider FX. No difference in brain activation during cognitive performance between ecstasy (3,4-methylenedioxymethamphetamine) users and control subjects: a [H2(15)O]-positron emission tomography study. J Clin Psychopharmacol 2001;21:66–71.
22. MacInnes N, Handley SL, Harding GF. Former chronic methylenedioxymethamphetamine (MDMA or ecstasy) users report mild depressive symptoms. J Psychopharmacol 2001;15:181–186.
23. Kalechstein AD, Newton TF, Longshore D, et al. Psychiatric comorbidity of methamphetamine dependence in a forensic sample. J Neuropsychiatry Clin Neurosci 2000;12:480–484.
24. Fergusson DM, Lynskey MT, Horwood LJ. Comorbidity between depressive disorders and nicotine dependence in a cohort of 16-year-olds. Arch Gen Psychiatry 1996;53:1043–1047.
25. Brown RA, Lewinsohn PM, Seeley JR, Wagner EF. Cigarette smoking, major depression, and other psychiatric disorders among adolescents. J Am Acad Child Adolesc Psychiatry 1996;35:1602–1610.
26. Dierker LC, Avenevoli S, Merikangas KR, Flaherty BP, Stolar M. Association between psychiatric disorders and the progression of tobacco use behaviors. J Am Acad Child Adolesc Psychiatry 2001;40:1159–1167.

27. Bovasso GB. Cannabis abuse as a risk factor for depressive symptoms. Am J Psychiatry 2001;158:2033–2037.
28. Brook DW, Brook JS, Zhang C, Cohen P, Whiteman M. Drug use and the risk of major depressive disorder, alcohol dependence, and substance use disorders. Arch Gen Psychiatry 2002;59:1039–1044.
29. Chen CY, Wagner FA, Anthony JC. Marijuana use and the risk of major depressive episode. Epidemiological evidence from the United States National Comorbidity Survey. Soc Psychiatry Psychiatr Epidemiol 2002;37:199–206.
30. Patton GC, Coffey C, Carlin JB, Degenhardt L, Lynskey M, Hall W. Cannabis use and mental health in young people: cohort study. Br Med J 2002;325:1195–1198.
31. Vaillant GE. The Natural History of Alcoholism: Causes, Patterns and Pathways to Recovery. Cambridge, MA: Harvard University Press, 1983.
32. McLellan AT, Luborsky L, Woody GE, O'Brien CP, Druley KA. Predicting response to alcohol and drug treatments. Role of psychiatric severity. Arch Gen Psychiatry 1983;40:620–625.
33. McLellan AT, Luborsky L, O'Brien CP. Alcohol and drug abuse treatment in three different populations: is there improvement and is it predictable? Am J Drug Alcohol Abuse 1986;12:101–120.
34. Rounsaville BJ, Dolinsky ZS, Babor TF, Meyer RE. Psychopathology as a predictor of treatment outcome in alcoholics. Arch Gen Psychiatry 1987;44:505–513.
35. Schaefer MR, Sobieraj K, Hollyfield RL. Severity of alcohol dependence and its relationship to additional psychiatric symptoms in male alcoholic inpatients. Am J Drug Alcohol Abuse 1987;13:435–447.
36. Powell BJ, Penick EC, Nickel EJ, et al. Outcomes of co-morbid alcoholic men: a 1-year follow-up. Alcohol Clin Exp Res 1992;16:131–138.
37. Bjork JM, Dougherty DM, Moeller FG. Symptomatology of depression and anxiety in female "social drinkers". Am J Drug Alcohol Abuse 1999;25:173–182.
38. Mueller TI, Lavori PW, Keller MB, et al. Prognostic effect of the variable course of alcoholism on the 10-year course of depression. Am J Psychiatry 1994;151:701–706.
39. Hasin DS, Tsai W-Y, Endicott J, et al. Five-year course of major depression: effects of comorbid alcoholism. J Affect Disord 1996;41:63–70.
40. Barraclough B, Bunch J, Nelson B, Sainsbury P. A hundred cases of suicide: clinical aspects. Br J Psychiatry 1974;125:355–373.
41. Robins E. The Final Months: A Study of the Lives of 134 Who Committed Suicide. New York: Oxford University Press, 1981.
42. Tondo L, Baldessarini RJ, Hennen J, et al. Suicide attempts in major affective disorder patients with comorbid substance use disorder. J Clin Psychiatry 1999;60(Suppl 2):S63–S69; discussion 75–76, 113–116.
43. Grant BF, Hasin DS. Suicidal ideation among the United States drinking population: results from the National Longitudinal Alcohol Epidemiologic Survey. J Stud Alcohol 1999;60:422–429.
44. Aharonovich E, Liu X, Nunes E, Hasin DS. Suicide attempts in substance abusers: effects of major depression in relation to substance use disorders. Am J Psychiatry 2002;159:1600–1602.
45. Davis LL, Rush JA, Wisniewski SR, et al. Substance use disorder comorbidity in major depressive disorder: an exploratory analysis of the Sequenced Treatment Alternatives to Relieve Depression cohort. Compr Psychiatry 2005;46:81–89.
46. Curran GM, Flynn HA, Kirchner J, Booth BM. Depression after alcohol treatment as a risk factor for relapse among male veterans. J Subst Abuse Treat 2000;19:259–265.
47. Hasin DS, Liu X, Nunes E, McCloud S, Samet S, Endicott J. Effects of major depression on remission and relapse of substance dependence. Arch Gen Psychiatry 2002;59:375–380.
48. Kahler CW, Ramsey SE, Read JP, Brown RA. Substance-induced and independent major depressive disorder in treatment-seeking alcoholics: associations with dysfunctional attitudes and coping. J Stud Alcohol 2002;63:363–371.
49. DSM-IV. Diagnostic and Statistical Manual of Mental Disorders. Washington, DC: American Psychiatric Association, 1994.

50. Hesselbrock VM, Tennen H, Stabenau J, Hesselbrock M. Affective disorder in alcoholism. Int J Addict 1983;18:435–444.
51. Jaffe JH, Ciraulo DA. Alcoholism and depression. In: Meyer RE, ed. Psychopathology and Addictive Disorders. New York: Guilford, 1986:293–320.
52. Khantzian EJ. Psychopathology, psychodynamics, and alcoholism. In: Pattison EM, Kaufman E, eds. Encyclopedia Handbook of Alcoholism. New York: Gardner, 1982:581–597.
53. Behar D, Winokur G, Berg CJ. Depression in the abstinent alcoholic. Am J Psychiatry 1984;141:1105–1107.
54. Beck AT. Depression Inventory. Philadelphia: Philadelphia Center for Cognitive Therapy, 1978.
55. Schuckit M. Alcoholic patients with secondary depression. Am J Psychiatry 1983;140:711–714.
56. Merikangas KR, Gelernter CS. Comorbidity for alcoholism and depression. Psychiatr Clin North Am 1990;13:613–632.
57. Ross HE, Glaser FB, Germanson T. The prevalence of psychiatric disorders in patients with alcohol and other drug problems. Arch Gen Psychiatry 1988;45:1023–1031.
58. Abraham HD, Fava M. Order of onset of substance abuse and depression in a sample of depressed outpatients. Compr Psychiatry 1999;40:44–50.
59. Hesselbrock MN, Meyer RE, Keener JJ. Psychopathology in hospitalized alcoholics. Arch Gen Psychiatry 1985;42:1050–1055.
60. Hen CW, Overall JE, Kaufman E. Predicting the post treatment depressive state of an alcoholic patient. Int J Addict 1990;25:1263–1273.
61. Kay DC. The search for psychopathic states in alcoholics and other drug abusers. In: Fann WE, Karacan I, Pokorny AD, Williams RL, eds. Phenomenology and Treatments of Alcoholism. New York: Spectrum, 1980:269–304.
62. Ciraulo DA, Creelman WL, Shader RI, O'Sullivan R. Cyclic antidepressants. In: Ciraulo DA, Shader RI, Greenblatt DJ, Creelman WL, eds. Drug Interactions in Psychiatry. Baltimore, MD: Williams & Wilkins, 1995:29–64.
63. Tanaka E. Toxicological interactions involving psychiatric drugs and alcohol: an update. J Clin Pharm Ther 2003;28:81–95.
64. Ciraulo DA, Shader RI, Greenblatt DJ. SSRI drug-drug interactions. In: Ciraulo DA, Shader RI, Greenblatt DJ, Creelman WL, eds. Drug Interactions in Psychiatry. Baltimore, MD: Williams & Wilkins, 1995:64–90.
65. Naranjo CA, Kadlec KE, Sanhueza P, Woodley-Remus D, Sellers EM. Fluoxetine differentially alters alcohol intake and other consummatory behaviors in problem drinkers. Clin Pharmacol Ther 1990;47:490–498.
66. Ciraulo DA, Barnhill JG, Jaffe AJ, Ciraulo AM, Tarmey MF. Intravenous pharmacokinetics of 2-hydroxyimipramine in alcoholics and normal controls. J Stud Alcohol 1990;51:366–372.
67. Thase ME, Salloum IM, Corneliis JD. Comorbid alcoholism and depression: treatment issues. J Clin Psychiatry 2001;63(Suppl 20):S32–S41.
68. Mason BJ. Dosing issues in the pharmacotherapy of alcoholism. Alcohol Clin Exp Res 1996;20(Suppl 7):10A–16A.
69. Ciraulo DA, Barnhill JG, Jaffe JH. Clinical pharmacokinetics of imipramine and desipramine in alcoholics and normal volunteers. Clin Pharmacol Ther 1988;43:509–518.
70. Ciraulo DA, Jaffe JH. Tricyclic antidepressants in the treatment of depression associated with alcoholism. J Clin Psychopharmacol 1981;1:146.
71. Mason BJ, Kocsis MD. Despiramine treatment of alcoholism. Psychopharmacol Bull 1991;27:155–161.
72. Nunes EV, McGrath PJ, Quitkin FM, et al. Imipramine treatment of alcoholism with comorbid depression. Am J Psychiatry 1993;150:963–965.
73. McGrath PJ, Nunes EV, Stewart JW, et al. Imipramine treatment of alcoholics with primary depression: a placebo-controlled clinical trial. Arch Gen Psychiatry 1996;53:232–240.
74. Mason BJ, Kocsis MD, Ritvo EC, Cutler RB. A double-blind, placebo-controlled trial of desipramine for primary alcohol dependence stratified on the presence or absence of major depression. JAMA 1996;275:803–804.

75. Hyatt MC, Bird MA. Amitriptyline augments and prolongs ethanol-induced euphoria. J Clin Psychiatry 1987;7:277–278.
76. Lejoyeux M. Use of serotonin (5-hydroxytryptamiine) reuptake inhibitors in the treatment of alcoholism. Alcohol Alcohol 1996;31(Suppl 1):S69–S75.
77. Sellers EM, Higgins GA. Opportunities for treatment of psychoactive substance use disorders with serotonergic medications. J Clin Psychiatry 1991;52(Suppl 12):S49–S54.
78. Leonard BE. The comparative pharmacology of new antidepressants. J Clin Psychiatry 1993;54(Suppl 8):S3–S5.
79. Loo H, Malka R, Defrance R, et al. Tianeptine and amitriptyline. Controlled double-blind trial in depressed alcoholic patients. Neuropsychobiology 1988;19:79–85.
80. Cornelius JR, Salloum IM, Cornelius MD, et al. Fluoxetine trial in suicidal depressed alcoholics. Psychopharmacol Bull 1993;29:195–199.
81. Kranzler HR, Burleson JA, Korner P. Placebo-controlled trial of fluoxetine as an adjunct to relapse prevention in alcoholics. Am J Psychol 1995;152:391–397.
82. Cornelius JR, Salloum IM, Ehler JG, et al. Fluoxetine in depressed alcoholics. A double-blind, placebo-controlled trial. Arch Gen Psychiatry 1997;54:700–705.
83. Cornelius JR, Salloum IM, Thase ME, et al. Fluoxetine versus placebo in depressed alcoholic cocaine abusers. Psychopharmacol Bull 1998;34:117–121.
84. Cornelius JR, Salloum IM, Haskett RF, et al. Fluoxetine versus placebo in depressed alcoholics: a 1-year follow-up study. Addict Behav 2000;25:307–310.
85. Cornelius JR, Bukstein OG, Birmaher B, et al. Fluoxetine in adolescents with major depression and an alcohol use disorder: an open-label trial. Addict Behav 2001;26:735–739.
86. Cornelius JR, Clark DB, Bukstein OG, et al. Acute phase and five-year follow-up study of fluoxetine in adolescents with major depression and a comorbid substance use disorder: a review. Addict Behav 2005;30(9):1824–1833.
87. Riggs PD, Mikulich SK, Coffman LM, Crowley TJ. Fluoxetine in drug-dependent delinquents with major depression. J Child Adolesc Psychopharmacol 1997;7:87–95.
88. Roy A. Placebo-controlled study of sertraline in depressed recently abstinent alcoholics. Biol Psychiatry 1998;44:633–637.
89. Pettinati HM, Volpicelli JR, Luck G. Double-blind clinical trial of sertraline treatment for alcohol dependence. J Clin Psychopharmacol 2001;21:143–153.
90. Moak DH, Anton RF, Latham PK, et al. Sertraline and cognitive behavioral therapy for depressed alcoholics: results of a placebo-controlled trial. J Clin Psychopharmacol 2003;23:553–562.
91. Gual A, Balcells M, Torres M, et al. Sertraline for the prevention of relapse in detoxicated alcohol dependent patients with a comorbid depressive disorder: a randomized controlled trial. Alcohol Alcohol 2003;38:619–625.
92. Kranzler HR, Mueller T, Cornelius J, et al. Sertraline treatment of co-occurring alcohol dependence and major depression. J Clin Psychopharmacol 2006;26(1):13–20.
93. Tiihonen J, Ryynanen OP, Kauhanen HP, Hakola HP, Salaspuro M. Citalopram in the treatment of alcoholism: a double-blind placebo-controlled study. Pharmacopsychiatry 1996;29:27–29.
94. Naranjo CA, Poulos CX, Bremner KE, Lanctot KL. Citalopram decreases desirability, liking, and consumption of alcohol in alcohol-dependent drinkers. Clin Pharmacol Ther 1992;51:729–739.
95. Balldin J, Berggren U, Engel J, et al. Effect of citalopram on alcohol intake in heavy drinkers. Alcohol Clin Exp Res 1994;18:1133–1136.
96. Naranjo CA, Knoke DM, Bremner KE. Variations in response to citalopram in men and women with alcohol dependence. J Psychiatry Neurosci 2000;25:269–275.
97. Muhonen LH, Lonnqvist J, Juva K, Alho H. Double-blind, randomized comparison of memantine and escitalopram for the treatment of major depressive disorder comorbid with alcohol dependence. J Clin Psychiatry 2008a;69(3):392–399.
98. Muhonen LH, Lahti J, Sinclair D, Lonnqvist J, Alho H. The treatment of alcohol dependence in patients with co-morbid major depressive disorder – predictors for the outcomes with memantine and escitalopram medication. Subst Abuse Treat Prev Policy 2008b;3:20.

99. Muhonen LH, Lonnqvist J, Lahti J, Alho H. Age at onset of first depressive episode as a predictor for escitalopram treatment of major depression comorbid with alcohol dependence. Psychiatry Res 2009;167(1–2):115–122.
100. Pettinati HM. Antidepressant treatment of co-occurring depression and alcohol dependence. Biol Psychiatry 2004;56(10):785–792.
101. Gopalakrishnan R, Ross J, O'Brien C, Oslin D. Course of late-life depression with alcoholism following combination therapy. J Stud Alcohol Drug 2009;70(2):237–241.
102. Pettinati HM, Oslin DW, Kampman KM, et al A double-blind, placebo-controlled trial combining sertraline and naltrexone for treating co-occurring depression and alcohol dependence. Am J Psychiatry (http://ajp.psychiatryonline.org/) AJP in Advance, published March 15, 2010 (doi: 10.1176/appi.ajp.2009.08060852). Accessed April 29, 2010.
103. Nierenberg AA, Adler LA, Peselow E, Zornberg G, Rosenthal M. Trazodone for antidepressant-associated insomnia. Am J Psychiatry 1994;151:1069–1072.
104. Le Bon O, Murphy JR, Staner L, et al. Double-blind, placebo-controlled study of the efficacy of trazodone in alcohol post-withdrawal syndrome: polysomnographic and clinical evaluations. J Clin Psychopharmacol 2003;23:377–383.
105. Pettinati HM. The use of selective serotonin reuptake inhibitors in treating alcoholic subtypes. J Clin Psychiatry 2001;62(Suppl 20):S26–S31.
106. Pettinati HM, Kranzler HR, Madaras J. The status of serotonin-selective pharmacotherapy in the treatment of alcohol dependence. Recent Dev Alcohol 2003;16:247–262.
107. Johnson BA, DiClemente CC, Cloninger CR, et al. Ondansetron for reduction of drinking among biologically predisposed alcoholic patients. JAMA 2000;284:963–971.
108. Lader MH. Tolerability and safety: essentials in antidepressant pharmacotherapy. J Clin Psychiatry 1996;57(Suppl 2):39–44.
109. Roy-Byrne PP, Pages KP, Russo JE, et al. Nefazodone treatment of major depression in alcohol-dependent patients: a double-blind, placebo-controlled trial. J Clin Psychopharmacol 2000;20:129–136.
110. Hernandez-Avila CA, Modesto-Lowe V, Feinn R, Kranzler HR. Nefazodone treatment of comorbid alcohol dependence and major depression. Alcohol Clin Exp Res 2004;28(3):433–440.
111. Liappas J, Paparrigopoulos T, Tzavellas E, Rabavilas A. Mirtazapine and venlafaxine in the management of collateral psychopathology during alcohol detoxification. Prog Neuropsychopharmacol Biol Psychiatry 2004;29(1):55–60.
112. Altintoprak AE, Zoriu N, Coskunol H, Akdeniz F. Effectiveness and tolerability of mirtazapine and amitriptyline in alcoholic patients with co-morbid depressive disorder: a randomized, double-blind study. Hum Psychopharmacol 2008;23(4):313–319.
113. Yoon SJ. Pae CU. Kim DJ, et al. Mirtazapine for patients with alcohol dependence and comorbid depressive disorders: a multicentre, open label study. Prog Neuropsychopharmacol Biol Psychiatry 2006;30(7):1196–1201.
114. Garcia-Portilla MP, Bascaran MT. Saiz PA, et al. Effectiveness of venlafaxine in the treatment of alcohol dependence with comorbid depression [Spanish]. Actas Esp Psiquiatr 2005;33(1):41–45.
115. Goodwin FK. Clinic Psychiatric News 1994:11.
116. Ostracher MJ, Perlis RH, Nierenberg AA, et al. Impact of substance use disorders on recovery from episodes of depression in bipolar disorder patients: prospective data from the Systematic Treatment Enhancement Program for Bipolar Disorder (STEP-BD). Am J Psychiatry 2010;167(3):289–297.
117. Salloum IM, Cornelius JR, Daley DC, et al. Efficacy of valproate maintenance in patients with bipolar disorder and alcoholism: a double-blind placebo-controlled study. Arch Gen Psychiatry 2005;62:37–45.
118. Brown ES, Garza M, Carmody TJ. A randomized, double-blind, placebo-controlled add-on trial of quetiapine in outpatients with bipolar disorder and alcohol uses disorders. J Clin Psychiatry 2008;69(5):701–705.
119. Reich LH, Davies RK, Himmelhoch JM. Excessive alcohol use in manic depressive illness. Am J Psychiatry 1974;131:83–86.

120. Brady KT, Sonne SC, Anton R, Ballenger JC. Valproate in the treatment of acute bipolar affective episodes complicated by substance abuse: a pilot study. J Clin Psychiatry 1995;56:118–121.
121. Albanese MJ, Clodfelter RC, Jr., Khantzian EJ. Divalproex sodium in substance abusers with mood disorder. J Clin Psychiatry 2000;61:916–921.
122. Kemp DE, Gao K, Ganocy SJ, et al. A 6-month, double-blind, maintenance trial of lithium monotherapy versus the combination of lithium and divalproex for rapid-cycling bipolar disorder and co-occurring substance abuse or dependence. J Clin Psychiatry 2009;70(1):113–121.
123. Rubio G, Lopez-Munoz F, Alamo C. Effects of lamotrigine in patients with bipolar disorder and alcohol dependence. Bipolar Disord 2006;8(3):289–293.
124. Hertzman M. Divalproex sodium to treat concomitant substance abuse and mood disorders. J Subst Abuse Treat 2000;18:371–372.
125. Goldberg JF, Garno JL, Leon AC, Kocis JH, Portera L. A history of substance abuse complicates remission from acute mania in bipolar disorder. J Clin Psychiatry 1999;60:733–740.
126. Johnson BA, Ait-Daoud N, Bowden CL, et al. Oral topiramate for treatment of alcohol dependence: a randomised controlled trial. Lancet 2003;361:1677–1685.
127. Gawin FH, Kleber HD. Abstinence symptomatology and psychiatric diagnosis in cocaine abusers. Clinical observations. Arch Gen Psychiatry 1986;43:107–113.
128. Brower KJ, Maddahian E, Blow FC, Beresford TP. A comparison of self-reported symptoms and DSM-III-R criteria for cocaine withdrawal. Am J Drug Alcohol Abuse 1988;14:347–356.
129. Lowenstein DH, Massa SM, Rowbotham MC, Collins SD, McKinney HE, Simon RP. Acute neurologic and psychiatric complications associated with cocaine abuse. Am J Med 1987;83:841–846.
130. Ford JD, Gelernter J, DeVoe JS, et al. Association of psychiatric and substance use disorder comorbidity with cocaine dependence severity and treatment utilization in cocaine-dependent individuals. Drug Alcohol Depend 2009;99(1–3):193–203.
131. Tang YL, Kranzler HR, Gelernter J, et al. Comorbid psychiatric diagnoses and their association with cocaine-induced psychosis in cocaine-dependent subjects. Am J Addict 2007;16(5):343–351.
132. Kleinman PH, Miller AB, Millman RB, et al. Psychopathology among cocaine abusers entering treatment. J Nerv Ment Dis 1990;178:442–447.
133. Brown RA, Monti PM, Myers MG, et al. Depression among cocaine abusers in treatment: relation to cocaine and alcohol use and treatment outcome. Am J Psychiatry 1998;155:220–225.
134. Gawin FH, Kleber HD, Byck R, et al. Desipramine facilitation of initial cocaine abstinence. Arch Gen Psychiatry 1989;46:117–121.
135. Weiss RD. Relapse to cocaine abuse after initiating desipramine treatment. JAMA 1988;260:2545–2546.
136. Ziedonis DM, Kosten TR. Depression as a prognostic factor for pharmacological treatment of cocaine dependence. Psychopharmacol Bull 1991;27:337–343.
137. Nunes EV, McGrath PJ, Quitkin FM, et al. Imipramine treatment of cocaine abuse: possible boundaries of efficacy. Drug Alcohol Depend 1995;39:185–195.
138. McDowell D, Nunes EV, Seracini AM, et al. Desipramine treatment of cocaine-dependent patients with depression: a placebo-controlled trial. Drug Alcohol Depend 2005;80(2):209–221.
139. Gonzalez G, Feingold A, Oliveto A, et al. Comorbid major depressive disorder as a prognostic factor in cocaine-abusing buprenorphine-maintained patients treated with desipramine and contingency management. Am J Drug Alcohol Abuse 2003;29:497–514.
140. Brown ES, Nejtek VA, Perantie DC, et al. Lamotrigine in patients with bipolar disorder and cocaine dependence. J Clin Psychiatry 2003;64(2):197–201.
141. Brown ES, Perantie DC, Dhanani N, et al. Lamotrigine for bipolar disorder and comorbid cocaine dependence: a replication and extension study. J Affect Disord 2006;93(1–3):219–222.
142. Schmitz JM, Averill P, Stotts AL, et al. Fluoxetine treatment of cocaine-dependent patients with major depressive disorder. Drug Alcohol Depend 2001;63:207–214.

143. McDowell DM, Levin FR, Seracini AM, Nunes EV. Venlafaxine treatment of cocaine abusers with depressive disorders. Am J Drug Alcohol Abuse 2000;26:25–31.
144. Kampman KM, Leiderman D, Holmes T, et al. Cocaine Rapid Efficacy Screening Trials (CREST): lessons learned. Addiction 2005;100(Suppl 1):102–111.
145. Poling J, Oliveto A, Petry N, et al. Six-month trial of bupropion with contingency management for cocaine dependence in a methadone-maintained population. Arch Gen Psychiatry 2006;63(2):219–228.
146. Kampman KM, Pettinati H, Lynch KG, et al. A pilot trial of topiramate for the treatment of cocaine dependence. Drug Alcohol Depend 2004;75:233–240.
147. Gonzalez G, Desai R, Sofuoglu M, et al. Clinical efficacy of gabapentin versus tiagabine for reducing cocaine use among cocaine dependent methadone-treated patients. Drug Alcohol Depend 2007;87(1):1–9.
148. Bisaga A, Aharonovich E, Garawi F, et al. A randomized placebo-controlled trial of gabapentin for cocaine dependence. Drug Alcohol Depend 2006;81(3):267–274.
149. Brady KT, Sonne SC, Malcolm RJ, et al. Carbamazepine in the treatment of cocaine dependence: subtyping by affective disorder. Exp Clin Psychopharmacol 2002;10:276–285.
150. Elkashef A, Fudala PJ, Gorgon L, et al. Double-blind, placebo-controlled trial of selegiline transdermal system (STS) for the treatment of cocaine dependence. Drug Alcohol Depend 2006;85(3):191–197.
151. Dackis CA, Kampman KM, Lynch KG, et al. A double-blind, placebo-controlled trial of modafinil for cocaine dependence. Neuropsychopharmacology 2005;30(1):205–211.
152. Ciraulo DA, Knapp C, Rotrosen J, et al. Nefazodone treatment of cocaine dependence with comorbid depressive symptoms [Clinical Trial. Journal Article. Randomized Controlled Trial. Research Support, N.I.H., Extramural. Research Support, Non-U.S. Gov't. Research Support, U.S. Gov't, P.H.S.]. Addiction 2005;100(Suppl 1):23–31.
153. Gawin FH. New uses of antidepressants in cocaine abuse. Psychosomatics 1986;27(Suppl 11):S24–S29.
154. Johnson BA, Roache JD, Ait-Daoud N, et al. A preliminary randomized, double-blind, placebo-controlled study of the safety and efficacy of ondansetron in the treatment of cocaine dependence. Drug Alcohol Depend 2006;84(3):256–263.
155. Albanese MJ, Suh JJ. Risperidone in cocaine-dependent patients with comorbid psychiatric disorders. J Psychiatr Pract 2006;12(5):306–311.
156. Brodie JD, Figueroa E, Dewey SL. Treating cocaine addiction: from preclinical to clinical trial experience with gamma-vinyl GABA. Synapse 2003;50(3):261–265.
157. Brodie JD, Figueroa E, Laska EM, Dewey SL. Safety and efficacy of γ-vinyl GABA (GVG) for the treatment of methamphetamine and/or cocaine addiction. Synapse 2004;55(2):122–125.
158. Brodie JD, Case BC, Figueroa E, et al. Randomized, double-blind, placebo-controlled trial of vigabatrin for the treatment of cocaine dependence in Mexican Parolees. Am J Psychiatry 2009;166(11):1269–1277.
159. Meyer RE. New pharmacotherapies for cocaine dependence revisited. Arch Gen Psychiatry 1992;49:900–904.
160. Lima MS, Reisser AA, Soares BG, Farrell M. Antidepressants for cocaine dependence. Cochrane Database Syst Rev 2003;2:CD002950.
161. Batki SL, Manfredi LB, Jacob P, III, Jones RT. Fluoxetine for cocaine dependence in methadone maintenance: quantitative plasma and urine cocaine/benzoylecgonine concentrations. J Psychopharmacol 1993;13:243–250.
162. Rounsaville BJ, Weissman MM, Kleber H, Wilber C. Heterogeneity of psychiatric diagnosis in treated opiate addicts. Arch Gen Psychiatry 1982;39:161–166.
163. Brooner RK, King VL, Kidorf M, Schmidt CW, Jr., Bigelow GE. Psychiatric and substance use comorbidity among treatment-seeking opioid abusers. Arch Gen Psychiatry 1997;54:71–80.
164. Dean AJ, Bell J, Christie MJ, Mattick RP. Depressive symptoms during buprenorphine vs. methadone maintenance: findings from a randomized, controlled trial of opioid dependence. Eur Psychiatry 2004;19(8):510–513.

165. Nunes EV, Sullivan MA, Levin FR. Treatment of depression in patients with opiate dependence. Biol Psychiatry 2004;56:793–802.
166. Woody GE, Luborsky L, McLellan AT, et al. Psychotherapy of opiate addicts: does it help? Arch Gen Psychiatry 1983;40:639–645.
167. Woody GE, O'Brien CP, Rickels K. Depression and anxiety in heroin addicts: a placebo-controlled study of doxepin in combination with methadone. Am J Psychiatry 1975;132:447–450.
168. Titievsky J, Seco G, Barranco M, Kyle EM. Doxepin as adjunctive therapy for depressed methadone maintenance patients: a double-blind study. J Clin Psychiatry 1982;43:454–456.
169. Kleber HD, Weissman MM, Rounsaville BJ, Wilber CH, Prusoff BA, Riordan CE. Imipramine as treatment for depression in addicts. Arch Gen Psychiatry 1983;40:649–653.
170. Nunes EV, Quitkin FM, Donovan SJ, et al. Imipramine treatment of opiate-dependent patients with depressive disorders. A placebo-controlled trial. Arch Gen Psychiatry 1998;55:153–160.
171. Maany I, Dhopesh V, Arndt IO, et al. Increase in desipramine serum levels associated with methadone maintenance. Am J Psychiatry 1989;146:1611–1613.
172. Maxwell JC, McCance-Katz EF. Indicators of buprenorphine and methadone use and abuse: what do we know? Am J Addict 2009;19(1):73–88.
173. Vazquez V, Gury C, Laquille X. Methadone: from pharmacokinetic profile to clinical pharmacology. Encephale 2006;32(4 Pt 1):478–486.
174. Petrakis I, Carroll KM, Nich C, et al. Fluoxetine treatment of depressive disorders in methadone-maintained opioid addicts. Drug Alcohol Depend 1998;50:221–226.
175. Dean AJ, Bell J, Mascord DJ, et al. A randomized, controlled trial of fluoxetine in methadone maintenance patients with depression. J Affect Disord 2002;72:85–90.
176. Hamilton SP, Nunes EV, Janai M, Weber L. The effect of sertraline on methadone plasma levels in methadone-maintained patients. Am J Addict 2000;9:63–69.
177. Carpenter KM, Brooks AC, Vosburg SK, Nunes EV. The effect of sertraline and environmental context on treating depression and illicit substance use among methadone maintained opiate dependent patients: a controlled clinical trial. Drug Alcohol Depend 2004;74:123–134.
178. Stein MD, Herman DS, Solomon DA, et al. Adherence to treatment of depression in active injection drug users: the minerva study. J Subst Abuse Treat 2003;26:87–93.
179. Woody GE, McLellan AT, Luborsky L, et al. Severity of psychiatric symptoms as a predictor of benefits from psychotherapy: the Veterans Administration-Penn study. Am J Psychiatry 1984;141:1172–1177.
180. Woody GE, McLellan AT, Luborsky L, O'Brien CP. Twelve-month follow-up of psychotherapy for opiate dependence. Am J Psychiatry 1987;144:590–596.
181. Kosten TR, Rounsaville BJ, Kleber HD. A 2.5-year follow-up of depression, life crises, and treatment effects on abstinence among opioid addicts. Arch Gen Psychiatry 1986;43:733–738.
182. Kanof PD, Aronson MJ, Ness R. Organic mood syndrome associated with detoxification from methadone maintenance. Am J Psychiatry 1993;150:423–428.
183. Keller MB. Long-term outcome of episodes of major depression. JAMA 1984;252:788–792.
184. Kofoed L, Kania J, Walsh T, Atkinson RM. Outpatient treatment of patients with substance abuse and coexisting psychiatric disorders. Am J Psychiatry 1986;143:867–872.
185. O'Malley SS, Jaffe AJ, Chang G, et al. Naltrexone and coping skills therapy for alcohol dependence. Arch Gen Psychiatry 1992;49:881–887.
186. Volpicelli JR, Alterman AI, Hayashida M, O'Brien CP. Naltrexone in the treatment of alcohol-dependence. Arch Gen Psychiatry 1992;49:876–880.
187. Pelc I, Verbanck P, Le Bon O, et al. Efficacy and safety of acamprosate in the treatment of detoxified alcohol-dependent patients. Br J Psychiatry 1997;171:73–77.
188. McLellan AT, Alterman AI. Patient treatment matching: a conceptual and methodological review with suggestions for future research. In: Pickens RW, Leukefeld CG, Schuster CR, eds. Improving Drug Abuse Treatment. Rockville, MD: National Institute on Drug Abuse, 1991:114–135.

189. Haertzen CA. Development of scales based on patterns of drug effects, using the addiction research center inventory. Psychol Rep 1966;18:163–194.
190. Sarid-Segal O, Knapp CM, Ciraulo AM, et al. Decreased EEG sensitivity to alprazolam in subjects with a parental history of alcoholism. J Clin Pharmacol 2000;40:84–90.
191. Akiskal HS. Subaffective disorders: dysthymic, cyclothymic, and bipolar II disorders in the "borderline" realm. Psychiatr Clin North Am 1981 Apr;4(1):25–46.

Antidepressant Treatments in PTSD

Janet E. Osterman, Brandon Z. Erdos, Mark Oldham, and Ana Ivkovic

Posttraumatic Stress Disorder (PTSD)

Posttraumatic stress disorder (PTSD) is a clinical syndrome with a high degree of morbidity that may follow a traumatic event. PTSD is characterized by three symptom clusters: (1) reexperiencing of the traumatic event; (2) avoidance of reminders of the traumatic event and emotional numbing; and (3) hyperarousal symptoms (1). PTSD results in significant distress and morbidity. For example, following an assault a person may experience intrusive thoughts of the assault, suffer from nightmares of threat or assault, or experience flashbacks of all or some portions of the assault. Avoidance of reminders is common and may include, for example, avoidance of the site of the assault or similar places, avoidance of people who are similar to the perpetrator, or avoidance of conversations about community or domestic violence. Following a traumatic event, emotional numbing such as a sense of being unable to have loving feelings, feeling detached from others, or having decreased interest may occur. Difficulty falling asleep, being easily startled, irritability, and hypervigilance are common hyperarousal symptoms (see DSM-IV for criteria) (1).

Acute Stress Disorder

Acute stress disorder (ASD) provides a diagnostic category for symptoms between the event and the 1 month criterion for PTSD (1). ASD is characterized by dissociative, reexperiencing, avoidance, and hyperarousal symptoms that must begin between 2 days and 4 weeks following the index event. Dissociative symptoms, including derealization, depersonalization, being in a daze, numbing, and amnesia, frequently predominate. Some preliminary studies suggest that the presence of

---

J.E. Osterman (✉)
Department of Psychiatry, Boston University School of Medicine and Boston Medical Center, Dowling 7 850 Harrison Avenue, Boston, MA 02118, USA
e-mail: osterman@bu.edu

D.A. Ciraulo and R.I. Shader (eds.), *Pharmacotherapy of Depression*,
DOI 10.1007/978-1-60327-435-7_7,

ASD is predictive for developing PTSD (2–4), while many studies show that peri-traumatic dissociation is a risk factor for PTSD (5–7).

Disorders of Extreme Stress or Complex PTSD

Disorders of extreme stress (DES) or complex PTSD has been proposed by van der Kolk, Herman, and others (8, 9) to define a posttraumatic clinical syndrome characterized by problems in self-regulation of affect and impulses, disordered interpersonal functioning, somatization, as well as alterations in attention or consciousness, perceptions of the perpetrator, self-perceptions, and meaning systems. These symptoms are currently described as associated features of PTSD in DSM-IV (1). Findings from the field trials for DSM-IV found that adult survivors of childhood sexual abuse were 4.4 times more likely to suffer from DES. Adults who suffered both childhood sexual and physical abuse were 14.4 times more likely to suffer from this symptom complex (9). A recent study by de Jong et al. suggests that DES may be a cultural finding as this symptom complex was not found in several non-western populations (10).

Epidemiology of Trauma and PTSD

Prevalence of Traumatic Events

Prevalence of traumatic events is a common experience. The National Comorbidity Survey (11) reveals that 60.7% of men and 51.2% of women in the United States have experienced a traumatic event that meets the DSM-IV stressor criteria. The DSM-IV (1) defines a traumatic event as one in which the person experiences, witnesses, or is confronted with actual or threatened death or serious injury, or a threat to the physical integrity of oneself or others and responds to this event with intense fear, helplessness, or horror. The National Comorbidity Survey (11) found that experiencing one or more traumatic events was not uncommon. Both genders reported similar prevalence rates for a single traumatic event (26%) and two traumatic events (14%); however, men had nearly twice the prevalence rates for three events (9.5 vs. 5%) and four events (10.2 vs. 6.4%).

The most common traumatic events for both genders were witnessing someone severely injured or killed, being in a fire, flood, or natural disaster, or being in a life-threatening accident. Men more often were involved in these common traumatic events with 35.6% being witness to life threat, 18.9% experiencing a fire, flood, or natural disaster, and 25% being involved in a life-threatening accident; while 14.5% of women witnessed life threat, 15.2% experienced fire, flood, or natural disaster, and 13.8% were in a life-threatening accident. Men reported higher proportions of physical attack (11.1 vs. 6.9%), combat (6.4 vs. 0%), and being threatened with a weapon, held captive or kidnapped (19 vs. 6.8%). Women suffered more frequently from rape (9.2 vs. 0.7%), sexual molestation (12.3 vs. 2.8%), childhood neglect (3.4 vs. 2.1%), and childhood physical abuse (4.8 vs. 3.2%) (4). In general, men are more at risk from strangers while women and girls are more at risk from family or acquaintances.

Although more than half the population in the United States suffered a traumatic event in their lifetime, only 7.8% of those traumatized had a lifetime prevalence of PTSD (see Table 1). Women, although suffering fewer lifetime traumatic events, were more likely to suffer from PTSD (10.4%) when compared to men with a 5.0% prevalence rate. Events that were reported to be most disturbing more frequently resulted in PTSD. Rape for both men and women was the most disturbing trauma and most likely to result in PTSD with 65% of men and 45.9% of women developing PTSD following rape. Other traumatic events for men that resulted in PTSD included combat, childhood neglect or physical abuse; and for women, included sexual molestation, physical attack, being threatened by a weapon, held captive, or kidnapped, and childhood physical abuse. Women were more likely to have experienced one of the traumatic events identified as most disturbing and resulting in PTSD (67.6% compared to 44.6% of men). Excluding rape and childhood neglect, women had a greater exposure to high-impact events and a greater likelihood of developing PTSD following exposure, accounting for the 2:1 probability that women will develop PTSD (11).

Comorbid/Cooccurring Disorders

Comorbid/Cooccurring disorders are common in people who suffer from PTSD (11–13) (see Table 2). Data from the National Comorbidity Survey (11) reveal that 88.3% of men with PTSD and in 79% of women PTSD suffered from another disorder.

Table 1 Prevalence of trauma experiences from the National Co-morbidity Study (10)

Trauma type	Men (%)	Women (%)
Witness to life threat	35.6	14.5
Fire, flood, other natural disaster	18.9	15.2
Accident	25.0	13.8
Physical attack	11.1	6.9
Combat	6.4	0
Threatened with weapon, held captive, or kidnapped	19.0	6.8
Rape	0.7	9.2
Sexual molestation	2.8	12.3
Childhood neglect	2.1	3.4
Childhood physical abuse	3.2	4.8

Adapted from Kessler et al. (10)

Table 2 Co-morbidty and PTSD from the National Co-morbidity Study (10)

Co-morbid disorder	Men (%)	Women (%)
Major depressive disorder	47.9	48.5
Dysthymia	21.4	23.3
Alcohol abuse or dependence	51.9	27.9
Drug abuse or dependence	26.9	26.9
Simple phobia	31.4	29
Social phobia	27.6	28.4
Generalized anxiety disorder	16.8	15.0
Agoraphobia	16.1	22.4
Panic disorder	7.3	12.6
Conduct disorder	43.3	15.4

Adapted from Kessler et al. (10)

Men and women with PTSD were most likely to suffer from three or more comorbid disorders. This is in sharp contrast to men and women with other psychiatric disorders, who were much less likely to have any comorbid disorder. The most common comorbid disorders for men with PTSD were alcohol abuse or dependence (51.9%), major depressive disorder (47.9%), conduct disorder (43.3%), simple phobia (31.4%), drug abuse or dependence (26.9%), social phobia (27.6%), dysthymia (21.4%), generalized anxiety disorder (16.8%), and agoraphobia (16.1%). The most common comorbid disorders for women with PTSD were major depressive disorder (48.5%), simple phobia (29%), social phobia (28.4%), alcohol abuse or dependence (27.9%), drug abuse or dependence (26.9%), dysthymia (23.3%), and agoraphobia (22.4%).

The question of whether or not people with PTSD suffer from a comorbid disorder is confounded by the overlap in the diagnostic nomenclature for PTSD, other anxiety disorders, and major depressive disorder (12). Symptoms of diminished interest, sleep disturbances, irritability, difficulty concentrating, and restricted affect are shared between major depressive disorder and PTSD. Arousal and avoidance symptoms are common in PTSD and other anxiety disorders including generalized anxiety disorders, simple phobia, social phobia, and agoraphobia.

An additional question that is often difficult to sort out clinically is which disorder is the primary disorder. The National Comorbidity Survey (11) attempted to answer this by assessing the age at which the disorders were found. The survey results suggested that PTSD was primary when major depressive disorder and substance abuse disorders were comorbid. In women, but not men, conduct disorder was secondary to PTSD. PTSD was likely to be primary when an anxiety disorder was present, although the findings were less robust than for affective and substance abuse disorders. In the clinical setting, it is often difficult to determine whether PTSD or another disorder is the primary disorder. Unfortunately, assessing a family history is not revealing as family history of an affective disorder is a risk factor for PTSD (14), and a family history of substance abuse is a risk factor for childhood abuse or neglect (15, 16). The age of the index traumatic event is the most reliable indicator for which disorder is primary. However, this does not preclude that the comorbid disorder may have developed independently in a particular patient. The question of primary disorder or comorbid disorder is relevant in the medication management as many comorbid disorders are chronic, recurring disorders associated with significant morbidity and are typically treated with maintenance medication.

The National Comorbidity Survey Replication study of 4,141 participants evaluated the relationship between childhood physical and sexual abuse and anxiety disorders revealing gender differences in response to abuse. Women with childhood physical abuse had strong associations with PTSD and specific phobia while sexual abuse was associated with PTSD, social anxiety disorder, and panic disorder. Both physical and sexual abuse were linked to PTSD and social anxiety disorder in sampled men (17).

The relationship between suicidal behaviors and thoughts and PTSD with or without major depressive disorder was assessed in a national household survey of 3,085 adult women. Lifetime comorbidity of PTSD and major depressive disorder revealed a higher prevalence of suicidal ideation than in either PTSD or major depressive disorder. Suicide attempts were higher in people with comorbid PTSD and major depressive disorder than in major depressive disorder alone (18). Thus, suicide safety assessment is critical in patients with a history of trauma and PTSD.

Neurobiology of PTSD

Over the past decade, much has been learned about the neurobiological underpinnings of PTSD. However, questions remain, stimulating ongoing research into the biological, neuroendocrine, and neurochemical mechanisms of psychological trauma and PTSD. An area of common interest to PTSD and other anxiety disorders is the biology of fear (19–23). Fear and conditioned fear memories have been understood to be a component of PTSD and were the initial basis for the development of behavioral treatment of PTSD (24). The current state of knowledge indicates that while fear conditioning is an important factor, PTSD is due to more complicated neurobiological mechanisms. Investigations of fear and PTSD suggest that both likely share common pathways and neuroanatomic sites with complex interactions between multiple sites including the amygdala, the hippocampus, the pre-frontal cortex, and the hypothalamic-pituitary-adrenal (HPA) axis (19–23, 25–28). Neuroimaging studies reveal increased amygdala and anterior paralimbic activity in response to trauma-related stimuli (29) and decreased reactivity in the anterior cingulate and orbitofrontal cortices (30).

The amygdala, the "fear center" of the brain, has been shown to be intimately involved in both fear and PTSD (19, 21–23). During a fear response, the amygdala has been shown to activate downstream brain nuclei and pathways leading to increased startle response, increased release of catecholamines, and activation of the sympathetic nervous system. At the same time, projections from the central nucleus of the amygdala to the bed nucleus of the stria terminalis result in activation of the HPA axis. All of these result in preparation of the body for a "freeze, flight, or fight" response and then subsequent negative feedback loop to attenuate this response (31).

Yehuda et al. (25, 26, 32–34) have reported that subjects with PTSD experience a dysregulation of the HPA axis, resulting in hypocortisolemia, but paradoxically high corticotrophin-releasing factor levels in the cerebral spinal fluid (CSF). Additionally, subjects with PTSD may have an exaggerated suppression of cortisol in response to dexamethasone. Recent studies have demonstrated that low cortisol levels at the time of trauma resulted in a greater likelihood of developing PTSD. This, in turn, has prompted research examining the possible therapeutic benefits of hydrocortisone administration soon after the traumatic event (35). Subjects with PTSD appear to have an exaggerated suppression of cortisol in response to dexamethasone. These findings suggest that there is an increased sensitivity of the negative-feedback system of the HPA axis. Yehuda (25, 26, 32) has hypothesized that PTSD is facilitated by a failure to turn off the normal stress response at the time of the trauma, resulting in a cascade of neuroendocrine and neurochemical alterations that lead to the development of PTSD symptoms.

Recently, much attention has been given to hippocampal changes and the development of PTSD. Elevated cortisol levels at the time of trauma have been proposed to result in hippocampal damage that has been found in subjects with PTSD (32, 36, 37). More specifically, a recent study comparing veterans with combat trauma and PTSD vs. age-matched controls without PTSD demonstrates that PTSD is associated with selective volume loss of the CA3/dentate gyrus subfields of the hippocampus (38). This study supports previous findings that chronic stress suppresses hippocampal neurogenesis and dendritic branching. However, findings in a study of twin pairs discordant for trauma exposure suggest that a smaller hippocampus is not the result of trauma, but may be a risk factor for developing PTSD subsequent to a traumatic event (39). Treatments with several medications, including paroxetine, sertraline, and phenytoin, have shown neurogenesis and increased hippocampal volume in subjects with PTSD (40, 41). Other neuroanatomical structures implicated in PTSD are the amygdala and prefrontal cortex. Although there is no evidence for structural changes in the amygdala with PTSD, imaging studies have shown that subjects with PTSD have an amygdala that is both hyperresponsive to reminders of trauma and hypersensitive to threatening cues. The prefrontal cortex appears to modulate stress responsiveness via its inhibitory effect on the amygdala (35).

Corticotropin releasing hormone (CRH) has been found to be higher in the CSF of veterans with PTSD when compared with that of a healthy community sample (42). Abnormalities in other neuroendocrine systems have also been reported. Dysregulation of the hypothalamic-pituitary-7thyroid axis with elevations in levels of tri-iodothyronine (T3) and thyroxine (T4) in subjects with PTSD have been reported (33), although these results are not consistent (43).

In addition to the neuroendocrine abnormalities observed, neurotransmitters such as norepinephrine, serotonin, and glutamate play a role in PTSD (22, 25, 34, 36, 44, 45). Subjects with PTSD have elevated circulating levels of norepinephrine and increased adrenergic receptor reactivity. Yohimbine, a centrally acting α_2-adrenergic antagonist, has been shown to exacerbate anxiety, panic, and PTSD like symptoms in subjects (22, 45, 46). Medications such as selective serotonin reuptake inhibitors (SSRIs) and dual action antidepressants that increase both serotonin and norepinephrine at the synapse have been shown to be effective in the management of some of the symptoms of PTSD (36). The excitatory neurotransmitter glutamate seems to play a role in the pathophysiology of PTSD via its effect on the HPA axis. Pretreatment with a glutamatergic *N*-methyl-D-aspartate (NMDA) antagonist has been shown to decrease stress-responsiveness, as measured by ACTH release, in some studies (47). Neuropeptide Y may also be involved in promoting recovery from PTSD. Combat veterans without PTSD have been shown to have higher plasma levels of NPY than veterans with PTSD (48).

Glutamatergic and GABA systems are integrally involved in the encoding and recovery of memories and appear to have a role in PTSD, especially in the disturbances of memory (36). Norepinephrine and low cortisol as well as hippocampal dysfunction and amygdala activation have also been implicated in the memory problems common in PTSD (36, 45). Animal and human studies have shown that chronic stress results in dendritic atrophy in the hippocampus and medial prefrontal cortex, as well as decreased neurogenesis (38). Although glutamate has been shown to play an important role in memory formation and may, when elevated, facilitate the encoding of traumatic memories, higher than normal levels of glutamate following traumatic experiences can result in hippocampal damage and subsequent memory problems (36). This has prompted research into preventative treatment modalities targeting NMDA receptors. van der Kolk et al., in their study of memory for traumatic experiences, found that such memories are qualitatively different from memories of everyday events (49–51). Traumatic memories typically have a substantial sensorimotor or affective quality with little or no narrative component and occur as nightmares, flashbacks, or intrusions accompanied by increased autonomic activity.

Another neurobiological consideration for the development of PTSD is the role of genetics and neurocircuitry of fear inhibition on a more general level. A recent review article on this subject summarizes findings that suggest that the rostral regions of the anterior cingulate gyrus of the ventromedial prefrontal cortex are associated with the inhibition of fear (52). The exaggerated fear responses seen in PTSD may be due to a weakened inhibitory control of the amygdala by the prefrontal cortex. Despite several studies to date, little remains known about the genetic mechanisms of PTSD (52). One particular protein that has received increasing attention is FKBP5, which regulates the sensitivity of the glucocorticoid receptor that is overly active in PTSD. Data suggest that the interaction of an index trauma with stress-related genes alters amygdala regulation of fear, increasing risk of developing PTSD later in life.

Accumulating evidence suggests that people with PTSD suffer from a global neurobiological dysregulation that primarily involve neuroendocrine, serotonergic, and adrenergic systems. Dysfunction of several brain regions including the hippocampus, amygdala, prefrontal and cingulate cortex, and cerebellum have been implicated in this disorder.

Pharmacotherapy for PTSD

Antidepressant Treatment

Several reviews and current American Psychiatry Association treatment guidelines consider serotonin-reuptake inhibitors as the first line agents in the medication treatment of PTSD due to efficacy and safety (25, 53–62). Double-blind, placebo-controlled studies have found that several SSRIs (fluoxetine (63–66), paroxetine (67–69), and sertraline (70–75)) have efficacy in the treatment of PTSD. However, the effect sizes have been fairly small (0.3–0.5), and, for the most part, the studies were short-term (12 weeks or fewer) (53, 76). SSRIs are also effective in the treatment of some of the common comorbid disorders associated with PTSD, including major depressive disorder, anxiety disorders, and substance abuse disorders (76–78). Sertraline and paroxetine have acquired FDA approval for the treatment of PTSD.

SSRI Antidepressants

Fluoxetine

Fluoxetine was found to be effective in the treatment of PTSD in four double-blind, placebo-controlled studies (63–66). A 5-week double-blind, placebo-controlled trial reported efficacy in total PTSD symptoms and in the numbing and hyperarousal clusters but not in the reexperiencing and avoidant symptoms (63). A subgroup analysis revealed that efficacy for PTSD symptoms was robust for the community sample, but the veteran sample did not show significant differences between fluoxetine and placebo. This study used flexible dosing (20 mg–60 mg/day) with an average dose of 40 mg/day in the fluoxetine group. Depression symptoms also improved in the fluoxetine group. Three fluoxetine treatment-emergent side effects reached significance, headache, diarrhea, and sweating.

In a 12-week double-blind, placebo-controlled study, 53 civilians were randomly assigned to fluoxetine (20 mg–60 mg/day) or placebo (64). This study of primarily female subjects (91%) found that fluoxetine significantly improved PTSD symptoms and overall functioning. A subsequent report of an analysis of PTSD symptoms and the 3 PTSD symptom subscales reported efficacy across all subscales with the strongest response in the symptoms of avoidance and numbing (78).

A double-blind, placebo-controlled trial of fluoxetine was conducted in subjects from several war-torn areas in Europe, Israel, and South Africa (65). The subjects were predominantly male (81%), white (91%), experienced multiple combat-related events (48%) and/or were a survivor of war or witness to wars (47%), and/or witnessed another person's death (33%). Random assignment resulted in 226 subjects being treated with fluoxetine in dosages titrated from 20 mg to 80 mg/day (mean dose, 57 mg) and 75 subjects receiving placebo. In clinician-rated measures, fluoxetine resulted in significant improvement in total PTSD scores, as well as the intrusive and hyperarousal subscales, but not the avoidance and numbing subscale. These findings were statistically significant by week 6 and maintained significance through the 12-week study. In addition, clinician-administered measures of depression found significant improvement in depression symptoms in the fluoxetine treated sample, while the patient-rated measures for both PTSD and depression failed to show a difference between placebo and fluoxetine. Fluoxetine was well tolerated with no treatment-emergent side effects reaching statistical significance; however, the fluoxetine treated group had a slight decrease in erythrocyte count.

A placebo-controlled trial (66) of fluoxetine in 144 predominantly male combat veterans recruited in Bosnia-Herzegovina, Croatia, and Yugoslavia used flexible dosing (20–80 mg/day) in a 12-week acute phase treatment. The acute phase was followed by a 24-week relapse prevention phase of responders, as defined by a 50% reduction in PTSD symptoms, a Clinical Global Impression of Severity (CGI) of ≤2, and the absence of at least one core symptom of PTSD on the Clinician Administered PTSD scale (CAPS). Subjects in this study were less than 7 years posttrauma and showed a significant improvement with fluoxetine treatment (56.4%) when compared with placebo (32.4%). It should be noted that high doses appeared to be effective with mean dose of 65 ± 17.6 mg. The second phase randomized responders to fluoxetine or placebo with continued treatment resulting in overall better functioning, continued symptom reduction, and relapse prevention. These two international studies (65, 66) contradict prior studies of American combat veterans with chronic, severe PTSD who failed to show any benefit from treatment with fluoxetine (63, 79). The differences between these studies of combat veterans were in geography and length of time from combat to treatment, with earlier treatment appearing to have greater efficacy.

Another study by this international research group recruited 411 subjects from 43 sites in the United States. Fixed dosing of fluoxetine (20 mg, 40 mg/day) were compared with placebo (80). The reduction in PTSD as measured by the CAPS revealed improvement in all groups, failing to show a significant difference. The placebo response rate was nearly 37% with the fluoxetine treatment response of 43%.

Paroxetine

Paroxetine has also been found efficacious in the treatment of PTSD. A 12-week double-blind, placebo-controlled trial of 551 subjects with chronic PTSD randomly assigned subjects to a fixed daily dose of 20 or 40 mg paroxetine or placebo (67). Sixty-two percent of the subjects receiving a 40-mg dose of paroxetine and 54% receiving 20-mg had significant global improvement. There was a significant reduction in total PTSD symptoms and across all three symptom subscales. Paroxetine was well tolerated with treatment-emergent side effects of asthenia, diarrhea, abnormal ejaculation, impotence, nausea, and somnolence reaching significance compared to placebo.

A double-blind, placebo-controlled study randomly assigned subjects to flexible dosages (20 mg–50 mg/day; mean dose 27.6 mg) or placebo (68). PTSD symptoms in paroxetine treated subjects were significantly improved at weeks 4, 8, and 12. Subjects in the paroxetine group were significantly improved in overall functioning in occupational, social, and family life. Paroxetine was well tolerated with nausea, dry mouth, asthenia, and abnormal ejaculation, significant treatment-emergent side effects.

A placebo-controlled trial in 52 subjects using a flexible dose design reported significant improvement in the paroxetine group when compared with placebo, showing efficacy in global improvement, reduction in CAPS scores, reduction in dissociation, and improvement in interpersonal problems. A 12-week maintenance phase found continued improvement in the paroxetine group (69). Two open-label studies, in Bosnia (81) and Japan (82), found that paroxetine improved symptoms of PTSD.

Sertraline

Sertraline has been investigated in several double-blind, placebo-controlled trials (70–72, 74, 75, 83, 84). A double-blind, placebo-controlled study of 187 subjects with PTSD using flexible dosing (50 mg–200 mg/day) reported that sertraline resulted in greater improvement in PTSD symptoms and global functioning. Treatment with sertraline resulted in a 53% reduction in total PTSD symptoms (71). Significant efficacy was found in two of three symptoms clusters, avoidance and numbing and increased arousal, but not in the reexperiencing/intrusion cluster. Sertraline was well tolerated with only insomnia reaching significance when compared with placebo.

A second 12-week double-blind, placebo-controlled study in 200 subjects reported that sertraline achieved greater reduction in PTSD symptoms (60 vs. 38% in placebo group) (72). Across the three symptom clusters, reexperiencing/intrusions symptoms were reduced by 50%, avoidance and numbing symptoms by 47%, and increased arousal by 40%. Sertraline treatment resulted in marked improvement in quality of life and functional measures with 58% of subjects within 10% of community norms (74). When compared with placebo, sertraline was reported to have significant side effects of insomnia, diarrhea, nausea, fatigue, and decreased appetite (72). A 24-week open-label continuation phase found 25% of improvements in PTSD symptoms occurred after 12 weeks of treatment (85). In addition, 54% of nonresponders in the initial 12-week study responded with continuation of sertraline treatment (73). The 24-week continuation phase resulted in an additional 20% improvement in quality of life and functioning. A follow-up study enrolled continuation phase responders in a double-blind, placebo-controlled maintenance study for an additional 28 weeks (70). Sertraline was dosed flexibly from 50 mg to 200 mg/day. Continued treatment with sertraline resulted in lower relapse rates (5% compared to the 26% in the placebo group) with significant findings across all three PTSD symptom clusters. Subjects who received placebo were 6.4 times more likely to relapse with significant recurrences of PTSD symptoms and accompanying reductions in quality of life and functioning, although with fewer symptoms and improved quality of life than at initial study entry.

A double-blind, placebo-controlled trial of sertraline assessed efficacy in 395 PTSD sufferers as a result of adult interpersonal trauma, defined as physical or sexual assault, when compared to those with childhood abuse. Flexible dosing of sertraline (50 mg–200 mg/day) showed greater efficacy for both types of trauma when compared with placebo (74).

Two studies did not support efficacy of sertraline, both studies included only combat veterans. One study, conducted 10 years prior to publication, of 169 male Vietnam veterans in a 12-week double-blind, placebo-controlled trial found no difference between sertraline and placebo groups (83). The authors suggest that the negative finding in this and other studies may be due to the chronicity of the veteran cohort, a particularly treatment-refractory population A 10-week placebo-controlled pilot study of 42 Israeli male and female veterans found a nonsignificant improvement in symptoms concluding that larger studies would be needed to determine whether sertraline would have efficacy (84).

Sertraline treatment of cooccurring PTSD and alcohol dependence was reported in two papers of a study of 94 adults (51 men, 43 women) (76, 77). Participants were titrated up to a dose of 150 mg of sertraline and outcomes determined by several standardized PTSD and alcohol use measures. This study included a 1-h cognitive-behavioral therapy (CBT) session that focused only on alcohol use and not on PTSD symptoms. Approximately 50% of patients had significant improvement in PTSD symptoms and in global response (alcohol use and PTSD); the alcohol-only responders were predominantly male (90.9%). Global improvements appeared to be related to improvement in PTSD symptoms, especially the hyper-arousal cluster, positively impacting alcohol consumption (77). However, the efficacy of sertraline in PTSD symptoms in this group was not significant (76). Cluster analysis revealed that sertraline treatment was most effective for alcohol use in subjects with less severe alcohol dependence and early-onset PTSD in contrast to those with more severe alcohol dependence and later onset PTSD. Subjects treated with sertraline had significant decreases in number of drinks/day, number of drinking days, and percent of heavy drinking days when compared with placebo. The authors of this preliminary study suggest that cooccurring PTSD symptoms impact alcohol dependence and treatment of PTSD may be beneficial for patients suffering from both alcohol dependence and PTSD (77).

Citalopam/Escitalopram

Citalopram and escitalopram have not been studied in double-blind, placebo-controlled trials for the treatment of PTSD. One case report (86) and one open label study (87) suggest that citalopram is well tolerated and reduces PTSD symptomatology. An open label study of escitalopram in 25 veterans with PTSD reported decreased PTSD symptoms, especially in avoidance, numbing, and hyper-arousal symptoms (88). Further study is warranted to determine efficacy.

Fluvoxamine

Fluvoxamine has been studied only in open-label trials with all reporting improvement in some or all clusters of PTSD symptoms (89–92). An open-label study of 15 veterans with combat-related PTSD resulted in nearly a 50% drop-out rate due to side effects (92).

SNRI Antidepressants

Venlafaxine

One open-label trial (93) and two randomized-controlled clinical trials (94, 95) support the use of venlafaxine for the treatment of PTSD. A 6-week open-label study randomized 32 Bosnian refugees living in the US to sertraline, paroxetine, or venlafaxine treatment (93). Sertraline was dosed at 50 mg for 14 days and then increased to 100 mg if tolerated while the paroxetine group received a fixed dose of 20 mg. Venlafaxine was initiated at 37.5 mg twice daily for 2 weeks and increased to 75 mg twice daily as tolerated. All three treatment groups reported a significant decline in the number of PTSD symptoms, although all remained sufficiently symptomatic at the end of the study to meet diagnostic criteria for PTSD. In addition, both sertraline and paroxetine, but not venlafaxine, significantly decreased depressive symptoms and increased overall functioning. Sertraline and paroxetine were better tolerated than venlafaxine, which had a high dropout rate. None of the subjects dropped out of sertraline and paroxetine treatment. This study is limited by its design as a brief trial and low dosages.

A 12-week double-blind trial compared the efficacy of extended release venlafaxine (venlafaxine ER) with sertraline and with placebo (94). The 538 subjects in this study received flexible doses of venlafaxine ER (37.5 mg–300 mg/day), sertraline (50 mg–200 mg/day), or placebo. Both medication treatments were significantly effective when compared with placebo and both were well tolerated. This study group conducted a second 6-month double-blind, placebo-controlled trial to assess the efficacy of flexibly dosed venlafaxine ER for the treatment of PTSD (95). Three hundred and twenty-nine subjects were randomly assigned to venlafaxine ER or placebo with 112 in each arm completing the trial. Outcome measures included the CAPS and its subclusters (reexperiencing, avoidance and numbing, hyperarousal), Clinical Global Impression-Severity Illness (CGI-I) scale, Hamilton Rating Scale for depression, and Global Assessment of Functioning mean scores. Venlafaxine ER showed statistically significant improvement when compared with placebo in total CAPS scores and two subclusters, reexperiencing, and avoidance and numbing. All other assessments found venlafaxine ER with significantly greater efficacy than placebo. In addition, the medication group showed greater improvement in resilience and stress vulnerability as well as in measure of quality of life and functionality. Mean dosage was high with the average daily dose of 181.7 mg/day. The most common adverse events were headache, nausea, dizziness, dry mouth, constipation, fatigue, insomnia, and increased sweating.

Duloxetine

A naturalistic 8-week study of 20 predominately Caucasian (95%), Vietnam veterans (80%) with chronic, combat-related treatment resistant PTSD and comorbid major depressive disorder reported that duloxetine reduced symptoms of PTSD and comorbid major depression (96). Following a 6-day washout period, subjects were started on 30 mg of duloxetine, increased up to 120 mg daily in a flexible dosing regimen (average ~105 mg). PTSD Checklist scores, Hamilton Anxiety Scale, Montgomery Åsberg Depression Rating Scale, and CGI-I improved significantly from baseline. The most common side effects were increased dream activity without nightmares, sleep disturbance, and increased fatigability. The results of this small open label study of combat-related PTSD limit conclusions about efficacy. The risk of hepatic dysfunction and current limited research show no advantage of duloxetine over treatment with an SSRI or venlafaxine.

Novel Antidepressants

Nefazadone

Nefazadone, an SSRI and 5-HT_2 antagonist, may have efficacy for the treatment of PTSD. A small 12-week placebo-controlled trial found that subjects treated with nefazadone had significant decreases in the overall CAPS scores; however, subcluster analysis could not be determined due to the sample size. Depression and dissociative symptoms improved significantly with medication compared to placebo (97). A second double-blind 12-week study compared nefazadone with sertraline, using the CAPS, CAPS subscales, scales for depression and anxiety, disability, sleep quality, and CGI-I (98). No significant differences were found between nefazadone and sertraline efficacies for PTSD and its comorbid depression and anxiety. Both of these controlled studies have small sample sizes, limiting conclusions. Given the black box warning of the risk hepatic failure and the current level of research data, nefazadone provides no significant advantage when compared with the SSRI antidepressants.

Trazadone

Trazadone is an SSRI and 5-HT_2 antagonist, and is commonly used as a hypnotic as it is highly sedating. One open-label study of trazodone as monotherapy found only mild effectiveness for PTSD symptoms (99). Trazadone is often used in combination with SSRIs as a hypnotic with a dosage range of 25–500 mg at bedtime.

Mirtazapine

A small 8-week double-blind, placebo-controlled pilot study found mirtazapine, in dosages up to 45 mg/day, reduced symptoms of PTSD (100). Primary outcome measures including the Short Posttraumatic Stress Disorder Rating Scale and the Global Improvement Item determined that mirtazapine was more effective than placebo (65 vs. 20%). Secondary outcome measures revealed effectiveness for anxiety.

An 8-week open-label pilot study of mirtazapine was conducted in Korea and followed by a 24-week open continuation phase with 12 of 15 subjects phase one completer enrolled (101). Twice as many subjects had decreased PTSD symptoms as measured by the short rating interview at week 24 when compared with that of week 8. There was no significant statistical difference over time in measures of depression or other measures of PTSD, including a more detailed interview assessment. A second open-label, 12-week trial of 13 war veterans with PTSD reported statistically significant improvement of PTSD symptoms (102). Subjects were in active treatment and their treating psychiatrist had determined that mirtazapine was clinically indicated for non-PTSD symptoms. Mirtazapine was started at 15 mg/day and titrated up to 45 mg/day using a flexible dosing regimen; all concurrent psychotropics were allowed except for other antidepressants. The investigators found a statistically significant improvement in the Mississippi Scale for Combat-Related PTSD with improvements in the total CAPS score and Hospital Anxiety and Depression Scale. At present, the small sample sizes and study designs limit conclusions about the use of mirtazapine in the treatment of PTSD.

Buproprion

Buproprion was reported to reduce hyperarousal symptoms of PTSD in one small open-label study (103). Buproprion was well tolerated but appeared to be most helpful to comorbid symptoms of depression than for PTSD. A placebo-controlled trial of 30 subjects with PTSD found no differences between groups in treating symptoms of PTSD (104).

Monoamine Oxidase Inhibitors (MOA-Is)

Phenelzine, an irreversible monoamine oxidase inhibitor (MAO-I), has been found to be effective in the treatment of PTSD in two randomized studies (105, 106). A review of the MAO-I literature noted that 82% of subjects with PTSD obtained moderate to good improvement with the greatest symptom reductions in reexperiencing and insomnia (107). Avoidant/numbing and hyperarousal symptoms as well as symptoms of depression and anxiety did not improve. MAO-I medications raised clinician concern for patients who will not comply with dietary restrictions, which may result in a hypertensive crisis following ingestion of foods or beverages high in tyramine. Similarly, for substance abusing patients, the risk of a serotonin syndrome with the use of some medications (meperidine), prescribed or illicit, is of concern. These concerns limit the extent to which MAO-I's are used. However, meclobemide, a reversible MAO-A inhibitor, does not share these problems and has been shown in an open-label study to reduce both reexperiencing and avoidant

PTSD symptoms (108). There is conflicting evidence for the effectiveness of brofaromine, a reversible MAO-I, in the treatment of PTSD. Brofaromine may provide some benefit for less severe symptoms of PTSD (109). A large, multicentered double-blind, placebo-controlled trial reported no efficacy of brofaromine (110). Moclobemide and brofaromine are unavailable in the United States.

Tricyclic and Tetracyclic Antidepressants

Randomized clinical trials found that imipramine (105) and amitriptyline (111), but not despiramine (112), were effective for the treatment of PTSD. An analysis of 15 case reports and both open-label and randomized clinical trials found that 45% of subjects treated with tricyclic and tetracyclic antidepressants (TCAs) reported improvement in PTSD symptoms (107). These finding were less robust than the comparison of MOA-Is. Overall, the TCAs were more effective for reexperiencing symptoms than the avoidant/numbing or hyperarousal symptoms. The side effects of TCAs, due to blockade of muscarinic cholinergic receptors (dry mouth, constipation, urinary retention, mydraisis), blockade of histamine H_1 (sedation, weight gain), and α_1 receptor blockade (orthostatic hypotension), are not well tolerated by many patients with PTSD. Given their side effect profile and efficacy status, TCAs hold no advantage over SSRIs or MAO-I's. However, the efficacy may not be as negative as is suggested by these studies, which were performed primarily in combat veterans with PTSD, because combat veterans did not respond as well as community subjects in some PTSD treatment studies with SSRI (63, 79, 83, 84). TCAs may have a role in the patient who is refractory or unable to tolerate SSRIs or MAO-I's. In general, the tertiary amine TCAs, which have more serotonergic effects, have shown greater efficacy in the treatment of PTSD than the secondary amine TCAs, which have both serotonergic and norepinephrine effects.

Summary of Antidepressant Treatment of PTSD

SSRIs are the first line treatment for PTSD, having the most robust and replicated findings of efficacy for PTSD (see Table 3). In general, SSRIs are well tolerated. Treatment studies of fluoxetine, sertraline, and paroxetine indicate that all are effective in the treatment of PTSD. Other SSRIs have been studied only in small, open-label studies but given their mechanism of action, should have efficacy and may be selected if better tolerated by the patient. SSRIs have several advantages in the treatment of PTSD including efficacy in the treatment of disorders that may be comorbid with PTSD including major depressive disorder and other anxiety disorders (generalized anxiety disorder, social phobia, and panic disorder). In addition, some early studies suggest that SSRIs may be helpful in the treatment of comorbid alcohol disorders. If an SSRI is not effective, a change within class to another SSRI or to venlafaxine, an SNRI is warranted. Venlafaxine is well tolerated and effective for the treatment of depression and anxiety. Current data about duloxetine for PTSD

Table 3 Antidepressant medications in treatment of PTSD

Treatment choice	Type and strength of evidence
First-line treatment: SSRI	
[a]Sertraline 50–200 mg	RCT +++
[a]Paroxetine 10–60 mg	RCT +++
Fluoxetine 20–80 mg	RCT +++
Second-line treatment: SNRI	
Venlafaxine XR 37.5–300 mg	RCT ++
Third-line treatment	
Mitrazpine 15–45 mg	RCT +
Imipramine 150–300 mg	RCT +

Strength +++ (strong); ++ (moderate); + (weak)
[a]Has FDA approval

treatment is insufficient. MAO-I's and tertiary TCAs may have some role in treating nonresponders or patients intolerant of SSRIs or SNRIs. Novel antidepressants including mirtazapine, buproprion, nefazadone, and trazadone have little data to date to support their use for the treatment of PTSD. Trazadone may have a role as a sedative-hypnotic to treat sleep disorders commonly associated with PTSD. Given the concerns of serious hepatotoxicity with nefazadone, there is no advantage in using this medication.

The evidence to date indicates that while antidepressant medications, in particular the SSRIs, decrease the severity of PTSD symptoms, roughly one third will respond early, one third will respond to a longer trial, and one third will receive little benefit. In addition, discontinuation of medication treatment is likely to result in relapse.

Nonantidepressant Somatic Therapies

Anxiolytics/Hypnotics

Sleep disturbances are common in people with PTSD, including initial insomnia, frequent awakenings, nightmares, and terminal insomnia. As such, treatment of these sleep problems is essential. Some patients will respond to antidepressant treatment, while others will continue with sleep disturbance and anxiety. The role of benzodiazepines in treatment of persisting anxiety and/or sleep disturbances in PTSD continues to be debated. Unfortunately, these data are extremely limited and do not provide clinicians with sufficient information to make evidenced-based decisions about use of sedative/hypnotics. A small randomized, controlled trial of alprazolam in ten subjects had no effect on PTSD symptoms (113). Short-term treatment with temazepam in a randomized, controlled trial with 22 subjects following an acute trauma had no significant impact on PTSD symptoms (114). A single blind study of clonazepam as a PTSD in six subjects with combat-related PTSD reported improvement in initial insomnia, an increase in length of time asleep, and early awakening but reported no benefit for nightmares or frequent awakenings (115). These few open-label studies of benzodiazepines have a subject size that is too small to be meaningful, yet appear to form the basis recommending against the use of benzodiazepines as an adjunctive treatment.

PTSD treatment guidelines vary in their recommendations regarding adjunctive benzodiazepines in the treatment of PTSD ranging from guarded support (e.g., (54)) to no support (e.g., (55)). However, clinical practice appears to suggest that this is in sharp contrast to clinical practice (116). The question of the disparity of clinical practice and treatment recommendations indicates that further study of benzodiazepines is warranted. In addition, nearly all reviews advocate caution based on the comorbidity with substance use disorders, although there is no indication that the vast majority of patients prescribed adjunctive benzodiazepines for treatment of PTSD misused these prescribed medications.

For patients with persisting anxiety or sleep disturbance in the early aftermath of a traumatic event who have not benefited from acute psychological interventions, judicious short-term use of a benzodiazepine may calm the patient sufficiently to allow engagement in psychological interventions. In addition, patients with chronic sleep disturbance or excessive persisting daytime anxiety who have not benefited from other interventions (e.g., sleep hygiene, cognitive-behavioral treatment, or anxiety management treatment) may respond to a long acting benzodiazepine such as clonazepam. However, the presence of a current comorbid substance use disorder must be assessed and may preclude use of benzodiazepine treatment. In general, the shortest possible course of benzodiazepines as an adjunctive and not as monotherapy for PSTD is recommended (117). Trazadone may be a preferred alternative for sleep.

Buspirone in a small open-label trial of eight subjects with PTSD found some improvement in symptoms of PTSD (118), but the sample size and open label design do not warrant its recommendation for the treatment of PTSD.

Mood Stabilizers

The theoretical premise for the use of anticonvulsants is based upon the kindling theory, which suggests that symptoms of PTSD begin with an irritable limbic focus that expands to recruit larger areas of the brain, resulting in more symptoms (36). The anticonvulsants appear to raise the neuronal threshold for arousal by stimulating GABA receptors and increasing chloride conductance. Thus, it was hypothesized that intrusive thoughts and hyperarousal symptoms would diminish.

Older Agents

Two randomized, placebo-controlled trials of valproic acid as monotherapy did not show efficacy in PTSD (119, 120). An 8-week randomized, placebo-controlled trial in 82 veterans found no significant changes between divalproex and placebo on

CAPS scores (total and subscales). In addition, six other standardized scores evaluating anxiety, depression, or global improvement showed no difference (119). A recent small randomized, placebo-controlled trial of divalproex reported no significant differences between groups on the CAPS total score; however, the placebo group had a significant decrease in avoidance/numbing scores as well as a greater global improvement (120). Two open-label studies of carbamazepine in veterans with complex PTSD, anger, substance abuse, and Axis II disorders reported improvements in impulse control (121, 122). An open-label study of phenytoin in nine adult male subjects with PTSD found a reduction in total PTSD symptoms and all three symptom clusters as measured by the CAPS (123). There were no improvements in depression or anxiety symptoms.

These older anticonvulsants may cause a range of side effects including sedation, dizziness, nausea, and vomiting. However, two potentially serious adverse reactions associated with carbamazepine treatment, blood dyscrasia (aplastic anemia and agranulocytosis), and hepatitis require monitoring during treatment. Carbamazepine has a black box warning for the blood dyscrasia. Valproic acid has been found to elevate cholesterol and carries black box warnings for hepatotoxicity, pancreatitis, and is a Class D teratogen, thus contraindicated during pregnancy. Phenytoin and carbamazepine should also be used with caution during pregnancy.

Lithium has been investigated in two open-label trials in combat veterans with both studies reporting improvements in emotional control and hyperarousal symptoms (124, 125). Its use in the treatment of PTSD remains unclear.

Newer Agents

Several newer anticonvulsant medications have been investigated for the treatment of PTSD. A retrospective, open-label study of gabapentin reported fewer sleep disturbances and decreased frequency of nightmares (126). A small, 12-week double-blind study of lamotrigine found improvement in reexperiencing and avoidance/numbing symptoms (127). Two small, randomized, controlled trials of topiramate suggest that it may provide mild relief from PTSD as monotherapy or as an adjunct. A small 12-week randomized, controlled trial of topiramate monotherapy in 19 subjects compared with 19 subjects treated with placebo reported improvements in only reexperiencing symptoms but not in total CAPS score, Davidson Trauma Scale, or CGI (128). A small 7-week randomized, controlled trial of adjunctive topiramate compared with adjunctive placebo found no significant benefit across a number of measures (CAPS, CGI-S, Beck Depression Inventory, and Traumatic Dissociation Scale) and showed high treatment arm drop-out rate of 55% compared to 25% in the placebo arm (129). A retrospective review of 23 patients with partial or nonresponse to antidepressant therapy were treated with adjunctive levetiracetam for 9.7 ± 3.7 weeks with six subjects moving into in full remission and 13 with some improvement (130). A 12-week multicenter double-blind study of 232 subjects found no efficacy of tiagabine in the treatment of PTSD across many standardized measures including the CAPS, CGI-I, and the Montgomery-Åsberg Depression Rating Scale (131). This is the only study of the mood stabilizing class that was a large double-blind trial with sufficient power to assess efficacy, raising questions of the efficacy in the treatment of PTSD of drugs that target the GABA system.

All of these newer agents share side effects of somnolence, fatigue, dizziness, and ataxia, but lamotrigine has been associated with serious rashes that may have a fatal or disfiguring outcome (Stevens–Johnson syndrome). The development of a rash while taking lamotrigine warrants immediate discontinuation, although this does not ensure that Stevens–Johnson syndrome will be averted as noted in the black box warning. The current data for this class of medications is sufficiently weak or negative such that its use is not warranted. Further data are needed to determine whether this group of medications holds any advantage as an adjunctive or monotherapy for PTSD.

Antipsychotics

As with several other psychopharmacologic interventions in current clinical use for treating symptoms of PTSD, there are few studies that have investigated the use of either typical or atypical neuroleptics. A data analysis from two large outcome studies examined the role of neuroleptics in PTSD, finding that patients with more severe PTSD symptoms (particularly intrusive symptoms) were commonly treated with a neuroleptic medication. However, treatment outcomes were not different when compared with that of neuroleptic-free patients (132). Several open and randomized, controlled trials indicate that atypical antipsychotic medications may have a role in treating PTSD for targeted symptoms (133–152). The quality and quantity of the currently available randomized-controlled studies of atypical antipsychotics for the treatment of PTSD are limited with the best evidence for comorbid psychosis. Given the potential for metabolic syndrome with the atypical antipsychotic class and tardive dyskinesia, these medications should be used with caution and for the shortest time possible.

Risperidone

A 6-week open-label trial of risperidone in 26 male veterans with psychosis and combat-related PTSD found risperidone effective in reducing psychotic symptoms as well as PTSD symptoms (133). A 12-week open-label study found that adding risperidone to SSRI treatment in 17 combat veterans with chronic PTSD had no effect on objective measures of nightmares or sleep; however, patient logs at 6 weeks indicated a reduction in trauma-related dreams and frequency of awakenings (134). A 5-week prospective, randomized, placebo-controlled study of adjunctive risperidone in 37 combat veterans with PTSD and comorbid psychotic symptoms reported a modest reduction in the Positive and Negative Syndrome Scale (PANSS) in the treatment arm, but had no effect for PTSD with total CAPS scores showing no difference when compared with that of placebo (135). A 6-week double-blind, placebo-controlled study of 15 combat veterans with high arousal symptoms of PTSD found risperidone reduced irritability, aggression, and intrusive thoughts (136). A small 16-week double-blind, placebo-controlled, parallel group design was used to assess the response to adjunctive risperidone vs. placebo for combat-related PTSD (137). Outcomes were measured using CAPS, the Hamilton scales for anxiety and for depression, and the Positive subscale of the Positive and Negative Syndrome Scale (PANSS-P). Subjects treated with risperidone showed significant improvement in PTSD, anxiety, and the PANSS-P but not depression. The only CAPS subscale that showed significant improvement compared to placebo was the hyperarousal scale.

Two small studies assessed the efficacy of risperidone in women with PTSD. Twenty-one women with PTSD related to childhood abuse were randomized to risperidone, flexibly dosed from 0.5 mg to 8 mg/day, or to placebo (138). The medication group had a significant reduction in PTSD with the greatest effects seen in the reexperiencing and hyperarousal subscales. A study randomized 20 women with PTSD due to sexual assault or domestic violence to risperidone or placebo after washout of other medications (139). Scores for PTSD, anxiety, and depression in the risperidone group showed a significant difference from baseline at week 6 and continued through the 11-week study, while the placebo group showed no difference in any symptoms. A study of civilians with PTSD assessed the efficacy of adjunctive risperidone to sertraline treatment (140). The initial phase treated 34 subjects with those showing less than a 70% reduction in CAPS ($n=25$) randomized to risperidone or placebo. All subjects showed improvement on sertraline. Of the 20 completers of phase two, there were no significant differences between the risperidone and control group.

Quetiapine

Two open-label and one retrospective studies of adjunctive treatment with quetiapine reported improvement in PTSD symptoms (141–143). A 6-week open trial of quetiapine in 18 combat veterans reported significantly improved CAPS scores with good tolerability (141). An 8-week open-label study of eight men and seven women with PTSD reported that the addition of quetiapine to existing antidepressant treatment resulted in a 42% improvement in PTSD with efficacy across all three symptoms clusters and decreased levels of disability and impairment (142). A retrospective chart review of veterans with treatment-resistant combat-related PTSD showed improvement in all three symptom clusters of PTSD, but most strongly in the hyperarousal cluster (143).

Olanzapine

In an 8-week open trial of combat veterans, olanzapine improved PTSD, depression, and anxiety (144). However, the drop-out rate was higher than in other trials of atypical antipsychotics. A 10-week double-blind, placebo-controlled study of olanzapine did not show a significant difference at the end of 10 weeks of treatment (145). This finding is in contrast to a 12-week double-blind, placebo-controlled study of adjunctive olanzapine for 19 Vietnam veterans whose PTSD symptoms were minimally treated by an SSRI (146). This study concluded that adjunctive olanzapine significantly improved symptoms of PTSD, sleep disturbances, and depression when compared with placebo. In addition, the improvement in PTSD was correlated with improvements in sleep with the authors attributing improvements in PTSD to improved sleep. Despite these improvements, global functioning did not significantly improve in the medication group compared to placebo. In addition, the mean weight gain was 13 pounds, thus raising concerns about metabolic syndrome associated with atypical antipsychotics.

Aripiprazole

In a 12-week prospective study of aripiprazole with a mean daily dose 12.95 mg as a monotherapy for PTSD, 8 of 22 subjects dropped out due to distressing side effects. Using missing data analysis, the authors reported a significant 20% decrease in CAPS (147). A 16-week, open-label study of 32 subjects with PTSD, using an intention-to-treat analysis, found aripiprazole improved endpoint CAPS scores (from 82.7±23.1 to 51.4±31.4) as well scores on the Beck Anxiety Inventory, Social Adjustment Scale, Medical Outcome Study Short Form, and Beck Depression Inventory (148). However, it should be noted that the standard deviation in CAPS scores is sufficiently high as to leave open the question of effectiveness for PTSD. In a recent open-label, flexible-dose trial of adjunctive aripiprazole, 53% of the 17 subjects responded to aripiprazole with a 20% reduction in total CAPS score (149). With an average aripiprazole dose of 13.06 mg at the end of 12 weeks, total CAPS scores subscales of assessing reexperiencing and avoidance/numbing symptoms, and PANSS scores were significantly improved. The preliminary results on the effectiveness of aripiprazole merit further study, given the improved cardiometabolic profile of aripiprazole over other atypical antipsychotics.

Other Antipsychotics

A 6-week open-label trial of both typical (fluphenazine) and atypical (olanzapine, risperidone, or quetiapine) antipsychotics as monotherapy for inpatient treatment-refractory combat veterans reported improvement in both psychotic symptoms and

PTSD symptoms in all treatment groups (150). A metaanalysis of olanzapine and risperidone included 192 subjects (seven studies) randomized to medication or placebo with improvement in PTSD symptoms and in particular the symptom of intrusions (151). Ziprasidone has only been described in case studies of male combat veterans (152).

Other Treatments

Various classes of medications with sympatholytic effects (α_2 adrenoreceptor agonists, α_1 adrenoreceptor antagonists, β-adrenoreceptor antagonists), NMDA, GABA, and other specific receptor agonist or antagonists have been investigated for the management of targeted symptom clusters in PTSD or prevention of PTSD.

α_2 Adrenoreceptor Agonists

Clonidine has been reported in open label studies in adults (153, 154) and children (155, 156) to reduce PTSD symptoms including reexperiencing and hyperarousal symptoms. Harmon and Riggs (155) caution the use of clonidine in children noting cardiac concerns. Clonidine is sedating, and this side effect may be helpful for managing sleep disturbances. Clonidine is used to treat menopausal symptoms, particularly night sweats, and thus may be an excellent choice for the symptomatically menopausal women with PTSD. An 8-week, double-blind study of guanfacine, an α_2 agonist, in 63 Vietnam veterans, failed to show any difference compared to placebo for PTSD, sleep, or mood (157).

α_1 Adrenoreceptor Antagonists

Prazosin improved sleep quality and decreased nightmares in an initial placebo-controlled study of ten male Vietnam veterans (158) and in a subsequent 8-week, placebo-controlled trial of 34 male Vietnam veterans) (159).There was no between-group differences in CAPS scores in the second study. A retrospective chart review of 23 refugees with PTSD treated with prazosin reported significant improvement in total CAPS scores and CGI-C scores 8 weeks after treatment initiation (160). A small open study of prazosin for nightmares and non-nightmare distressed awakenings reported decreases in sleep difficulty and significant improvements in both trauma-related nightmares as well as non-nightmare distressed awakenings (161). A 12-week, open study of 12 noncombat males and females with PTSD found the α_1-antagonist doxazosin improved CAPS scores, including items related to sleep and distressing dreams, as well as MADRS and CGI scores (162).

Various Antagonists/Agonists

Two placebo-controlled trials of cyproheptadine, a histamine 1 (H_1) and serotonin 2 (5-HT_2) receptor antagonist, reported no improvement in sleep or nightmares (163, 164) with one group reporting an exacerbation of sleep disturbance (163). Baclofen, a GABA-B receptor agonist, was studied for PTSD in an open label study of 14 male veterans with chronic PTSD (165). Following an 8-week trial with doses titrated to a maximum of 80 mg of the 11 completers, the mean CAPS scores were reduced, although the mean score remained about the threshold for PTSD. Glutamatergic neurotransmission dysfunction has been postulated as a factor leading to PTSD with the suggestion that enhanced transmission at the NMDA subtype of glutamate receptors might reduce PTSD symptoms. D-cycloserine, a partial agonist at the glycine regulatory site on the NMDA receptor, was studied double-blind, placebo-controlled, cross-over trial using a daily dose of 50 mg (166). Both D-cycloserine and placebo improved symptoms of numbing and avoidance as well as anxiety.

Prevention Medication

Nonselective β-adrenoreceptor antagonists have been explored for PTSD prevention following trauma. Propranolol, a β-blocker, has been investigated in two double-blind, placebo-controlled pilot studies (167, 168) and one retrospective study (169). One pilot study investigated if propranolol might have a role in prevention of PTSD (167). Of 31 completers, 11 were treated with propranolol for 10 days following the index event with initiation of treatment within the first 6 h. At the 1 month and 3 month follow-up assessments, there was no significant difference in PTSD scores. The propranolol group exhibited less physiological arousal to script-driven imagery at the 3-month follow-up. A study using a similar design found that of 11 subjects with an elevated heart rate who accepted 40 mg of propranolol three times a day for 7 days compared to eight similar subjects who refused treatment had lower levels of PTSD symptoms at 2 months, but did not show a significant reduction in having PTSD (168). A retrospective study of Operation Iraqi Freedom/ Operation Enduring Freedom soldiers who sustained burn injuries compared 31 patients who had received propranolol as part of their burn treatment with 34 matched control burn patients (169). There was no difference in rates of PTSD in those soldiers receiving propranolol when compared with those with no propranolol. A recent retrospective chart review of a 363 pediatric burn cohort who had been in a prior randomized, placebo-controlled trial assessed propranolol administration for ASD, reporting no between-group differences (170). A double-blind, randomized controlled trial started within the first 48 h following an injury requiring admission to a surgical trauma unit compared 14 days of propranolol or gabapentin to placebo as a prevention for PTSD. No significant benefit of propranolol or gabapentin was found at 1, 4, and 8 months on outcome measures of symptoms of depression and PTSD (171).

The adrenergic medications are commonly used in the treatment of hypertension and may result in hypotension in normotensive persons. In addition, propranolol is contraindicated in persons with asthma and chronic obstructive pulmonary disease, should be used with caution in patients with type 2 diabetes mellitus, as it can mask the signs of hypoglycemia, and has been reported to induce or exacerbate major depressive episodes. These data to-date do not support the theoretical construct of preventing an amygdala-based conditioned response as a means of preventing PTSD or of enhanced transmission at the NMDA receptor. More research is needed to determine whether any medication might interrupt the neurobiological cascade that follows trauma and leads to PTSD.

Repetitive Transcranial Magnetic Stimulation

Repetitive transcranial magnetic stimulation (rTMS) has been studied in a double-blind, placebo-controlled trial of 30 civilian subjects, randomized to right or left dorsolateral prefrontal cortex stimulation or to sham. Subjects received high frequency (20 Hz) rTMS administered 10 times over the course of 2 weeks. Both left and right rTMS improved subject scores on the PTSD Checklist and Treatment Outcome PTSD Scale as early as day 5 with sustained improvements at 3 months. Right rTMS had a greater effect on the core symptoms of PTSD, Hamilton Anxiety Rating Scale, and Controlled Oral Word Association Test. Left rTMS improved Hamilton Depression Rating Scale scores (172).

Psychosocial Treatments

In addition to pharmacotherapy, psychosocial treatments of PTSD are indicated. According to published treatment guidelines for PTSD (53, 54, 60, 62), both exposure-based therapies and pharmacotherapy are efficacious for the treatment of PTSD. Among the exposure-based therapies, CBT is given the highest rating with eye movement desensitization and reprocessing (EMDR) an alternative treatment option. A recent study investigated the effect of augmenting sertraline treatment for chronic PTSD with prolonged exposure (173). Following 10 weeks of treatment with sertraline, dosed from 25 to 200 mg/day as tolerated, 31 subjects were randomized to sertraline plus ten sessions of prolonged exposure therapy and 34 to sertraline alone. As in other studies of sertraline, treatment response was seen in PTSD, depression, and anxiety symptoms. Treatment with sertraline alone for five additional weeks resulted in no further improvement, whereas the addition of prolonged exposure resulted in improvements in PTSD but not depression or anxiety. Further analysis revealed that this augmentation effect was found only in medication partial responders but not in subjects who had excellent response to medication. In addition, medication partial responders who had an additional response to prolonged exposure suffered more severe PTSD symptoms at the end of 15 weeks of treatment than those who were excellent medication responders. The authors argue for further study of combined psychopharmacology and exposure-based treatments to determine whether single treatment or combined treatment offers the best clinical practice for the treatment of this chronic disorder.

References

1. American Psychiatric Association. Diagnostic and statistical manual of mental disorders, 4th edition: DSM-IV. Washington: American Psychiatric Association; 1994:427–432.
2. Brewin CR, Andrews B, Rose S, Kirk M. Acute stress disorder and posttraumatic stress disorder in victims of violent crime. Am J Psychiatry 1999;156:360–366.
3. Harvey AG, Bryant RA. Two-year prospective evaluation of the relationship between acute stress disorder and posttraumatic stress disorder following mild traumatic brain injury. Am J Psychiatry 2000;157:626–628.
4. Brewin CR, Andrews B, Rose S. Diagnostic overlap between acute stress disorder and PTSD in victims of violent crime. Am J Psychiatry 2003;160:783–785.
5. Cardeña E, Spiegel D. Dissociative reactions to the San Francisco Bay Area earthquake of 1989. Am J Psychiatry 1993;150:474–478.
6. Kooppman C, Classen C, Spiegel D. Predictors of posttraumatic stress symptoms among survivors of the Oakland/Berkeley, California, Firestorm. Am J Psychiatry 1994;151:888–894.
7. Osterman JE, Hopper J, Heran WJ, Keane TM, van der Kolk BA. Awareness under anesthesia and the development of posttraumatic stress disorder. Gen Hosp Psychiatry 2001;23:198–204.
8. Herman JL. Complex PTSD: A syndrome in survivors of prolonged and repeated trauma. J Trauma Stress 1992;5:377–391.
9. van der Kolk BA, Roth S, Pelcovitz D. Complex PTSD: Results of the PTSD field trials for DSM IV. Washington DC. American Psychiatric Association; 1993.
10. De Jong JTVM, Komproe IH, Spinazzola J, van der Kolk B, van Ommeren M. DESNOS in four post conflict settings: Cross-cultural construct equivalence. J Traumatic Stress 2005;18:13–23.
11. Kessler RC, Sonnega A, Bromet E, Hughes M, Nelson CB. Posttraumatic stress disorder in the National Comorbidity Survey. Arch Gen Psychiatry 1995;52:1048–1060.
12. Keane TM, Kaloupek DG. Comorbid psychiatric disorders in PTSD: Implications for research. Ann N Y Acad Sci 1997;821:24–34.
13. Brady KT, Killeen TK, Brewerton T, Lucerini S. Comorbidity of psychiatric disorders and posttraumatic stress disorder. J Clin Psychiatry 2000;61(Suppl 7):22–32.
14. Davidson JRT, Connor KM. Family studies of PTSD: A review, in risk factors in posttraumatic stress disorder. Washington: American Psychiatric Press; 1999:79–91.
15. Besinger BA, Garland AF, Litrownik AJ, Landsverk JA. Caregiver substance abuse among maltreated children placed in out-of-home care. Child Welfare 1999;78:221–239.
16. Chaffin M, Kelleher K, Hollenberg J. Onset of physical abuse and neglect: Psychiatric, substance abuse, and social risk factors from prospective community data. Child Abuse Negl 1996;20:191–203.
17. Cougle JR, Timpano KR, Sachs-Ericsson N, Keough ME, Riccardi CJ. Examining the unique relationships between anxiety disorders and childhood physical and sexual abuse in the National Comorbidity Survey-Replication. Psychiatry Res 2010;177:150–155. Epub 2010 Apr 9.
18. Cougle JR, Resnick H, Kilpatrick DG. PTSD, depression, and their comorbidity in relation to suicidality: Cross-sectional and prospective analyses of a national probability sample of women. Depress Anxiety. 2009;26:1151–1157.

19. LeDoux JE. Emotion circuits in the brain. Ann Rev Neurosci 2000;23:155–158.
20. Armony JL, LeDoux JE. How the brain processes emotional information. Ann N Y Acad Sci 1997;821:259–270.
21. Charney DS, Deutch AY, Krystal JH, Southwick SM, Davis M. Psychobiologic mechanisms of posttraumatic stress disorder. Arch Gen Psychiatry 1993;50:294–305.
22. Garakani A, Mathew SJ, Charney DS. Neurobiology of anxiety disorders and implications for treatment. Mt Sinai J Med 2006;73:941–949.
23. Southwick SM, Krystal JH, Morgan AC, Johnson D, Nagy L, Nicolaou A, Heninger GR, Charney DS. Abnormal noradrenergic function in post traumatic stress disorder. Arch Gen Psychiatry 1993;50:266–274.
24. Keane TM, Fairbank JA, Caddell JM, Zimmering RT. Implosive (flooding) therapy reduces symptoms of PTSD in Vietnam combat veterans. Behav Ther 1989;20:245–260.
25. Yehuda R. Post-traumatic stress disorder. N Engl J Med 2002;364:108–114.
26. Yehuda R. Sensitization of the hypothalamic-pituitary-adrenal axis in posttraumatic stress disorder. Ann N Y Acad Sci 1997;821:57–75.
27. Bremner JD, Vythilingam M, Vermetten E, Southwick SM, McGlashan T, Nazeer A, Khan S, Vaccarino LV, Soufer R, Garg PK, Ng CK, Staib LH, Duncan JS, Charney DS. MRI and PET study of deficits in hippocampal structure and function in women with childhood sexual abuse and posttraumatic stress disorder. Am J Psychiatry 2003;160:924–932.
28. Lanius RA, Bluhm R, Lanius U, Pain C. A review of neuroimaging studies in PTSD: Heterogeneity of response to symptom provocation. J Psychiatr Res 2006;40:709–729.
29. Lieberzon I, Taylor SF, Amdur R, et al. Brain activation in PTSD in response to trauma-related stimuli. Bio Psychiatry 1999;45:817–826.
30. Shin LM, McNally RJ, Kosslyn SM, et al. Regional cerebral blood flow during script-driven imagery in childhood sexual abuse-related PTSD: A PET investigation. Am J Psychiatry 1999;56:575–584.
31. LeDoux JE, Iwata J, Cicchetti P, Reis DJ. Different projections of the central amygdaloid nucleus mediate autonomic and behavioral correlates of conditioned fear. J Neurosci 1988;8:2517–2529.
32. Yehuda R. Biology of posttraumatic stress disorder. J Clin Psychiatry 2000;61(Suppl 7): 14–21.
33. de Kloet CS, Vermetten E, Geuze E, Kavelaar A, Heijnen CJ, Westenberg HGM. Assessment of HPA-axis function in posttraumatic stress disorder: Pharmacological and non-pharmacological challenge tests, a review. J Psychiatr Res 2006;40:550–567.
34. Newport DJ, Nemeroff CB. Neurobiology of posttraumatic stress disorder. Curr Opin Neurobiol 2000;10:211–218.
35. Heim C, Nemeroff CB. Neurobiology of posttraumatic stress disorder. CNS Spectr 2009;14 (1 Suppl 1):13–24.
36. Hageman I, Andersen HS, Jorgensen MB. Post traumatic stress disorder: A review of psychobiology and pharmacotherapy. Acta Psychiatr Scand 2001;104:411–422.
37. McEwen BS. Effects of adverse experiences for brain structure and function. Biol Psychiatry 2000;48:721–731.
38. Wang Z, Neylan T. Magnetic resonance imaging of hippocampal subfields in posttraumatic stress disorder. Arch Gen Psych 2010;67:296–303.
39. Gilbertson MW, Shenton ME, Ciszewski A, Kasai K, Lasko NB, Orr SP, Pitman RK. Smaller hippocampal volume predicts pathologic vulnerability to psychological trauma. Nat Neurosci 2002;5:1242–1247.
40. Bremner JD, Elzinga B, Schmahl C, Vermetten E. Structural and functional plasticity of the human brain in posttraumatic stress disorder. Prog Brain Res 2008;167:171–186.
41. Bossini L, Tavanti M, Lombardelli A, Calossi S, Polizzotto NR, Galli R, Vatti G, Pieraccini F, Castrogiovanni P. Changes in hippocampal volume in patients with post-traumatic stress disorder after sertraline treatment. J Clin Psychopharmacol 2007;27:233–235.
42. Bremner J, Licinio J, Darness A, et al. Elevated CRF cortico-tropin-releasing factor concentrations in posttraumatic stress disorder. Am J Psychiatry 1997;154:624–629.

43. Olff M, Guzelcan Y, de Vries GJ, Assies J, Gersons BPR. HPA-and HPT-axis alterations in chronic posttraumatic stress disorder. Psychoneuroendocrinology 2006;31:1220–1230.
44. Southwick SM, Bremner JD, Rasmusson A, Morgan CA III, Arnsten A, Charney DS. Role of norepinephrine in the pathophysiology and treatment of posttraumatic stress disorder. Bio Psychiatry 1999;46:1192–1204.
45. Southwick SM, Krystal JH, Bremner JD, Morgan CA III, Nicolaou AL, Nagy LM, Johnson DR, Heninger GR, Charney DS. Noradrenergic and serotonergic function in posttraumatic stress disorder. Arch Gen Psychiatry 1997;54:749–758.
46. Bremner JD, Innis RB, Ng CK, Staib LH, Salomon RM, Bronen RA, Duncan J, Southwick SM, Krystal JH, Rich D, Zubal G, Dey H, Soufer R, Charney DS. Positron emission tomography measurement of cerebral metabolic correlates of yohimbine administration in combat-related posttraumatic stress disorder. Arch Gen Psychiatry 1997;54:246–254.
47. Jezova D. Control of ACTH secretion by excitatory amino acids: Functional significance and clinical implications. Endocrine 2005;28:287–293.
48. Yehuda R, Brand S, Yang RK. Plasma neuropeptide Y concentrations in combat exposed veterans: Relationship to trauma exposure, recovery from PTSD, and coping. Biol Psychiatry 2006;59:660–663.
49. van der Kolk BA, Fisler R. Dissociation and the fragmentary nature of traumatic memories: Overview and exploratory study. J Trauma Stress 1995;8:505–525.
50. Osterman JE, van der Kolk BA. Awareness during anesthesia and post-traumatic stress disorder. Gen Hosp Psychiatry 1998;20:274–281.
51. van der Kolk, BA, Hopper, JW, Osterman, JE. Exploring the nature of traumatic memory: Bridging clinical knowledge and laboratory method. J Aggress Maltreat Trauma 2001;4:9–31.
52. Jovanovic T, Ressler K. How the neurocircuitry and genetics of fear inhibition may inform our understanding of PTSD. Am J Psychiatry 2010;167(6):648–662.
53. Ballenger JC, Davidson JRT, Lecrubier Y, Nutt DJ, Foa EB, Kessler RC, McFarlane AC, Shalev AY. Consensus statement on posttraumatic stress disorder from the International Consensus Group on Anxiety and Depression. J Clin Psychiatry 2004;65:55–62.
54. Foa EB, Keane TM, Friedman MJ, Cohen JA. Effective treatments for PTSD: Practice guidelines from the International Society for Traumatic Stress Studies, 2nd edition. New York: Guilford; 2009.
55. Stein DJ, Ipser JC, Seedat S. Pharmacotherapy for post traumatic stress disorder (PTSD). Cochrane Database Syst Rev 2006;(1):CD002795.
56. Schoenfeld FB, Marmar CR, Neylan TC. Current concepts in pharmacotherapy for posttraumatic stress disorder. Psychiatry Serv 2004;55:519–531.
57. Cooper J, Carty J, Creamer M. Pharmcotherapy for posttraumatic stress disorder: Empirical review and clinical recommendations. Aust N Z J Psychiatry 2005;29:395–401.
58. Davidson JR. Pharmacologic treatment of acute and chronic stress following trauma. J Clin Psychiatry 2006;67(Suppl 2):34–39.
59. Anis GM, Kohn SR, Henderson M, Brown NL. SSRIs versus non-SSRIs in post-traumatic stress disorder: An update with recommendations. Drugs 2004;64:383–404.
60. Ursano RJ, Bell C, Eth S, Friedman M, Norwood A, Pfefferbaum B, Pynoos JD, Zatzick DF, Benedek DM, McIntyre JS, Charles SC, Altshuler K, Cook I, Cross CD, Mellman L, Moench LA, Norquist G, Twemlow SW, Woods S, Yager J. Practice guideline for the treatment of patients with acute stress disorder and posttraumatic stress disorder. Am J Psychiatry 2004;161(11 Suppl):3–31.
61. Davis LL, Frazier EC, Williford RB. Long-term pharmacotherapy for post-traumatic disorder. CNS Drugs 2006;20:465–467.
62. Ursano RJ, Bell C, Spencer E, Friedman M, Norwood A, Pfefferbaum B, Pynoos RS, Zatzick DF. Practice guide lines for the treatment of patients with Acute Stress Disorder and Posttraumatic Stress Disorder. 2010 American Psychiatric Publishing, Inc. http://www.psychiatryonline.com/pracGuide/pracGuideTopic_11.aspx.

63. van der Kolk BA, Dreyfuss D, Michaels M, Shera D, Berkowitz R, Fisler R, Saxe G. Fluoxetine in post-traumatic stress disorder. J Clin Psychiatry 1994;35:517–522.
64. Connor KM, Sutherland SM, Tupler LA, Malik ML, Davidson JR. Fluoextine in post-traumatic stress disorder. Randomized double-blind study. Br J Psychiatry 1999;175:17–22.
65. Martenyi F, Brown EB, Zhang H, Prakash A, Koke SC. Fluoxetine versus placebo in post-traumatic stress disorder. J Clin Psychiatry 2002;63:199–206.
66. Martenyi F, Soldatenkova V. Fluoxetine in the acute treatment and relapse prevention of combat-related post-traumatic stress disorder: Analysis of the veteran group of a placebo-controlled, randomized clinical trial. Eur Neuropsychopharmacol 2006;16:340–349.
67. Marshall RD, Beebe KL, Oldham M, Zanielli R. Efficacy and safety of paroxetine treatment for chronic PTSD: A fixed dose, placebo-controlled study. Am J Psychiatry 2001;158:1982–1988.
68. Tucker P, Zaninelli R, Yehuda R, Ruggiero L, Dillingham K, Pitts CD. Paroxetine in the treatment of chronic posttraumatic stress disorder: Results of a placebo-controlled, flexible-dosage trial. J Clin Psychiatry 2001;62:860–868.
69. Marshall RD, Lewis-Fernandez R, Blanco C, Simpson HB, Lin SH, Vermes D, Garcia W, Schneier F, Neria Y, Sanchez-Lacay A, Liebowitz MR. A controlled trial of paroxetine for chronic PTSD, dissociation, and interpersonal problems in mostly minority adults. Depress Anxiety 2007;24:77–84.
70. Davidson J, Pearlstein T, Londborg P, Brady KT, Rothbaum B, Bell J, Maddock R, Hegel MT, Farfel G. Efficacy of sertraline in preventing relapse of posttraumatic stress disorder: Results of a 28-week double-blind, placebo-controlled study. Am J Psychiatry 2001;158:1974–1981.
71. Brady K, Pearlstein T, Asnis GM, Baker D, Rothbaum B, Sikes CR, Farfel GM. Efficacy and safety of sertraline treatment of posttraumatic stress disorder: A randomized controlled trial. JAMA 2000;283:1837–1844.
72. Davidson JRT, Rothbaum BO, van der Kolk BA, Sikes CR, Farfel GM. Multicenter, double-blind comparison of sertraline and placebo in the treatment of posttraumatic stress disorder. Arch Gen Psychiatry 2001;58:485–492.
73. Rapport MH, Endicott J, Cleary CM. Posttraumatic stress disorder and quality of life: Results across 64 weeks of sertraline treatment. J Clin Psychiatry 2002;63:59–65.
74. Stein DJ, van der Kolk BA, Austin C, Fayyad R, Clary C. Efficacy of sertraline in posttraumatic stress disorder secondary to interpersonal trauma or childhood abuse. Ann Clin Psychiatry 2006;18:243–249.
75. Charney DS, Grothe DR, Smith SL, Brady KT, Kaltsounis-Puckett J, Wright CW, Laird LK, Rush AJ. Overview of psychiatric disorders and the role of newer antidepressants. J Clin Psychiatry 2002;63:3–9.
76. Brady KT, Sonne S, Anton RF, Randall CL, Back SE, Simpson K. Sertraline in the treatment of co-occurring alcohol dependence and post-traumatic stress disorder. Alcohol Clin Exp Res 2005;29:395–401.
77. Back SE, Brady KT, Sonne SC, Verduin ML. Symptom improvement in co-occurring PTSD and alcohol dependence. J Nerv Ment Dis 2006;194:690–696.
78. Meltzer-Brody S, Connor KM, Churchill E, Davidson JR. Symptom-specific effects of fluoxetine in post-traumatic stress disorder. Int Clin Psychopharmacol 2000;15:227–231.
79. Hertzberg MA, Feldman ME, Beckham JC, Kudler HS, Davidson JR. Lack of efficacy for fluoxetine in PTSD: A placebo controlled trial in combat veterans. Ann Clin Psychiatry 2000;12:101–105.
80. Martenyi F, Brown EB, Caldwell CD. Failed efficacy of fluoxetine in the treatment of post-traumatic stress disorder: results of a fixed-dose, placebo-controlled study. J Clin Psychopharmacol 2007;27:166–170.
81. Kucukalic A, Bravo-Mehmedbasic A, Dzubur-Kulenovic A. Paroxetine in the treatment of post traumatic stress disorder: Our experiences. Bosn J Basic Med Sci 2008;8:76–79.
82. Kim Y, Asukai N, Konishi T, Kato H, Hirotsune H, Maeda M, Inoue H, Narita H, Iwasaki M. Clinical evaluation of paroxetine in post-traumatic stress disorder (PTSD): 52-week, non-comparative open-label study for clinical use experience. Psychiatry Clin Neurosci 2008;62:646–652.

83. Friedman MJ, Marmar CR, Baker DG, Sikes CR, Farfel GM. Randomized, double-blind comparison of sertraline and placebo for posttraumatic stress disorder in a Department of Veterans Affairs setting. J Clin Psychiatry 2007;68:711–720.
84. Zohar J, Amital D, Miodownik C, Kotler M, Bleich A, Lane RM, Austin C. Double-blind placebo-controlled pilot study of sertraline in military veterans with posttraumatic stress disorder. J Clin Psychopharmacol 2002;22:190–195.
85. Londborg PD, Hegel MT, Goldstein S, Goldstein D, Himmelhoch JM, Maddock R, Patterson WM, Rausch J, Farfel GM. Sertraline treatment of posttraumatic stress disorder: Results of 24 weeks of open-label continuation treatment. J Clin Psychiatry 2001;62:325–331.
86. Khouzam HR, el-Gabalawi F, Donnelly NJ. The clinical experience of citalopram in the treatment of post-traumatic stress disorder: A report of two Persian Gulf War veterans. Mil Med 2001;166:921–923.
87. Seedat S, Lockhat R, Kaminer D, Zungu-Dirwayi N, Stein DJ. An open trial of citalopram in adolescents with post-traumatic stress disorder. Int Clin Psychopharmacol 2001;16:21–25.
88. Robert S, Hamner MB, Ulmer HG, Lorberbaum JP, Durkalski VL. Open-label trial of escitalopram in the treatment of posttraumatic stress disorder. J Clin Psychiatry 2006;67:1552–1556.
89. Escalona R, Canive JM, Calais LA, Davidson JR. Fluvoxamine treatment in veterans with combat-related post-traumatic stress disorder. Depress Anxiety 2002;15:29–33.
90. Tucker P, Smith KL, Marx B, Jones D, Miranda R, Lensgraf J. Fluvoxamine reduces physiologic reactivity to trauma scripts in posttraumatic stress disorder. J Clin Psychopharmacol 2000;20:367–372.
91. Neylan TC, Metzler TJ, Schoenfeld FB, Weiss DS, Lenoci M, Best SR, Lipsey TL, Marmar CR. Fluvoxamine and sleep disturbances in posttraumatic stress disorder. J Trauma Stress 2001;14:461–467.
92. Marmar CR, Schoenfeld F, Weiss DS, Metzler T, Zatzick D, Wu R, Smiga S, Tecott L, Neylan T. Open trial of fluvoxamine treatment for combat-related posttraumatic stress disorder. J Clin Psychiatry 1996;57(Suppl 8):66–70; discussion 71–72.
93. Smajkic A, Weine S, Djuric-Bijedic Z, Boskaili E, Lewis J, Pavkovic I. Sertraline, paroxetine, and venlafaxine in refugee posttraumatic stress disorder with depressive symptoms. J Trauma Stress 2001;14:445–452.
94. Davidson J, Rothbaum BO, Tucker P, Asnis G, Benattia I, Musgnung JJ. Venlafaxine extended release in posttraumatic stress disorder: A sertraline- and placebo-controlled study. J Clin Psychopharmacol 2006;26:259–267.
95. Davidson J, Baldwin D, Stein DJ, Kuper E, Benattia I, Ahmed S, Pedersen R, Musgnung J. Treatment of posttraumatic stress disorder with venlafaxine extended release: A 6-month randomized controlled trial. Arch Gen Psychiatry 2006;63:1158–1165.
96. Walderhaug E, Kasserman S, Aikins D, Vojvoda D, Nishimura C, Neumeister A. Effects of duloxetine in treatment-refractory men with posttraumatic stress disorder. Pharmacopsychiatry 2010;43:45–49.
97. Davis LL, Jewell ME, Ambrose S, Farley J, English B, Bartolucci A, Petty F. A placebo controlled study of nefazodone for the treatment of chronic posttraumatic stress disorder: A preliminary study. J Clin Psychopharmacol 2004;24:292–297.
98. McRae AL, Brady KT, Mellman TA, Sonne SC, Killeen TK, Timmerman MA, Bayles-Dazet W. Comparison of nefazadone and sertraline for the treatment of posttraumatic stress disorder. Depress Anxiety 2004;19:190–196.
99. Hertzberg MA, Feldman ME, Beckham JC, Davidson JRT. Trial of trazodone for posttraumatic stress disorder using multiple baseline group design. J Clin Psychopharmacol 1996;16:294–298.
100. Davidson JR, Weisler RH, Butterfield MI, Casat CD. Connor KM, Barnett S, van Meter S. Mirtazapine vs. placebo in posttraumatic stress disorder: A pilot trial. Biol Psychiatry 2003;53:188–191.
101. Kim W, Pae CU, Chae JH, Jun TY, Bahk WM. The effectiveness of mirtazapine in the treatment of post-traumatic stress disorder: A 24 week continuation study. Psychiatry Clin Neurosci 2005;59:743–747.

102. Alderman CP, Condon JT, Gilbert AL. An open-label study of mirtazapine as treatment for combat-related PTSD. Ann Pharmacother 2009;43(7):1220–1226.
103. Canive JM, Clark RD, Calais LA, Qualls C, Tuason VB. Buproprion treatment in veterans with posttraumatic stress disorder: An open study. J Clin Psychopharmacol 1998;18:379–383.
104. Becker ME, Hertzberg MA, Moore SD, Dennis MF, Bukenya DS, Beckham JC. A placebo-controlled trial of bupropion SR in the treatment of chronic posttraumatic stress disorder. J Clin Psychopharmacol 2007;27:193–197.
105. Frank JB, Kosten TR, Giller EL Jr, Dan E. A randomized clinical trial of phenelzine and imipramine for posttraumatic stress disorder. Am J Psychiatry 1988;145:1289–1291.
106. Kosten TR, Frank JB, Dan E, McDougle CJ, Giller EL Jr. Pharmacotherapy for posttraumatic stress disorder using phenelzine or imipramine. J Nerv Ment Dis 1991;179:366–370.
107. Southwick SM, Yehuda R, Giller El, Charney DS. Use of tricyclics and monoamine oxidase inbibitors in the treatment of PTSD: A quantitative review. In MM Murburg, editor. Catecholamine function in post-traumatic stress disorder: Emerging concepts. Washington: American Psychiatric Press; 1994:149–155.
108. Neal LA, Shapland W, Fox C. An open trial of moclobemide in the treatment of post-traumatic stress disorder. Int Clin Psychopharmacol 1997;12:231–237.
109. Katz RJ, Lott MH, Arbus P, Crocq L, Herlobsen P, Lingjaerde O, Lopez G, Loughrey GC, MacFarlane DJ, McIvor R, et al. Pharmacotherapy of post-traumatic stress disorder with a novel psychotropic. Anxiety 1994;95:169–174.
110. Baker DG, Diamond BI, Gillette G, Hamner M, Katzelnick D, Keller T, Mellman TA, Pontius E, Rosenthal M, Tucker P, et al. A double-blind, randomized, placebo-controlled, multi-center study of brofaromine in the treatment of post-traumatic stress disorder. Psychopharmacology 1995;122:386–389.
111. Davidson JRT, Kudler H, Smith R, Mahoney SL, Lipper S, Hammett E, Saunders WB, Cavenar JL Jr. Treatment of posttraumatic stress disorder with amitriptyline and placebo. Arch Gen Psychiatry 1990;47:259–266.
112. Reist C, Kaufman CD, Haier RJ, Sangdahl C, DeMet EM, Chicz-DeMet A, Nelson JN. A controlled trial of desipramine in 18 men with posttraumatic stress disorder. Am J Psychiatry 1989;146:513–516.
113. Braun P, Greenberg D, Dasberg H, Lerer B. Core symptoms of posttraumatic stress disorder unimproved by alprazolam treatment. J Clin Psychiatry 1990;51:236–238.
114. Mellman TA, Bustamante V, David D, Fins AI. Hynoptic medication in the aftermath of trauma. J Clin Psychiatry 2002;63:1183–1184.
115. Cates ME, Bishop MH, Davis LL, Lowe JS, Woolley TW. Clonazepam for treatment of sleep disturbances associated with combat-related posttraumatic stress disorder. Ann Pharmacother 2004;38:1395–1359.
116. Mellman TA, Clark RE, Peacock WJ. Prescribing patterns for patients with ttraumatic stress disorder. Psychiatr Serv 2003;23:15–20.
117. Davidson JR. Use of benzodiazepines in social anxiety disorder, generalized anxiety disorder, and posttraumatic stress disorder. J Clin Psychiatry 2004;65(Suppl 5):29–33.
118. Duffy JD, Malloy PF. Efficacy of buspirone in the treatment of posttraumatic stress disorder: An open trial. Ann Clin Psychiatry 1994;6:33–37.
119. Davis LL, Davidson JRT, Ward LC, Bartolucci A, Bowden CL, Petty F. Divalproex in the treatment of posttraumatic stress disorder: A randomized, double-blind, placebo-controlled trial in a veteran population. J Clin Psychopharmacol 2008;28:84–88.
120. Hamner MB, Faldowski RA, Robert S, Ulmer HG, Horner MD, Lorberbaum JP. A preliminary controlled trial of divalproex in posttraumatic stress disorder. Ann Clin Psychiatry. 2009;21:89–94.
121. Wolf ME, Alavi A, Mosnaim AD. Posttraumatic stress disorder in Vietnam veterans: Clinical and EEG findings; possible therapeutic effects of carbamazepine. Biol Psychiatry 1988;23:642–644.
122. Lipper S, Davidson JR, Grady TA, Edinger JD, Hammett EB, Mahorney SL, Cavenar JO Jr. Preliminary study of carbamazepine in posttraumatic stress disorder. Psychosomatics 1986;27:849–854.

123. Bremner DJ, Mletzko T, Welter S, Siddiq S, Reed L, Williams C, Heim CM, Nemeroff CB. Treatment of posttraumatic stress disorder with phenytoin: An open-label pilot study. J Clin Psychiatry 2004;65:1559–1564.
124. Sutherland SM, Davidson JRT. Pharmacotherapy of posttraumatic stress disorder. Psychiatr Clin North Am 1994;17:409–423.
125. Viola J, Ditzler T, Batzer W, Harazin J, Adams D, Lettich L, Berigan T. Pharmacologic management of posttraumatic stress disorder: Clinical summary of a five-year retrospective study, 1990–1995. Mil Med 1997;162:616–619.
126. Hamner MB, Brodrick PS, Labbate LA. Gabapentin in PTSD: A retrospective, clinical series of adjunctive therapy. Ann Clin Psychiatry 2002;13:141–146.
127. Hertzberg MA, Butterfield MI, Feldman ME, Beckham JC, Sutherland SM, Connor KM, Davidson JR. A preliminary study of lamotrigine for the treatment of posttraumatic stress disorder. Bio Psychiatry 1999;45:1226–1229.
128. Tucker P, Trautman RP, Wyatt DB, Thompson J, Wu SC, Capece JA, Rosenthal NR. Efficacy and safety of topiramate monotherapy in civilian posttraumatic stress disorder: A randomized, double-blind, placebo-controlled study. J Clin Psychiatry 2007;68:201–206.
129. Lindley SE, Carlson EB, Hill K. A randomized, double-blind, placebo-controlled trial of augmentation topiramate for chronic combat-related posttraumatic stress disorder. J Clin Psychopharmacol 2007;27:677–681.
130. Kinrys G, Wygant LE, Pardo TB, Melo M. Levetiracetam for treatment – refractory posttraumatic stress disorder. J Clin Psychiatry 2006;67:211–214.
131. Davidson JR, Brady K, Mellman TA, Stein MB, Pollack MH. The efficacy and tolerability of tiagabine in adult patients with post-traumatic stress disorder. J Clin Psychopharmacol 2007;27:85–88.
132. Sernyak MJ, Kosten TR, Fontana A, Rosenheck R. Neuroleptic use in the treatment of posttraumatic stress disorder. Psychiatr Q 2001;72:197–213.
133. Kozari-Kovaci D, Pivac N, Muck-Seler D, Rothbaum BO. Risperidone in psychotic combat-related posttraumatic stress disorder: An open trial. J Clin Psychiatry 2005;66:922–927.
134. David D, De Faria L, Mellman TA. Adjunctive risperidone treatment and sleep symptoms in combat veterans with chronic PTSD. Depress Anxiety 2006;23:489–491.
135. Hamner MB, Faldowski RA, Ulmer HG, Frueh BC, Huber MG, Arana GW. Adjunctive risperidone treatment in post-traumatic stress disorder: A preliminary controlled trial of effects on comorbid psychotic symptoms. Int Clin Psychopharmacol 2003;18:1–8.
136. Monnelly EP, Ciraulo DA, Knapp C, Keane T. Low-dose risperidone as adjunctive therapy for irritable aggression in posttraumatic stress disorder. J Clin Psychopharmacol 2003;23:193–196.
137. Bartzokis G, Lu PH, Turner J, Mintz J, Saunders CS. Adjunctive risperidone in the treatment of chronic combat-related posttraumatic stress disorder. Biol Psychiatry 2005;57:474–479.
138. Reich DB, Winternitz S, Hennen J, Watts T, Stanculescu C. A preliminary study of risperidone in the treatment of posttraumatic stress disorder related to childhood abuse in women. J Clin Psychiatry 2004;65:1601–1606.
139. Padala PR, Madison J, Monnahan M, Marcil W, Price P, Ramaswamy S, Din AU, Wilson DR, Petty F. Risperidone monotherapy for post-traumatic stress disorder related to sexual assault and domestic abuse in women. Int Clin Psychopharmacol 2006;21:275–280.
140. Rothbaum BO, Killeen TK, Davidson JR, Brady KT, Connor KM, Heekin MH. Placebo-controlled trial of risperidone augmentation for selective serotonin reuptake inhibitor-resistant civilian posttraumatic stress disorder. J Clin Psychiatry 2008;69:520–525.
141. Hamner MB, Deitsch SE, Brodrick PS, Ulmer HG, Lorberbaum JP. Quetiapine treatment in patients with posttraumatic stress disorder: An open trial of adjunctive therapy. J Clin Psychopharmacol 2003;23:15–20.
142. Ahearn EP, Mussey M, Johnson C, Krohn A, Krahn D. Quetiapine as an adjunctive treatment for post-traumatic stress disorder: An 8-week open-label study. Int Clin Psychopharmacol 2006;21:29–33.
143. Sokolski KN, Denson TF, Lee RT, Reist C. Quetiapine for treatment of refractory symptoms of combat-related post-traumatic stress disorder. Mil Med 2003;168:486–489.

144. Petty F, Brannan S, Casada J, Davis LL, Gajewski V, Kramer GL, Stone RC, Teten AL, Worchel J, Young KA. Olanzapine treatment for post-traumatic stress disorder: An open-label study. Int Clin Psychopharmacol 2001;16:331–337.
145. Butterfield MI, Becker ME, Connor KM, Sutherland S, Churchill LE, Davidson JR. Olanzapine in the treatment of posttraumatic stress disorder: A pilot study. Int Clin Psychopharmacol 2001;16:197–203.
146. Stein MB, Kline NA, Matloff JL. Adjunctive olanzapine for SSRI-resistant combat- related PTSD: A double-blind, placebo-controlled study. Am J Psychiatry 2002;159:1777–1779.
147. Villarreal G, Calais LA, Canive JM, Lundy SL, Pickard J, Toney G. Prospective study to evaluate the efficacy of aripiprazole as a monotherapy in patients with severe chronic post-traumatic stress disorder: An open trial. Psychopharmacol Bull 2007;40:6–18.
148. Mello MF, Costa MC, Schoedl AF, Fiks JP. Aripiprazole in the treatment of posttraumatic stress disorder: An open-label trial. Rev Bras Psiquiatr 2008;30:358–361.
149. Robert S, Hamner MB, Durkalski VL, Brown MW, Ulmer HG. An open-label assessment of aripiprazole in the treatment of PTSD. Psychopharmacol Bull 2009;42:69–80.
150. Pivac N, Kozaric-Kovacic D. Pharmacotherapy of treatment-resistant combat-related post-traumatic stress disorder with psychotic features. Croat Med J 2006;47:440–451.
151. Pae CU, Lim HK, Peindl K, Ajwani N, Serretti A, Patkar AA, Lee C. The atypical antipsychotics olanzapine and risperidone in the treatment of posttraumatic stress disorder: A meta-analysis of randomized, double-blind, placebo-controlled clinical trials. Int Clin Psychopharmacol 2008;23:1–8.
152. Siddiqui Z, Marcil WA, Bhatia SC, Ramaswamy S, Petty F. Ziprasidone therapy for post-traumatic stress disorder. J Psychiatry Neurosci 2005;30:430–431.
153. Kolb LC, Burris BC, Griffiths S. Propranolol and clonidine in the treatment of posttraumatic stress disorders of war. In B van der Kolk, editor. Post-traumatic stress disorder: Psychological and biological sequelae. Washington: American Psychiatric Press; 1984.
154. Kinzie JD, Leung P. Clonidine in Cambodian patients with posttraumatic stress disorder. J Nerv Ment Dis 1989;177:546–550.
155. Harmon RJ, Riggs PD. Clonidine for posttraumatic stress disorder in preschool children. J Am Acad Child Adolesc Psychiatry 1996;35:1247–1249.
156. Lustig SL, Botelho C, Lynch L, Nelson SV. Eichelberger WJ. Vaughan BL. Implementing a randomized clinical trial on a pediatric psychiatric inpatient unit at a children's hospital: The case of clonidine for post-traumatic stress. Gen Hosp Psychiatry 2002;24:422–429.
157. Neylan TC, Lenoci M, Samuelson KW, Metzler TJ, Henn-Haase C, Hierholzer RW, Lindley SE, Otte C, Schoenfeld FB, Yesavage JA, Marmar CR. No improvement of posttraumatic stress disorder symptoms with guanfacine treatment. Am J Psychiatry 2006;163:2186–2188.
158. Raskind MA, Peskind ER, Kanter ED, Petrie EC, Radant A, Thompson CE, Dobie DJ, Hoff D, Rein RJ, Straits-Troster K, Thomas RG, McFall MM. Reduction of nightmares and other PTSD symptoms in combat veterans by prazosin: A placebo-controlled study. Am J Psychiatry 2003;160:371–373.
159. Raskind MA, Peskind ER, Hoff DJ, Hart KL, Holmes HA, Warren D, Shofer J, O'Connell J, Taylor F, Gross C, Rohde K, McFall ME. A parallel group placebo-controlled study of prazosin for trauma nightmares and sleep disturbance in combat veterans with post-traumatic stress disorder. Biol Psychiatry 2007;61:928–934.
160. Boynton L, Bentley J, Strachan E, Barbato A, Raskind M. Preliminary findings concerning the use of prazosin for the treatment of posttraumatic nightmares in a refugee population. J Psychiatr Pract 2009;15:454–459.
161. Thompson CE, Taylor FB, McFall ME, Barnes RF, Raskind MA. Nonnightmare distressed awakenings in veterans with posttraumatic stress disorder: Response to prazosin. J Trauma Stress 2008;21:417–420.
162. De Jong J, Wauben P, Huijbrechts I, Oolders H, Haffmans J. Doxazosin treatment for post-traumatic stress disorder. J Clin Psychopharmacol 2010;30:84–85.
163. Clark RD, Canive JM, Calais LA, Qualls C, Brugger RD, Vosburgh TB, Cyproheptadine treatment of nightmares associated with posttraumatic stress disorder. J Clin Psychopharmacol 1999;19:486–487.

164. Jacobs-Rebhun S, Schnurr PP, Friedman MJ, Peck R, Brophy M, Fuller D. Posttraumatic stress disorder and sleep difficulty. Am J Psychiatry 2000;157:1525–1526.
165. Drake RG. Davis LL. Cates ME. Jewell ME. Ambrose SM. Lowe JS. Baclofen treatment for chronic posttraumatic stress disorder. Ann Pharmacother 2003;37:1177–1181.
166. Heresco-Levy U, Kremer I, Javitt DC, Goichman R, Reshef A, Blanaru M, Cohen T. Pilot-controlled trial of D-cycloserine for the treatment of post-traumatic stress disorder. Int J Neuropsychopharmacol 2002;5:301–307.
167. Pitman RK, Sanders KM, Zusman RM, Healy AR, Cheema F, Lasko NB, Cahill L, Orr SP. Pilot study of secondary prevention of posttraumatic stress disorder with propranolol. Biol Psychiatry 2002;51:189–192.
168. Vaiva G, Ducrocq F, Jezequel K, Averland B, Lestavel P, Brunet A, Marmar CR. Immediate treatment with propranolol decreases posttraumatic stress disorder two months after trauma [see comment]. Biol Psychiatry 2003;54:947–994 [erratum appears in Biol Psychiatry. 2003 15;54(12):1471].
169. McGhee LL, Maani CV, Garza TH, Desocio PA, Gaylord KM, Black IH. The effect of propranolol on posttraumatic stress disorder in burned service members. J Burn Care Res 2009;30(1):92–97.
170. Sharp S, Thomas C, Rosenberg L, Rosenberg M, Meyer W 3rd. Propranolol does not reduce risk for acute stress disorder in pediatric burn trauma. J Trauma 2010;68(1):193–197.
171. Stein MB, Kerridge C, Dimsdale JE, Hoyt DB. Pharmacotherapy to prevent PTSD: Results from a randomized controlled proof-of-concept trial in physically injured patients. J Trauma Stress 2007;20:923–932.
172. Boggio PS, Rocha M, Oliveira MO, Fecteau S, Cohen RB, Campanhã C, Ferreira-Santos E, Meleiro A, Corchs F, Zaghi S, Pascual-Leone A, Fregni F. Noninvasive brain stimulation with high-frequency and low-intensity repetitive transcranial magnetic stimulation treatment for posttraumatic stress disorder. J Clin Psychiatry. 2009 http://www.mindcarecentres.com/knowledgecentre/journalcentre.aspx?category=POST-TRAUMATIC STRESS. Dec 29, 2009.
173. Rothbaum BO, Cahill SP, Foa EB, Davidson JRT, Compton J, Connor KM, Astin MC, Hahn CG. Augmentation of sertraline with prolonged exposure in the treatment of posttraumatic stress disorder. J Trauma Stress 2006;19:625–638.

Diagnosis and Treatment of Depression During Pregnancy and Lactation

Daniel Shaw

Depression and Pregnancy

Over the past decade there has been increasing interest in women's mental health and the problems of treating mood disorders throughout the reproductive cycle (1). In particular there has been increasing awareness that depression during pregnancy is highly prevalent and poses risks to both mother and fetus and infant (1, 2). The number of articles and reviews increases each year often with findings that contradict previous evidence. As the field grows it raises more questions than answers about how to balance competing mental health needs and risks during the perinatal period.

The psychopharmacologic treatment of depression during pregnancy presents several challenges. The clinician has to balance health and safety of the mother, fetus, and newborn. To do this the clinician must understand the evidence-based data and have a framework for discussing the risks, the benefits, and the treatment alternatives. This framework has to be integrated with the patient's own history of depression, response to medication, attitudes towards depression and towards pregnancy, attitudes about taking medication, and anxiety about treatment.

In making treatment recommendations the clinician must take into account the nature of the depression: its severity, the degree to which it interferes with functioning and inter-personal relationships, the degree of co-morbid anxiety, and any co-morbid disorder. Is the mother at risk because of potential for suicide or poor self-care or anorexia? Is the social network supportive? Is there risk of diminished social network or support because of depression? The level and nature of stress experienced by the mother is also a factor. Stress both contributes to and exacerbates depression. Though these are all factors in treating depression in non-pregnant women, they acquire greater salience in pregnancy where the fetus and newborn are now part of the equation.

This chapter will discuss the salient literature related to prevalence of depression, the risk depression poses to mother, fetus, and newborn, the risks and benefits of psychopharmacological interventions, and the considerations for breast-feeding.

D. Shaw (✉)
Department of Psychiatry, Boston University School of Medicine, Boston MA, USA
e-mail: dshaw@bu.edu

D.A. Ciraulo and R.I. Shader (eds.), *Pharmacotherapy of Depression*,
DOI 10.1007/978-1-60327-435-7_8,

The Risk of Being Depressed During Pregnancy

Depression is a highly prevalent disorder. Lifetime prevalence (NCS-R) is 16.2%, and prevalence for women is almost twice that of men. The 1-month prevalence for women is 3.9% (3). Depression is a complicated disorder that is highly co-morbid. Co-morbidity for anxiety is 57.5% and for substance-abuse disorders it is 8.5%. The implications of this, for perinatal depression, are significant. Substance abuse poses a significant threat to the fetus and newborn resulting in increased mortality. Anxiety during pregnancy is a significant source of stress for the fetus and newborn (4), the effects of which will be discussed in a later section.

Depression is highly disabling. Role functioning is impaired 35.1 days of the year compared to 15 days for most chronic conditions (3). The implications are significant for pregnancy where role functioning involves a high level of self-care in order to care for the developing fetus.

There are two different methods that have been used to define the prevalence of depression during pregnancy rating scales and population studies. Self-report scales such as the Edinburgh Depression Scale or the Beck Depression Inventory (BDI) or the Center for Epidemiologic Studies Depression Scale (CES-D) have been employed primarily in obstetric clinics to define symptoms of depression. These do not provide a diagnosis, and a cut-off score is used to define depression. Another group of rating scales is structured diagnostic interviews such as the PRIME-MD, or the Schedule for Affective Disorders (SAD) or Research Diagnostic Criteria (RDC) have been employed in the same settings to give a definitive diagnosis. The populations range from a few 100 to 1,400. A third approach is population studies which examine large databases of several hundred to several thousand subjects and include both case-controlled and cohort studies.

The results have varied widely. The EDS and BDI and the CES-D capture both major and minor depression, and often cannot differentiate between them. Studies before 2003, which employed the BDI or EDS, were reviewed by Bennet (5) who found that the point prevalence for significant levels of depressive symptoms ranged from 2 to 51% with an average of 17%. Studies done since 2005 (6–9) have also reported prevalence rates from 9 to 20.5%.

When structured interview schedules (SADS or RDC) are employed, the average prevalence of MDD in the third trimester is 4.5% and minor depression ranged from 0.5 to 16% (5). Extrapolating data from all studies the prevalence of depression (major and minor) ranged from 7.4% in the first trimester to 12% in the third trimester (5). The lower first trimester rate may be an artifact, fewer first trimester studies were available, and women may not come for prenatal care till late in first trimester. It is also possible that depressed women may delay getting care till further along in pregnancy. By the second trimester the rate has risen to 12% (5).

Using PRIME-MD in a prospective point prevalence survey of 1,795 Swedish women Andersson (10) found the second trimester prevalence for MDD to be 3.3% and minor depression 6.9%. This rate is supported by an Agency for Healthcare Research and Quality (AHRQ) meta-analysis of studies, which employed structured interviews. The rate for MDD increased from 3.1% in the first trimester to 4.9% in the third trimester. The rate for major+minor depression ranged from 8.5 to 11%. These results are consistent with the NCS 1-month prevalence for MDD of 3.9%.

Population studies reviewing data from HMOs and other registers have reported somewhat higher prevalence. These studies reflect ICD 9 depression diagnostic codes and as such would include MDD as well as dysthymia and neurotic depression (roughly equivalent to depressive disorder NOS). Prevalence ranged from 6.9 (11) to 14% (12).

For many women depression during pregnancy is a continuation of pre-conception depression. Fifty-six percent of those identified as depressed during pregnancy were depressed during the 39 weeks before conception.

Vesga-Lopez (13), in a community epidemiological survey [random sample interviewed door to door], found a prevalence rate for MDD during pregnancy of 8.4%, which was not significantly different from the 8.1% rate in the non-pregnant sample. The most striking finding was an increased rate for postpartum women of 9.3% (AOR 1.52, CI 1.07–2.15). This rate is considerably higher than the AHQR rate though it does confirm the rise in prevalence postpartum.

It is difficult to reconcile the wide range of prevalence. Though structured interview-based studies all report similar depression rates consistent with the general prevalence they do not capture the range of debilitating symptoms of depression. Self-report scales such as the EDS report higher rates because they are capturing any depressive symptom at a moment in time. Symptoms that may be normal to pregnancy (fatigue, loss of libido, worry, and sleep disturbance loss of energy) overlap with the neuro-vegetative symptoms of depression (1). There is also overlap with symptoms of medical conditions common to pregnancy such as anemia, thyroid dysfunction, and gestational diabetes (14).

The wide range of prevalence may also reflect differences in demographics, reproductive events, history of depression, and other confounding factors. Differences may also result from women's willingness to report symptoms due to cultural factors. Edge (15) noted that Black Caribbean women living in England reported much lower rates of depression than were actually present. This was a reflection of a number of cultural factors and factors related to the health care delivery system, differences may also be reflected in pregnancy risk status. For women on a high-risk obstetrics ward the prevalence of MDD was 20% (16).

Though the reported rates vary widely it is clear that depression is at least as prevalent during pregnancy as in women of reproductive age. There is a possibility that prevalence may rise in second and third trimesters, and postpartum though this needs further investigation.

Though it has been difficult to define the incidence of depression in pregnancy, an AHRQ meta-analysis found that a new episode of major or minor depression during pregnancy occurs in 14.5% of women, and a new episode of major depressive episodes occurs in 7.5% of women. Thirty-three percent of episodes during pregnancy are first episodes (17). One study (11) reported that 41% of women who were depressed during pregnancy were not depressed during the 39 weeks prior to conception. Kitamura (18), in a relatively small study in Japan $n=290$, reported an incidence rate for MDD of 5.6%.

The implications from these data are significant. Case finding during pregnancy achieves importance not only because of high prevalence but also because of the impact of depression on the mother, the fetus, and the newborn. Since prevalence may rise at each trimester and new cases appear in significant numbers, depression screening should be done at least once each trimester and postpartum (19).

Risk Factors for Developing Depression During Pregnancy

The risk of developing depression is the intersection of environmental factors and endogenous factors. Endogenous factors include gender, previous episodes of depression, genetic predisposition, and personality traits such as neuroticism (a simple definition is predisposition to respond with emotional upset, excessive anxiety, and depression to adversity) (20, 21).

Environmental risk factors for depression are primarily stress-related. Risk of depression increases with adversity, such as job loss, marital difficulties, loss of a close personal relationship, and health problems (3, 21). Weaker factors are lower SES and lower levels of social support, never married, or divorced (22). Environmental factors are presumed to be superimposed on a predisposition to depression (1, 21, 22).

Hormonal factors may play a role, particularly fluctuations in estrogen levels and HPA axis alterations (23). This is an area that is still being investigated with no definitive findings. There is a suggestion that gonadal hormones play a role in modulating the serotonin system. In premenstrual dysphoric disorder, for example, where there is no evidence of alteration in gonadal steroid levels, symptoms may be related to alterations in serotonin system sensitivity. This effect may extend to the vulnerability to depression during pregnancy.

The primary risk factor for developing depression during pregnancy is the previous history of depression. More than three previous major depressive episodes predict an 80% risk of relapse (21, 24). This is consistent with a fourfold increase in the risk of depression during pregnancy with previous history of depression (25). Depression in the year before pregnancy also increases the risk fourfold of developing depression during pregnancy (25, 26). Environmental factors may increase this association; Lovisi (27) found a sevenfold increase in risk of depression in Brazilian women with low SES and multiple stress factors and previous history of depression.

Subsyndromal symptoms are also predictors of increased rate of MDD and decreased interval to relapse of MDD (28). Between 10 and 20% of pregnant women have subsyndromal symptoms (2, 5, 29). This suggests that these women are at increased risk for an episode of MDD during pregnancy or postpartum.

Discontinuing antidepressant medication is a major risk factor for recurrence. The relapse rate in pregnant women who discontinue medication is 68% (30), similar to the 70% risk of relapse in the general population (31).

Environmental risk factors have been extensively explored in pregnancy and their contribution to depression is profound. Social relationships exert a significant effect. Not having a partner (10, 32–34), and loss of an intimate relationship through divorce or death, increases the risk of depression (27). Poor social support or social conflict increases the risk of developing depressive symptoms (35). A particularly stressful aspect of social relationships is verbal and/or physical abuse (27, 36, 37). The incidence of abuse ranges from 1 to 20% of all pregnant women and rises during pregnancy (38). Verbal and physical abuse probably plays a role in onset or exacerbation of depression.

Pregnancy itself can be a stressor. A poor pregnancy outcome in the past or an unplanned pregnancy are often experienced as stressful life events (39) increasing the risk of depression (34, 40–42). Anxiety about the pregnancy (43) and negative attitudes towards the pregnancy are also associated with increased risk of depression (8, 18, 44). High-risk pregnancy increases the risk of developing depression. Forty-nine percent of women with high-risk pregnancy on an obstetrics ward had depressive symptoms and 18% met criteria for MDD (16).

Other stressful factors such as lower SES (32), financial difficulties (27), and two or more stressful events in the past year (25, 45) are also associated with increased risk of depression, consistent with the findings in the general population (22).

The broad range of risk factors reflects the biopsychosocial nature of depression. Though depression may not be present at the time of evaluation, presence of these risk factors should signal increased clinician alertness. This is particularly true if there is a history of depression or anxiety, or a tendency to worry or emotional reactivity. Screening for risk factors is part of screening for depression and should occur at least once a trimester.

The Risk to the Mother of Untreated Depression

Depression poses a significant risk to wellbeing and functional capacity. Depression in the general population is associated with increased medical utilization, decreased productivity, and increased disability days (15, 46–49). It impairs both role function and self-care (3, 49). It is also associated with adverse relationships with family and friends.

These findings extend to pregnancy as well. In pregnancy the presence of depression also leads to an increased number of disability days and impaired role function (49). Pregnancy requires increased attention to health status, and poor health behaviors increase rates of fetal mortality and morbidity. Depression interferes with a woman's capacity to attend to her health putting herself and her fetus at risk. A history of depression and other psychiatric disorders is associated with inadequate prenatal care (50) and reduced participation in prenatal care programs (51). Depressed women who do attend prenatal care have more complaints of nausea and vomiting and have more frequent visits to the doctor than women who are free of depression and/or anxiety (49). Antibiotic use is increased when depression is present during pregnancy (32).

Depression is associated with poor health outcomes including lower-than-expected weight gain, decreased appetite, and greater likelihood of using drugs or alcohol (52–54). Rates of smoking are increased in depressed pregnant women (53, 54). Women who are depressed are significantly less likely to be able to stop smoking (55).

Depression in pregnancy results in a reduced health quality of life (56). This encompasses a broad group of problems ranging from physical role to general health to social functioning to emotional functioning.

Depression and/or anxiety during pregnancy also may increase the risk of pre-eclampsia. A Finnish cohort study (57) reported adjusted OR of 2.5 (1.4–5.4) for depression and adjusted OR of 3.2 (1.4–7.4) for anxiety. Andersson (49) did not find an association. The OR was 1.37 (0.57–3.27). Using a chart review from a cohort study of 2,600 women, Qiu et al. (58) found that the risk of pre-eclampsia was increased almost twofold in women who are moderately depressed throughout pregnancy compared to non-depressed controls. Women who have severe depression had a threefold increased risk of developing pre-eclampsia. Caseness was defined by chart review, and it is possible that many depressed women were classified as controls. Though this may have skewed the result, a similar study in Peru using PHQ9 scores found a similar pattern of dose-related increased risk of pre-eclampsia in depressed pregnant women (59). The weight of the evidence at this point is that the risk of pre-eclampsia is significantly increased by the presence of MDD.

A supportive social network is important for the wellbeing and functioning of the mother during pregnancy and postpartum. Depression during pregnancy also has a negative impact on the family members (48, 60). As a result there is increase of stress and compromised support network and isolation. Depression also has a direct impact on socialization, and people with depression often isolate themselves.

Suicide is a significant risk factor in depression. Pregnancy affords some protection against suicide, for suicide rates are reduced in perinatal depression compared to the non-pregnant population (61). Two large cohort studies (62, 63) found that the suicide rate was between 1/3 and 1/2 the expected rate. Nonetheless rates of suicidal ideation are increased during pregnancy (61). In spite of reduced risk of suicide the clinician needs to be vigilant about this issue for suicide accounts for 28% of maternal deaths and is the leading cause of maternal death during pregnancy (64).

Depression during pregnancy is related to an increased risk of verbal and physical abuse (65). It also contributes to an increased risk of being hit by ones partner in the first postpartum year (66).

Depression during pregnancy poses significant risks to the mother's wellbeing, and by extension to the fetus and newborn. Since many of these risks are related to reduced functional capacity and reduced quality of health care, the importance of screening for and treating depression cannot be underestimated.

Risk of Untreated Depression to the Fetus and to Pregnancy Outcome

Untreated depression during pregnancy may have adverse effects on pregnancy outcome, and adverse effects on the fetus, new born, and infant. One risk that has been reported is pre-term labor and delivery, defined as delivery before the 37th week. Another is the risk of fetal growth restriction (FGR), resulting in newborns that are small for gestational age (13) i.e., in the 10th percentile for weight. Another is the risk of poor neonatal adaptation as reflected in Apgar scores and neonatal distress. A fourth adverse outcome of untreated maternal depression is stress to the fetus. This is conceptualized as fetal programming which becomes evident in the neonate, infant, and child who have developmental delays, behavioral difficulties, and cognitive deficits.

The Effect of Untreated Depression on Pregnancy Outcome

In 2005 the prevailing view, presented in several articles and books, was that untreated depression and anxiety pose a significant risk to pregnancy outcome. Specifically, depression poses an increased risk of premature labor, premature delivery, and infants who are SGA (19, 67–69). Since then several reviews (70–73) and several articles have presented conflicting results so that it is no longer clear that depression portends an adverse outcome.

The Risk of Pre-Term Labor/Delivery

Pre-term labor or birth has been investigated in several large cohort studies (74–79) which have yielded mixed results. A prospective study (74) of African American women, primarily with low SES, found a twofold increase in the risk of pre-term birth in women who scored in the upper 10th percentile of the CES-D. Dayan (75) prospectively followed 634 women in France and found that untreated depression, as well as anxiety, was associated with pre-term labor – OR 2.1 (1.1–4.1). When depression was associated with a BMI below 19, the OR rose to 6.9 (1.8–26.2). Pre-term labor under-represents negative outcome for pregnancy for it only predicts 50% of the cases of pre-term delivery (80). This finding was refined in a later study by Dayan (76) who followed 681 women – this time examining pre-term birth. The OR for pre-term birth in depressed women was 3.3 (1.2–9.2), higher than the rate for pre-term labor.

Suri (77), in a prospective study of 80 women (only 19 of whom were non-depressed controls), did not find an association between pre-term birth and depression. The authors said they were surprised by this findings. It is possible the study did not have enough power to prevent a type II error.

Complicating the picture are two Scandinavian studies. A Swedish study, using PRIME-MD, found no association with pre-term birth in 1,492 women (49). The same population of depressed women had increased nausea and vomiting and prolonged sick leave during pregnancy indicating probable increase in stress.

Berle (78) gave the Hospital Anxiety/Depression Scale (HADS) to 680 Norwegian women and found no correlation between pre-term birth and symptoms of anxiety or depression. Women with higher levels of psychosocial stress attended clinic less often and had a significantly higher rate of pre-term delivery. As a result the study was skewed toward healthier women with lower stress levels. In addition the authors note that their study may have suffered from a type II error.

In a group of 613 Chinese women living in Hong Kong, Chung et al. (81) found no increase in the risk of pre-term labor or delivery. The authors noted that there was also no relationship for depression and FGR; however, they commented that the statistical power was not adequate to prevent a type II error and they would have had to examine 6,000 subjects.

Wisner et al. (82) studied the impact of untreated depression and depression treated with SSRIs. She found that there is a dose effect for depression so that the risk of pre-term birth is increased twofold for depression that continues through pregnancy vs. depression that is present for two trimesters or less. Women who were continuously depressed but untreated had more severe depression and lower GAF scores than the women who had partial depression.

Further support for depression's association with increased risk of pre-term birth comes from a study by Li et al. using an insurance database. Mothers with a first trimester CESD score of ≥22 had a greater than twofold increase in the risk of pre-term birth. Furthermore there is a dose effect. The risk is greater for more severe depression than for moderate depression where CESD scores are between 16 and 21.

Compared to depression or anxiety alone, co-morbid depression and anxiety symptoms are likely to increase the risk of pre-term birth. The presence of anxiety may account for an increase in stress factors such as daily hassles, relationship difficulties, and greater sleep disturbance (83).

Though the evidence is conflicted, more and more information is appearing that depression, particularly more severe depression, increases the risk of pre-term birth.

Effect of Untreated Depression on the Course of Labor

Depressed women had an increase in rates of epidural anesthesia and cesarean section (49, 81). This may be related to a posited reduced tolerance for pain, secondary to depression, and reduced tolerance for stress, secondary to both anxiety and depression. Anxiety may also impair uterine contractility (81).

The Impact of Untreated Depression on Fetal Development

There is conflicting evidence that depression contributes to growth restriction (FGR) or small for gestational age (13). Several cohort studies, all employing different methods of assessing depression (PRIME+MD, CESD, EDS), found no correlation with depression and FGR (49, 81, 84). The populations included Danish women (84), Chinese women (81), and Swedish women (49) and women in the UK (85). These studies all had large *N*s ranging from 613 (81) to 10,967 in the ALSPAC study in the UK (85). It also appears that anxiety does not contribute to FGR (78).

Kelly (86), using a population-based study of all deliveries in California in 1 year, found a significant correlation with psychiatric diagnoses as well as substance use disorders and low birth weight. Unfortunately diagnoses were only at delivery, depression was not segregated from psychiatric diagnoses, and confounders were not assessed.

Rahman (87), in a cohort study in a single district in rural Pakistan, found an association with prenatal depression and low birth weight. Hoffman (88) studying at women with lower SES found a weak association with fetal growth restriction and depression.

Oberlander (12) in a case-controlled study of 203,500 hospital records used a propensity scale to define severity of depression. He found an association with increased severity of depression in untreated depressed women and pre-term birth as well as fetal growth restriction.

For both pre-term labor/delivery and FGR, the conflicting findings may reflect a difference between populations and the quality of prenatal care. In the Scandinavian countries prenatal care may be far better, pre-term birth is less frequent so that the effect of depression is diluted. It is possible that some of the findings of adverse outcome may be a result of depression, amplifying already tenuous prenatal care.

The studies that did find an association with pre-term labor/delivery or FGR were primarily in populations where mothers were of low SES and/or had many stressors (86–88) or had more severe depression (12). A further confounder is maternal anemia, which can contribute to FGR. This was not examined in the studies discussed. Further complicating the issue, as noted, is the possibility that some of the studies were under-powered.

These ambiguities leave clinicians with uncertainty about how to evaluate the risks of untreated depression to pregnancy outcome. Depression amplifies factors that may mitigate good prenatal care and this, rather than a direct effect of depression, may be the mediator for pre-term labor/delivery and FGR. Severity of depression and the presence of co-morbid disorders such as anxiety and substance misuse probably play a role as well.

The Impact of Stress and Anxiety on the Fetus

Though pregnancy outcome may not be affected directly by depression there are several studies that point to stress and anxiety having an adverse effect on the fetus, the neonate, the infant, and child. A few of these studies focus on depression, most focus on stress and anxiety. Stress is a broadly defined term encompassing adverse events, anxiety, or some aspects of depression as well as all other psychiatric diagnoses. Often stress or anxiety is measured without addressing depression. Because of the high co-morbidity of depression and anxiety, and the likelihood of depression contributing to stress, it would not be surprising if depression was a factor in the stress-focused studies.

Effect of Stress on the Fetus

The uterine artery resistance index is increased in women with high anxiety levels as measured by the State Trait Anxiety Index (STAI) (89). This may contribute to fetal growth restriction (90).

Fetuses of depressed mothers demonstrate more activity on stimulation in the fifth month. This is followed by a decline in response in the ensuing months. The implication is that heightened motor activity may represent a heightened alarm reaction followed by either adaptation or exhaustion (91).

Effect of Depression or Stress on the Neonate

Depression in the year before birth is associated with an increased rate of SIDS (92). Lower Apgar scores are associated with anxiety but not depression (78), but the authors noted that the prevalence of depression (2.8%) was very low and the *N* for depressed women was only 19 vs. 71 for anxious women. Several other studies did not find an association with lower Apgar scores and depression (49, 77, 81). Nonetheless some infants born to mothers with untreated depression have increased risk of admission to NICU (12, 81).

Neonates of mothers with high levels of anxiety, depression, and anger have higher levels of norepinephrine, lower dopamine and serotonin levels, and spend more time in deep sleep and less time in quiet alert states (90). Motor organization is lower as is autonomic instability (90). This is confounded by another study by Field (93), where women with just depression alone were evaluated – their offspring had less time in deep sleep, more time in disorganized sleep, and increased fussing and crying. The reason for this contradiction may be a difference in the symptom profile, for these women were not evaluated for anxiety.

The Effect of Stress on Development

Prepartum depression is reflected in increased negative responses to stressors in the infant (94, 95) and increased crying (95); infants of mothers with prepartum depression also exhibit decreased consolability when crying (96) and negative temperament (a combination of distress, sadness, fear, shyness, and frustration) (94).

Large prospective studies such as the Avon Longitudinal Study of Parents and Children (ALSPAC) have demonstrated an association with prenatal depression and cognitive behavioral and emotional outcomes into the teens. Children of mothers who had high levels of anxiety in the third trimester are at increased risk of having behavioral problems at ages 4 and 7 (97, 98). Antenatal depression, but not post-partum depression, is associated with a twofold increased risk of antisocial behavior and a fourfold risk of violent behavior by age 16 (99).

The risk of a child having ADHD is increased with increased maternal stress (97, 100).

This area of concern is unfolding slowly. There is a suggestion that antenatal depression, as opposed to postpartum depression, contributes significantly to adverse emotional behavioral and cognitive outcomes. Postpartum depression and environmental factors have a significant confounding effect the development and emotional/behavioral stability. Multiple confounders make this a very difficult area to study. Many more studies with consistent methodologies are needed before definitive associations can be made.

Fetal Programming and Its Relationship to Developmental Outcome

Finding of the relationship between prenatal stress/anxiety/depression is explained by the fetal programming hypothesis. The hypothesis states that factors that stress the fetus, particularly at sensitive periods during development, will disrupt programming of physiological/neurological set points. The result will not become evident until the environment changes later in life. The organism's equilibrating responses will be negatively affected because the programmed set points cannot adapt readily. The resulting maladaptive responses predispose to disease or behavioral/temperamental disorganization. This hypothesis is derived from studies in animals, primarily rats who were subjected to antenatal stress. Stress-related changes in the HPA axis adversely affected behavioral, emotional, and cognitive development (100).

Prenatal Stress and Outcome: Animal Studies

Prenatal stress can adversely affect offspring's ability to learn and to attain developmental milestones. Offspring of stressed dams exhibit depressive and anxiety-related behaviors and appear behaviorally inhibited, exhibiting less exploratory behavior (101). Additionally they exhibit behavioral hyper-arousal, problems with attention, and impaired cognitive functioning (102).

This appears to be mediated by the HPA axis. Cortisol levels are increased in stressed dams. Cortisol levels are also increased in fetuses and CRH may be hypersecreted. These changes may persist till adulthood. These offspring have exaggerated cortisol responses to stress and changes in the circadian rhythm of cortisol secretion (101).

Cortisol Stress and Fetal Programming

In humans the HPA axis has been implicated in adverse pregnancy outcome. Elevated maternal cortisol releasing hormone (CRH) levels in the third trimester are correlated with pre-term labor and fetal growth restriction. CRH plays a role in stimulating synthesis of estrogen by the fetus, which in turn interacts with prostaglandins and oxytocin to stimulate myometrial contractility (103).

Elevated CRH also influences cortisol levels (44). Elevated maternal cortisol at 32 weeks as well as depression and anxiety are associated with negative affect and motor activity, an aspect of infant temperament. This is elicited when a 2-month-old is presented with novel stimuli (95).

Depression is known to influence the HPA in the direction of increased cortisol levels and alterations in the cortisol circadian rhythm. The same correlation persists into pregnancy (44), where elevated cortisol levels are associated not only with depression but also with anxiety and "daily hassles." Though stress was correlated with elevated cortisol, only cortisol, and not stress, was correlated with fetal growth restriction (44).

The studies of fetal programming are intriguing and promising. At this time the field cannot deliver on the promise because of wide variation in the studies. There is wide variation in sample size and wide variation in the definition of maternal stress. Stress is defined at one end by self-report of "daily hassles" and pregnancy specific worries (104) and at the other end by depression, defined by CES-D. Anxiety is defined by the well-validated STAI or by the more generic pregnancy specific worries (105). There is a debate as to the best time of day to take levels, and how to account for disruptions in circadian rhythm related to depression (106). Till these problems are resolved the field remains intriguing but not definitive.

The weight of the evidence appears to associate stress and depression with adverse perinatal outcome. The effect of stress may be a reflection of the size of the studies or the particular group studied. When population studies are used to investigate the effects of psychosocial difficulties the findings from smaller studies sometimes disappear. It is clear that depression confers an increased risk of adverse outcome. It is likely that it contributes to an increased risk of pre-term birth and to behavioral and developmental problems for the children of mothers with antenatal depression. These factors may have different weights in discussion with pregnant women and their families, for environmental factors, as well as treating depression, may alter developmental outcome. There are no studies examining the impact of well-treated depression on pre-term birth or other adverse outcomes.

Treating Depression During Pregnancy

Decisions on how to treat depression during pregnancy take into account a network of factors in which no one factor is definitive. In addition to competing risk/benefit factors the preferences of mother and father and other involved family members must be considered.

Decisions are made based on the factors related to mother, fetus, newborn, and the developmental outcomes. Maternal factors involve understanding of the mother's history of depression and response to treatment, particularly to antidepressants. Risk to the fetus includes teratogenic risk, possibility of intra-uterine death, spontaneous abortion, and fetal growth restriction. Postnatal concerns are neonatal toxicity, developmental problems in infants, and behavioral problems in young children.

There are several variables that impact pregnancy outcomes such as maternal weight and nutritional status, use of abusable substances, use of medication including over the counter drugs, stressful events, and patient's adherence to the medication regimens. These problems are exacerbated by depression.

Pharmacologic Treatment of Depression During Pregnancy

Taking antidepressants is often complicated by stigma and cultural conflicts (15) that lead to problems with adherence and response. This is compounded by anxiety about taking medication during pregnancy by mother, family members, and the other health providers (15). Warnings by regulatory agencies add to anxiety (107). When discussing medication use during pregnancy, the physician should have a clear understanding of how pregnant women and their families perceive taking medication so that discussions can proceed with appropriate reassurance, working through of conflicts, and understanding of the risks and benefits of treatment.

The Risks and Benefits of Pharmacologic Treatment During Pregnancy

The risks of untreated depression, and the benefits of treating depression, have been discussed in the previous sections. This section will focus on the risks of using psychotropic agents during pregnancy. The risk analysis starts with an evaluation of the current mental status. Is the mother depressed or is she euthymic but has a history of depression? What is the severity? Is suicide risk present? What is the impact of the current episode, or past episodes, on appetite and sleep and interpersonal relationships? Is the primary and social network maintained or does depression result in isolation? Has role functioning been impaired?

For women with a first episode of depression the question is always when, if at all, to start antidepressants. It is essential that depression be effectively treated because dominating the analysis of all the debatable risks of untreated depression is the markedly increased risk of postpartum depression (9).

Co-morbid disorders are highly prevalent in depression, particularly substance misuse and anxiety. These have particular relevance in pregnancy. Depressive symptoms increase the risk of relapse of substance misuse whether it is nicotine, alcohol, or heroin. Anxiety adds to the stress load on the fetus, and anxiety and depression increase the risk of postpartum depression (108).

Each woman with a history of depression has a distinct profile of depression and its course. There are several predictors of outcome. The greater the number of episodes, the greater the risk of relapse in the face of stress (21). Other factors are the presence of dysthymia, the nature of the episodes, resilience during episodes, and response to medication, interval to relapse when medication is stopped, speed and quality of response when medication is restarted. Family history, particularly history of postpartum depression and bipolar disorder, is also important.

Women often abruptly stop medication early in pregnancy (109) usually when they first learn they are pregnant (4). This runs the risk of withdrawal symptoms, which are stressful not only to mother but also to the fetus (110). It also increases the risk for relapse.

There are a few general principles for prescribing medication. Coordination among members of the multidisciplinary team involving a psychiatrist and other mental health clinicians, obstetrician, primary care provider, and pediatrician is essential for decision making (4). A single medication, even at higher doses, is preferred over poly-pharmacy. History of previous response to medication is a helpful guide (4). Medications, which have higher levels of protein binding, are less likely to cross the placenta. Sertraline is 99% protein bound and citalopram is 80% protein bound (111). Medications with fewer metabolites and fewer drug interactions are preferred (4).

The choice of medication is confounded by the FDA system for categorizing the risk of different medications. It is often inconsistent and confusing (1). It consists of five categories A, B, C, D, and X. In Category A are medications considered safe to use during pregnancy. Category C, which includes most psychotropic medications, consists of medications for which human studies are lacking and "risk cannot be ruled out." Almost all tricycles and SSRIs are classified as pregnancy category C. Maprotiline, however, is category B. Paroxetine is category D "positive evidence of risk." Most benzodiazepines (BDPs) are categorized as category D and a few hypnotic BDPs as category X (112).

Risk of Malformations

The incidence of congenital malformations in the United States is estimated to between 1 and 3 or 4% (14, 110). Formation of the major organ systems is complete by the end of the first trimester. Each organ system has a critical period during which development takes place. That is the period of greatest susceptibility. Neural tube folding and closure is complete by week 4. Formation of the heart and great blood vessels takes place by 9 weeks after conception. Formation of the lip and palate is completed by 12 weeks (1).

Neuronal migration and differentiation continues through pregnancy. After the first trimester the impact on brain and nervous system becomes evident in long-term behavioral sequelae, behavioral teratogenesis (14).

Very few of the SSRIs and TCAs are associated with teratogenic risk (107, 113, 114). The SSRI, most significantly associated with teratogenic risk, is paroxetine. Several studies (115–117) have supported the association with septal defects and with right ventricular outflow defects. The FDA has issued a public health advisory related to this.

The risk of cardiac malformations with paroxetine appears to be significant enough to warrant consideration during pre-conception counseling. Nonetheless, the risk for cardiac defects is small, approximately 2/1,000 live births (4). If a woman has been exposed during the first trimester fetal echocardiography should be preformed (4). The use of paroxetine is further complicated by troublesome withdrawal symptoms and the need for a slow taper (118). These considerations suggest that paroxetine should not be a first choice in women of child-bearing age.

An increased risk of omphalocele may be associated with sertraline though this is not consistent across studies (114–116). An association between craniosynostosis and SSRIs as a class and also anencephaly and SSRIs appeared in one large case-controlled study (114) but not in others (115, 116). No single SSRI is associated with these malformations.

The risk of omphalocele, craniosynostosis, and anencephaly is extremely small. At baseline, omphalocele is 1/5,000 births, craniosynostosis 1/1,800 births, and anencephaly 1/1,000 births (116). For SSRIs taken during the first trimester odds ratios for these defects range from 2.4 to 2.8 (114), yielding a 2–3-fold increase in these birth defects (114) These findings (114, 115) are confounded by the fact the statistical analysis in each of these studies required over 40 operations to achieve significance (114, 116). This increases the likelihood that the finding is due to chance (114, 119).

The question of teratogenic effects is further confounded by three other recent studies. Einarson (107) collected data on paroxetine taken in the first trimester from eight teratogen services worldwide and combined them with previously published cases. This created a pool of over 3,379 exposed infants who were compared to an equal number of unexposed infants. The study controlled for smoking, alcohol use, socioeconomic status, and demographics. The rate of cardiovascular defects was 0.7% in both groups. The study had enough power to detect a twofold increase. The study is skewed by the population, which consists of women who called a teratogen service. They are primarily well educated and older and have a higher SES. This reduces generalizability.

Berard (120) in another large population study found no association with SSRIs and congenital anomalies. Paroxetine did not have an increase in cardiovascular defects. When adjusting for dose >25 mg a day, however, paroxetine triggered a twofold increase in congenital malformations and a threefold increase in cardiac malformations, mostly septal defects.

Oberlander (121) examined a large population database in British Columbia. No increase in malformation rates was noted for SSRIs or benzodiazepines (BDP) alone. There was a significant increase in malformation rate when BDP and SSRIs were taken together. There was no dose effect as reported by Berard (120).

Adding confusion to the issue is a cohort study using large Danish registries. Pedersen et al. (122) found no increase in the risk of major malformations. They did find statistically significant increases in the risk of septal defects, but not other cardiac malformations, for sertraline and citalopram but not for paroxetine or fluoxetine. This contradicts the findings in other large studies discussed previously. TCAs and venlafaxine were taken by too few women for analysis. It should be noted that the absolute difference between drugs with significant effect and rates of no drugs was small, 0.9% for sertraline vs. 0.5% for unexposed infants. The use of two SSRIs was associated with a fourfold increase in the rate of septal defects.

Venlafaxine does not demonstrate an increased rate of malformations (116, 121, 123). The *N* for these studies is not large and they may not have been adequately powered to detect differences in rare malformations.

Tricyclics (TCA) and bupropion are not associated with congenital malformations (95, 113, 116, 124). Clomipramine is the exception and has been associated with increased rate of VSD and ASD in one large population study (115). The only study examining the phenylpiperazines, trazodone, and nefazodone (125) had a small *N*. There was no evidence of an increased rate of malformations for these medications; again the *N* was not large enough to detect differences in rare malformations.

Mirtazapine was studied prospectively by Djulis (126). Of 99 infants exposed in the first trimester, 2% had major malformations, which did not differ from the control unexposed group. The reliability of this finding is limited by the small *N*. As the authors note it would take 800 cases to detect a twofold increase in common malformations. It would take thousands to detect the same increase in rare malformations. Lennenstal (123), combining three Swedish databases, found no increase in the rate of malformation in 141 exposures. The authors also noted that the power was too small to detect infrequent or rare malformations.

Information on monoamine oxidases (MAOIs) is limited to one small ($n=21$) study (127), where an increased rate of congenital malformations was noted. Because of the risks of hypertensive crisis, MAOIs are relatively contraindicated particularly if general anesthesia is required at delivery (127) or if terbutaline or other tocolytic medications are used to forestall early labor (1).

The suggestion of an association of SSRIs with major malformations is not supported because the findings across studies are so inconsistent. Different malformations appear in different studies, sometimes for the same drug. This is particularly true for paroxetine, where some studies support the association with septal defects and others do not. This confounds the risk benefit analysis and makes it difficult to make a reasonable association of a drug with outcome. Though the evidence is just as conflicted for paroxetine as it is for other SSRIs, the FDA issued an advisory regarding paroxetine and septal defects. In 2006 the risk of septal defects triggered reclassifying paroxetine from pregnancy category C to category D.

In this climate it is difficult to translate the findings into clinical practice or recommendations. Since each of the commonly used SSRIs has been implicated in at least one study it is difficult to determine which drug carries a lower risk. A reasonable approach in the treatment discussion with the mother and her family can include the fact that the risk is very small and the support in the literature is inconsistent. The relatively small risk needs to be evaluated in the context of much larger risks related to depression itself.

The risk analysis is scant comfort if the outcome for your patient's baby is a birth defect. "The stark reality is that pregnancy in the context of a history of affective illness often leaves the mother, the baby, and their doctors between Scylla and Charybdis" (128).

Concerns about the risk of malformations often lead women, or those who treat them early in pregnancy, to recommend stopping antidepressants and then restart them later (129). For many women with histories of depression this strategy is perilous. Not only is there a high rate of risk of relapse but also restarting medication often does not result in a return to baseline (30).

Risk of Spontaneous Abortion

There is a suggestion that antidepressants and SSRIs in particular may increase the rate of spontaneous abortion (SA). The findings are inconsistent with one prospective study of SSRIs (130) showing no increase in stillbirth or spontaneous abortion. Bupropion had a significantly higher rate of spontaneous abortion than controls (131). Neither TCAs (132) nor citalopram (133) demonstrated a difference in SA rates. Trazodone and nefazodone had marginally significant increases in SA (125).

Hemel's (134) review of available literature found 6 out of 15 articles with extractible data that were analyzed for confounders. The rate of spontaneous abortion with all antidepressants was 12.4%. The comparison group's SA rate was 8.7%. The overall relative risk (RR) was 1.45 (1.19–1.77). TCAs did not demonstrate a significant increase in RR but SSRIs and N/SRIs did. This analysis may be distorted because the SA rate in the general population is 12–15% (135). Because of difficulties in collecting and reporting data the true rate of SA is difficult to measure. None of the studies controlled for reproductive history. Confounders also were difficult to control for.

Pre-term Birth and Fetal Growth Restriction (or Small for Gestational Age)

Other aspects of pregnancy outcome also show an increased rate with SSRI/SNRI exposure. Many population studies show an increased rate of pre-term birth (95, 115, 136) or risk of SGA (95, 115, 137). This finding is not consistent, for Hendrick (138) found no increase in pre-term birth or SGA for a cohort of middle class women with no confounders such as smoking or alcohol use. Malm (139), using a Finnish registry, did not find an increase in pre-term birth or SGA. There was no effect of TCAs on either birth weight or gestational age (95, 113). There was no association with SGA and treated depression but there may be an association for untreated depression (12).

The impact of SSRIs varies with degree of exposure. In the same study that considered the impact of depression, Wisner et al. (82) studied the effect of SSRIs on pregnancy outcome. SSRIs that were continued through pregnancy increased the rate of pre-term birth (PTB) OR5.43 (CI 1.98–14.84) compared to women with no SSRI exposure. The risk was also significantly increased compared to women who had taken SSRIs for any two trimesters or less. This very large risk is twice that of the risk of PTB as a result of depression alone as reported in the same study. However, the women who took SSRIs had more severe depression than those who were depressed but did not take SSRIs, or for those women who had only partial SSRI use.

When SSRI use is compared to women with a psychiatric history but no SSRI use during pregnancy, the risk of pre-term birth is increased twofold. This is from a large (more than 50,000 subject obstetrical database) prospective cohort study using a questionnaire during the second trimester, and interviews about medication use and chart review immediately postpartum. Birth-weight was unaffected by SSRI use. As with many other studies, the effect of depression on pregnancy outcome could not be separated from SSRI use. Women who take SSRIs during pregnancy generally tend to have more severe depression and compromised functioning (140).

The weight of the current evidence leans towards increased risk for PTB for women who take SSRIs throughout pregnancy. Nonetheless there are several confounders, chief among them severity of depression and co-morbid disorders, particularly anxiety and substance misuse. These factors independently increase the risk of PTB. These confounders have a large impact on the decision algorithm when the risk of PTB is considered.

Impact of Antidepressants on the Neonate

Neonatal Adaptation

The most well-defined problem affecting prescribing antidepressants during pregnancy is the impact of all SSRIs on neonatal adaptation. Poor neonatal adaptation (PNA) is a pattern of symptoms noted in some babies born to mothers who use antidepressants during the later stages of pregnancy. It is often referred to as a neonatal abstinence syndrome (NAS), and is theorized to be a withdrawal effect similar to the NAS seen with withdrawal from opiates or barbiturates (141). It is characterized by: jitteriness, poor muscle tone, weak or absent cry, respiratory distress, hypoglycemia, low Apgar score, and seizures (142–144). Some studies have also included neonatal jaundice in their evaluations (12, 136). Incidence rates can range from 10% to a high of 30% of exposed infants (12, 136, 145). Two percent of exposed infants have special care admissions (12). The RR for NAS is 3.0 (CI 2.0–4.4) (146).

The rate of NAS/PNA for non-exposed infants is 6–9% (136). Because symptoms can last longer than the usual 1–2 days of postpartum infant observation, it is important to observe infants and educate mothers about potential symptoms.

Treatment is primarily supportive measures and when needed respiratory support. Phenobarbital can be given for severe irritability, rigidity, or seizures (115).

Respiratory distress is the most consistent finding in several studies (12, 95, 123, 137). This is particularly true for third-trimester exposure (95). Respiratory distress typically starts within 3 days after birth and is self-limiting. A variable, but small number of infants will require time in a specialized care nursery or NICU (136, 139). Oberlander (12) found that when severity of depression was factored into analysis of all symptoms of NAS only respiratory distress was related to SSRI use.

Persistent Pulmonary Hypertension

Chambers found a sixfold increase in persistent pulmonary hypertension (PPHTN) in the newborn, but only for women who took SSRIs during the second half of pregnancy. Women who took TCAs or who stopped antidepressants in the first 20 weeks of pregnancy did not have infants with an increased rate of PPHTN. The baseline rate for this rare disorder is 1/1,000. Putative mechanisms are related to higher levels of circulating serotonin which has vasoconstrictive properties and which stimulates proliferation of smooth muscle cells, the chief pathological finding in PPHTN (147).

Since the initial study by Chambers, two more studies of this rare outcome have been published. They reflect the difficulty is ascertaining the true risk.

Andrade et al. (148) used a case-controlled study of an HMO research database. The study found no difference in rate between SSRI use in each trimester and unexposed neonates. As the authors note, the study was powered to detect sixfold difference but not a twofold difference. It is possible that this is a type 2 error and there is an increased risk, though not as large as reported by Chambers and Kallen (see below).

Using the Swedish birth registry of all infants born in Sweden between 1977 and 2005, Kallen et al. (149) found an increased RR of 2.4 (CI 1.2–4.3) for all infants for whom information on exposure was available. Unfortunately medication status in the registry was only available for the first trimester and many women taking SSRIs who were prescribed by outpatient prescribers were not recorded. Where information on SSRI exposure for the last trimester was available (2,413 women of the 7,587 cases in first trimester), the RR was 3.6 (CI 1.2–8). This study was adequately powered to detect a small increase in risk. The result is midway between Chambers and Andrade. It is confounded by the probability that many women had medication prescribed but were not entered into the database. Though the lower rate of SSRI for the third trimester is consistent with most studies and clinical experience, it is possible that a large number of women still taking SSRIs in the third trimester were missed. Furthermore comparison with Andrade and Chambers is confounded by the lower PHTN rate of 0.05% for the Swedish study compared to the rate in the United States of 1–2%. This study was powered to detect a very small (twofold) increase in risk. As such it lends weight to the possible risk of PHTN in the newborn. There is enough of a suggestion of increased risk of PHTN in the newborn to recommend including it in the risk analysis where appropriate.

Non-SSRIs

Trazodone and nefazodone (the two phenylpiperazine antidepressants) have not been evaluated with respect to NAS or PNA. Einarson et al. (125) followed a cohort of 147 women on these drugs and found no increase in malformation or problematic pregnancy outcomes. The *N* was substantial but the study may not have been powered enough to give definitive answers.

TCAs, compared to SSRIs, confer a slightly increased risk for respiratory distress, hypoglycemia and neonatal convulsions (95, 136), and temperature-regulation disorders (95). Anticholinergic effects of TCAs present an additional challenge to the neonate. Functional bowel obstruction and urinary retention have been reported (14). Apgar scores are not adversely affected by TCAs (113).

There is an increased risk of neonatal convulsions with clomipramine (CMI), and the risk is slightly increased with TCAs as well (136). These are withdrawal seizures, which are related to declining blood levels of CMI (150).

There are very limited data on duloxetine. Eyal and Yaeger (151) report a single case of a woman on 90 mg of duloxetine who came to their attention in her 36th week. Dose was reduced to 60 mg with no relapse of depression. The neonate had classic signs of PNA, particularly respiratory distress. Whether this is typical for duloxetine or a random finding awaits further study. Briggs (152) reported a case of a mother who took duloxetine through the second half of pregnancy. The baby was born full term and of normal weight. Apgars at 1 and 5 min were 8 and 9, respectively.

Umbilical Cord Levels

Umbilical cord blood levels of SSRIs are significantly lower than in maternal serum. Ratios range from 0.29 to 0.89, and sertraline levels are significantly lower than fluoxetine (153). Though levels are lower serotonin turnover is higher in the fluoxetine or citalopram exposed fetus (154). For exposed infants there is a negative correlation between lowered 5HIAA levels in cord blood and PNA scores and there is a positive correlation between 5-HIAA levels and lower Apgar scores at 15 min seen in exposed children (154).

Managing NAS

Interventions to reduce risk of NAS/PNA are very limited. The only intervention is to taper SSRIs gradually late in the last trimester. The regulatory agencies in the United States and Canada have weighed in judiciously on this issue. Though there were reports of a Health Canada recommendation to taper during the last 2 weeks or the third trimester (145), an update has not advised any specific interventions (155). The FDA has suggested, but not recommended, a taper during the last trimester (156).

The suggestion to taper has been guardedly supported in some discussions of treatment (145), but only after women discuss the risks and benefits with their doctors and taper as gradually as possible over several weeks. A very gradual taper is recommended because of the risk of withdrawal syndromes on abrupt discontinuation (145, 157, 158). Miller (159) suggests that the taper should start at 35 weeks and reduce by 25% of current dose every 2 weeks. This gives time for only two dose reductions, which may not be enough if doses are higher than 20 mg of citalopram or 50 mg of sertraline. For fluoxetine, with its long half-life, the taper would have to start 6–8 weeks before the estimated due date (EDD). Starting a taper sooner than 2 weeks before the EDD may expose the mother to a prolonged period without protection against depressive relapse. As noted above the relapse rate for medication discontinued during pregnancy is 68% (30). The timing of the taper is also complicated by the unpredictability of onset of labor and birth. There are no studies of taper (146).

If a decision is made to discontinue antidepressants, Miller (159) has suggested some practical criteria for a taper. The mother's mood should be euthymic. The mother should have insight and be able to seek help if she becomes depressed. There should be minimal stress, good social support, and a history of a depression characterized by mild severity, no refractory episodes, or high-risk episodes.

Clearly the risk of NAS/PNA (30%) with its transient symptoms and infrequent neonatal nursery admissions (2%) has to be weighed against the risk of relapse (68%) and the marked increase in the risk of postpartum depression in untreated depression. The extended period of time for a withdrawal-free taper may pose unconscionable risks for the mother's wellbeing.

Developmental Risks

Behavioral teratology associated with SSRI use in pregnancy has been addressed in a small number of studies. Casper (160), in a small prospective study, found that exposed infants had lower scores on the Bayley Scale of Infant Development (BSID). The major findings were a slight delay in psychomotor development, subtle changes in fine motor control, and very mild tremulousness.

Misri (161) found no increase in internalizing behavior at age 4 for children exposed to SSRIs in pregnancy. Internalizing behavior is defined as emotional reactivity, depressed mood, anxiety, irritability, and withdrawal.

Oberlander (162) studied externalizing behavior, defined as non-compliance, disruptive acts, verbal/physical aggression, and emotional outbursts, in a small cohort of 4-year-old children who were exposed to SSRIs during pregnancy. There was no difference in externalizing behaviors between these children and non-exposed children. However, *N* in this study was very small, 22 exposed and 14 not exposed.

Nulman (163) looking at 40 children whose mothers were taking fluoxetine in pregnancy and 46 who were taking TCAs found no difference with matched pairs on measures of cognition , language development, or temperament at age 15–71 months. There was, however, a negative association for severity of maternal depression and IQ, and a positive association with number of episodes of depression and delayed language development.

In a large study utilizing a Danish registry, Pedersen et al. (164) conducted a prospective case-controlled study. Women exposed to SSRIs in the second or third trimester were interviewed by telephone about their children's developmental milestones at 6 and 19 months. The control group was women who were depressed during pregnancy but not taking medication for depression. Gross motor delays at 6 months in the exposed group resolved by 19 months. Delays in attention remained at 19 months. Though these delays had statistical significance, they were within the normal range and were not clinically significant. There were no direct observations of the infants, and postpartum depression was not adequately controlled for. Postpartum depression has a significant adverse impact on attention and development.

As noted in a review of studies available through the end of 2009 (165), there are several problems with all the studies. None carry the analysis through the first school years when cognitive and developmental delays often become evident. Only Nulman's studies controlled for maternal IQ. The majority of the studies used the gold standard BSID. This scale has reduced classification accuracy in younger groups. As was the case with the Pedersen study, the impact of postpartum maternal depression was not taken into account in several of the studies, and severity of depression was not evaluated.

It is reassuring that a significant majority of these studies did not demonstrate an association between behavioral teratology or developmental delays and SSRIs taken during pregnancy. Nonetheless more studies and meta-analyses would certainly help define this important area.

Prescribing Antidepressants During Pregnancy

When an expectant mother has decided to take antidepressants there are several considerations in choosing a drug. Considerations include the individual patient's responses to medication, potential toxicity and side effects of the drug for both mother and fetus, and efficacy of the drug. The goal of treatment is remission of symptoms if possible.

The risks and benefits of each of the antidepressants have already been discussed.

Dosing Considerations During Pregnancy

There are several pharmacokinetic changes that occur during pregnancy that impact the metabolism of the antidepressants. Rates of absorption are altered by an increase in gastric acidity, a decrease in gastric motility, and changes in the activity of CP450 enzymes in the gut wall. This results in increased degradation of the drug in the stomach and decreased absorption from the gut (166, 167). Hepatic blood flow is diminished (168), and there are estrogen-induced changes in hepatic CYP450 enzymes (167). Metabolic activity of CYP2D6 (169), 2C9, and 3A3/4 is increased during pregnancy (166) and activity of CYP 1A2 and CYP 2C19 is decreased (166). The result is increased metabolism of drugs such as fluoxetine, which is metabolized primarily by 2D6 and 3A3/4. Citalopram has a complex metabolic pathway via CYP 2D6 28%, 3A3/4 (34%), and 2C19 37%. Because of polymorphisms in 2D6 and 2C19 as well as age-related changes in 3A3/4, it is difficult to predict which women will need to have the dose of citalopram, or other SSRIs for that matter, increased during pregnancy.

The volume of distribution is altered during pregnancy because of an increase in body water. This alters drug distribution, and peak serum concentrations of many drugs are decreased. Pregnancy-induced decreases in albumin increase free drug concentration by reducing protein binding. Since free drug is the moiety available for drug action the effects may cancel each other out (168). Nonetheless for each woman drug distribution may differ depending on the nutritional status and the weight changes during pregnancy.

The glomerular filtration rate increases as well. This primarily affects drugs that are almost exclusively excreted by the kidneys such as lithium (168). It has minimal effect on antidepressants.

There have been a few case series examining changes in dosage during pregnancy. Dose increases were required for a majority of women taking TCAs. To restore euthymia and bring blood levels back to the therapeutic range the average dose had to be increased by 70–80%, usually after week 20. Some patients do not exhibit a decline in blood levels till the third trimester (170, 171).

SSRIs exhibit a similar profile. After week 20, 70–80% of women relapse and require dose increases, usually 1.8 times the dose at conception (172, 173). In spite of declines in levels of SSRIs not all women require dose increases. Though trough levels for citalopram (174) and fluoxetine (175) were ½ postpartum levels, only 2 of 19 women suffered a relapse of depressive symptoms and required a dose increase.

The ratio of metabolites to parent drug increases after the 20th week. L/D ratios of citalopram shift to the less active D stereoisomer starting at the 20th week. This returns to baseline 2 weeks postpartum (173). Similarly there is an increase in DM-citalopram and norfluoxetine metabolites after the 20th week, which returns to baseline by the second week postpartum (175).

Measuring blood levels in the first, second, and third trimesters may provide some guidance, but not all women suffer a depressive relapse. The best approach is careful clinical observation and a strong therapeutic alliance. Doses may have to be decreased in postpartum weeks 2–4.

Other Somatic Treatments

Electroconvulsive Therapy

Electroconvulsive therapy (ECT) is an important treatment option in many situations. ECT is recommended when medication is not feasible or depression has been unresponsive to many medication trials. It is also recommended in depression with high risk of malnutrition or suicide or where waiting 4 weeks for medication to take effect is too risky (176). It is an effective therapy – 80–90% of treated patients show improvement (177) and 50% of treatment-resistant depressions respond (178).

The American Psychiatric Association (70) has endorsed ECT for use in all three trimesters of pregnancy, though during the first 8 weeks of pregnancy the teratogenic effects of anesthesia must be considered. Nonetheless the APA considers that the risk from anesthesia is unlikely to be greater than that from medication. Fetal heart rate should be monitored during and after treatment. High-risk pregnancy, where there is a risk of induction of premature labor, may be a relative contraindication (179).

Numerous case reports of a positive outcome with harm to neither mother nor fetus have been published (180). Ecchevarria (181) reviewed all cases reported in the literature from 1942 to 1992 – a total of 318 case reports. There were 28 cases where complications were reported – arrhythmias, vaginal bleeding, uterine contractions, and premature labor and miscarriage. There were three cases of neonatal death and one of respiratory distress. Confounding factors were not reported. Additional cases have been reported since then with fetal heart rate deceleration, and cases of uterine contractions requiring tocolytic medication (182).

It is difficult to assess the true significance of these outcomes. Case reports are often skewed towards negative outcomes. ECT is usually given to women who are extremely depressed. Some case reports describe psychotic depression or schizophrenia and high risk of self-harm or anorexia (180, 181, 183, 184). Other reports have not included clinical description at the time ECT was given (182, 185, 186).

The outcome of these cases was variable with some pregnancies carried to term without complication (180, 186) and some ending in miscarriage (181) or pre-term birth (183).

Theoretically, ECT could induce early labor. ECT releases oxytocin whose level peaks a few minutes after the seizure (187). Oxytocin increases uterine tone and can stimulate uterine contraction. Other hormones released during ECT such as vasopressin, cortisol, or an increase in parasympathetic tone do not have an effect on the uterus or fetus (187). Walker (187) recommends having tocolytic agents on hand and recommends measuring fetal heart rate during ECT and shortly afterward as well.

The severity of depression and related psychosis makes the choice clear – the risk to the fetus would be far greater if ECTs were not given. Since there is little evidence to support the safety of ECT during pregnancy, and little evidence to contraindicate its use, ECT should be reserved for those cases where the mother's life is in danger, or depression is so severe that self-care and mother's health are at risk.

Transcranial Magnetic Stimulation

Transcranial magnetic stimulation (TCMS) (188) is a promising new treatment which has been approved by the FDA for treatment of Major Depressive Disorder. Theoretically, it should not affect the fetus. Magnetic pulses stimulate the prefrontal cortex only and reach only to the uppermost layers of the cortex. It is unlikely that pulses reach as far as the fetus. Pulses can be targeted unlike ECT. No seizure is induced which decreases the risk of pre-term labor. No sedation or anesthesia is required as the case with ECT. There is no adverse cognitive posttreatment effect. This treatment needs to be studied in pregnancy but, like many interventions for depression during pregnancy, the off-label use of a treatment becomes the initial clinical trial.

Managing Mood Disorders in the Postpartum Period

Postnatal depression presents a different set of challenge for the perinatal clinician. Not only must the clinician deal with treating mood disorders but also deal with the question of breast-feeding and its impact on the infant.

Postpartum Blues and Postpartum Depression

Onset Prevalence and Risk Factors

During the first few weeks postpartum 50–80% of women will experience postpartum blues, a short-lived episode of depressed mood, tearfulness emotional lability, irritability, and anxiety (189). This subsides in a matter of hours to 2–3 days (189). Twenty-five percent of this group will develop postpartum depression (190).

The first challenge in treating postpartum depression is recognition. Many common postpartum experiences, such as lack of sleep, fatigue, irritability, and difficulty concentrating are components of the criteria for an MDE (191). This overlap contributes to the low rate of recognition, for symptoms of depression are dismissed as normal for new baby care.

Prolonged postpartum blues lasting more than a week suggest the presence of a clinically significant mood disorder, but this is frequently dismissed as just postpartum blues (192, 193). Providers and mothers and significant others collude in not recognizing postpartum depression (194). In a review of the literature, Dennis outlined several factors contributing to poor recognition. Maternal factors resonate with provider reluctance to diagnose depression. Shame and concerns about stigma are prominent factors. Many cultures, including many Americans, separate somatic symptoms from emotional problems. Health providers are then considered inappropriate for dealing with emotional problems. Lack of knowledge about postpartum depression on the part of providers and mothers prevents recognition in many cases (194).

Women do not disclose depressive symptoms to their families because they are afraid of being perceived as burdensome or they would "give the family a bad name" (194). There are also cultural factors such as the perception that being able to endure and persevere through depression is a sign being a "strong black woman" (15). Another is the "myth of happy mothering" (195). This is a common myth that mothers who are happy in their new role and are fulfilled in mothering are good mothers (195).

Lack of recognition poses a public health problem. Postpartum depression is highly prevalent and detrimental to the child's development and the mother's ability to function.

The prevalence of depression postpartum is increased over the prepartum rate though some studies have shown that the 1-month prevalence is only slightly higher than during pregnancy (11). It is also not statistically higher than during pregnancy (2, 196) or than in the general population (2). This is confounded by Vesga-Lopez's (13) community survey, which is the gold standard for assessing prevalence. Additionally, 50% of new episodes occur postpartum (11, 197).

For the majority of women, the onset of depression usually occurs within the first few weeks or months after delivery (198). However, for some mothers, the onset of depressive symptoms occurred after 12 weeks and others much later, between 6 and 12 months (198).

A systematic review of 30 studies evaluating the prevalence and incidence of postpartum depression found that the prevalence of major and minor depressions began to rise following delivery with the highest increase being 12.9% at 3 months. The prevalence then declined slightly in the 4th–7th month (9.9–10.6%), and declined even further to 6.6% in the 8th–12th month (2). As such, the presence of depressive symptoms remains fairly high for the first 6 months postpartum before it starts to decline.

The public health implications are significant. Since the rate of postpartum depression is higher than the general population and rises for the first 3 months, there are a large number of infants exposed to maternal depression and its adverse effect on development.

A range of risk factors has been associated with postpartum depression, similar to the risk factors for depression during pregnancy. A core risk factor is depression during pregnancy or any history of depression prior to pregnancy (11, 199–201). Other core risk factors are: antenatal anxiety, major life events, lack of practical/emotional support, or lack of partner support (201). Pregnancy, labor, delivery, and new motherhood may be stressors that contribute to the onset of depression (11).

Thoughts or concerns about dying during the first month and difficulty falling asleep during first month (200) postpartum can also be indicators of potential postpartum depression. These may represent subsyndromal depressive symptoms.

Additional stressors contributing to postpartum depression include physical abuse before, during, or after pregnancy, loss of a partner, chronic conflict with a partner, rejection of the pregnancy by mother or partner, traumatic events during pregnancy, and financial stress during pregnancy (196). These are similar to risk factors for MDD during pregnancy.

Hormonal changes may play a role in the onset of postpartum depression though this association has not been definitely established. Within a few days after delivery daily levels of estrogen fall rapidly, along with progesterone and cortisol and human chorionic gonadotropin (192). Though withdrawal of estrogen is thought to precipitate postpartum depression (202, 203) the results are equivocal (192, 204). Withdrawal of estrogen and other hormones may not exert a direct effect but, as with the onset of depression in the general population and during pregnancy, the change in hormone balance may alter the modulation of serotonin receptors in vulnerable women (23, 192, 205, 206).

Risk Posed by Postpartum Depression to Mother and Infant

Morbidity for mother and child has been well documented. Mothers who have postpartum depression which resolves have a twofold risk of another episode within 5 years (23). Mothers may suffer from difficulty with parenting. They may experience difficulty with attachment and bonding, they may provide mechanical care, they may be more irritable (207), and have thoughts of harming their infant and fear being alone. They exhibit less verbal and play-time interaction with their infants (207).

Infant and child development is also adversely affected. The infants sleep poorly and cry more frequently and for longer duration (208–210). Children of mothers with postpartum depression are at increased risk of behavioral inhibition (211).

Infants of mothers with postpartum depression have poorer performance on cognitive tasks at 18 months and boys perform significantly less well than girls (210). By 5 years cognitive performance deficits were no longer evident but the children were reported to have more behavioral problems (212). The effect at 18 months was thought to be mediated by mother's speech, which was less infant-focused and more negative.

The magnitude of the effect on child behavioral problems is not modest. Beck (213) in her 1999 meta-analysis found a moderate effect size ($r=0.29$, $d=0.61$).

Treating Postpartum Depression

The adverse effects of depression on both mother and child highlight the importance of treating postpartum depression effectively. American College of Obstetricians and Gynecologists (4) recommends continuing antidepressants started during pregnancy and starting antidepressants promptly at the onset of postpartum depression. Unfortunately these recommendations are not often implemented. Less than 25% of depressed women seek treatment (214, 215). There are several barriers to women's acceptance of medication.

Dennis (194) in her 2008 review identified several barriers to pharmacological treatment. As is the case in the general population many women believe their symptoms will resolve spontaneously. They also are concerned about stigma and fear addiction to antidepressants. In addition they are concerned about potential long-term as yet unknown harm from antidepressants. Among breast-feeding women acceptability of medication was particularly low because of fear of transmitting drugs to their baby.

A variety of psychotherapies have proved effective in postpartum depression (194, 216). A Cochrane review (194) identified Inter-personal Psychotherapy (IPT) and Cognitive Behavioral Therapy (CBT) as being effective. Prevention strategies include psychoeducation, support groups, and psychosocial interventions (216).

Pharmacodynamic considerations in the postpartum impact the dose of antidepressant. For some patients the prepartum dose had to be changed. The blood level declines to pre-conception levels for most patients between 2 weeks and 2 months (173–175). Metabolism does not return to baseline till 12 weeks when, for example, L/D ratios of citalopram return to normal (173).

If postpartum depression is left untreated there are significant risks to mother, infant, and to the relationship. If postpartum depression is treated the primary risk factors involve breast-feeding. The concerns about infant exposure to antidepressants will be dealt with in the next section.

Breast-Feeding

Breast-feeding is considered the best source of nutrition for the newborn infant, and it is recommended as the only source of nutrition for the infant during the first 6 months of life (217). The benefits of breast-feeding are many: lower rates of infectious diseases (218–220), lower rates of metabolic disease (221), and lower rates of atopic diseases (222).

At least 60% of women initiate breast-feeding (223) and at least 5–10% of those women will have symptoms of depression requiring treatment. Based on these figures, approximately a quarter of a million women will be breast-feeding and will be candidates for taking antidepressants (224).

Treatment of women with postpartum depression who are considering breast-feeding presents several challenges. The clinician must weigh the risk of stopping antidepressants for at least 6 months against the potential adverse effects for the infant from drug excreted into mother's milk. The goal is to minimize the infant's exposure as much as possible while maintaining a level of medication adequate to effectively treat the mother's depression and prevent relapse.

Antidepressants, as is the case with most drugs, are transferred in to milk by passive diffusion. Thus, levels in milk vary as blood levels in the mother rise or fall (225). Maternal blood levels vary with several factors including body weight, albumin levels, and hepatic function, particularly function of the CYP 450 system (166, 167). Thus, as pharmacodynamics return to pre-pregnancy status over the first month postpartum (173) concentration of antidepressants in milk will rise in concert with an increase in the mother's blood level. It should be noted, however, that changes in blood levels do not occur in all women during pregnancy (see Section "Dosing Considerations During Pregnancy") and so each patient needs be evaluated individually.

The standard index for evaluating the amount of milk that reaches the infant is the milk plasma ratio (M/P) (168, 225). An M/P ratio of less than 1 indicates that transfer into breast milk is relatively low (168, 225, 226). Several antidepressants are reported to have M/P ratios higher than 1. Tables 1 and 2 summarize data from two reviews (225, 226) and one pooled analysis (227) of M/P ratios. As can be seen individual M/P ratios vary widely from study to study. The intra-drug differences are not necessarily dose-related.

Furthermore, not all studies report whether they sampled foremilk or hind milk. Paroxetine in one study (228) was sampled from foremilk only. This would give a lower level than hindmilk or pooled foremilk and hindmilk. The lack of differentiation for sampling times and foremilk vs. hindmilk makes it difficult to wrest clinical utility from the reported research (229). Furthermore, a single breast-milk

Table 1 From Gentile (225)

Drug	*N*	M/P range	Dose range (mg)
Paroxetine	67	0.09–3.33	20–50
Fluoxetine	71	0.28–3.29	20–60
Norfluoxetine[a]	70	0.08–1.4	
Sertraline	79	0.53–2.3 ± 1.3[b]	50–200
DM sertraline[c]	27	0.6–1.64 ± 0.19[b]	
Citalopram	45	0.93–2.24	20–60
DM citalopram	43	0.9–6.3[b]	
Escitalopram	8	1.7–2.7	10–20
Fluvoxamine	6	0.29–1.59	50–200

[a]One study with an *N* of 1 did not measure norfluoxetine
[b]Not all studies reported means with SD, two studies did not report DM-CIT
[c]Several studies did not measure DM-SER independently

Table 2 From Gentile (226); Weissman (227) (227–228)

Drug	*N*	M/P range	Dose range
Venlafaxine*	14	2.5–4.8	
O-DM VLFX		2.7–3.8	
Bupropion**	1	7.1	300
Desipramine**	1	1.2	175
Imipramine**	4	1.1–2.0 mean 1.4	75–200 mg
Notriptyline**	35	0–2.4 mean 0.6	50–150 mg
Amitriptyline**	5	0–1.6 mean 0.8	75–175 mg

* From Gentile 2005 (226)
** From Weissman 2004 (227)

measurement is problematic and exhibits greater variability than multiple samples (230, 231). For these reasons sampling of breast-milk is generally not clinically useful.

Another guide for clinicians is the relative infant dose (RID) as a percent of the mother's weight adjusted dose (226, 232). The notional safety limit is a conservative 10%. Newborns have 20% or more of the maternal capacity to clear drug, and this reaches adult levels at 6 months (225). This calculation is not reported consistently. When it is reported the RID for most antidepressants is well below 10%. Mirtazapine is reported as 3.9–4.4% depending on the sampling of foremilk or hind milk (which has a higher concentration of mirtazapine) (231). The RID for fluoxetine is reported as 6.8% (230), 10.8% (233), and 3–10% (234). Inter-individual differences can be quite wide. For one infant RID was 12% (230). Spigset (235) reported a range of 0.7–5.9% for the RID.

Measurement of blood levels in infants is unreliable and a single level may not be meaningful. The timing of the sample in relation to breast-feeding and the amount of breast milk taken in each feeding can influence the level. For example, sertraline exhibits a twofold gradient between foremilk and hind milk (236). Peak levels in breast milk are variable for each drug often lagging 2 h behind maternal peak levels and different drugs peak at different intervals (227). For fluoxetine, the peak breast milk level is usually 8 h (226). The intra-patient level may also vary (227). The solution to these problems is to take several samples over a prolonged period of time and calculate the AUC (227). This is highly invasive and distressing to the infant and not practical. Additionally, infant levels are often less than 2 ng/ml, and are undetectable by commercial labs.

Even when research quality assays are used undetectable levels can occur in situations that make no sense. Berle (237) phenotyped mothers and infants for a number of CYP450 enzymes. In a mother and infant pair both homozygous for the poor metabolizer phenotype and genotype (homozygous for the inactivating CYP450*4 genotype) the infant had undetectable levels of paroxetine in spite of robust levels in mother and in breast milk. Other genotypes ranging from homozygous for the high metabolizer allele (CYP4502D6*1) to heterozygous for high and normal metabolizer alleles also exhibited inconsistent infant levels. This study, unlike many others, calculated fore and hind milk gradients and took multiple samples of serum from infants in order to calculate AUC for infant levels.

Serotonin transporter blockade is another measure of infant exposure. In 14 mother–infant breast-feeding pairs, where mothers were taking sertraline, maternal platelet 5HT levels were significantly reduced. The infants showed no reduction in 5HT platelet levels. The infant blood levels were at or below the level of detection.

From this data, inconsistent as it is, it appears that most infants have virtually no detectible levels of antidepressant and suffer no consequences from the drug they ingest. Nonetheless some infants do have greater exposure and require more careful monitoring.

At this time the only meaningful method for assessing the effects of infant exposure is clinical. Several studies and reviews have evaluated infant clinical response (204, 224, 225, 228, 236, 238, 239), Heikkenen (175) found very few adverse effects. Some of these were probably not related to the drug. There are, for example, occasional case reports of adverse impact with fluoxetine which were transient and for which there were no long-term sequelae. One of the few severe reports was of an infant who required 3 days in the NICU. The baby was feverish, somnolent, and unresponsive (240).

Long-term studies need to be done particularly to assess the neuro-behavioral impact of antidepressants in breast-feeding. Heikennen (175) followed infants up to 1 year using neurological exams, pediatrician exams, and Gesell developmental schedules (which screen for gross and fine motor function, speech development, and social behavior). All of the infants were classified as reaching normal milestones. There do not appear to be any adverse neuro-developmental sequelae for children of mothers who take TCAs and breast feed (163).

Lee (6) did a study comparing 31 breastfeeding women with MDD on citalopram, 12 depressed and breast-feeding women not in medication, and 31 women with no psychiatric disorder who were breast-feeding. No differences in infant outcome were noted.

Two infants whose mother's were taking venlafaxine had normal neuro-behavioral development when followed for first 6 months (241).

Choosing a Drug

Though use of the M/P has become the standard of care (232) its clinical utility appears limited. Other guidelines are the American Academy of Pediatrics guidelines (242) (summarized in Ragan, K) (232), which rates antidepressants globally as "unknown but may be of concern." Hale's lactation risk categories (243) list most TCAs and SSRIs or dual action ADs as L2 (safer) with the exception of doxepin L5 (contraindicated) and maprotiline, citalopram, bupropion, venlafaxine, and mirtazapine which are listed as L3 (moderately safe).

Ragan (232) reviewed the 2005 PDR and found it was not very helpful. Most drugs have no comment. According to the PDR (2007) fluoxetine and duloxetine are not recommended, caution is advised for paroxetine and sertraline and desipramine. For venlafaxine and bupropion, the PDR (2007) recommends deciding to discontinue either drug or nursing. For doxepin it should be noted that the contraindicated finding is based on one case report of infant respiratory depression (4, 159).

A useful guide is the web site Drugs and Lactation Database (LactMed), (http://toxnet.nlm.nih.gov/cgi-bin/sis/htmlgen?LACT) from the National Library of Medicine. It reviews the data available for every drug.

The final decision rests on strictly clinical data. The American College of Obstetrics and Gynecologists (ACOG) 2008 (4) and American Academy of Pediatrics (232) both recommend not drawing serum levels in the neonate. Similarly assays for breast milk do not have much clinical utility.

A clinical approach would first evaluate the impact on the mother of discontinuing medication. How likely is relapse in the first 6 months of breast-feeding (the length of time breast-feeding has a significant positive effect on the infant). How likely is a depressed mother to use or resume using cigarettes, alcohol, or drugs? How well will the mother respond to non-pharmacologic treatment? How does a relapse of depression affect the mother's relationship with her support system? How will a relapse affect care of her baby.

If antidepressant medications are continued the question of weaning or not breast-feeding need to be addressed. After all breast-feeding is a recommendation not a requirement.

If both medication and breast-feeding continue, a practical approach was outlined by Newport (216) and by Ragan (232). Use medication for which there has been a prior positive response. If the infant has been exposed to a particular drug during pregnancy that drug should be continued postpartum. Monotherapy is preferred even if higher doses are needed. Use medication with established clinical data.

The exception to the suggestion of using established drugs is duloxetine (152). If a mother has responded to duloxetine during or before pregnancy continuation during breast-feeding can be considered. There is only one case report for this drug. The RID was 8.2% and the M/P was 1.2. The infant showed no adverse effects from 0 to 32 days.

If the mother has a first episode of depression available evidence suggests that sertraline might be a reasonable choice. Most of the infant blood levels in a pooled analysis (227) were zero. There have been no case reports of adverse infant reactions to breast-feeding with sertraline on board. However, the *N* for sertraline, though higher than most reported SSRIs, is still quite low, and even if it appears safer the exposed infant should be monitored carefully for signs of a medication effect.

Guidelines to Consider in Deciding on Continuing Medication (These Guidelines Are Adapted from di Scalea (244))

1. A risk/benefit analysis
   - (a) Mother – risk of relapse of depression with and without medication
   - (b) Infant – risk of adverse effects from ingestion of drug in milk
   - (c) Mother–infant pair – risk of disruption of breast-feeding
   - (d) A discussion with mother and father regarding the risks and benefits of medication and the alternatives
2. For mild to moderate depression psychotherapy should be considered as the first line treatment
3. For moderate to severe depression antidepressants should be considered, particularly for women who have not responded to psychotherapy alone
4. Clinical factors that impact the decision to use medication and weigh heavily on the side of using antidepressants are
   - (a) Presence of suicidal ideation and/or psychotic symptoms
   - (b) Bipolar depression
   - (c) Impaired self-care and/or anorexia with significant weight loss
   - (d) Previous history of relapse when medication has been discontinued
   - (e) Was medication started during or before pregnancy? Was the response robust?
   - (f) History of break through depression particularly if severe
   - (g) The presence of markedly impaired relationships and withdrawal from social support
   - (h) Depressive symptoms that interfere with adequate care of the infant
     - a. Impaired maternal bonding
     - b. Severe anxiety that interferes with caring for the infant

   c. Withdrawal, constriction of emotional responses, or irritability and anger in response to infant demands

5. If the infant exhibits possible adverse effects such as irritability , jitteriness, poor sleep, and feeding difficulties consider the following:
   (a) Rule out other causes in consultation with the pediatrician
   (b) Try breast-feeding at of trough levels (this is often impractical)
   (c) Weigh the risks of discontinuing medication vs. the lower risk of discontinuing breastfeeding
   (d) If medication is discontinued monitor closely for depressive relapse, compromised functioning, anxiety which impairs functioning, and adverse maternal responses to the infant

6. For first episode depression consider sertraline.

Conclusion

How is a clinician to thread his/her way through the briar patch of conflicting evidence? There are few, if any, thorn-free paths. Some aspects of treatment are clear. Depression is debilitating for most people. Being depressed during pregnancy poses more problems for the mother than for the general population because of increased demands and expectations and stressors. Though this may not be true for every woman it is true for the majority. Each patient has to be assessed individually based on her own clinical profile.

Untreated depression may or may not pose a risk to the fetus or the course of pregnancy. The data on risk to the fetus in the first trimester are so confounded and contradictory that it provides little clear guidance. What is clear is that the risks for malformations are very small, compared to the risk of untreated depression for the mother. This is also true for the risk of pulmonary hypertension in the newborn. It is also clear that there is a withdrawal syndrome that affects up to 30% of all infants. Though this is often troubling to the mother and family in risk benefit discussions, it does not appear to pose a significant threat to the infant, and only a very small proportion have to spend time in the NICU.

Whatever risks for pregnancy outcome may or may not be present it is clear that the risk for postpartum depression is markedly increased for any woman with a history of depression or onset of depression during pregnancy. Considering the adverse effect of postpartum depression on infant and child development, and on inter-personal relationships, screening for, and treating, depression and anxiety is an essential part of perinatal care.

Medication is a core modality in the treatment of depression Though many women are reluctant to continue or start antidepressants for fear of harming their baby, the weight of the evidence is that untreated, or partially treated depression is more harmful than the risks of medication.

Each pregnant woman deserves careful evaluations for depression and anxiety and ongoing discussions with her perinatal clinicians about how to best treat her depression both prepartum and postpartum.

The guidelines for treating depression during pregnancy are similar to the guidelines for breastfeeding. These are based on the ACOG recommendations for 2009 (245) and the author's clinical experience.

1. Screening for depression and anxiety should be done at the first prenatal visit and every trimester thereafter, as well as 6 weeks, 3, 6 months, and 1 year postpartum.
2. The decision to treat with medication is first and foremost a shared decision on the part of the mother, father, and family (if involved). It is a risk benefit decision colored by personal preferences on the part of the mother. It involves extensive discussions with concerned parties at several points during pregnancy. Other members of the mental health team as well as the obstetrical clinician should be involved. In our perinatal psychiatric clinic we have a bi-weekly mental health rounds as well as frequent hallway consultations.
3. If the mother to be is not currently depressed but there is history of depression, then careful monitoring is in order. If there are significant stressors, or anxiety is present, then therapy is recommended. Stress and anxiety as well as a history of depression increase the risk of depression during pregnancy.
4. Parameters *C, and D* which are outlined above in the section on breast-feeding apply equally when treating antenatal depression.
5. In addition to the factors outlined above additional factors that weight the risk equation more heavily on the medication side are:
   (a) A history of at least one episode of depression pre-pregnancy
      a. If this was mild–moderate then a trial of psychotherapy is warranted.
   (b) A history of postpartum depression.
6. Choosing an antidepressant.
   (a) No single SSRI is considered safer or more effective than any other.
   (b) Bupropion is probably the safest antidepressant. There is no evidence that it has increased risk of malformation, pre-eclampsia, or pre-term birth. There are no reports of NAS.
   (c) Mirtazapine, venlafaxine, and duloxetine appear safe but the studies are not large enough to confirm this.
   (d) TCAs are not associated with malformations or any risks to pregnancy. The NAS, though uncommon, can be troublesome.
   (e) If the mother plans to breastfeed, then sertraline is a first choice.

Treating perinatal depression poses many challenges on the clinician, challenges not usually present in general psychiatric practice. In addition to clinical skill it requires more time and coordination of care. Perinatal depression is a major public health risk, and return on this investment is warranted by prevention of adverse effects on mother, child, and family and improved outcomes for mother, infant, and family.

References

1. Cohen LS, Nonacs R. Mood and Anxiety Disorders During Pregnancy and Postpartum. Washington, DC: American Psychiatric Publishing; 2005.
2. Gavin NI, Gaynes BN, Lohr KN, Meltzer-Brody S, Gartlehner G, Swinson T. Perinatal depression: a systematic review of prevalence and incidence. Obstet Gynecol. 2005;106(5 Pt 1):1071–83.
3. Kessler RC, Berglund P, Demler O, Jin R, Koretz D, Merikangas KR, et al. The epidemiology of major depressive disorder: results from the National Comorbidity Survey Replication (NCS-R). JAMA. 2003;289(23):3095–105.
4. ACOG Practice Bulletin: Clinical management guidelines for obstetrician-gynecologists number 92, April 2008 (replaces practice bulletin number 87, November 2007). Use of psychiatric medications during pregnancy and lactation. Obstet Gynecol. 2008;111(4): 1001–20.
5. Bennett HA, Einarson A, Taddio A, Koren G, Einarson TR. Prevalence of depression during pregnancy: systematic review. Obstet Gynecol. 2004;103(4):698–709.
6. Lee A, Woo J, Ito S. Frequency of infant adverse events that are associated with citalopram use during breast-feeding. Am J Obstet Gynecol. 2004;190(1):218–21.
7. Evans J, Heron J, Francomb H, Oke S, Golding J. Cohort study of depressed mood during pregnancy and after childbirth. BMJ. 2001;323(7307):257–60.
8. Limlomwongse N, Liabsuetrakul T. Cohort study of depressive moods in Thai women during late pregnancy and 6-8 weeks of postpartum using the Edinburgh Postnatal Depression Scale (EPDS). Arch Womens Ment Health. 2006;9(3):131–8.
9. Rich-Edwards JW, Kleinman K, Abrams A, Harlow BL, McLaughlin TJ, Joffe H, et al. Sociodemographic predictors of antenatal and postpartum depressive symptoms among women in a medical group practice. J Epidemiol Community Health. 2006;60(3):221–7.
10. Andersson L, Sundstrom-Poromaa I, Bixo M, Wulff M, Bondestam K, aStrom M. Point prevalence of psychiatric disorders during the second trimester of pregnancy: a population-based study. Am J Obstet Gynecol. 2003;189(1):148–54.
11. Dietz PM, Williams SB, Callaghan WM, Bachman DJ, Whitlock EP, Hornbrook MC. Clinically identified maternal depression before, during, and after pregnancies ending in live births. Am J Psychiatry. 2007;164(10):1515–20.
12. Oberlander TF, Warburton W, Misri S, Aghajanian J, Hertzman C. Neonatal outcomes after prenatal exposure to selective serotonin reuptake inhibitor antidepressants and maternal depression using population-based linked health data. Arch Gen Psychiatry. 2006;63(8):898–906.
13. Vesga-Lopez O, Blanco C, Keyes K, Olfson M, Grant BF, Hasin DS. Psychiatric disorders in pregnant and postpartum women in the United States. Arch Gen Psychiatry. 2008;65(7):805–15.
14. Nonacs R, Cohen LS. Depression during pregnancy: diagnosis and treatment options. J Clin Psychiatry. 2002;63(Suppl 7):24–30.
15. Edge D, Rogers A. Dealing with it: Black Caribbean women's response to adversity and psychological distress associated with pregnancy, childbirth, and early motherhood. Soc Sci Med. 2005;61(1):15–25.
16. Brandon AR, Trivedi MH, Hynan LS, Miltenberger PD, Labat DB, Rifkin JB, et al. Prenatal depression in women hospitalized for obstetric risk. J Clin Psychiatry. 2008;69(4):635–43.
17. Gaynes BN, Gavin N, Meltzer-Brody S, Lohr KN, Swinson T, Gartlehner G, et al. Perinatal depression: prevalence, screening accuracy, and screening outcomes. Evid Rep Technol Assess (Summ). 2005(119):1–8.
18. Kitamura T, Yoshida K, Okano T, Kinoshita K, Hayashi M, Toyoda N, et al. Multicentre prospective study of perinatal depression in Japan: incidence and correlates of antenatal and postnatal depression. Arch Womens Ment Health. 2006;9(3):121–30.

19. American College of Obstetricians and Gynecologists Committee on Health Care for Undeserved Woman. ACOG Committee Opinion No. 343: psychosocial risk factors: perinatal screening and intervention. Obstetrics & Gynecology 2006;108:469–477.
20. Eysenck SG, Eysenck HJ, Barrett P. A revised version of the psychoticism scale. Person Indiv Dif. 1985;6:21–9.
21. Kendler KS, Gardner CO, Prescott CA. Toward a comprehensive developmental model for major depression in women. Am J Psychiatry. 2002;159(7):1133–45.
22. Fava M, Kendler KS. Major depressive disorder. Neuron. 2000;28(2):335–41.
23. Steiner M, Dunn E, Born L. Hormones and mood: from menarche to menopause and beyond. J Affect Disord. 2003;74(1):67–83.
24. Mueller TI, Leon AC, Keller MB, Solomon DA, Endicott J, Coryell W, et al. Recurrence after recovery from major depressive disorder during 15 years of observational follow-up. Am J Psychiatry. 1999;156(7):1000–6.
25. Marcus SM, Flynn HA, Blow FC, Barry KL. Depressive symptoms among pregnant women screened in obstetrics settings. J Womens Health (Larchmt). 2003;12(4):373–80.
26. McGrath PJ, Stewart JW, Petkova E, Quitkin FM, Amsterdam JD, Fawcett J, et al. Predictors of relapse during fluoxetine continuation or maintenance treatment of major depression. J Clin Psychiatry. 2000;61(7):518–24.
27. Lovisi GM, Lopez JR, Coutinho ES, Patel V. Poverty, violence and depression during pregnancy: a survey of mothers attending a public hospital in Brazil. Psychol Med. 2005;35(10):1485–92.
28. Judd LL, Akiskal HS, Maser JD, Zeller PJ, Endicott J, Coryell W, et al. Major depressive disorder: a prospective study of residual subthreshold depressive symptoms as predictor of rapid relapse. J Affect Disord. 1998;50(2–3):97–108.
29. Lee AM, Lam SK, Sze Mun Lau SM, Chong CS, Chui HW, Fong DY. Prevalence, course, and risk factors for antenatal anxiety and depression. Obstet Gynecol. 2007;110(5): 1102–12.
30. Cohen LS, Altshuler LL, Harlow BL, Nonacs R, Newport DJ, Viguera AC, et al. Relapse of major depression during pregnancy in women who maintain or discontinue antidepressant treatment. JAMA. 2006;295(5):499–507.
31. Kupfer DJ, Frank E, Perel JM, Cornes C, Mallinger AG, Thase ME, et al. Five-year outcome for maintenance therapies in recurrent depression. Arch Gen Psychiatry. 1992;49(10):769–73.
32. Field T, Hernandez-Reif M, Diego M. Risk factors and stress variables that differentiate depressed from nondepressed pregnant women. Infant Behav Dev. 2006;29(2):169–74.
33. Eshbaugh EM. Predictors of depressive symptomatology among low-income adolescent mothers. Arch Womens Ment Health. 2006;9(6):339–42.
34. Larsson C, Sydsjo G, Josefsson A. Health, sociodemographic data, and pregnancy outcome in women with antepartum depressive symptoms. Obstet Gynecol. 2004;104(3):459–66.
35. Westdahl C, Milan S, Magriples U, Kershaw TS, Rising SS, Ickovics JR. Social support and social conflict as predictors of prenatal depression. Obstet Gynecol. 2007;110(1):134–40.
36. Rodriguez MA, Heilemann MV, Fielder E, Ang A, Nevarez F, Mangione CM. Intimate partner violence, depression, and PTSD among pregnant Latina women. Ann Fam Med. 2008;6(1):44–52.
37. Martin SL, Li Y, Casanueva C, Harris-Britt A, Kupper LL, Cloutier S. Intimate partner violence and women's depression before and during pregnancy. Violence Against Women. 2006;12(3):221–39.
38. ACOG Committee Opinion No. 343: psychosocial risk factors: perinatal screening and intervention. Obstet Gynecol. 2006;108(2):469–77.
39. Geller G. Pregnancy as a stressed life event. CNS Spectr. 2004;9(3):186–97.
40. Fatoye FO, Adeyemi AB, Oladimeji BY. Emotional distress and its correlates among Nigerian women in late pregnancy. J Obstet Gynaecol. 2004;24(5):504–9.
41. Brier N. Anxiety after miscarriage: a review of the empirical literature and implications for clinical practice. Birth. 2004;31(2):138–42.

42. Song D, Sands RG, Wong YL. Utilization of mental health services by low-income pregnant and postpartum women on medical assistance. Women Health. 2004;39(1):1–24.
43. Kazi A, Fatmi Z, Hatcher J, Kadir MM, Niaz U, Wasserman GA. Social environment and depression among pregnant women in urban areas of Pakistan: importance of social relations. Soc Sci Med. 2006;63(6):1466–76.
44. Diego MA, Jones NA, Field T, Hernandez-Reif M, Schanberg S, Kuhn C, et al. Maternal psychological distress, prenatal cortisol, and fetal weight. Psychosom Med. 2006;68(5):747–53.
45. Rubertsson C, Wickberg B, Gustavsson P, Radestad I. Depressive symptoms in early pregnancy, two months and one year postpartum-prevalence and psychosocial risk factors in a national Swedish sample. Arch Womens Ment Health. 2005;8(2):97–104.
46. Wells KB, Stewart A, Hays RD, Burnam MA, Rogers W, Daniels M, et al. The functioning and well-being of depressed patients. Results from the Medical Outcomes Study. JAMA. 1989;262(7):914–9.
47. Lepine JP, Gastpar M, Mendlewicz J, Tylee A. Depression in the community: the first pan-European study DEPRES (Depression Research in European Society). Int Clin Psychopharmacol. 1997;12(1):19–29.
48. Ormel J, Vonkorff M, Oldehinkel AJ, Simon G, Tiemens BG, Ustun TB. Onset of disability in depressed and non-depressed primary care patients. Psychol Med. 1999;29(4):847–53.
49. Andersson L, Sundstrom-Poromaa I, Wulff M, Astrom M, Bixo M. Implications of antenatal depression and anxiety for obstetric outcome. Obstet Gynecol. 2004;104(3):467–76.
50. Kim HG, Mandell M, Crandall C, Kuskowski MA, Dieperink B, Buchberger RL. Antenatal psychiatric illness and adequacy of prenatal care in an ethnically diverse inner-city obstetric population. Arch Womens Ment Health. 2006;9(2):103–7.
51. Tough SC, Siever JE, Johnston DW. Retaining women in a prenatal care randomized controlled trial in Canada: implications for program planning. BMC Public Health. 2007;7:148.
52. Zuckerman B, Amaro H, Bauchner H, Cabral H. Depressive symptoms during pregnancy: relationship to poor health behaviors. Am J Obstet Gynecol. 1989;160(5 Pt 1):1107–11.
53. Kelly R, Zatzick D, Anders T. The detection and treatment of psychiatric disorders and substance use among pregnant women cared for in obstetrics. Am J Psychiatry. 2001;158(2):213–9.
54. Kelly RH, Danielsen BH, Golding JM, Anders TF, Gilbert WM, Zatzick DF. Adequacy of prenatal care among women with psychiatric diagnoses giving birth in California in 1994 and 1995. Psychiatr Serv. 1999;50(12):1584–90.
55. Blalock JA, Robinson JD, Wetter DW, Cinciripini PM. Relationship of DSM-IV-based depressive disorders to smoking cessation and smoking reduction in pregnant smokers. Am J Addict. 2006;15(4):268–77.
56. Nicholson WK, Setse R, Hill-Briggs F, Cooper LA, Strobino D, Powe NR. Depressive symptoms and health-related quality of life in early pregnancy. Obstet Gynecol. 2006;107(4):798–806.
57. Kurki T, Hiilesmaa V, Raitasalo R, Mattila H, Ylikorkala O. Depression and anxiety in early pregnancy and risk for preeclampsia. Obstet Gynecol. 2000;95(4):487–90.
58. Qiu C, Williams MA, Calderon-Margalit R, Cripe SM, Sorensen TK. Preeclampsia risk in relation to maternal mood and anxiety disorders diagnosed before or during early pregnancy. Am J Hypertens. 2009;22(4):397–402.
59. Qiu C, Sanchez SE, Lam N, Garcia P, Williams MA. Associations of depression and depressive symptoms with preeclampsia: results from a Peruvian case-control study. BMC Womens Health. 2007;7:15.
60. Edge D. Ethnicity, psychosocial risk, and perinatal depression--a comparative study among inner-city women in the United Kingdom. J Psychosom Res. 2007;63(3):291–5.
61. Lindahl V, Pearson JL, Colpe L. Prevalence of suicidality during pregnancy and the postpartum. Arch Womens Ment Health. 2005;8(2):77–87.
62. Marzuk PM, Tardiff K, Leon AC, Hirsch CS, Portera L, Hartwell N, et al. Lower risk of suicide during pregnancy. Am J Psychiatry. 1997;154(1):122–3.

63. Gissler M, Hemminki E, Lonnqvist J. Suicides after pregnancy in Finland, 1987-94: register linkage study. BMJ. 1996;313(7070):1431–4.
64. Oates M. Perinatal psychiatric disorders: a leading cause of maternal morbidity and mortality. Br Med Bull. 2003;67:219–29.
65. Dunn LL, Oths KS. Prenatal predictors of intimate partner abuse. J Obstet Gynecol Neonatal Nurs. 2004;33(1):54–63.
66. Radestad I, Rubertsson C, Ebeling M, Hildingsson I. What factors in early pregnancy indicate that the mother will be hit by her partner during the year after childbirth? A nationwide Swedish survey. Birth. 2004;31(2):84–92.
67. Sarid-Segal O. Diagnosis and Teatment of Depression During Pregnancy and Lactation. In: Ciraulo DA, Shader RI, editors. Pharmacotherapy of Depression. Totowa, NJ: Humana Press; 2004.
68. Petrillo LF, Nonacs RM, Viguera AC, Cohen LS. Course of Psychiatric Illness During Pregnancy and Postpartum. In: Cohen LS, Nonacs RM, editors. Mood and Anxiety Disorders During Pregnancy and Postpartum. Washington, DC: American Psychiatric Publishing; 2005.
69. Bonari L, Bennett H, Einarson A, Koren G. Risks of untreated depression during pregnancy. Can Fam Physician. 2004;50:37–9.
70. Rice F, Jones I, Thapar A. The impact of gestational stress and prenatal growth on emotional problems in offspring: a review. Acta Psychiatr Scand. 2007;115(3):171–83.
71. Alder J, Fink N, Bitzer J, Hosli I, Holzgreve W. Depression and anxiety during pregnancy: a risk factor for obstetric, fetal and neonatal outcome? A critical review of the literature. J Matern Fetal Neonatal Med. 2007;20(3):189–209.
72. Littleton HL, Breitkopf CR, Berenson AB. Correlates of anxiety symptoms during pregnancy and association with perinatal outcomes: a meta-analysis. Am J Obstet Gynecol. 2007;196(5):424–32.
73. Ross LE, McLean LM. Anxiety disorders during pregnancy and the postpartum period: a systematic review. J Clin Psychiatry. 2006;67(8):1285–98.
74. Orr ST, James SA, Blackmore Prince C. Maternal prenatal depressive symptoms and spontaneous preterm births among African-American women in Baltimore, Maryland. Am J Epidemiol. 2002;156(9):797–802.
75. Dayan J, Creveuil C, Herlicoviez M, Herbel C, Baranger E, Savoye C, et al. Role of anxiety and depression in the onset of spontaneous preterm labor. Am J Epidemiol. 2002;155(4):293–301.
76. Dayan J, Creveuil C, Marks MN, Conroy S, Herlicoviez M, Dreyfus M, et al. Prenatal depression, prenatal anxiety, and spontaneous preterm birth: a prospective cohort study among women with early and regular care. Psychosom Med. 2006;68(6):938–46.
77. Suri R, Altshuler L, Hellemann G, Burt VK, Aquino A, Mintz J. Effects of antenatal depression and antidepressant treatment on gestational age at birth and risk of preterm birth. Am J Psychiatry. 2007;164(8):1206–13.
78. Berle JO, Mykletun A, Daltveit AK, Rasmussen S, Holsten F, Dahl AA. Neonatal outcomes in offspring of women with anxiety and depression during pregnancy. A linkage study from The Nord-Trondelag Health Study (HUNT) and Medical Birth Registry of Norway. Arch Womens Ment Health. 2005;8(3):181–9.
79. Dole N, Savitz DA, Hertz-Picciotto I, Siega-Riz AM, McMahon MJ, Buekens P. Maternal stress and preterm birth. Am J Epidemiol. 2003;157(1):14–24.
80. Lockwood CJ. The diagnosis of preterm labor and the prediction of preterm delivery. Clin Obstet Gynecol. 1995;38(4):675–87.
81. Chung TK, Lau TK, Yip AS, Chiu HF, Lee DT. Antepartum depressive symptomatology is associated with adverse obstetric and neonatal outcomes. Psychosom Med. 2001;63(5):830–4.
82. Wisner KL, Sit DK, Hanusa BH, Moses-Kolko EL, Bogen DL, Hunker DF, et al. Major depression and antidepressant treatment: impact on pregnancy and neonatal outcomes. Am J Psychiatry. 2009;166(5):557–66.
83. Field T, Diego M, Hernandez-Reif M, Figueiredo B, Deeds O, Ascencio A, et al. Comorbid depression and anxiety effects on pregnancy and neonatal outcome. Infant Behav Dev. 2010;33(1):23–9.

84. Hedegaard M, Henriksen TB, Sabroe S, Secher NJ. The relationship between psychological distress during pregnancy and birth weight for gestational age. Acta Obstet Gynecol Scand. 1996;75(1):32–9.
85. Evans J, Heron J, Patel RR, Wiles N. Depressive symptoms during pregnancy and low birth weight at term: longitudinal study. Br J Psychiatry. 2007;191:84–5.
86. Kelly RH, Russo J, Holt VL, Danielsen BH, Zatzick DF, Walker E, et al. Psychiatric and substance use disorders as risk factors for low birth weight and preterm delivery. Obstet Gynecol. 2002;100(2):297–304.
87. Rahman A, Creed F. Outcome of prenatal depression and risk factors associated with persistence in the first postnatal year: prospective study from Rawalpindi, Pakistan. J Affect Disord. 2007;100(1–3):115–21.
88. Hoffman S, Hatch MC. Depressive symptomatology during pregnancy: evidence for an association with decreased fetal growth in pregnancies of lower social class women. Health Psychol. 2000;19(6):535–43.
89. Teixeira JM, Fisk NM, Glover V. Association between maternal anxiety in pregnancy and increased uterine artery resistance index: cohort based study. BMJ. 1999;318(7177):153–7.
90. Field T, Diego M, Hernandez-Reif M, Schanberg S, Kuhn C, Yando R, et al. Pregnancy anxiety and comorbid depression and anger: effects on the fetus and neonate. Depress Anxiety. 2003;17(3):140–51.
91. Emory EK, Dieter JN. Maternal depression and psychotropic medication effects on the human fetus. Ann N Y Acad Sci. 2006;1094:287–91.
92. Howard LM, Kirkwood G, Latinovic R. Sudden infant death syndrome and maternal depression. J Clin Psychiatry. 2007;68(8):1279–83.
93. Field T, Diego M, Hernandez-Reif M, Figueiredo B, Schanberg S, Kuhn C. Sleep disturbances in depressed pregnant women and their newborns. Infant Behav Dev. 2007;30(1):127–33.
94. Huot RL, Brennan PA, Stowe ZN, Plotsky PM, Walker EF. Negative affect in offspring of depressed mothers is predicted by infant cortisol levels at 6 months and maternal depression during pregnancy, but not postpartum. Ann N Y Acad Sci. 2004;1032:234–6.
95. Davis EP, Glynn LM, Schetter CD, Hobel C, Chicz-Demet A, Sandman CA. Prenatal exposure to maternal depression and cortisol influences infant temperament. J Am Acad Child Adolesc Psychiatry. 2007;46(6):737–46.
96. Zuckerman B, Bauchner H, Parker S, Cabral H. Maternal depressive symptoms during pregnancy, and newborn irritability. J Dev Behav Pediatr. 1990;11(4):190–4.
97. O'Connor TG, Heron J, Golding J, Beveridge M, Glover V. Maternal antenatal anxiety and children's behavioural/emotional problems at 4 years. Report from the Avon Longitudinal Study of Parents and Children. Br J Psychiatry. 2002;180:502–8.
98. O'Connor TG, Heron J, Golding J, Glover V. Maternal antenatal anxiety and behavioural/emotional problems in children: a test of a programming hypothesis. J Child Psychol Psychiatry. 2003;44(7):1025–36.
99. Hay DF, Pawlby S, Waters CS, Perra O, Sharp D. Mothers' antenatal depression and their children's antisocial outcomes. Child Dev. 2010;81(1):149–65.
100. Van den Bergh BR, Marcoen A. High antenatal maternal anxiety is related to ADHD symptoms, externalizing problems, and anxiety in 8- and 9-year-olds. Child Dev. 2004;75(4):1085–97.
101. Newport DJ, Stowe ZN, Nemeroff CB. Parental depression: animal models of an adverse life event. Am J Psychiatry. 2002;159(8):1265–83.
102. Talge NM, Neal C, Glover V. Antenatal maternal stress and long-term effects on child neurodevelopment: how and why? J Child Psychol Psychiatry. 2007;48(3–4):245–61.
103. Wadhwa PD, Garite TJ, Porto M, Glynn L, Chicz-DeMet A, Dunkel-Schetter C, et al. Placental corticotropin-releasing hormone (CRH), spontaneous preterm birth, and fetal growth restriction: a prospective investigation. Am J Obstet Gynecol. 2004;191(4):1063–9.
104. Huizink AC, Robles de Medina PG, Mulder EJ, Visser GH, Buitelaar JK. Stress during pregnancy is associated with developmental outcome in infancy. J Child Psychol Psychiatry. 2003;44(6):810–8.

105. DiPietro JA, Novak MF, Costigan KA, Atella LD, Reusing SP. Maternal psychological distress during pregnancy in relation to child development at age two. Child Dev. 2006;77(3):573–87.
106. Egliston KA, McMahon C, Austin MP. Stress in pregnancy and infant HPA axis function: conceptual and methodological issues relating to the use of salivary cortisol as an outcome measure. Psychoneuroendocrinology. 2007;32(1):1–13.
107. Einarson A, Pistelli A, DeSantis M, Malm H, Paulus WD, Panchaud A, et al. Evaluation of the risk of congenital cardiovascular defects associated with use of paroxetine during pregnancy. Am J Psychiatry. 2008;165(6):749–52.
108. Miller RL, Pallant JF, Negri LM. Anxiety and stress in the postpartum: is there more to postnatal distress than depression? BMC Psychiatry. 2006;6:12.
109. Einarson A. Abrupt discontinuation of psychotropic drugs following confirmation of pregnancy: a risky practice. J Obstet Gynaecol Can. 2005;27(11):1019–22.
110. Einarson A, Selby P, Koren G. Abrupt discontinuation of psychotropic drugs during pregnancy: fear of teratogenic risk and impact of counselling. J Psychiatry Neurosci. 2001;26(1):44–8.
111. Rosenbaum JF, Tollefson GD. Fluoxetine. In: Schatzberg AF, Nemeroff CB, editors. The American Psychiatric Textbook of Psychopharmacology, Third edition. Washington, DC: American Psychiatric Publishers; 2004.
112. www.safefetus.com.
113. Simon GE, Cunningham ML, Davis RL. Outcomes of prenatal antidepressant exposure. Am J Psychiatry. 2002;159(12):2055–61.
114. Alwan S, Reefhuis J, Rasmussen SA, Olney RS, Friedman JM. Use of selective serotonin-reuptake inhibitors in pregnancy and the risk of birth defects. N Engl J Med. 2007;356(26):2684–92.
115. Kallen B. The safety of antidepressant drugs during pregnancy. Expert Opin Drug Saf. 2007;6(4):357–70.
116. Louik C, Lin AE, Werler MM, Hernandez-Diaz S, Mitchell AA. First-trimester use of selective serotonin-reuptake inhibitors and the risk of birth defects. N Engl J Med. 2007;356(26):2675–83.
117. Bar-Oz B, Einarson T, Einarson A, Boskovic R, O'Brien L, Malm H, et al. Paroxetine and congenital malformations: meta-Analysis and consideration of potential confounding factors. Clin Ther. 2007;29(5):918–26.
118. Rosenbaum JF, Zajecka J. Clinical management of antidepressant discontinuation. J Clin Psychiatry. 1997;58(Suppl 7):37–40.
119. Greene MF. Teratogenicity of SSRIs – serious concern or much ado about little? N Engl J Med. 2007;356(26):2732–3.
120. Berard A, Ramos E, Rey E, Blais L, St-Andre M, Oraichi D. First trimester exposure to paroxetine and risk of cardiac malformations in infants: the importance of dosage. Birth Defects Res B Dev Reprod Toxicol. 2007;80(1):18–27.
121. Oberlander TF, Warburton W, Misri S, Riggs W, Aghajanian J, Hertzman C. Major congenital malformations following prenatal exposure to serotonin reuptake inhibitors and benzodiazepines using population-based health data. Birth Defects Res B Dev Reprod Toxicol. 2008;83(1):68–76.
122. Pedersen LH, Henriksen TB, Vestergaard M, Olsen J, Bech BH. Selective serotonin reuptake inhibitors in pregnancy and congenital malformations: population based cohort study. BMJ. 2009;339:b3569.
123. Lennestal R, Kallen B. Delivery outcome in relation to maternal use of some recently introduced antidepressants. J Clin Psychopharmacol. 2007;27(6):607–13.
124. Cole JA, Modell JG, Haight BR, Cosmatos IS, Stoler JM, Walker AM. Bupropion in pregnancy and the prevalence of congenital malformations. Pharmacoepidemiol Drug Saf. 2007;16(5):474–84.
125. Einarson A, Bonari L, Voyer-Lavigne S, Addis A, Matsui D, Johnson Y, et al. A multicentre prospective controlled study to determine the safety of trazodone and nefazodone use during pregnancy. Can J Psychiatry. 2003;48(2):106–10.

126. Djulus J, Koren G, Einarson TR, Wilton L, Shakir S, Diav-Citrin O, et al. Exposure to mirtazapine during pregnancy: a prospective, comparative study of birth outcomes. J Clin Psychiatry. 2006;67(8):1280–4.
127. Gracious BL, Wisner KL. Phenelzine use throughout pregnancy and the puerperium: case report, review of the literature, and management recommendations. Depress Anxiety. 1997;6(3):124–8.
128. Rubinow DR. Antidepressant treatment during pregnancy: between Scylla and Charybdis. Am J Psychiatry. 2006;163(6):954–6.
129. Bonari L, Koren G, Einarson TR, Jasper JD, Taddio A, Einarson A. Use of antidepressants by pregnant women: evaluation of perception of risk, efficacy of evidence based counseling and determinants of decision making. Arch Womens Ment Health. 2005;8(4):214–20.
130. Kulin NA, Pastuszak A, Sage SR, Schick-Boschetto B, Spivey G, Feldkamp M, et al. Pregnancy outcome following maternal use of the new selective serotonin reuptake inhibitors: a prospective controlled multicenter study. JAMA. 1998;279(8):609–10.
131. Chun-Fai-Chan B, Koren G, Fayez I, Kalra S, Voyer-Lavigne S, Boshier A, et al. Pregnancy outcome of women exposed to bupropion during pregnancy: a prospective comparative study. Am J Obstet Gynecol. 2005;192(3):932–6.
132. McElhatton PR, Garbis HM, Elefant E, Vial T, Bellemin B, Mastroiacovo P, et al. The outcome of pregnancy in 689 women exposed to therapeutic doses of antidepressants. A collaborative study of the European Network of Teratology Information Services (ENTIS). Reprod Toxicol. 1996;10(4):285–94.
133. Sivojelezova A, Shuhaiber S, Sarkissian L, Einarson A, Koren G. Citalopram use in pregnancy: prospective comparative evaluation of pregnancy and fetal outcome. Am J Obstet Gynecol. 2005;193(6):2004–9.
134. Hemels ME, Einarson A, Koren G, Lanctot KL, Einarson TR. Antidepressant use during pregnancy and the rates of spontaneous abortions: a meta-analysis. Ann Pharmacother. 2005;39(5):803–9.
135. Garcia-Enguidanos A, Calle ME, Valero J, Luna S, Dominguez-Rojas V. Risk factors in miscarriage: a review. Eur J Obstet Gynecol Reprod Biol. 2002;102(2):111–9.
136. Kallen B. Neonate characteristics after maternal use of antidepressants in late pregnancy. Arch Pediatr Adolesc Med. 2004;158(4):312–6.
137. Kallen B, Otterblad Olausson P. Antidepressant drugs during pregnancy and infant congenital heart defect. Reprod Toxicol. 2006;21(3):221–2.
138. Hendrick V, Smith LM, Suri R, Hwang S, Haynes D, Altshuler L. Birth outcomes after prenatal exposure to antidepressant medication. Am J Obstet Gynecol. 2003;188(3):812–5.
139. Malm H, Klaukka T, Neuvonen PJ. Risks associated with selective serotonin reuptake inhibitors in pregnancy. Obstet Gynecol. 2005;106(6):1289–96.
140. Lund N, Pedersen LH, Henriksen TB. Selective serotonin reuptake inhibitor exposure in utero and pregnancy outcomes. Arch Pediatr Adolesc Med. 2009;163(10):949–54.
141. Theis JG, Selby P, Ikizler Y, Koren G. Current management of the neonatal abstinence syndrome: a critical analysis of the evidence. Biol Neonate. 1997;71(6):345–56.
142. Cohen LS, Heller VL, Bailey JW, Grush L, Ablon JS, Bouffard SM. Birth outcomes following prenatal exposure to fluoxetine. Biol Psychiatry. 2000;48(10):996–1000.
143. Koren G, Matsui D, Einarson A, Knoppert D, Steiner M. Is maternal use of selective serotonin reuptake inhibitors in the third trimester of pregnancy harmful to neonates? CMAJ. 2005;172(11):1457–9.
144. Einarson TR, Koren G, Einarson A. Problems with maternal antidepressant treatment and neonatal outcomes study. Arch Gen Psychiatry. 2007;64(7):866; author reply 7–8.
145. Kalra S, Einarson A, Koren G. Taking antidepressants during late pregnancy. How should we advise women? Can Fam Physician. 2005;51:1077–8.
146. Moses-Kolko EL, Bogen D, Perel J, Bregar A, Uhl K, Levin B, et al. Neonatal signs after late in utero exposure to serotonin reuptake inhibitors: literature review and implications for clinical applications. JAMA. 2005;293(19):2372–83.
147. Chambers CD, Hernandez-Diaz S, Van Marter LJ, Werler MM, Louik C, Jones KL, et al. Selective serotonin-reuptake inhibitors and risk of persistent pulmonary hypertension of the newborn. N Engl J Med. 2006;354(6):579–87.

148. Andrade SE, McPhillips H, Loren D, Raebel MA, Lane K, Livingston J, et al. Antidepressant medication use and risk of persistent pulmonary hypertension of the newborn. Pharmacoepidemiol Drug Saf. 2009;18(3):246–52.
149. Kallen B, Olausson PO. Maternal use of selective serotonin re-uptake inhibitors and persistent pulmonary hypertension of the newborn. Pharmacoepidemiol Drug Saf. 2008;17(8):801–6.
150. Cowe L, Lloyd DJ, Dawling S. Neonatal convulsions caused by withdrawal from maternal clomipramine. Br Med J (Clin Res Ed). 1982;284(6332):1837–8.
151. Eyal R, Yaeger D. Poor neonatal adaptation after in utero exposure to duloxetine. Am J Psychiatry. 2008;165(5):651.
152. Briggs GG, Ambrose PJ, Ilett KF, Hackett LP, Nageotte MP, Padilla G. Use of duloxetine in pregnancy and lactation. Ann Pharmacother. 2009;43(11):1898–902.
153. Hendrick V, Stowe ZN, Altshuler LL, Hwang S, Lee E, Haynes D. Placental passage of antidepressant medications. Am J Psychiatry. 2003;160(5):993–6.
154. Laine K, Heikkinen T, Ekblad U, Kero P. Effects of exposure to selective serotonin reuptake inhibitors during pregnancy on serotonergic symptoms in newborns and cord blood monoamine and prolactin concentrations. Arch Gen Psychiatry. 2003;60(7):720–6.
155. http://www.hc_sc.ca/ahc-asc/media/advisories-avis/_2004/2004_44-eng.php. [cited 2008 6–13].
156. www.fda.gov/ohrms/dockets/ac/04/slides/2004-4050S1_11_Levin.ppt. [cited 2008 6–13].
157. Pearson KH, Nonacs RM, Viguera AC, Heller VL, Petrillo LF, Brandes M, et al. Birth outcomes following prenatal exposure to antidepressants. J Clin Psychiatry. 2007;68(8):1284–9.
158. van Geffen EC, Hugtenburg JG, Heerdink ER, van Hulten RP, Egberts AC. Discontinuation symptoms in users of selective serotonin reuptake inhibitors in clinical practice: tapering versus abrupt discontinuation. Eur J Clin Pharmacol. 2005;61(4):303–7.
159. Miller LJ, Bishop JR, Fischer JH, Geller SE, Macmillan C. Balancing risks: dosing strategies for antidepressants near the end of pregnancy. J Clin Psychiatry. 2008;69(2):323–4.
160. Casper RC, Fleisher BE, Lee-Ancajas JC, Gilles A, Gaylor E, DeBattista A, et al. Follow-up of children of depressed mothers exposed or not exposed to antidepressant drugs during pregnancy. J Pediatr. 2003;142(4):402–8.
161. Misri S, Reebye P, Kendrick K, Carter D, Ryan D, Grunau RE, et al. Internalizing behaviors in 4-year-old children exposed in utero to psychotropic medications. Am J Psychiatry. 2006;163(6):1026–32.
162. Oberlander TF, Reebye P, Misri S, Papsdorf M, Kim J, Grunau RE. Externalizing and attentional behaviors in children of depressed mothers treated with a selective serotonin reuptake inhibitor antidepressant during pregnancy. Arch Pediatr Adolesc Med. 2007;161(1):22–9.
163. Nulman I, Rovet J, Stewart DE, Wolpin J, Pace-Asciak P, Shuhaiber S, et al. Child development following exposure to tricyclic antidepressants or fluoxetine throughout fetal life: a prospective, controlled study. Am J Psychiatry. 2002;159(11):1889–95.
164. Pedersen LH, Henriksen TB, Olsen J. Fetal exposure to antidepressants and normal milestone development at 6 and 19 months of age. Pediatrics. 2010;125(3):e600–8.
165. Gentile S, Galbally M. Prenatal exposure to antidepressant medications and neurodevelopmental outcomes: A systematic review. J Affect Disord. 2010.
166. Anderson GD. Pregnancy-induced changes in pharmacokinetics: a mechanistic-based approach. Clin Pharmacokinet. 2005;44(10):989–1008.
167. Redmond GP. Physiological changes during pregnancy and their implications for pharmacological treatment. Clin Invest Med. 1985;8(4):317–22.
168. Loebstein R, Lalkin A, Koren G. Pharmacokinetic changes during pregnancy and their clinical relevance. Clin Pharmacokinet. 1997;33(5):328–43.
169. Wadelius M, Darj E, Frenne G, Rane A. Induction of CYP2D6 in pregnancy. Clin Pharmacol Ther. 1997;62(4):400–7.
170. Wisner KL, Perel JM, Wheeler SB. Tricyclic dose requirements across pregnancy. Am J Psychiatry. 1993;150(10):1541–2.

171. Altshuler LL, Hendrick VC. Pregnancy and psychotropic medication: changes in blood levels. J Clin Psychopharmacol. 1996;16(1):78–80.
172. Hostetter A, Stowe ZN, Strader JR, Jr., McLaughlin E, Llewellyn A. Dose of selective serotonin uptake inhibitors across pregnancy: clinical implications. Depress Anxiety. 2000;11(2):51–7.
173. Sit DK, Perel JM, Helsel JC, Wisner KL. Changes in antidepressant metabolism and dosing across pregnancy and early postpartum. J Clin Psychiatry. 2008;69(4):652–8.
174. Heikkinen T, Ekblad U, Kero P, Ekblad S, Laine K. Citalopram in pregnancy and lactation. Clin Pharmacol Ther. 2002;72(2):184–91.
175. Heikkinen T, Ekblad U, Palo P, Laine K. Pharmacokinetics of fluoxetine and norfluoxetine in pregnancy and lactation. Clin Pharmacol Ther. 2003;73(4):330–7.
176. Hirshfield RM, Bowden CL, Gitlin MJ, Keck PE, Suppes T, Thase ME, et al. Work Group on Bipolar Disorder. 2002 [cited 2008 6/22/2008]; Second:Available from: http://www.psychiatryonline.com/content.aspx?aid=50051.
177. Kaplan, SB. Kaplan and Sadock's Synopsis of Psychiatry: Behavioral Sciences/Clinical Psychiatry. Sadock B, Sadock V, editors, Tenth Edition. Philadelphia: Lippincott Williams & Wilkins.
178. Avery D, Winokur G. The efficacy of electroconvulsive therapy and antidepressants in depression. Biol Psychiatry. 1977;12(4):507–23.
179. Remick RA, Maurice WL. ECT in pregnancy. Am J Psychiatry. 1978;135(6):761–2.
180. Yellowlees PM, Page T. Safe use of electroconvulsive therapy in pregnancy. Med J Aust. 1990;153(11–12):679–80.
181. Echevarria Moreno M, Martin Munoz J, Sanchez Valderrabanos J, Vazquez Gutierrez T. Electroconvulsive therapy in the first trimester of pregnancy. J ECT. 1998;14(4):251–4.
182. Pinette MG, Santarpio C, Wax JR, Blackstone J. Electroconvulsive therapy in pregnancy. Obstet Gynecol. 2007;110(2 Pt 2):465–6.
183. Kasar M, Saatcioglu O, Kutlar T. Electroconvulsive therapy use in pregnancy. J ECT. 2007;23(3):183–4.
184. Bozkurt A, Karlidere T, Isintas M, Ozmenler NK, Ozsahin A, Yanarates O. Acute and maintenance electroconvulsive therapy for treatment of psychotic depression in a pregnant patient. J ECT. 2007;23(3):185–7.
185. Forssman H. Follow-up study of sixteen children whose mothers were given electric convulsive therapy during gestation. Acta Psychiatr Neurol Scand. 1955;30(3):437–41.
186. Loke KH, Salleh R. Electroconvulsive therapy for the acutely psychotic pregnant patient: a review of 3 cases. Med J Malaysia. 1983;38(2):131–3.
187. Walker R, Swartz CM. Electroconvulsive therapy during high-risk pregnancy. Gen Hosp Psychiatry. 1994;16(5):348–53.
188. Kim DR, Gonzalez J, O'Reardon JP. Pregnancy and depression: exploring a new potential treatment option. Curr Psychiatry Rep. 2009;11(6):443–6.
189. Gurel S, Gurel H. The evaluation of determinants of early postpartum low mood: the importance of parity and inter-pregnancy interval. Eur J Obstet Gynecol Reprod Biol. 2000;91(1):21–4.
190. Josefsson A, Berg G, Nordin C, Sydsjo G. Prevalence of depressive symptoms in late pregnancy and postpartum. Acta Obstet Gynecol Scand. 2001;80(3):251–5.
191. Nonacs RM. Postpartum Mood Disorders. In: Cohen LS, Nonacs RM, editors. Mood and Anxiety Disorders During Pregnancy. Washington, DC: American Psychiatric Publishing; 2005.
192. Noble RE. Depression in women. Metabolism. 2005;54(5 Suppl 1):49–52.
193. McQueen K, Montgomery P, Lappan-Gracon S, Evans M, Hunter J. Evidence-based recommendations for depressive symptoms in postpartum women. J Obstet Gynecol Neonatal Nurs. 2008;37(2):127–36.
194. Dennis CL. Psychosocial and psychological interventions for prevention of postnatal depression: systematic review. BMJ. 2005;331(7507):15.

195. Barr JA. Postpartum depression, delayed maternal adaptation, and mechanical infant caring: a phenomenological hermeneutic study. Int J Nurs Stud. 2008;45(3):362–9.
196. Prevalence of self-reported postpartum depressive symptoms – 17 states, 2004-2005. MMWR Morb Mortal Wkly Rep. 2008;57(14):361–6.
197. Yonkers KA, Ramin SM, Rush AJ, Navarrete CA, Carmody T, March D, et al. Onset and persistence of postpartum depression in an inner-city maternal health clinic system. Am J Psychiatry. 2001;158(11):1856–63.
198. Cooper PJ, Murray L. Course and recurrence of postnatal depression. Evidence for the specificity of the diagnostic concept. Br J Psychiatry. 1995;166(2):191–5.
199. O'Hara MW. Social support, life events, and depression during pregnancy and the puerperium. Arch Gen Psychiatry. 1986;43(6):569–73.
200. Chaudron LH. Treating pregnant women with antidepressants: the gray zone. J Womens Health (Larchmt). 2007;16(4):551–3.
201. Robertson E, Grace S, Wallington T, Stewart DE. Antenatal risk factors for postpartum depression: a synthesis of recent literature. Gen Hosp Psychiatry. 2004;26(4):289–95.
202. Hendrick V, Altshuler LL, Suri R. Hormonal changes in the postpartum and implications for postpartum depression. Psychosomatics. 1998;39(2):93–101.
203. Halbreich U, Endicott J. Possible involvement of endorphin withdrawal or imbalance in specific premenstrual syndromes and postpartum depression. Med Hypotheses. 1981;7(8):1045–58.
204. Wisner KL, Stowe ZN. Psychobiology of postpartum mood disorders. Semin Reprod Endocrinol. 1997;15(1):77–89.
205. Joffe H, Cohen LS. Estrogen, serotonin, and mood disturbance: where is the therapeutic bridge? Biol Psychiatry. 1998;44(9):798–811.
206. Harris B, Lovett L, Smith J, Read G, Walker R, Newcombe R. Cardiff puerperal mood and hormone study. III. Postnatal depression at 5 to 6 weeks postpartum, and its hormonal correlates across the peripartum period. Br J Psychiatry. 1996;168(6):739–44.
207. Righetti-Veltema M, Bousquet A, Manzano J. Impact of postpartum depressive symptoms on mother and her 18-month-old infant. Eur Child Adolesc Psychiatry. 2003;12(2):75–83.
208. Miller AR, Barr RG, Eaton WO. Crying and motor behavior of six-week-old infants and postpartum maternal mood. Pediatrics. 1993;92(4):551–8.
209. Armstrong KL, O'Donnell H, McCallum R, Dadds M. Childhood sleep problems: association with prenatal factors and maternal distress/depression. J Paediatr Child Health. 1998;34(3):263–6.
210. Grace SL, Evindar A, Stewart DE. The effect of postpartum depression on child cognitive development and behavior: a review and critical analysis of the literature. Arch Womens Ment Health. 2003;6(4):263–74.
211. Moehler E, Kagan J, Parzer P, Brunner R, Reck C, Wiebel A, et al. Childhood behavioral inhibition and maternal symptoms of depression. Psychopathology. 2007;40(6):446–52.
212. Murray L, Hipwell A, Hooper R, Stein A, Cooper P. The cognitive development of 5-year-old children of postnatally depressed mothers. J Child Psychol Psychiatry. 1996;37(8):927–35.
213. Beck CT. The effects of postpartum depression on maternal-infant interaction: a meta-analysis. Nurs Res. 1995;44(5):298–304.
214. McIntosh J. Postpartum depression: women's help-seeking behaviour and perceptions of cause. J Adv Nurs. 1993;18(2):178–84.
215. Robinson S, Young J. Screening for depression and anxiety in the post-natal period: acceptance or rejection of a subsequent treatment offer. Aust N Z J Psychiatry. 1982;16(2):47–51.
216. Newport DJ, Hostetter A, Arnold A, Stowe ZN. The treatment of postpartum depression: minimizing infant exposures. J Clin Psychiatry. 2002;63(Suppl 7):31–44.
217. Work Group on Breastfeeding: Breastfeeding and the use of human milk. Pediatrics. 1997:1035–9.
218. Takala AK, Eskola J, Palmgren J, Ronnberg PR, Kela E, Rekola P, et al. Risk factors of invasive Haemophilus influenzae type b disease among children in Finland. J Pediatr. 1989;115(5 Pt 1):694–701.

219. Aniansson G, Alm B, Andersson B, Hakansson A, Larsson P, Nylen O, et al. A prospective cohort study on breast-feeding and otitis media in Swedish infants. Pediatr Infect Dis J. 1994;13(3):183–8.
220. Wright AL, Holberg CJ, Martinez FD, Morgan WJ, Taussig LM. Breast feeding and lower respiratory tract illness in the first year of life. Group Health Medical Associates. BMJ. 1989;299(6705):946–9.
221. Mayer EJ, Hamman RF, Gay EC, Lezotte DC, Savitz DA, Klingensmith GJ. Reduced risk of IDDM among breast-fed children. The Colorado IDDM Registry. Diabetes. 1988;37(12):1625–32.
222. Halken S, Host A, Hansen LG, Osterballe O. Effect of an allergy prevention programme on incidence of atopic symptoms in infancy. A prospective study of 159 "high-risk" infants. Allergy. 1992;47(5):545–53.
223. Wright A, Schanler R. The resurgence of breastfeeding at the end of the second millennium. J Nutr. 2001;131(2):421S–5S.
224. Epperson CN, Terman M, Terman JS, Hanusa BH, Oren DA, Peindl KS, et al. Randomized clinical trial of bright light therapy for antepartum depression: preliminary findings. J Clin Psychiatry. 2004;65(3):421–5.
225. Gentile S, Rossi A, Bellantuono C. SSRIs during breastfeeding: spotlight on milk-to-plasma ratio. Arch Womens Ment Health. 2007;10(2):39–51.
226. Gentile S. The safety of newer antidepressants in pregnancy and breastfeeding. Drug Saf. 2005;28(2):137–52.
227. Weissman AM, Levy BT, Hartz AJ, Bentler S, Donohue M, Ellingrod VL, et al. Pooled analysis of antidepressant levels in lactating mothers, breast milk, and nursing infants. Am J Psychiatry. 2004;161(6):1066–78.
228. Misri S, Kim J, Riggs KW, Kostaras X. Paroxetine levels in postpartum depressed women, breast milk, and infant serum. J Clin Psychiatry. 2000;61(11):828–32.
229. Larsen LA, Ito S, Koren G. Prediction of milk/plasma concentration ratio of drugs. Ann Pharmacother. 2003;37(9):1299–306.
230. Bergman K, Sarkar P, O'Connor TG, Modi N, Glover V. Maternal stress during pregnancy predicts cognitive ability and fearfulness in infancy. J Am Acad Child Adolesc Psychiatry. 2007;46(11):1454–63.
231. Suri R, Stowe ZN, Hendrick V, Hostetter A, Widawski M, Altshuler LL. Estimates of nursing infant daily dose of fluoxetine through breast milk. Biol Psychiatry. 2002;52(5): 446–51.
232. Ragan K, Stowe Z, Newport DJ. Use of Antidepressants and Mood Stabilizers in Breast-feeding Woman. In: Cohen LS, Nonacs RM, editors. Mood and Anxiety Disorders During Pregnancy and Postpartum. Washington, DC: American Psychiatric Publishing; 2005.
233. Taddio A, Ito S, Koren G. Excretion of fluoxetine and its metabolite, norfluoxetine, in human breast milk. J Clin Pharmacol. 1996;36(1):42–7.
234. Yoshida K, Smith B, Craggs M, Kumar RC. Fluoxetine in breast-milk and developmental outcome of breast-fed infants. Br J Psychiatry. 1998;172:175–8.
235. Spigset O, Carieborg L, Ohman R, Norstrom A. Excretion of citalopram in breast milk. Br J Clin Pharmacol. 1997;44(3):295–8.
236. Stowe ZN, Owens MJ, Landry JC, Kilts CD, Ely T, Llewellyn A, et al. Sertraline and desmethylsertraline in human breast milk and nursing infants. Am J Psychiatry. 1997;154(9):1255–60.
237. Berle JO, Steen VM, Aamo TO, Breilid H, Zahlsen K, Spigset O. Breastfeeding during maternal antidepressant treatment with serotonin reuptake inhibitors: infant exposure, clinical symptoms, and cytochrome p450 genotypes. J Clin Psychiatry. 2004;65(9):1228–34.
238. Stowe ZN, Cohen LS, Hostetter A, Ritchie JC, Owens MJ, Nemeroff CB. Paroxetine in human breast milk and nursing infants. Am J Psychiatry. 2000;157(2):185–9.
239. Baab SW, Peindl KS, Piontek CM, Wisner KL. Serum bupropion levels in 2 breastfeeding mother-infant pairs. J Clin Psychiatry. 2002;63(10):910–1.
240. Hale TW, Shum S, Grossberg M. Fluoxetine toxicity in a breastfed infant. Clin Pediatr (Phila). 2001;40(12):681–4.

241. Ilett KF, Hackett LP, Dusci LJ, Roberts MJ, Kristensen JH, Paech M, et al. Distribution and excretion of venlafaxine and O-desmethylvenlafaxine in human milk. Br J Clin Pharmacol. 1998;45(5):459–62.
242. American Academy of Pediatrics Committee on Drugs. Transfer of drugs and other chemicals into human milk (2001;108:776). Pediatrics. 2001;108(4):1029.
243. ACOG PBN. Use of psychiatric medications during pregnancy and lactation. In: Hale TW, editor. Medications in Mother's Milk. Obstetrics & Gynecology. 2007;110:1179–1198.
244. di Scalea TL, Wisner KL. Pharmacotherapy of postpartum depression. Expert Opin Pharmacother. 2009;10(16):2593–607.
245. Yonkers KA, Wisner KL, Stewart DE, Oberlander TF, Dell DL, Stotland N, et al. The management of depression during pregnancy: a report from the American Psychiatric Association and the American College of Obstetricians and Gynecologists. Gen Hosp Psychiatry. 2009;31(5):403–13.

Antidepressant Treatment of Pediatric Depression

Ricardo M. Vela, Carol A. Glod, Timothy M. Rivinus, and Rebecca Johnson

Introduction

Since the publication of the first edition of this book 6 years ago, antidepressant treatment of children and adolescents has been fraught with controversy. The efficacy of these agents in the young population has been questioned. Their potential role in triggering suicidal behavior prompted the FDA to require black box warnings and strict government guidelines for patient monitoring. These measures appear to have deterred clinicians from prescribing these medications, and, as we will discuss later, may have contributed to an increase, rather than a decrease, in suicide rates in the young. Therefore, more than ever, clinicians need knowledge of the efficacy and safety of these medications in order to use their best judgment in making informed decisions about the treatment of pediatric depression.

Despite the rapid growth of knowledge in the field of clinical pharmacology in the last two decades, there has been a paucity of systematic research on the antidepressant treatment of child and adolescent depression (1). Research findings of antidepressants in adults cannot be applied directly to children and adolescents, who have different developmental, biochemical, neurobiological, pharmacokinetic, and pharmacodynamic characteristics. The purpose of this chapter is to review the current literature on the effectiveness of antidepressants in youth, critically review the available safety data, and make recommendations for clinicians who pharmacologically treat children and adolescents who suffer from depression.

R.M. Vela (✉)
Department of Child and Family Services, Harvard Medical School, Boston, MA USA
e-mail: rvela@northsuffolk.org

D.A. Ciraulo and R.I. Shader (eds.), *Pharmacotherapy of Depression*,
DOI 10.1007/978-1-60327-435-7_9, © Springer Science+Business Media, LLC 2011

Epidemiology

Depression is a common psychiatric disorder, particularly in adolescents. Epidemiological studies of children and adolescents have found a prevalence of depression ranging from 0.4 to 2.5% in children, and from 0.4 to 8.3% in adolescents, depending on the methodology and sample studied (2–9). Lifetime prevalence rate in adolescents (i.e., prevalence during the span of adolescent years) has been reported to be between 15 and 20% (2, 4, 9). The reported data on dysthymic disorder in the pediatric population is more limited. Point prevalence rates range between 0.6 and 1.7% in children and between 1.6 and 8.0% in adolescents (3–6).

Rates of major depression in the pediatric age group vary developmentally with age (5). The female-to-male ratio in boys and girls under 12 years is 1:1, but in adolescents it is 2:1 – a ratio that persists into adulthood (6, 9, 10). The cause of this disparity is yet to be elucidated scientifically, although genetic, biological, cognitive, and socio-cultural factors have been proposed (11–13).

Diagnosis and Course

Diagnostic criteria for major depression and dysthymic disorder in children and adolescents are similar to adult criteria; in children and adolescents, however, mood may be irritable instead of depressed. In ordinary clinical practice, symptom presentation in children and adolescents – corresponding to diagnostic criteria for major depression – may be quite different than that of adults (see Table 1). Children and adolescents tend to show more mood reactivity than adults, often confusing parental observations and not infrequently making their assessment more difficult. In addition, depressed children tend to have symptoms of separation anxiety, phobias, somatic complaints, and behavior problems more frequently than adults (7).

Although dysthymic disorder is milder in terms of symptom severity than major depressive disorder, it should not be construed as a benign form of depression. About 70% of children with dysthymic disorder will develop a superimposed major depressive episode during the course of illness, which has been termed "double depression." Children and adolescents with "double depression" have more severe and longer major depressive episodes, a higher incidence of co-morbid disorders, increased suicidality, and more pronounced social impairment in contrast with children with "single" major depression. Fifty percent of children and adolescents with dysthymic disorder have other psychiatric diagnoses; these co-morbidities include anxiety disorders (40%), conduct disorders (30%), attention-deficit hyperactivity disorder (ADHD) (24%), and enuresis/encopresis (15%). In addition, about 15% of children and adolescents with dysthymic disorder have two or more psychiatric diagnoses (7).

About 40–70% of children and adolescents with major depression have co-morbid psychiatric disorders. Twenty to fifty percent have two or more co-morbid diagnoses. The most common co-morbid diagnoses are dysthymic disorder (30%),

Table 1 DSM-IV diagnostic criteria for major depressive disorder and examples of corresponding childhood clinical presentation

DSM-IV diagnostic criteria	Childhood clinical presentation
Depressed mood	Looks or feels "unwell" or "sad"; cries easily or is often irritable and negative
Anhedonia	"Nothing is fun"; gives up on peers; excessively bored; decreased interest in extracurricular activities
Sleep disturbance	Stays up late; unwilling to sleep alone
Weight changes or changes in appetite	Failure to achieve expected weight gain or newly picky with food or uninterested in eating or overeating to deal with emotions
Decrease in concentration or indecisiveness	Loss of interest in school; decreased academic performance; newly distractible or forgetful
Suicidal ideation/thoughts of death	Suicidal ideation, writing or talk (sometimes projected toward parent or others, as "...you wish I were dead," "nobody likes me" "nobody would miss me"); morbid diary entries, morbid confessionals to friends or preoccupation with nihilism, the occult – including dressing in black – or death and dying. Suicidal gestures (secret overdoses; cutting or other self-mutilation) or acts (reckless driving, pathological intoxication, unprotected sex)
Psychomotor agitation	New onset of hyperactivity; recklessness or destructive or impulsive and dangerous acts
Decreased energy	Daytime fatigue; sleeping in school; excessive school absenteeism
Worthlessness or guilt	Self-depreciation or guilt; "I'm stupid"; "I can't do anything right"; "I hate myself"; "it's all my fault"

anxiety disorders (80%), disruptive disorders (10–80%), substance abuse (20–30%), and personality disorders (60%) (7, 11).

It is often difficult to differentiate between major depression and bipolar disorder. The initial presentation of major depression in children and adolescents with bipolar disorder is varied. For example, what appears to be MDD may be a manifestation of the depressive phase of Bipolar I Disorder in a youngster who has not yet developed mania, which is not uncommon. In fact, about 20% of youths with MDD go on to develop manic episodes by adulthood (14–19). Factors that predict future development of mania in children and adolescents include rapid onset of depression, psychomotor retardation, psychotic features, and a family history of bipolar disorder. In contrast to adults, changes in mood, behavior, and energy are notably erratic and labile, rather than persistent. In the pediatric population, mania may present with more atypical symptoms such as irritability, rather than euphoria, or with a more mixed symptom profile (19). Some researchers require the presence of elevated mood to distinguish bipolar disorder from severe mood dysregulation (20). Rather than being a cyclical disorder with alternating acute episodes of mania and depression, juvenile bipolar disorder presents with chronic difficulties with mood regulation, emotional instability, and erratic/explosive behavior. Reduced need for sleep – a pathognomonic sign of mania in adults – occurs in less than half of bipolar children and adolescents. About 44% of children with bipolar-I continue to have manic episodes past the age of 18 years (21). The term "bipolar disorder not otherwise specified" has been used to describe youth with bipolar disorder who do not have the classic adult presentation (22, 23). Symptoms of MDD may also appear in Bipolar II Disorder (hypomania without full mania) and as part of a mixed episode of BD (concurrent symptoms of both mania and depression). The DSM-V task force has proposed the term Temper Dysregulation Disorder with Dysphoria for a disorder characterized by severe, recurrent, intense, temper outbursts in response to common stressors, grossly out of proportion to the situation (23).

Consequences of untreated depression include difficulty in peer and family relationships, worsening school performance and school dropout, alcohol and substance abuse, and suicide (24, 25).

In the following sections, we will objectively review the current literature and clinical perspective on the effectiveness of antidepressants in youth, critically appraise the available safety data, and make recommendations for clinicians who work with children and adolescents suffering from major depression.

Research on Antidepressants in Child and Adolescent Depression

Tricyclic antidepressants, which had been the mainstay of treatment in adult MDD until the 1990s, were not found to be effective in double-bind, placebo-controlled studies of child and adolescent MDD (26). Reports of sudden deaths and evidence of cardiotoxicity in children and adolescents taking tricyclic antidepressants discouraged clinicians from prescribing these medications. There have been no randomized clinical trials of monoamine oxidase inhibitors in depressed children and adolescents, and compliance with dietary restrictions limit suitability for treatment (27). With the introduction of fluoxetine – which proved to be an effective and safer antidepressant for adults – new hopes for an effective and safe agent in children emerged. Below, we will summarize the published double-blind placebo-controlled clinical trials of the second-generation antidepressants for pediatric depression. The term "second-generation antidepressants," when used in this chapter, encompasses the selective serotonin reuptake inhibitors (SSRIs) (i.e., fluoxetine, sertraline, paroxetine, citalopram, and escitalopram) as well as venlafaxine, bupropion, nefazodone, and mirtazapine.

Fluoxetine

The first double-blind, placebo-controlled study of adolescents with MDD did not find significant differences between placebo and fluoxetine, in a very small sample that had a high placebo and medication response rate (28). Data suggesting the effectiveness of fluoxetine in the treatment of major depression in children and adolescents was initially based on two prospective double-blind placebo-controlled clinical trials by Emslie and collaborators (29, 30). In the first of these trials, 96 children and adolescents (aged 7–17 years, mean age 12.2 years) with non-psychotic major depressive disorder were randomized to receive either 20 mg/day of fluoxetine or placebo. Based on Clinical Global Impression-Improvement (CGI-I), response rates in the fluoxetine treatment group were significantly greater than that of the placebo group (56 vs. 33%, respectively). Significant differences were also observed using the Children's Depression Rating Scale-Revised (CDRS-R) after 5 weeks of treatment; full remission of depressive symptoms (in the CDRS-R) occurred in relatively low proportions (31% of patients randomized to fluoxetine vs. 23% given placebo) (29).

In the second study conducted by Emslie and collaborators, 122 children and 97 adolescents were randomly assigned to fluoxetine or placebo, again using a fixed dose of 20 mg of fluoxetine. Response to treatment was assessed using the CDRS-R. Fluoxetine treatment was associated with significantly greater improvements in the CDRS-R compared to placebo, beginning after 1 week of treatment. Significantly more fluoxetine-treated patients (41%) than placebo-treated patients (20%) met the prospectively defined criteria for remission. Based on the *a priori* outcome measure definition of response – which was defined as a 30% or greater improvement in CDRS-R score – the difference in percentage of patients responding to fluoxetine (65.1%) vs. placebo (53.5%) was not statistically significant. Fluoxetine, however, would have been statistically significant superior to placebo if response had been defined as ≥20, ≥40, ≥50, or ≥60% reduction in CDRS-R total score. Headache was the only unsolicited (but not by checklist) adverse event reported significantly in fluoxetine- than placebo-treated patients (30).

Further evidence emerged from a large randomized multi-center trial of 378 children and adolescents funded by the National Institute of Mental Health in the US. The Treatment for Adolescents with Depression Study (TADS) Team studied the effectiveness of fluoxetine alone, fluoxetine in combination with cognitive–behavioral therapy (CBT), CBT alone, and placebo (31). Response rate was quantified using the Clinical Global Impressions Improvement (CGI-I) Scale. Compared with placebo, the most effective treatment was fluoxetine and CBT (71% response rate), followed by medication alone (61%), while the response rate to CBT alone (43%) failed to reach statistical significance when compared with placebo (35%), based on ratings from the Children's Depression Rating Scale-Revised (CDRS-R) total scores (31). There were five suicide attempts reported on fluoxetine, and one attempt on placebo. Overall, 24 (5.5%) of the 439 patients experienced a suicide-related adverse event: 12% on fluoxetine alone, 8% on fluoxetine with CBT, 4.5% on CBT alone, and 5% on placebo (31).

Sertraline

Wagner and collaborators (32) combined two international, multi-center, double-blind placebo-controlled clinical trials of a total of 376 children and adolescents

(6–17 years) with MDD; subjects were randomly assigned to receive either a flexible dose of sertraline (50–200 mg/day) or placebo for 10 weeks. They found modest, but statistically significant, superior response rates with sertraline (69%) compared with placebo (59%), based on a 40% decrease in the CDRS-R total score at study end point (32). When overall mean response rates were compared, a small – but statistically significant – difference emerged (2.7 points on a 113-point CDRS-R scale). Significantly more sertraline patients withdrew from the study compared with placebo (9 vs. 3%); however, the details of the adverse effects were not reported. Adverse events occurring in more than 5% of sertraline-treated patients with an incidence of at least two times that of placebo included insomnia, diarrhea, anorexia, vomiting, agitation, urinary incontinence, and purpura (32). Overall, the authors of this trial concluded that sertraline presented a clinical as well as statistical difference.

Paroxetine

The first published, double-blind placebo-controlled clinical trials of paroxetine compared it to imipramine and placebo in a multicenter study of the treatment of adolescent major depression (33). A total of 275 adolescents were randomized into paroxetine, imipramine, and placebo. The two primary outcome measures were (1) endpoint response (defined *a priori* as a Hamilton Rating Scale [HAM-D] score ≤8 or a ≥50% reduction in baseline HAM-D score at the end of treatment) and (2) change from baseline in HAM-D total score. Paroxetine was not found to be superior to placebo in either of these two primary outcome measures. Of the five other depression-related variables declared *a priori*, paroxetine was superior to placebo in change in HAM-D depressed mood item ($p=0.001$), change in the Schedule for Affective Disorders and Schizophrenia for Adolescents-Lifetime version (K-SADS-L) depressed mood item ($p=0.05$), and CGI score of improved or very much improved ($p=0.02$). Imipramine was not superior to placebo in any of the seven variables.

Serious adverse events were more frequent with paroxetine than placebo (12.2 vs. 2.3%). Notably, 32% of imipramine-treated adolescents discontinued treatment due to adverse events, including cardiovascular effects (33). Of the paroxetine-treated patients who experienced severe adverse events, one reported headache during the medication taper, two experienced worsening depression, five showed emotional lability (which included suicidal ideation), two experienced conduct or hostility, and one developed euphoria.

Two other recent randomized multicenter, double-blind, placebo-controlled trials of paroxetine failed to find significant drug-placebo differences. Emslie and collaborators evaluated paroxetine (daily doses of 10–50 mg) in an 8-week trial of 206 subjects aged 7–17 years (34). Using the primary outcome of measure of change from baseline in the CDRS-R, they reported no differences in mean depression scores between paroxetine and placebo (22.6 vs. 23.3, respectively.) Overall – consistent with Keller's results – Emslie found more serious adverse events in paroxetine-treated children. In another study, Berard and collaborators conducted a 12-week international, multicenter, double-blind placebo-controlled clinical trials of 286 depressed adolescents aged 12–19 (35). MADRS response rates of 60.5% for paroxetine-treated and 58.2% for placebo-treated patients did not reach statistical significance. The authors noted that older adolescents treated with paroxetine had a greater response rate than younger adolescents, based on the Clinical Global Impression-Improvement (CGI-I) Scale. High rates of side effects were also reported for both groups (69 vs. 59%, paroxetine vs. placebo) (35).

Taken together, these three published multi-center trials of paroxetine fail to provide compelling evidence for the efficacy of this agent in children and adolescents with depression. High rates of side effects and more serious adverse events in patients receiving paroxetine lead to questions about the safety of this agent in pediatric patients. A review from the UK concluded that there was an "increase in rate of self-harm and potentially suicidal behavior" based on data – largely unpublished – from clinical trials of over 1,000 youth that found mood swings, increased crying, suicidal thoughts, and behavior twice as common (3.2 vs. 1.5%) in paroxetine-treated patients.

Venlafaxine

Studies of venlafaxine or venlafaxine-XR also have failed to find efficacy for these agents and have raised additional questions about their safety. A small published study of venlafaxine vs. placebo in 33 children and adolescents (8–17 years) that used a relatively low dose (75 mg) found no difference between medication and placebo (36). An 8-week study of venlafaxine ER vs. placebo in 334 children and adolescents with MDD (ages 7–17) failed to find major differences between drug and placebo (37). Using doses ranging from 37.5 to 225 mg, response rates in adolescents ranged from 43% in venlafaxine-treated subjects compared with 35% of placebo-treated subjects, which was reported as *statistically* significant ($p < 0.05$), although the clinical significance of this difference is unclear. Adverse events with an incidence greater than 5% on venlafaxine included anorexia and abdominal pain. However, hostility and suicide-related events (suicidal ideation, intentional injuries) occurred more often in venlafaxine than in the placebo group (37). In those followed for up to 6 months, venlafaxine-treated patients reported headache (53%), nausea (26%), infection (24%), abdominal pain (22%), vomiting (21%), and pharyngitis (19%). Overall, based on these data, venlafaxine and venlafaxine-XR do not appear effective and are not recommended for youth with MDD or generalized anxiety disorder (GAD).

Citalopram, Escitalopram

Wagner and collaborators (38) reported low but statistically significant response rates in 178 children and adolescents randomized to either citalopram or placebo (36 vs. 24%, respectively; $p<0.05$). Response was defined as a score of ≤28 on the CDRS-R. Treatment with citalopram led to a reduction of approximately 21 points (from 59 to 38 points) in mean CDRS-R scores, while scores were reduced about 16 points (58–32 points) in the placebo group; thus, depressed children and adolescents responded to citalopram, yet continued with a mild to moderate degree of depressive symptoms after 8 weeks of treatment (38). A limited discussion of side effects in this paper revealed treatment-emergent adverse events that occurred with a frequency greater than 5% and that exceeded placebo, which included rhinitis, nausea, abdominal pain, flu-like symptoms, fatigue, diarrhea, and back pain (38). Incidence of suicidal ideation or actions, or self-harm were not reported.

Von Knorring and collaborators (39) failed to find differences between citalopram and placebo in 160 subjects using K-SADS-P total scores as the major outcome measure. Although they found higher response rates than Wagner and collaborators, the average response rate to either drug or placebo was about 60%, without significant differences in the two groups. In another study, Wagner and colleagues reported negative results of a placebo-controlled study of escitalopram of 263 depressed children and adolescents aged 6–17 years on CDRS-R depression ratings or other measures (40). Using CGI scores as outcome measures, 63% of the subjects responded to escitalopram and 52% to placebo, failing to reach statistical significance in the whole sample. However, post-hoc analysis of only the adolescent age sample (12–17 years of age) showed significantly greater improvement in the escitalopram-treated group. Headaches and abdominal paid were the only adverse events reported by more than 10% of patients treated with escitalopram.

In a more recent study, Emslie and collaborators (41) published a double-blind, placebo-controlled trial of escitalopram in 312 adolescent subjects (ages 12–17 years) with major depression, 83% of whom completed the study. Subjects received either 10–20 mg/day of escitalopram or placebo. Significant improvement was reported in the escitalopram-treated group vs. the placebo group at end CDRS-R scores ($p=0.022$), using the last observation carried forward. However, overall improvement in mean depression scores using the CDRS-R revealed modest differences between groups at endpoint (–22 vs. –19 points, escitalopram vs. placebo). Remission rates (CDRS-R ≤28) at endpoint were 41.5% for escitalopram and 35.7% for placebo, not reaching statistical significance ($p=0.15$).

Other Second-Generation Antidepressants

No systematic placebo-controlled published studies are available for other antidepressants, including bupropion, fluvoxamine, or mirtazapine. There is, however, one preliminary study of bupropion and two studies of nefazodone, published only as abstracts. In a pilot double-blind placebo-controlled clinical trial, Glod and collaborators (42) reported that bupropion was significantly more effective than citalopram in adolescents with MDD; 80% responded to bupropion vs. 60% response to citalopram, however, neither was more effective than placebo. Emslie and collaborators (43) reported one positive 8-week study of 195 adolescents aged 12–17; obtaining CGI response ratings 62% of nefazodone-treated patients vs. 42% of those treated with placebo. Table 2 summarizes the published placebo-controlled research studies of the second-generation antidepressants.

In a critical review of six of the above studies, Jureidini and collaborators have raised serious concerns about the claims of efficacy of these antidepressants in youth, concluding that studies have "exaggerated" benefits and "downplayed" the harm of antidepressants (44). By contrast, more recently, Bridge and collaborators performed a meta-analysis of published and unpublished placebo-controlled, parallel-group trials of second-generation antidepressants in subjects younger than 19 years with MDD, obsessive-compulsive disorder (OCD), or non-OCD anxiety disorders (45). Based on the data from 13 trials with a total of 2,910 subjects with pediatric MDD, the pooled absolute rates of response were 61% (95% CI, 58–63%) in subjects treated with antidepressants and 50% (95% CI, 47–53%) in those treated with placebo, yielding a pooled risk difference of 11% (95% CI, 7–15%). Efficacy was found to be inversely proportional to the duration of depressive episode. Interestingly, although there was evidence for antidepressant treatment for adolescents across several antidepressant types, only fluoxetine outperformed placebo in depressed children under 12 years (45).

In a meta-analysis of randomized controlled trials of first and second-generation antidepressants in juvenile depression, involving over 3,000 subjects, Tsapakis and collaborators (46) found a modest drug/placebo response rate ratio. They concluded that antidepressants of all types showed limited efficacy, but fluoxetine may be more effective, especially in adolescents (46).

Discussion: Application of Antidepressant Research to Clinical Practice

Clinical depression in childhood, and particularly adolescence, is a major health concern. Left untreated, it can lead to declining school performance, impaired peer relationships, family discord and conflict, and the development of recurrent episodes of depression (24). Furthermore, untreated depression is associated with other high-risk behaviors including poor nutrition, alcohol and substance abuse and dependence, tobacco use, as well as intentional injuries and suicide (47, 48). It thus becomes imperative for clinicians to provide the best possible treatment to ameliorate this condition and prevent its complications.

In the United States, fluoxetine and escitalopram are the only antidepressants approved for advertisement in youth with MDD, while in the United Kingdom, the use of all antidepressants, with the exception of fluoxetine, has been discouraged.

Table 2 Double-blind, randomized, placebo-controlled trials of SSRIs and other second-generation antidepressants

Medication	Duration (weeks)	Age range (years)	Daily dose (mg/day)	*n*	Primary outcome measure	Response ratesMed vs. Placebo (%)	Statistical difference with Med > Placebo?	References
Citalopram	12	13–18	10–40	244	K-SADS items	60 vs. 61	No	(39)
Citalopram	8	7–17	20–40	178	CDRS-R	36 vs. 24	Yes	(38)
Escitalopram	8	6–17	10–20	268	CGI	63 vs. 52	No[a]	(40)
Escitalopram	8	12–17	10–20	312	CDRS-R	59 vs. 48	Yes	(41)
Fluoxetine	8	7–17	20	96	CGI	56 vs. 33	Yes	(29)
Fluoxetine	9	8–17	20	219	CDRS-R	41 vs. 20	Yes	(30)
Fluoxetine	13	12–17	10–40	221	CGI	61 vs. 35	Yes	(31)
Nefazodone	8	12–17	300–600	195	CGI	62 vs. 42	Yes	(43)[b]
Paroxetine	8	12–19	20–40	275	HDRS, K-SADS-L	63 vs. 46	Yes	(33)
Paroxetine	8	7–17	10–50	206	CDRS-R	23 vs. 23	No	(34)
Paroxetine	12	13–18	20–40	286	MADRS	61 vs. 58	No	(35)
Sertraline	10	6–17	25–200	376	CDRS-R	69 vs. 59	Yes	(32)
Venlafaxine	6	8–17	75	33	HDRS or CDRS	*Not reported*	No	(36)
Venlafaxine ER	8	7–17	37.5–225	334	HDRS or CDRS	44 vs. 38	No	(37)[b]

CGI Clinical Global Impression; *CDRS-R* Children's Depression Rating Scale-Revised; *HDRS* Hamilton Depression Rating Scale; *MADRS* Montgomery–Asberg Depression Rating Scale; *K-SADS* Kiddie-Schedule for Affective Disorders and Schizophrenia; *L* Lifetime Version

[a]Significant in adolescents only, not the total sample

[b]Data available only as published abstract

Nevertheless, as noted by Popper, "...FDA guidelines are meant to regulate advertising of pharmaceutical houses, not the clinical practice of clinicians (49)." It is in the face of incomplete medical knowledge, with a wide range of scientific unknowns about safety and the long-term developmental effects of drugs in the body, that we must practice pediatric psychopharmacology. Within this context we must make ethical and medical judgments to treat juvenile depression. This state of affairs, however, is not unique to child psychiatry. Many other pediatric medications are not FDA approved for advertisement in children, are logistically challenging to study, and lack adequate proof for effectiveness. For example, most medications used to treat seizures in children lack scientific proof of their effectiveness and are very difficult to research (e.g., placebo-controlled trials are unethical, outcome measurements are difficult). Yet, anticonvulsants are widely prescribed for seizures, and withholding them may be considered unethical or inhumane.

Clinicians prescribing antidepressants for children are faced with the decision to use or withhold medication. It is important to remember that withholding an antidepressant medication is not the same as giving a placebo, and the difference between medication and no medication is not comparable to the differential response of drug vs. placebo. MDD in children and adolescents has a high placebo response. Of course, it is considered unethical in clinical practice to give a placebo. Nevertheless active medications have a placebo component in addition to their biochemical pharmacodynamic effect. When these two effects are added we see the actual medication clinical response. Roughly, overall placebo response in antidepressant youth MDD trials is about 50%, response to active drug is 60%, and when CBT is added to active drug the treatment response rate is increased to about 70%.

Another important consideration to have in mind is that double-blind placebo-controlled clinical trials, although highly desirable, are not the only source that should guide a clinician to make decisions about antidepressants. Individual and shared experiences are very important guides to clinical practice. Research results, whether positive or negative, may not be generalizable to the particular population with which a clinician works. Moreover, every patient is clinically and genetically different. Based on clinical practice as well as on controlled studies, there appears to be a number of children and adolescents who unequivocally respond to antidepressant medications for MDD.

The Current Safety Controversy on Child and Adolescent Depression Treatment

Advisories, Warnings, and Regulations on Youth Suicide and Antidepressants

Concerns about the safety of antidepressant agents in the treatment of children and adolescents have generated a great deal of controversy among researchers, clinicians, and governmental regulatory agencies. In October 2003, the FDA issued the first public health advisory about reports of suicidal behavior and self-harm in youths treated with antidepressants. The United Kingdom Medicines and Healthcare Products Regulatory Agency (the equivalent of the US FDA) released a report on December 10, 2003, indicating that with the exception of fluoxetine, benefits of SSRIs and other second-generation antidepressants did not outweigh their potential risks. Further, the report states that these drugs were "not demonstrated" to be effective in MDD in children and adolescents, and may present "increased rates of self-harm and suicidal thoughts." In February 2004, the FDA held a preliminary review of antidepressants in youth and recommended a critical reanalysis of existing data. This was followed, on March 22, 2004, with a public health advisory warning strongly stating that the newer antidepressant drugs may be associated with an increased risk of suicidality, and advising physicians and families to closely monitor children with depression at the beginning of the treatment and during the dosing changes. On October 15, 2004, the FDA directed manufacturers of 10 second-generation antidepressant drugs to include a boxed warning ("black box") alerting health care providers to an increased risk of suicidality in children and adolescents being treated with these agents. In February 2005, the agency extended the warning to all antidepressant drugs. The FDA has also issued recommendations for very close monitoring for suicidal behavior in children and adolescents treated with any kind of antidepressant. Specifically these guidelines state that the prescribing clinician should have face-to-face contact with patient and family once a week during the first 4 weeks of treatment, every other week the following month, and monthly thereafter.

Evidence of Possible Antidepressant-Related Suicidal Ideation and Behavior

The FDA decision followed a meta-analysis on 24 randomized clinical trials involving 4,587 cases diagnosed mostly with major depression (16 trials), but with other diagnoses as well (OCD, four trials; GAD, two trials; social anxiety, one trial; and ADHD, one trial). A statistical greater pooled risk of cases involving suicidal ideation or non-fatal self-injurious behavior was found during exposure to SSRIs, compared to placebo. There were no completed suicides in any of these trials (50). In another study – this one a matched, case-controlled study of Medicaid beneficiaries who had received inpatient treatment for depression – antidepressant drug treatment was significantly associated with suicide attempts and suicide deaths in children and adolescents aged 6–18 years, although the same effect was not seen in adults. Medications with the highest odds ratio were sertraline, venlafaxine, and tricyclic antidepressants. The authors concluded that antidepressant drug treatment might be related to suicide attempts in children and adolescents (51). In contrast to these findings, another study used computerized health plan records to identify 65,103 patients (adults and children) with 82,285 episodes of antidepressant treatment during the 12½ years before June 2003 (52). ("Episode" was defined as an outpatient antidepressant prescription filled during the study period, no prior antidepressant prescription filled in the prior 180 days and a diagnosis of a depressive disorder made within 30 days of the index prescription.) The risk of suicide attempt was not significantly higher in the month after starting medication than in subsequent months. The risk of suicide attempt was highest in the month *before* starting antidepressant medication and declined progressively after medication was started. An increase in risk after starting treatment was seen only for the older drugs and not for the 10 newer antidepressants for which the FDA had initially issued a public health advisory warning.

Effect of FDA Warning on Antidepressant Prescribing and Suicide Rates

FDA warnings appear to have had an effect on antidepressant prescribing for youths. The number of antidepressant prescriptions for the pediatric population in the United States had increased about 10% from the beginning of July 2003 through March 2004. Following the strong FDA public health advisory warning that drugs may be associated with an increased risk of suicidality, from March 31 to June 30, 2005, the number of antidepressant prescriptions dispensed to patients aged 18 years and under decreased by 20%. The number of antidepressant prescriptions dispensed to adults remained fairly constant during this time period (53). Using a large pediatric cohort ($n = 65{,}349$) obtained from a national integrated claims database of managed care plans, Libby and collaborators found that following the FDA advisory in October 2003, the overall rate of diagnosis of depression declined and, among patients diagnosed, the proportion treated with antidepressants declined. Pediatricians and other primary care physicians – but not psychiatrists – were responsible for this reversal in diagnosis and treatment of depression (54).

Shaffer, in his presentation at the FDA Meeting on February 2, 2004, pointed to the fact that after a steady increase in suicide rates for 35 years, the rate of adolescent suicide had been decreasing consistently in many countries, coinciding with the increased exposure of adolescents to SSRI antidepressants (55). These trends could be related. After considering various alternative explanations, he concluded that more psychopharmacologic treatment, better recognition of adolescent depression, or some combination of these factors may have contributed to the declining rates of adolescent suicides. According to US vital statistics, in 2004, there was an increase of 18.2% in the suicide rate in children and adolescents up to 19 years of age compared with 2003 (56). (This represents a rate increase from 2.2 to 2.6 per 100,000 population.) Although there is no direct proof, this increase in suicide deaths roughly correlates with the decrease in antidepressant prescriptions written for children under 18 years of age following the FDA public health advisory warning. This is in agreement with the recent finding by Ludwig and collaborators using data from 26 countries for up to 25 years, which showed that an increase in SSRI sales of one pill per capita (adults and children) was associated with a *decline* in suicide mortality of around 5% (57). They also concluded that "these estimates imply a cost per statistical life far below most other government interventions to improve health outcomes." Furthermore, in a recent study, the authors examined US and Dutch data in prescription rates for SSRIs and suicide rates for children and adolescents, in order to assess whether the FDA and European Medicines Agency's warnings discouraged the use of antidepressants, and whether they led to increases in suicide rates as a result of untreated depression. The study found that SSRI prescriptions for youth decreased by about 22% in both the US and the Netherlands after the warnings were issued. Youth suicide rate increased by 49% in the Netherlands (from 2003 to 2005) and 14% in the US (from 2003 to 2004) (58).

Discussion: The Current Antidepressant-Suicide Controversy and Clinical Practice

In summary, meta-analyses of placebo-controlled studies of antidepressants for the treatment trials of major depression in children and adolescents indicate there is a statistically significant increase in suicidal ideation and suicidal attempts in research subjects receiving active medications as opposed to placebo. These increased rates of suicidal behavior are striking and unexpected, given the efforts in study designs to exclude high-risk candidates with histories of past and/or present suicidal behaviors, psychosis, or bipolar disorder (for a discussion see this excellent review by Baldessarini and collaborators) (59). On the other hand, aggregate and ecological studies seem to indicate that the increased use of second-generation antidepressants has turned around the previous steady increase of suicide in youth and probably has prevented the death of thousands of children and adolescents treated with these agents.

How do we reconcile these apparently contradictory findings in clinical practice? It appears that there are some vulnerable or predisposed minority of children who have an atypical response to antidepressants, by which, instead of decreasing suicidal ideation and risk for suicidal attempts, antidepressants actually increase these behaviors. These phenomena may occur mostly at the beginning of the treatment. (Those clinicians that have anecdotally observed the sudden emergence of suicidal ideation in their patients can attest their cases are convincing.) Other explanations for the increased occurrence of suicidal ideation and/or attempts have been offered. These include behavioral activation or manic switching; potential antidepressant side effects, such as insomnia, irritability, and agitation; and recruitment of trial subjects early in the course of illness, when suicidal behaviors are most common (59). This makes it very important to monitor the emergence of suicidal ideation, educate the patient and family of this possibility, and provide access to evaluation in case of this eventuality. Nevertheless, the FDA's recommendation of weekly face-to-face assessment of patients with their families for suicidal/homicidal behavior may be a hindrance to appropriate treatment from the practical point of view for primary care physicians and other clinicians with busy practices.

This may have deterred many clinicians from prescribing and deprived many children and adolescents from receiving effective and, in some cases, life-saving treatments. Thus, the FDA's "black box" warning on antidepressant treatment of children and adolescents and the guidelines for prescribers' close monitoring may have inadvertently and unintentionally produced the opposite effect of what they had intended for suicide prevention. From the results of aggregate studies, it can be inferred that the second-generation antidepressants overall prevent more suicides than they may possibly provoke. Moreover, antidepressant drug research trials data are mostly about suicidal ideation and nonlethal suicide attempts. These events may be a different phenomenon from completed suicide, as seem to be indicated by their different risk factors (59, 60).

Recommendations for Clinical Practice with Children and Adolescents with Major Depression

Specific antidepressant double-blind placebo-controlled clinical trials show variable results, ranging from statistically non-significant differences to a moderate advantage of antidepressants over placebo in the treatment of pediatric MDD. Recent meta-analysis of short-term studies in children and adolescents, however, show a more definitive – although modest – advantage of active medication when larger samples are pooled (50). When CBT is augmented to active medication, treatment efficacy increases about another 10%. The recent TORDIA study (61) evaluated the efficacy of four treatment strategies in 334 depressed adolescents with an SSRI-treatment failure/non-response. Interventions consisted of (1) switch to a second, different SSRI, such as paroxetine, citalopram, or fluoxetine; (2) switch to a different SSRI plus CBT; (3) switch to venlafaxine (150–225 mg); and (4) switch to venlafaxine plus CBT. The combination of CBT plus a change to another antidepressant was more effective than a medication change alone. In clinical practice, it is the authors' experience that CBT is a treatment modality difficult to access in the community. Nevertheless, Brent and collaborators have demonstrated that other forms of psychotherapy, such as non-directive supportive psychotherapy and systemic behavior family therapy, are also effective (62, 63). Interpersonal therapy (IPT) has also shown effectiveness (64–66), and treatment with phototherapy was shown to be effective in one trial (67). On the basis of available studies and clinical practice, we recommend the following treatment guidelines for children and adolescents with MDD.

Lack of significant improvement, defined as not more than 50% improved by week 4 of antidepressant treatment, suggests that patients will fail to remit (68). Instead, current data reveal that increasing the antidepressant dose, switching to another agent, and/or adding CBT are important short-term strategies for pediatric depression. Successful treatment with antidepressants is generally maintained for at least 1 year, depending on the initial depressive severity, co-morbidity, adherence, psychosocial issues, and other individual and family factors that impact treatment (69).

Treatment Guidelines

For mild to moderate MDD, first episode, without co-morbidity:

- Initial trial with CBT (or other available psychotherapy), weekly, for at least 6–12 weeks.
- If no response or worsening, consider adding antidepressant.
- Fluoxetine generally first-line.
- Avoid paroxetine, venlafaxine.
- Manage complications (academic, interpersonal, suicidal, and medical).

If a patient refuses psychotherapy or parent/child prefer medication:

- Consider antidepressant trial with clear parameters, outcome measures, and close weekly monitoring for worsening and suicidal ideation or self-harm behaviors.

For moderately severe to severe MDD, for chronic depression, for depression unresponsive to CBT (or other psychotherapies):

- Fluoxetine may be used as a first-line agent for children and adolescents; escitalopram may be used first line for adolescents aged 12–17 years.
- Avoid paroxetine, venlafaxine.
- Consider bipolarity (including family history, current cycling, and hypomania).
- Adequate dose for 4–8 weeks.
- Monitor carefully weekly for the first month.
- Informed consent with parents and child that discusses risks and benefits.
- Consider IPT or other psychotherapeutic modalities.
- Reevaluate diagnosis.

Other psychopharmacological and non-psychopharmacological treatment is indicated for:

- Dysthymia (CBT or other form of psychotherapy). Monitor closely for worsening of depression or development of superimposed MDD, and if so, treat with antidepressant. If co-morbid anxiety disorder is present use SSRI (treat anxiety).
- Seasonal MDD (phototherapy).
- Bipolar disorder (mood stabilizer) with cautious use of, or avoiding, antidepressants.
- MDD with psychotic features (treat psychosis with antipsychotic).
- MDD with attention-deficit/hyperactivity disorder (bupropion).
- MDD with obsessive-compulsive disorder (sertraline).

References

1. Vitiello B, Swedo S. Antidepressant medications in children. N Engl J Med. 2004;350(15):1489–91.
2. Lewinsohn PM, Duncan EM, Stanton AK, Hautzinger M. Age at first onset for nonbipolar depression. J Abnorm Psychol. 1986;95(4):378–83.

3. Kashani JH, Beck NC, Hoeper EW, Fallahi C, Corcoran CM, McAllister JA, et al. Psychiatric disorders in a community sample of adolescents. Am J Psychiatry. 1987;144(5):584–9.
4. Kashani JH, Carlson GA, Beck NC, Hoeper EW, Corcoran CM, McAllister JA, et al. Depression, depressive symptoms, and depressed mood among a community sample of adolescents. Am J Psychiatry. 1987;144(7):931–4.
5. Lewinsohn PM, Hops H, Roberts RE, Seeley JR, Andrews JA. Adolescent psychopathology: I. Prevalence and incidence of depression and other DSM-III-R disorders in high school students. J Abnorm Psychol. 1993;102(1):133–44.
6. Lewinsohn PM, Clarke GN, Seeley JR, Rohde P. Major depression in community adolescents: age at onset, episode duration, and time to recurrence. J Am Acad Child Adolesc Psychiatry. 1994;33(6):809–18.
7. Birmaher B, Ryan ND, Williamson DE, Brent DA, Kaufman J, Dahl RE, et al. Childhood and adolescent depression: a review of the past 10 years. Part I. J Am Acad Child Adolesc Psychiatry. 1996;35(11):1427–39.
8. Anderson JC, McGee R. Comorbidity of depression in children and adolescents. In: Reynolds WM, Johnson HF, editor. Handbook of depression in Children and Adolescents. New York: Plenum; 1994. p. 581–601.
9. Fleming JE, Offord DR. Epidemiology of childhood depressive disorders: a critical review. J Am Acad Child Adolesc Psychiatry. 1990;29(4):571–80.
10. Kessler RC, McGonagle KA, Zhao S, Nelson CB, Hughes M, Eshleman S, et al. Lifetime and 12-month prevalence of DSM-III-R psychiatric disorders in the United States. Results from the National Comorbidity Survey. Arch Gen Psychiatry. 1994;51(1):8–19.
11. Reinherz HZ, Stewart-Berghauer G, Pakiz B, Frost AK, Moeykens BA, Holmes WM. The relationship of early risk and current mediators to depressive symptomatology in adolescence. J Am Acad Child Adolesc Psychiatry. 1989;28(6):942–7.
12. Breslau N, Schultz L, Peterson E. Sex differences in depression: a role for preexisting anxiety. Psychiatry Res. 1995;58(1):1–12.
13. Rutter M. Age Changes in Depressive Disorders: Some Developmental Considerations. In: Garber DK, editor. The Developments of Emotional Regulation and Dysregulation New York: Cambridge University Press; 1991.
14. Geller B, Fox LW, Clark KA. Rate and predictors of prepubertal bipolarity during follow-up of 6- to 12-year-old depressed children. J Am Acad Child Adolesc Psychiatry. 1994;33(4):461–8.
15. Geller B, Zimerman B, Williams M, Bolhofner K, Craney JL. Bipolar disorder at prospective follow-up of adults who had prepubertal major depressive disorder. Am J Psychiatry. 2001;158(1):125–7.
16. Kovacs M. Presentation and course of major depressive disorder during childhood and later years of the life span. J Am Acad Child Adolesc Psychiatry. 1996;35(6):705–15.
17. Rao U, Ryan ND, Birmaher B, Dahl RE, Williamson DE, Kaufman J, et al. Unipolar depression in adolescents: clinical outcome in adulthood. J Am Acad Child Adolesc Psychiatry. 1995;34(5):566–78.
18. Strober M, Carlson G. Bipolar illness in adolescents with major depression: clinical, genetic, and psychopharmacologic predictors in a three- to four-year prospective follow-up investigation. Arch Gen Psychiatry. 1982;39(5):549–55.
19. McClellan J, Kowatch R, Findling RL. Practice parameter for the assessment and treatment of children and adolescents with bipolar disorder. J Am Acad Child Adolesc Psychiatry. 2007;46(1):107–25.
20. Rich BA, Schmajuk M, Perez-Edgar KE, Fox NA, Pine DS, Leibenluft E. Different psychophysiological and behavioral responses elicited by frustration in pediatric bipolar disorder and severe mood dysregulation. Am J Psychiatry. 2007;164(2):309–17.
21. Geller B, Tillman R, Bolhofner K, Zimerman B. Child bipolar I disorder: prospective continuity with adult bipolar I disorder; characteristics of second and third episodes; predictors of 8-year outcome. Arch Gen Psychiatry. 2008;65(10):1125–33.
22. National Institute of Mental Health research roundtable on prepubertal bipolar disorder. J Am Acad Child Adolesc Psychiatry. 2001;40(8):871–8.

23. DSM5. Available from: http://www.dsm5.org/ProposedRevisions/Pages?proposedrevision.aspx?rid=397.
24. Brent DA, Birmaher B. Clinical practice. Adolescent depression. N Engl J Med. 2002;347(9):667–71.
25. Kandel DB, Davies M. Adult sequelae of adolescent depressive symptoms. Arch Gen Psychiatry. 1986;43(3):255–62.
26. Hazell P, O'Connell D, Heathcote D, Henry D. Tricyclic drugs for depression in children and adolescents. Cochrane Database Syst Rev. 2002;(2):CD002317.
27. Ryan ND, Puig-Antich J, Rabinovich H, Fried J, Ambrosini P, Meyer V, et al. MAOIs in adolescent major depression unresponsive to tricyclic antidepressants. J Am Acad Child Adolesc Psychiatry. 1988;27(6):755–8.
28. Simeon JG, Dinicola VF, Ferguson HB, Copping W. Adolescent depression: a placebo-controlled fluoxetine treatment study and follow-up. Prog Neuropsychopharmacol Biol Psychiatry. 1990;14(5):791–5.
29. Emslie GJ, Rush AJ, Weinberg WA, Kowatch RA, Hughes CW, Carmody T, et al. A double-blind, randomized, placebo-controlled trial of fluoxetine in children and adolescents with depression. Arch Gen Psychiatry. 1997;54(11):1031–7.
30. Emslie GJ, Heiligenstein JH, Wagner KD, Hoog SL, Ernest DE, Brown E, et al. Fluoxetine for acute treatment of depression in children and adolescents: a placebo-controlled, randomized clinical trial. J Am Acad Child Adolesc Psychiatry. 2002;41(10):1205–15.
31. March J, Silva S, Petrycki S, Curry J, Wells K, Fairbank J, et al. Fluoxetine, cognitive-behavioral therapy, and their combination for adolescents with depression: treatment for Adolescents With Depression Study (TADS) randomized controlled trial. JAMA. 2004;292(7):807–20.
32. Wagner KD, Ambrosini P, Rynn M, Wohlberg C, Yang R, Greenbaum MS, et al. Efficacy of sertraline in the treatment of children and adolescents with major depressive disorder: two randomized controlled trials. JAMA. 2003;290(8):1033–41.
33. Keller MB, Ryan ND, Strober M, Klein RG, Kutcher SP, Birmaher B, et al. Efficacy of paroxetine in the treatment of adolescent major depression: a randomized, controlled trial. J Am Acad Child Adolesc Psychiatry. 2001;40(7):762–72.
34. Emslie GJ, Wagner KD, Kutcher S, Krulewicz S, Fong R, Carpenter DJ, et al. Paroxetine treatment in children and adolescents with major depressive disorder: a randomized, multicenter, double-blind, placebo-controlled trial. J Am Acad Child Adolesc Psychiatry. 2006;45(6):709–19.
35. Berard R, Fong R, Carpenter DJ, Thomason C, Wilkinson C. An international, multicenter, placebo-controlled trial of paroxetine in adolescents with major depressive disorder. J Child Adolesc Psychopharmacol. 2006;16(1–2):59–75.
36. Mandoki MW, Tapia MR, Tapia MA, Sumner GS, Parker JL. Venlafaxine in the treatment of children and adolescents with major depression. Psychopharmacol Bull. 1997;33(1):149–54.
37. Emslie GJ, Findling RL, Yeung PP, Kunz NR, Li Y. Venlafaxine ER for the treatment of pediatric subjects with depression: results of two placebo-controlled trials. J Am Acad Child Adolesc Psychiatry. 2007;46(4):479–88.
38. Wagner KD, Robb AS, Findling RL, Jin J, Gutierrez MM, Heydorn WE. A randomized, placebo-controlled trial of citalopram for the treatment of major depression in children and adolescents. Am J Psychiatry. 2004;161(6):1079–83.
39. von Knorring AL, Olsson GI, Thomsen PH, Lemming OM, Hulten A. A randomized, double-blind, placebo-controlled study of citalopram in adolescents with major depressive disorder. J Clin Psychopharmacol. 2006;26(3):311–5.
40. Wagner KD, Jonas J, Findling RL, Ventura D, Saikali K. A double-blind, randomized, placebo-controlled trial of escitalopram in the treatment of pediatric depression. J Am Acad Child Adolesc Psychiatry. 2006;45(3):280–8.
41. Emslie GJ, Ventura D, Korotzer A, Tourkodimitris S. Escitalopram in the treatment of adolescent depression: a randomized placebo-controlled multisite trial. J Am Acad Child Adolesc Psychiatry. 2009;48(7):721–9.

42. Glod CA, Lynch A, Berkowitz C, Hennen J, Baldessarini RJ. Bupropion vs. citalopram vs. placebo in adolescents with major depression. Biol Psychiatry. Abstract. 2004;(55):236S.
43. Emslie GJ, Findling RL, Rynn MA, Marcus RN, Fernandes LA, Damico MF. Efficacy and safety of nefazodone in the treatment of adolescents with major depressive disorder (Abstract). 42nd Annual Meeting of NCDEU, Orlando, FL, 17. 2002.
44. Jureidini JN, Doecke CJ, Mansfield PR, Haby MM, Menkes DB, Tonkin AL. Efficacy and safety of antidepressants for children and adolescents. BMJ. 2004;328(7444):879–83.
45. Bridge JA, Iyengar S, Salary CB, Barbe RP, Birmaher B, Pincus HA, et al. Clinical response and risk for reported suicidal ideation and suicide attempts in pediatric antidepressant treatment: a meta-analysis of randomized controlled trials. JAMA. 2007;297(15):1683–96.
46. Tsapakis EM, Soldani F, Tondo L, Baldessarini RJ. Efficacy of antidepressants in juvenile depression: meta-analysis. Br J Psychiatry. 2008;193(1):10–7.
47. Reeve A. Recognizing and treating anxiety and depression in adolescents. Normal and abnormal responses. Med Clin North Am. 2000;84(4):891–905.
48. Skegg K. Self-harm. Lancet. 2005;366(9495):1471–83.
49. Popper C. Psychiatric Pharmacosciences of Children and Adolescents. Washington, DC: American Psychiatric Press; 1987.
50. Hammad TA, Laughren TP, Racoosin JA. Suicide rates in short-term randomized controlled trials of newer antidepressants. J Clin Psychopharmacol. 2006;26(2):203–7.
51. Olfson M, Marcus SC, Shaffer D. Antidepressant drug therapy and suicide in severely depressed children and adults: A case-control study. Arch Gen Psychiatry. 2006;63(8):865–72.
52. Simon GE, Ludman EJ, Bauer MS, Unutzer J, Operskalski B. Long-term effectiveness and cost of a systematic care program for bipolar disorder. Arch Gen Psychiatry. 2006;63(5):500–8.
53. Rosack J. New data shows decline in antidepressant prescribing. Psychiatric News. 2005:1, 39.
54. Libby AM, Brent DA, Morrato EH, Orton HD, Allen R, Valuck RJ. Decline in treatment of pediatric depression after FDA advisory on risk of suicidality with SSRIs. Am J Psychiatry. 2007;164(6):884–91.
55. Shaffer D. www.fda.gov/ohrms/dockets/ac/04/slides/4006S1_03_Shaffer_files/outline.htm. 2004.
56. Hamilton BE, Minino AM, Martin JA, Kochanek KD, Strobino DM, Guyer B. Annual summary of vital statistics: 2005. Pediatrics. 2007;119(2):345–60.
57. Ludwig J, Marcotte DA. Antidepressants and Suicide. Cambridge, MA: National Bureau of Economic Research, 2003.
58. Gibbons RD, Brown CH, Hur K, Marcus SM, Bhaumik DK, Erkens JA, et al. Early evidence on the effects of regulators' suicidality warnings on SSRI prescriptions and suicide in children and adolescents. Am J Psychiatry. 2007;164(9):1356–63.
59. Baldessarini RJ, Pompili M, Tondo L. Suicidal risk in antidepressant drug trials. Arch Gen Psychiatry. 2006;63(3):246–8.
60. Ludwig J, Norberg K. Antidepressants and suicide. Cambridge, MA: National Bureau of Economic Research, 2003.
61. Brent D, Emslie G, Clarke G, Wagner KD, Asarnow JR, Keller M, et al. Switching to another SSRI or to venlafaxine with or without cognitive behavioral therapy for adolescents with SSRI-resistant depression: the TORDIA randomized controlled trial. JAMA. 2008;299(8):901–13.
62. Brent DA, Holder D, Kolko D, Birmaher B, Baugher M, Roth C, et al. A clinical psychotherapy trial for adolescent depression comparing cognitive, family, and supportive therapy. Arch Gen Psychiatry. 1997;54(9):877–85.
63. Birmaher B, Brent DA, Kolko D, Baugher M, Bridge J, Holder D, et al. Clinical outcome after short-term psychotherapy for adolescents with major depressive disorder. Arch Gen Psychiatry. 2000;57(1):29–36.
64. Mufson LH, Dorta KP, Olfson M, Weissman MM, Hoagwood K. Effectiveness research: transporting interpersonal psychotherapy for depressed adolescents (IPT-A) from the lab to school-based health clinics. Clin Child Fam Psychol Rev. 2004;7(4):251–61.

65. Mufson L, Gallagher T, Dorta KP, Young JF. A group adaptation of Interpersonal Psychotherapy for depressed adolescents. Am J Psychother. 2004;58(2):220–37.
66. Mufson L, Dorta KP, Wickramaratne P, Nomura Y, Olfson M, Weissman MM. A randomized effectiveness trial of interpersonal psychotherapy for depressed adolescents. Arch Gen Psychiatry. 2004;61(6):577–84.
67. Swedo SE, Allen AJ, Glod CA, Clark CH, Teicher MH, Richter D, et al. A controlled trial of light therapy for the treatment of pediatric seasonal affective disorder. J Am Acad Child Adolesc Psychiatry. 1997;36(6):816–21.
68. Tao R, Emslie G, Mayes T, Nakonezny P, Kennard B, Hughes C. Early prediction of acute antidepressant treatment response and remission in pediatric major depressive disorder. J Am Acad Child Adolesc Psychiatry. 2009;48(1):71–8.
69. Cheung A, Kusumakar V, Kutcher S, Dubo E, Garland J, Weiss M, et al. Maintenance study for adolescent depression. J Child Adolesc Psychopharmacol. 2008;18(4):389–94.

Managing Depression in Primary Care

Larry Culpepper and Peggy Johnson

Introduction

The need to manage depression more effectively in primary care is well established. Major depressive disorder is a common, chronic but episodic and costly condition for which primary care physicians provide the majority of care (1). Among nonpsychotic patients, symptom composition and severity differs little from adults presenting to psychiatrists (2). Patients who have chronic medical conditions such as diabetes or ischemic heart disease with concomitant major depression have poorer outcomes than do those without depression. In spite of its frequency and importance, recognition, evaluation, and management in primary care is often less than optimal, with up to 50% of depressed patients going unrecognized. In this chapter, we will focus on aspects of managing care of depression in primary care settings necessary.

Epidemiology

Major depression is the leading worldwide cause of disability as measured by the number of years lived with a disabling condition among persons age 5 and older (3). On the basis of 2001–2002 estimates, major depression occurs at some point in the lives of 16.2% (32.6–35.1 million) US adults and is present at some point during each year in 6.6% (13.1–14.2 million). The mean duration of an episode is 16 weeks. The prevalence of major depression usually ranges from 5 to 9% among adults seen in primary care settings.

P. Johnson (✉)
Department of Psychiatry, Boston University School of Medicine, 85 East Newton Street, Boston, MA, USA
e-mail: Peggy.johnson@bmc.org

D.A. Ciraulo and R.I. Shader (eds.), *Pharmacotherapy of Depression*,
DOI 10.1007/978-1-60327-435-7_10, © Springer Science+Business Media, LLC 2011

Diagnostic Screening in Primary Care

Patients with major depressive disorder present to primary care physicians in a variety of ways, including ones directly related to their mood, and others associated with a number of non-mood related problems. The latter include a variety of somatic complaints, and work, family, or other relationship problems. High utilization – especially for somatic symptoms not attributable to specific illness – might be a sign of underlying depressive illness, the likelihood of which increases as the number of such symptoms increases (4). Including these, common presentations associated with depression are:

- >5 Medical visits per year
- Multiple unexplained symptoms
- Fatigue
- Pain syndromes
- Sleep disturbance
- Weight gain or loss
- Dementia
- Irritable bowel syndrome
- Dampened effect
- Complaints of stress or mood disturbance
- Work or relationship dysfunction
- Changes in interpersonal relationships
- Decreased adherence to treatment recommendations and self-care

While many patients present with these conditions, depression is also common in other patients. Therefore screening of all adult primary care patients should be coupled with ongoing case identification based on recognition of the above presentations and of risk factors for depression.

Overview

The U.S. Preventive Services Task Force (USPSTF) recommends screening all adults for major depression (5). However, the Task Force qualifies this recommendation: screening is recommended only in practice settings that have the capacity to assure accurate diagnosis, effective treatment, and follow-up. In the absence of practice systems to actively manage patients who screen positive for depression, long-term outcomes are not improved by the detection of depression through screening. The Task Force concluded that the optimal interval for screening in adults is unknown.

The Task Force also concluded that the risks and benefits of routine screening of children and adolescents for depression are not known. It found that screening tests perform reasonably well in adolescents. In contrast, the impact of routine depression screening on patient outcome has not been studied in pediatric populations in primary care settings. Given that the prevalence of depression in children is about 1% and increases over teenage years to the adult rate, the positive predictive value of proposed instruments is low, and treatment is not as efficacious as in adults, screening (as opposed to case finding in those demonstrating symptoms or major risk factors) is of questionable benefit in children and adolescents, and conclusions from adult studies are likely not generalizable to these age groups (5).

For screening adults, a two-step process may be most efficient in primary care settings. In two-step screening processes the first step should have high sensitivity but can be of only moderate specificity to reduce the number of patients that proceed to the second step. The Task Force found that asking two questions is about as effective as longer instruments for the initial recognition (first step) of potentially depressed adults. These two questions are:

Over the past 2 weeks, have you felt down, depressed, or hopeless?
Over the past 2 weeks, have you felt little interest or pleasure in doing things?

If the response to either is "yes," progressing to a second more thorough set of screening questions can further reduce the number of false positives while gathering information to facilitate confirmation of the diagnosis by clinical interview. Case identification can use the same instruments as screening; starting with the second-step instrument may be most efficient.

In eight studies of depression screening evaluated by the Task Force (5), clinicians simply received the screening results; in seven of these, recognition of depression – especially major depression – increased by a factor of two to three compared with usual care. However, this increase in recognition did not result in increased treatment or improved patient outcomes. Although little data is available to quantitate them, the potential harms due to screening include false-positive screening results and the burden of further diagnostic work-up, adverse effects and costs of treatment for patients who are incorrectly diagnosed as depressed, and potential adverse effects of labeling.

Most screening instruments can be administered in less than 5 min and are easily interpreted. They generally have sensitivities (the percent of those who actually have major depression detected) of 80–90% but only fair specificities (the percent of those who are not depressed who score as such) in the 70–85% range (6). Given that about 5–10% of adults seen in primary care settings are depressed at the time, about 24–40% of those who screen positive actually have major depression. Some who screen false positive have dysthymia or minor depressive disorders that might benefit from closer monitoring or treatment. Still others may have other disorders such as an anxiety disorder, substance abuse, or grief reactions and some will have no disorder at all. Therefore the finding of a positive screen does not establish the diagnosis but requires further evaluation before a management plan is determined.

Screening Tools for Primary Care

The PHQ-9 (7), QIDS-C (clinician administered), QID-SR (patient self-rated) (8), and the Beck Depression Inventory (9) are brief instruments that have been validated both for the recognition of depression and as measures of severity, functional impairment, and change in these over time. These instruments have sensitivities and specificities for the detection of major depression of about 80% (10). For the elderly the Geriatric Depression Scale may be of particular benefit (11).

The PHQ-9 (7) (see Fig. 2) was developed in the late 90s specifically for use in primary care, and has been incorporated into a number of "toolkits" evaluated for effectiveness in the active management of major depression. It consists of a question for each of the nine symptoms used by the DSM-IV to establish diagnosis of major depression, plus a query regarding severity of functional impairment. The QIDS instrument was developed as part of a large NIMH funded study conducted in private primary care and psychiatric practices. It consists of 16 items and is slightly more complex in its scoring (8). The Beck comes in 13 and 21 item versions, the BDI (12), and the BDI-II (9). The items in it do not closely adhere to the DSM criteria; however, its clinical performance in screening for depression is similar to the PHQ-9 and QIDS. There is little evidence to recommend one screening instrument over another; so physicians should choose based on their personal preference, the patient population served, and the practice setting. Of note, the PHQ-9 and QIDS are available in numerous languages, and as part of larger practice toolkits proven beneficial in the community practice setting.

Risk Factors as a Screening Consideration

In addition to screening (evaluation of all including those not reporting symptoms) adult patients, physicians should consider case findings with either significant risks or presentations as listed above among their patients that are suggestive of depression. Case finding has not been evaluated separate from screening, but as with screening, it is likely to require active management of those determined to be depressed to be of benefit.

Risk factors for major depression include:

- Previous episodes of depression, current or past anxiety disorders, or substance abuse
- Recent bereavement or loss (e.g., death or divorce)
- Family history of depression
- Chronic medical illness
- Dysthymia
- Major trauma
- Stressful life events (job or geographic change)
- History of postpartum mood disorders
- Perimenopausal status
- Low income status
- Spouse with depressive illness

Of these, past history of depression, recent bereavement, and major trauma all convey major risk. Eighty-five percent of individuals will have a recurrence by 15 years following an initial lifetime episode of depression. A past history of a single episode of depression is associated with a 50% risk of recurrence within 5 years, two past episodes convey a 70% risk, and three or more episodes a 90% risk (13). Up to 30–40% of those experiencing or witnessing a major trauma develop major depression – a rate similar to that of developing post-traumatic stress disorder (14). Recent bereavement is a significant risk for depression, especially in the elderly.

The onset of depression is influenced by one's genetic makeup and family history, past and current stressful life events, and the interaction of these factors. Those with inherited biological vulnerability (e.g., through the short form of the serotonin transporter gene) have an increased risk of developing depression, and this is much more marked for those with both a childhood history of trauma or abuse, or a recent history of stressful life events (15). However, this relationship to stress (40–60% of first episodes of depression follow major life events) decreases as the number of past episodes increases. Chronic illness, including cardiac disease, diabetes, arthritis, and pain syndromes, all increase the risk of depression compared to those without any chronic illness. This relationship may be bi-directional and mediated by systems involved in the stress response, with major depression also resulting in an increased risk of a number of chronic illnesses (16).

Income relates to stress and depression as well, with the prevalence of depression increasing from about 5% in the highest income groups to 15% in the lowest (17). Interestingly, the risk of depression also doubles if a spouse experiences major depression (18).

Postpartum depression and premenstrual dysphoria are additional indicators of increased risk of depression. Women are also at increased risk of developing depression for the first time, or of having a recurrent episode of depression during the perimenopausal years (19, 20).

Assessment and Differential Diagnosis

For patients who screen positive for depression and for those for whom this diagnosis is suspected by initial clinical interview, further evaluation should:

- Verify the diagnosis through confirmation of symptom presence.
- Eliminate other potential causes for the symptoms.
- Assess severity.
- Assess suicidality.
- Assess other considerations pertinent to treatment selection and prognosis, including comorbidities, treatment history, and patient preferences.

Confirmation of diagnosis of major depression requires the presence of either or both anhedonia ("have you felt little interest or pleasure in doing things") or decreased mood ("have you felt down, depressed, or hopeless") over the past 2 weeks, at least five symptoms in total, and that symptoms significantly impair functioning (see Fig. 1). *The initial assessment also involves determining that other causes are not the source of symptoms prior to confirmation of diagnosis of major depression.*

DSM Criteria for Major Depression

A. Five (or more) of the following symptoms during the same 2-weeks and a change from previous functioning; at least one of the symptoms is either (1) depressed mood or (2) loss of interest or pleasure:

(1) depressed mood most of the day, nearly every day, as indicated by either subjective report (e.g., feels sad or empty) or observation made by others (e.g., appears tearful).

(2) markedly diminished interest or pleasure in all, or almost all, activities most of the day, nearly every day (as indicated by either subjective account or observation made by others)

(4) significant weight loss when not dieting or weight gain (e.g., a change of >5% of body weight in a month), or decrease or increase in appetite nearly every day.

(4) insomnia or hypersomnia nearly every day

(5) psychomotor agitation or retardation nearly every day (observable by others, not merely subjective feelings of restlessness or being slowed down)

(6) fatigue or loss of energy nearly every day

(7) feelings of worthlessness or excessive or inappropriate guilt (which may be delusional) nearly every day (not merely self-reproach or guilt about being sick)

(8) diminished ability to think or concentrate, or indecisiveness, nearly every day (either by subjective account or as observed by others)

(9) recurrent thoughts of death (not just fear of dying), recurrent suicidal ideation without a specific plan, or a suicide attempt or a specific plan for committing suicide

B. The symptoms do not meet criteria for a Mixed Bipolar Episode.

C. The symptoms cause clinically significant distress or impairment in social, occupational, or other important areas of functioning.

D. The symptoms are not due to the direct physiological effects of a substance (e.g., a drug of abuse, a medication) or a general medical condition (e.g., hypothyroidism).

E. The symptoms are not better accounted for by bereavement, i.e., after the loss of a loved one, the symptoms persist for longer than 2 months or are characterized by marked functional impairment, morbid preoccupation with worthlessness, suicidal ideation, psychotic symptoms, or psychomotor retardation.

Fig. 1 DSM criteria for major depression (90)

Potential other causes include other psychiatric illness (especially bipolar disorder and anxiety disorders), substance abuse, bereavement, medical illness, and medications.

Anxiety disorders at times present with symptoms that can be confused with depression. In addition, at least one anxiety disorder is comorbid with major depression in 50–60% of those with depression. Such comorbidity increases symptom severity, functional impairment, suicide risk, and the time required for response to treatment (21). When anxiety disorders are comorbid, they frequently develop several years before the first episode of major depression (22). In addition, while depression tends to be an episodic, recurrent disease, anxiety disorders tend to be chronic.

Few instruments have been developed for primary care screening of anxiety disorders. Remaining alert to and exploring further any history suggestive of generalized anxiety, panic attacks, social phobia, experiencing or witnessing major trauma (post traumatic stress disorder), or obsessive compulsive behaviors remains the best strategy for detection of anxiety disorders. For generalized anxiety disorder, the GAD-7 has recently been validated, and provides an instrument similar to the PHQ-9 for depression (23). Using this may help alert the family physician to generalized anxiety disorder, but might not detect other anxiety disorders.

Screening for substance abuse during the initial assessment of depressive symptoms is helpful in determining the correct diagnosis and in planning treatment. Major depressive disorder and alcoholism are distinct clinical entities rather than due to a common underlying pathologic state. While some depressed individuals may self-treat with alcohol (e.g., for accompanying insomnia), alcoholism is not a recognized complication of depression and the prevalence of alcoholism in patients with major depression is not increased over that in the general population (24). However, 10–30% of patients with alcoholism suffer from depression at the time of evaluation.

While bereavement is a normal process not requiring treatment, a major loss may lead to the development of a major depressive episode. A past history of depression leads to its frequent recurrence following a major loss, particularly for an individual with few social supports. In one study (25), at 2 months following the death of a spouse, almost nine out of ten were still grieving, while one out of five met criteria for major depression. At 2 years follow-up, the latter group had spent 76% of the intervening time with minor or major depression, were much more likely to remain functionally impaired, and to not remarry. At 2 months, the sadness associated with bereavement occurred in waves brought on by memories while that of depression was enduring and autonomous. Psychomotor retardation, feelings of worthlessness, and suicide plans also are uncommon with simple bereavement.

Finally, medical illness, particularly hypothyroidism, might be responsible for depressive symptoms. A screening TSH can be beneficial, particularly in those over the age of 40. A review of systems to recognize other comorbid medical illness may be helpful when considering treatment options. A number of chronic illnesses (e.g., congestive heart failure, renal disease, Alzheimer's disease, chronic pulmonary disease) have symptoms that overlap those of major depression. In such cases, symptoms remain valid for the diagnosis of major depression (26). Cognitive symptoms (negative thinking, difficulty concentrating) are highly reliable, affective symptoms (depressed mood, lack of interest or energy) are reliable, behavioral symptoms (impaired daily function) and physical symptoms (decreased appetite, weight loss, insomnia) are generally reliable but may be evaluated based on clinician judgment (27).

Bipolar Disorder

Bipolar disorder – because of its severity and the potential of antidepressants as monotherapy to precipitate a switch to mania or a mixed bipolar episode – should be considered before confirming the diagnosis of major depression. A history of early onset (before age 25), a family history suggestive of bipolar disorder, past treatment resistance or a rapid or exaggerated treatment response, decreased need for sleep, increased agitation or irritability should all raise suspicion of bipolar disorder. While the peak age of onset of major depression is in the mid to late 20s that of bipolar disorder is between the ages of 15 and 19 years. However, both can commence at any age, from early childhood into old age (28). In more than half of patients ultimately diagnosed with bipolar disorder, the first episodes of illness are depressive, and it is not uncommon for patients to have several depressive episodes prior to their first manic or hypomanic episode (29). Compared to those with major depression, those with bipolar disorder often have more severe depressive episodes and greater suicidal behavior. The Mood Disorder Questionnaire (MDQ) may be useful in further exploring this diagnostic possibility (30). However, its performance characteristics have not been determined within primary care settings for either screening or evaluation of the possibility of bipolar disorder in those considered to have unipolar depression (31). Given its performance in the general population and in psychiatric patients, it is likely to have a fairly high rate of false positive results and requires a clinical interview before a final diagnosis is determined.

Risk Assessment

About 31,000 people in the United States and one million worldwide die by suicide each year and 650,000 people in the United States are treated emergently following a suicide attempt (32). About 60% of completed suicides occur in those with histories of major depression. The risk of suicide in those with major depression compared to the general population is increased 20-fold (33). The lifetime rate of suicide attempts in those with major depression is estimated to be 8% with an increased risk in those with comorbid anxiety disorders (e.g., 25% with comorbid panic disorder and 38% in those with comorbid PTSD) (34).

In 2003 warnings about a possible association between antidepressant use and suicidal thinking and behavior were issued by the U.S. Food and Drug Administration and by several European regulators. A disturbing recent finding is that the resulting 22% decrease in SSRI prescriptions for youths in both the United States and the Netherlands was accompanied by a 14% increase in completed suicide in the same age group in the United States (2003–2004) and by a 49% increase in the Netherlands (2003–2005). This compares to a 33% decline in completed suicide in the United States accompanying a 91% increase in prescriptions during the preceding 5 years (1998–2003) and very similar changes in The Netherlands (35).

Despite its importance, there are no data to demonstrate that screening for suicide in primary care settings reduces completed suicide or attempts (36). In part, this is because suicidal actions are relatively uncommon, and we do not have instruments with adequate sensitivity and specificity to predict which patients with suicidal thoughts will attempt suicide. Depression scales measure depression severity better than suicide risk.

In primary care settings, recognition of the suicidal patient can be a challenge. Use of a depression screening and severity assessment instrument such as the PHQ-9 that includes a question about suicidal ideation ("Thought that you would be better off dead or hurting yourself in some way?") is helpful and can augment the clinician's interview.

Physicians might worry that asking about suicide would initiate suicidal ideation or actions, but this has not been demonstrated. In contrast, many patients seek the opportunity to discuss suicidal thoughts, and may not verbalize these issues without being prompted. The only clue for suicidality might be the initiation of an office visit. While some patients may be reluctant to initiate discussion of their intent to commit suicide, patients with suicidal ideation if asked usually will tell their physicians about such thoughts (37).

An understanding of the risk factors for suicide can be helpful in recognizing high risk patients, and in their assessment once identified. Patient characteristics that increase risk of suicide include:

Age, sex, and race: The risk of completed suicide increases with age; however, young adults attempt suicide more often than older adults (38). Women attempt suicide 4 times more often than men, but men are 3 times more likely to commit suicide (39). These differences relate more to the lethality of the method chosen (e.g., firearms) than to a difference across age or sex in completion rates for a particular method (40). About 90% of suicides in the United States are by white people, 72% by white men.

Marital and work status: Those never married are at highest risk, followed in descending order of risk by widowed, separated, or divorced individuals, those married without children, and those married with children. Unemployed and unskilled individuals are at higher risk of suicide than those employed and skilled; occupational failure may lead to higher risk. Physicians may be at increased risk; a meta-analysis of 25 studies found a suicide rate ratio for female physicians of 2.27 (95% CI 1.90–2.73) and for male physicians of 1.41 (95% CI 1.21–1.65) compared to the general population (41). Risk also increases in patients who live alone, have lost a loved one, or experienced a failed relationship within 1 year (42). The anniversary of a significant loss is also a time of increased risk.

Hopelessness: Hopelessness may mitigate the relationship between interpersonal losses, loneliness, low self esteem, and suicide and can persist with attendant continued high risk of suicide even when depression has remitted (32). In one multivariate model, hopelessness was 1.3 times more important than depression in explaining suicidal ideation (43).

Impulsivity: Particularly among adolescents and young adults, impulsivity increases the likelihood of acting on suicidal thoughts, and the combination of hopelessness, impulsivity, and dis-inhibition due to substance abuse may be particularly lethal (32).

Health: Suicide risk increases with medical illness including chronic pain, chronic disease, and recent surgery (32). However, HIV infection alone does not increase risk (44).

Past history: Half of suicide completers previously made an attempt and 1 out of 100 suicide attempt survivors die committing suicide within a year, a risk 100 times that of the general population (45). Abuse and other adverse childhood experiences may increase the risk of suicide in adults. This relationship appeared to be at least partially mediated by the presence of alcoholism, depression, and illicit drug use, which are also strongly associated with adverse events in childhood (32).

Family history and genetics: A family history of suicide increases the risk; a first-degree relative who committed suicide increases this risk sixfold. While it is not clear if genetic makeup leads to the underlying psychiatric disorder or to the suicide itself, the heritability of suicide is in the 30–50% range (32). Additionally, having a spouse who commits suicide increases the risk of suicide, showing the importance of environmental effects (46).

Access to means: The risk of suicide increases with access to weapons, especially firearms. In the United States, 57% of overall suicides and 62% in men are by firearm use; rates are increased four to tenfold in adolescents who live in a household with a gun (47). The second leading method of suicide in the United States is hanging for men and poisoning for women.

Protective factors: Social support and family connectedness is protective while family discord increases the risk of suicide (32). Parenthood – particularly for mothers – and pregnancy decrease the risk of suicide (48). Participating in religious activities and religiosity are associated with a lower risk of suicide.

The first step in assessing suicide risk is to evaluate the presence, frequency, intensity, duration and content of suicidal thoughts, any changes in chronic thoughts, and if or how the patient has been controlling these thoughts. This may be accomplished by asking the patient if he/she has thought of ending his/her life, or if he/she feels he/she would be better off dead, or has lost interest in living. Additional potentially helpful information might be derived from inquiring about expectations about death (e.g., thoughts of reuniting with a spouse), thoughts of punishment of others, escaping a painful situation, or of harming others.

For those with suicidal thoughts, the next step is to determine the characteristics of the patient's suicide plan (see Fig. 2) and any precipitating events such as the death of a loved one, breakup of a marriage, work, school or social failure, sexual identity crisis, or trauma. Further information that is helpful in determining appropriate management includes the patient's sense of hopelessness ("what the future looks like") any alcohol and substance history including binging, impulsivity, and family and social supports or stressors. Other important factors include whether the patient is engaged in and complying with treatment, and details of any previous suicide attempt.

With the above information in hand, the risk of suicide should be estimated. Consider it imminent (e.g., suicide might be attempted within the next 48 h) in patients who have an active plan or intent to harm themselves and have a lethal means readily accessible. Also at high risk are those who are psychotic (particularly

Evaluating a patient's suicide plan can be accomplished by asking about the following:

Has a plan been formulated or implemented, including a specific method, place, and time?
What is the anticipated outcome of the plan?
Are the means of committing suicide available or readily accessible?
Does the patient know how to use these means?
What is the lethality of the plan?
What is the patient's conception of lethality versus the objective lethality?
What is the likelihood of rescue?
Have any preparations been made (e.g., gathering pills, changing wills, suicide notes); how close has the patient come to completing the plan?
Has the patient practiced the suicidal act or has an actual attempt already been made?
What is the strength of the intent to carry out suicidal thoughts and plans, including the ability to control impulsivity?
What is the accessibility of support systems and recent stressors that may threaten the patient's ability to cope with difficulties and ability to participate in treatment planning?

Fig. 2 Evaluating a patient's suicide plan can be accomplished by asking the following

if they hear voices that are telling them to commit suicide), cognitively impaired, or lack judgment. Such patients usually require immediate hospitalization via ambulance. In such individuals, electroconvulsive therapy (ECT) may be lifesaving (32).

Patients in whom the risk of suicide is high but not imminent (e.g., those with a desire to commit suicide but who do not have a specific plan) need aggressive treatment, but not necessarily hospitalization. Interventions might include psychiatric treatment, control of substance use, mobilizing family and social supports, reducing access to firearms, medications, or other potentially lethal means, and ensuring frequent contact with helping professionals and supports. Contributing factors should be addressed including precipitating events, ongoing life difficulties, and comorbid mental disorders. Of note, contracting for safety has not been evaluated adequately; there is little evidence that such "contracts" are effective. Consequently, they may provide a false sense of security (32). Clear communication, maintaining a strong therapeutic alliance, and frequent re-evaluation are recommended. Supportive primary care counseling, referral to psychotherapy, and engagement of community, religious, and family supports can be helpful.

Symptom Severity Assessment

The PHQ-9 (7) and QIDS (49) are among instruments that provide a numeric score of severity and functional impairment (see Fig. 3 for PHQ-9 and interpretation) and have been validated for repeated use to measure change in severity over time. Having recurrent depression and comorbid psychiatric disorders are both associated with increased depression severity (50). Severity is categorized as:

- Mild: few, if any, symptoms in excess of those required to make the diagnosis and only minor impairment in occupational and/or social functioning.

a

PHQ-9

1.Over the *last 2 weeks*, how often have you been bothered by any of the following problems?

	Not at all	Several days	More than half the days	Nearly every day
	0	1	2	3
a. Little interest or pleasure in doing things				
b. Feeling down, depressed, or hopeless.				
c. Trouble falling/staying asleep, sleeping too much.				
d. Feeling tired or having little energy.				
e. Poor appetite or overeating.				
f. Feeling bad about yourself – or that you are a failure or have let yourself or your family down.				
g. Trouble concentrating on things, such as reading the newspaper or watching television.				
h. Moving or speaking so slowly that other people could have noticed. Or the opposite – being so fidgety or restless that you have been moving around a lot more than usual.				
i. Thoughts that you would be better off dead or of hurting yourself in some way.				

2. If you checked off any problem on this questionnaire so far, how difficult have these problems made it for you to do your work, take care of things at home, or get along with other people?

Not difficult at all	Somewhat difficult	Very difficult	Extremely difficult

b

Interpretation of PHQ-9 results

Score/ Symptom Level	Treatment
0-4 No depression	Consider other diagnoses
5-9 Minimal	▪ Consider other diagnoses ▪ If diagnosis is depression, watchful waiting is appropriate initial management
10-14 Mild	▪ Consider watchful waiting ▪ If active treatment is needed, medication or psychotherapy is equally effective; consider function score in choosing treatment
15-19 Moderate	▪ Active treatment with medication or psychotherapy is recommended ▪ Medication or psychotherapy is equally effective
20-27 Severe	▪ Medication treatment is recommended ▪ For many people, psychotherapy is useful as an additional treatment ▪ People with severe symptoms often benefit from consultation with a psychiatrist

Fig. 3 (**a**) PHQ-9. (**b**) Interpretation of PHQ-9 results (91)

- Moderate: symptoms or functional impairment between mild and severe.
- Severe: several symptoms in excess of those necessary to make the diagnosis and marked interference with occupational and/or social functioning. Severe is further subdivided into those with and without psychotic features. The latter generally are hallucinations or delusions.

Assessing severity at the time of diagnosis is important in determining both prognosis and treatment. It can also be helpful in timing follow-up contact. Increased severity has been shown consistently to be associated with worse outcomes and less likelihood of remission following treatment (51). Patients with severe depression also may take longer to respond to treatment (52). In addition, severe patients often are high utilizers of health care; in one study in family practice, severe symptoms were associated with a doubling of resource use (53). Perhaps most important, baseline assessment of severity provides a starting point for evaluating effectiveness of treatment and the need to adjust treatment if a patient does not respond adequately (see below).

For those with mild depression, watchful waiting with reassessment within a few weeks is appropriate. Patients with mild depression and significant stressors may benefit from counseling. For those with moderate severity depression either pharmacotherapy or psychotherapy is indicated. Since significant improvement with psychotherapy alone generally requires a longer interval of treatment than pharmacotherapy, pharmacotherapy is recommended for those with severe depression – either alone or in combination with psychotherapy.

Management of Depression

To be effective in improving outcomes, for many patients the management of major depressive disorder in primary care requires more than provision of medication or referral for psychotherapy and routine follow-up. Instead, evidence suggests that the optimal management program includes having a practice staff member serve as a case manager, treatment using medication or psychotherapeutic strategies proven effective, organized follow-up at which times treatment adherence and response are assessed and treatment adjusted if indicated, and access to psychiatric consultation or referral (54). The practice staff (e.g., office nurse) who serves as a case manager should have a systematic way of:

- Tracking and reminding patients of planned office visits.
- Making frequent contact with patients to provide education and self-management support.
- Monitoring treatment adherence and effectiveness, preferably using an objective measure such as the PHQ-9 or QIDS.

Several studies have evaluated such organized systems of depression treatment management and found them to be effective, particularly if they include a case manager and a strategy for collaboration with a psychiatric resource. In one study of a disease management program implemented in 3 HMOs, the rate of filling at least one prescription for an antidepressant increased from 32 to 82%, and of filling at least three prescriptions from 18 to 69% (55). Other studies have found similar improvements coupled with improvement in patient outcomes, although in some the degree of improvement was modest (54). A recent Cochrane Collaborative metaanalysis of 13 studies of case management of depression in primary care settings found that those receiving intervention had a relative risk of remission of 1.39, of response of 1.82, and of treatment adherence of 1.50 at 6–12 months (56. Common denominators of effective programs are assertive outreach and collaborative care to encourage recognition of depression (screening) and adequacy of treatment (frequent follow-up during the acute phase of treatment to encourage adherence and to make treatment adjustments as necessary). In contrast, multiple studies have demonstrated consistently that programs aimed solely at improving physician knowledge and skill (e.g., one study (57) used interactive discussions, expert demonstrations, role play, case reviews, and other techniques over a 3-month training interval) do not improve patient outcomes.

Maximizing Treatment Outcomes

Adherence and treatment outcomes are improved by engaging patients in understanding their illness and treatment options and their role in treatment management. Basic patient education includes messages that:

- Depression is common.
- Depression is a medical disease, not a character defect.
- Depression involves biological changes in the brain including depletion of key neurotransmitters called serotonin, catecholamines, and disturbances of the HPA axis.
- Treatment is effective for most patients; recovery is the rule, not the exception.
- The aim of treatment is complete and long-term remission, not just getting better but staying well.
- Be alert to early signs and symptoms of recurrence and seek treatment early if depression returns.

Attending to patient preference when choosing treatment improves adherence and outcomes (58). Patients who perceive more self-control in their health care have greater reduction in depressive symptoms, whether treated with psychotherapy or an antidepressant. While many patients are accepting of either medication or psychotherapy, for some, the time and expense associated with psychotherapy may make medications preferable, while others have concerns regarding medications or their side effects. Also of importance to treatment choice are the patient's cultural beliefs and sufficiency or lack of resources such as medical insurance, transportation, and child care. For the patient treated with an antidepressant, further patient education is critical. Based on a primary care study, the following educational messages are useful in improving adherence (59):

- Antidepressants work only if taken every day.
- Antidepressants are not addictive.
- Benefits from medication appear slowly.
- Mild side effects are common, and usually improve with time.
- Be alert for the emergence of agitation, irritability, or suicidality, and worsening depression and immediately report them to the physician.
- Continue antidepressants even after you feel better.
- If you're thinking about stopping the medication, call first.
- The goal of treatment is complete remission (e.g., a PHQ score of 4 or less); sometimes it takes a few tries.

Treatment Approaches

Treatment of depressive illnesses detected in primary care settings can be effective using either psychotherapy or medication (5). A review of 12 psychotherapy trials based on primary care settings found that psychotherapy resulted in similar outcomes to those obtained using antidepressants and better than a primary care physician's usual care (60). Lower relapse rates occur among patients receiving psychotherapy. In mild to moderate levels of depression, psychotherapy can be as effective as medication. With severe depression, antidepressant medication may be more helpful in the acute phases; and a combination of medication and psychotherapy may be particularly beneficial. Few studies have examined the effect of combining medications and psychotherapy. However, in one randomized trial of combination therapy, the combination resulted in a 73% response or remission, significantly better than either form of treatment alone (48%) (61).

There are numerous forms of psychotherapy, just as there are numerous medication options. Based on current professional guidelines and evidence reviews, problem-solving therapy, interpersonal psychotherapy, and pharmacotherapy are considered efficacious for major depression, with cognitive-behavioral and cognitive therapy also possibly efficacious (62). For women with a history of abuse, cognitive behavioral therapy may provide greater long-term benefit and resiliency than medication alone.

If the choice of treatment is medication, choice of antidepressant should be based on the patient's past response to treatment, comorbid psychiatric and medical conditions, and the physician's familiarity with specific antidepressants. A medication that previously resulted in treatment success and was well tolerated should be the initial choice if depression recurs (63). To date, clinical studies and systematic reviews have not demonstrated clear superiority with regard to clinical outcomes, quality of life outcomes, and overall treatment costs for any single class or individual antidepressant (64). Consequently, the SSRIs are usually the first choice in primary care because of less severe side effects and markedly less danger with overdose than the older heterocyclics. The latter antidepressants and the monoamine oxidase inhibitors may be lethal if overdosed and therefore should be avoided in patients who are suicidal. The selective serotonin reuptake inhibitors (SSRIs) appear to be much safer when taken in overdose and should be the drugs of choice in potentially suicidal depressed patients. Of note, the research regarding the efficacy of St. John's Wort is perplexing. While European (primarily German) trials consistently demonstrate efficacy similar to antidepressants, similar high quality studies in the United States have consistently demonstrated no difference in effect from placebo.

For patients who have comorbid cardiovascular disease or diabetes, the SSRIs may be the preferred agents, since, although not demonstrated conclusively, they may improve cardiac outcomes, including decrease in cardiac morbidity and mortality (65). Suggested mechanisms by which these outcomes might be improved include an antiplatelet aggregation effect similar to but through a different mechanism than aspirin (they may be used concomitantly with aspirin), improved cardiac beat-to-beat variability and decreased cardiac irritability, and improved adherence to lifestyle changes and treatment (66, 67). The SNRIs do not improve, and might decrease, cardiac beat-to-beat variability (68), and may have cardiac effects similar to the heterocyclics in overdose. Weight gain is a concern for many patients, including those with comorbid medical illness. Of the SSRIs, paroxetine has the highest rate of significant weight gain (20–25% of subjects reporting >7% increase from initial body weight) while other SSRIs/SNRIs are associated with weight gain in 5–10% of patients (69). Fluoxetine and paroxetine are strong inhibitors of the cytochrome P450 2D6 enzyme, and as such have greater potential than other SSRIs/SNRIs for drug interactions in those with chronic medical illness (70).

Nausea and occasionally diarrhea, agitation, restlessness, headache, and insomnia are common side effects with SSRIs. These usually subside after the first week or two of treatment, and usually do not recur with dose increase thereafter. They may be associated with a patient's genetic variation in drug metabolizing enzymes (71). Informing patients of these potential transient side effects can improve early adherence to treatment. Insomnia may occur either as a comorbid problem, symptom of depression, or treatment side effect. Treatment of insomnia with one of the non-benzodiazepine sleep medications may improve antidepressant adherence and other depressive symptoms.

Sexual side effects are not uncommon after several weeks or months of SSRI therapy and can lead to medication discontinuation. Since sexual dysfunction also may be comorbid or develop as a component of depression, a brief sexual function screen at the time of diagnosis or treatment initiation may be helpful. If sexual dysfunction is subsequently considered an antidepressant side effect, several interventions may be helpful (72). For patients using an antidepressant with a half-life in the 24–30 h range (e.g., citalopram, escitalopram, sertraline), a 12–16-h delay in a day's dosing can improve sexual function without precipitating discontinuation symptoms. For others, augmentation with bupropion or use of an erectile dysfunction medication may provide benefit (73).

Regardless of the specific treatment prescribed, an organized practice system for monitoring and managing depressed patients is essential to improving patient outcomes. The federally funded STAR-D study, involving patients in small primary care and psychiatric group practices, found that while only about 30% of patients attained remission from their initial medication treatment, this was increased to about 70% by active management during the acute phase of treatment (74). This management strategy included regular objective measurement of treatment response with a brief symptom severity scale (in this study the QIDS, although the PHQ-9 is equally useful) with treatment adjustment in those not responding or continuing to progress to remission. Treatment adjustments took into account patient preference for psychotherapy or pharmacotherapy. An increase to the maximum approved dosage of an antidepressant frequently results in further improvement (in the STAR-D trial, about two-thirds of patients required such dose increase).

Switching to a different antidepressant or to psychotherapy is a reasonable option for the patient who has not responded to initial treatment, or for whom side-effects are problematic. While referral for psychiatric consultation would be recommended in individuals who appear to be treatment resistant, there are several basic recommendations. For those with partial benefit from a treatment, augmentation (either with medication or psychotherapy) is a reasonable option. The STAR-D trial found that both augmentation and switching resulted in a further 20–30% of patients attaining remission with no one approach being markedly better (75). Augmentation in the STAR-D trial was with bupropion or buspirone; at a further step in the management protocol addition of thyroid supplementation or lithium were also demonstrated to be beneficial (76). A recent meta-analysis found that augmentation using an atypical antipsychotic might be beneficial in patients with treatment resistant depression (77).

Exercise at a dose consistent with public health recommendations can provide significant adjunctive therapeutic benefit, especially if the patient continues the exercise over time (78, 79). An exercise prescription is more likely to be effective if the physician helps the patient chose a form that they enjoy, set realistic goals, anticipate barriers including from symptoms of depression (fatigue, lack of motivation), and keep expectations realistic to avoid guilt or self-blame for not fully carrying out the exercise plan.

The treatment of depression in the context of substance abuse is particularly challenging though common in primary care settings. Few studies have evaluated integrated treatment strategies for patients with both major depression and substance abuse (80). However, several studies have found that alcohol, cocaine, and other substances dependencies are improved by treating comorbid depression. Even fewer studies have assessed the effect of treating substance abuse on comorbid depression.

Treatment Goals

The goal for the initial acute phase of treatment of depression is the attainment of remission of symptoms (for instance as indicated by a PHQ-9 score of <5). Once remission is attained, a continuation of treatment (the "continuation phase" of treatment) is required to prevent relapse. For patients in whom depressive episodes have been recurrent, the continuation phase of treatment is followed by a maintenance phase to prevent future recurrent episodes.

Initial remission of symptoms is important, since patients who respond to treatment (i.e., a >50% reduction in symptom severity) but continue to be symptomatic have persistent functional impairment and are at very high risk of relapse within a few months (81–83). In one study, personality disorder, recurrent depression, low self-esteem, and low satisfaction with social support were psychosocial predictors of not attaining remission (84). About two-thirds of patients who attain remission during the first 3–4 months of therapy but stop treatment at that point will relapse within the following year (85). This risk is reduced to about 20% if instead they continue treatment for at least an additional 4–6 months (63).

Patients with recurrent major depressive episodes are at high risk of further episodes, and this risk can be reduced substantially by indefinite continuation of antidepressant therapy at the dose required to obtain initial remission. Studies have demonstrated this benefit for at least the first 2 years of maintenance therapy, and the consensus of expert opinion is that long-term therapy is clearly indicated for those with at least three past episodes of depression and might be of benefit after two episodes for those with severe depression or depression marked by comorbidity or difficulty in attaining a treatment response (86, 87).

Several studies have identified the reasons for and timing of treatment discontinuation among patients treated for depression. In one survey about 40% stopped therapy by 3 months, with over 60% not informing their physician (59). In another, 55% stopped therapy because they were feeling better (at a mean of 11 weeks), while 23% stopped due to side effects (at a mean of 6.5 weeks). An additional group stopped for a number of reasons related to worry about taking medication or stigma related to depression (88). All of these concerns are potentially modifiable through initial patient education, reinforcement of such education as patients improve, and monitoring of treatment and treatment response though practice management systems as described above.

While not yet evidence based, a current research focus involves the concept of recovery as the ultimate goal of depression treatment. This concept includes not only attainment of remission of symptoms, but extends beyond it to the full recovery of functioning in all areas of life (e.g., work, family, social) and improvement in quality of life (89).

Conclusion

Depression is a treatable cause of pain, suffering, disability, and death. Its identification and treatment in primary care settings cannot be overstated. Judicious use of current screening tools, thorough assessment, and thoughtful treatment strategies are important in achieving desired outcomes.

References

1. Kessler RC, Berglund P, Demler O, Jin R, Koretz D, Merikangas KR, et al. The epidemiology of major depressive disorder: results from the National Comorbidity Survey Replication (NCS-R). JAMA. 2003;289(23):3095–105.
2. Gaynes BN, Rush AJ, Trivedi MH, Wisniewski SR, Balasubramani GK, Spencer DC, et al. Major depression symptoms in primary care and psychiatric care settings: a cross-sectional analysis. Ann Fam Med. 2007;5(2):126–34.
3. Murray CJL, Lopez AD, editors. A comprehensive assessment of mortality and disability from diseases, injuries, and risk factors in 1990 and projected to 2020. Cambridge: Harvard School of Public Health on behalf of the World Health Organization and the World Bank, Harvard University Press; 1996.
4. Kroenke K, Spitzer RL, Williams JB, Linzer M, Hahn SR, deGruy FV, III, et al. Physical symptoms in primary care. Predictors of psychiatric disorders and functional impairment. Arch Fam Med. 1994;3(9):774–9.
5. U.S. Preventive Services Task Force. Screening for depression: recommendations and rationale. Ann Intern Med. 2002;136(10):760–4.
6. Williams JW, Jr., Pignone M, Ramirez G, Perez Stellato C. Identifying depression in primary care: a literature synthesis of case-finding instruments. Gen Hosp Psychiatry. 2002;24(4):225–37.
7. Kroenke K, Spitzer RL, Williams JB. The PHQ-9: validity of a brief depression severity measure. J Gen Intern Med. 2001;16(9):606–13.
8. Rush AJ, Trivedi MH, Ibrahim HM, Carmody TJ, Arnow B, Klein DN, et al. The 16-Item Quick Inventory of Depressive Symptomatology (QIDS), clinician rating (QIDS-C), and self-report (QIDS-SR): a psychometric evaluation in patients with chronic major depression. Biol Psychiatry. 2003;54(5):573–83.
9. Beck AT, Steer RA, Ball R, Ranieri W. Comparison of Beck Depression Inventories -IA and -II in psychiatric outpatients. J Pers Assess. 1996;67(3):588–97.
10. Williams JW, Jr., Noel PH, Cordes JA, Ramirez G, Pignone M. Is this patient clinically depressed? JAMA. 2002;287(9):1160–70.
11. van Marwijk HW, Wallace P, de Bock GH, Hermans J, Kaptein AA, Mulder JD. Evaluation of the feasibility, reliability and diagnostic value of shortened versions of the geriatric depression scale. Br J Gen Pract. 1995;45(393):195–9.
12. Beck AT, Ward CH, Mendelson M, Mock J, Erbaugh J. An inventory for measuring depression. Arch Gen Psychiatry. 1961;4:561–71.
13. Mueller TI, Leon AC, Keller MB, Solomon DA, Endicott J, Coryell W, et al. Recurrence after recovery from major depressive disorder during 15 years of observational follow-up. Am J Psychiatry. 1999;156(7):1000–6.
14. Shalev AY, Freedman S, Peri T, Brandes D, Sahar T, Orr SP, et al. Prospective study of posttraumatic stress disorder and depression following trauma. Am J Psychiatry. 1998;155(5):630–7.
15. Caspi A, Sugden K, Moffitt TE, Taylor A, Craig IW, Harrington H, et al. Influence of life stress on depression: moderation by a polymorphism in the 5-HTT gene. Science. 2003;301(5631):386–9.
16. Katon W, Lin EH, Kroenke K. The association of depression and anxiety with medical symptom burden in patients with chronic medical illness. Gen Hosp Psychiatry. 2007;29(2):147–55.
17. Sturm R, Gresenz CR. Relations of income inequality and family income to chronic medical conditions and mental health disorders: national survey. BMJ. 2002;324(7328):20–3.
18. Hippisley-Cox J, Coupland C, Pringle M, Crown N, Hammersley V. Married couples' risk of same disease: cross sectional study. BMJ. 2002;325(7365):636.

19. Freeman EW, Sammel MD, Lin H, Nelson DB. Associations of hormones and menopausal status with depressed mood in women with no history of depression. Arch Gen Psychiatry. 2006;63(4):375–82.
20. Freeman EW, Sammel MD, Liu L, Gracia CR, Nelson DB, Hollander L. Hormones and menopausal status as predictors of depression in women in transition to menopause. Arch Gen Psychiatry. 2004;61(1):62–70.
21. Kessler RC, Chiu WT, Demler O, Merikangas KR, Walters EE. Prevalence, severity, and comorbidity of 12-month DSM-IV disorders in the National Comorbidity Survey Replication. Arch Gen Psychiatry. 2005;62(6):617–27.
22. Wittchen HU, Kessler RC, Pfister H, Lieb M. Why do people with anxiety disorders become depressed? A prospective-longitudinal community study. Acta Psychiatr Scand. 2000(406): 14–23.
23. Kroenke K, Spitzer RL, Williams JB, Monahan PO, Lowe B. Anxiety disorders in primary care: prevalence, impairment, comorbidity, and detection. Ann Intern Med. 2007;146(5): 317–25.
24. Depression in Primary Care. Volume 1. Detection and Diagnosis: US Department of Health and Human Services Public Health Service; 1993.
25. Zisook S, Dunn LB. Dementia and bereavement: adverse life experiences complicating depression in lateral life. Prim Care Companion J Clin Psychiatry. 2000;2(suppl 5):25–31.
26. Simon GE, Von Korff M. Medical co-morbidity and validity of DSM-IV depression criteria. Psychol Med. 2006;36(1):27–36.
27. Beekman A. Depression and medical illness in later life. Prim Care Companion J Clin Psychiatry. 2000;2(suppl 5):9–14.
28. Kupfer DJ, Frank E, Grochocinski VJ, Cluss PA, Houck PR, Stapf DA. Demographic and clinical characteristics of individuals in a bipolar disorder case registry. J Clin Psychiatry. 2002;63(2):120–5.
29. Post RM, Denicoff KD, Leverich GS, Altshuler LL, Frye MA, Suppes TM, et al. Morbidity in 258 bipolar outpatients followed for 1 year with daily prospective ratings on the NIMH life chart method. J Clin Psychiatry. 2003;64(6):680–90; quiz 738–9.
30. Hirschfeld RM. The mood disorder questionnaire: a simple, patient-rated screening instrument for bipolar disorder. Prim Care Companion J Clin Psychiatry. 2002;4(1):9–11.
31. Hirschfeld RM, Holzer C, Calabrese JR, Weissman M, Reed M, Davies M, et al. Validity of the mood disorder questionnaire: a general population study. Am J Psychiatry. 2003;160(1): 178–80.
32. Goldsmith S, Pellmar T, Kleinman A, Bunney W, editors. Reducing suicide: a national imperative. Washington: Institute of Medicine National Academies Press; 2002.
33. Harris EC, Barraclough B. Suicide as an outcome for mental disorders. A meta-analysis. Br J Psychiatry. 1997;170:205–28.
34. Bruce SE, Weisberg RB, Dolan RT, Machan JT, Kessler RC, Manchester G, et al. Trauma and posttraumatic stress disorder in primary care patients. Prim Care Companion J Clin Psychiatry. 2001;3(5):211–7.
35. Gibbons RD, Brown CH, Hur K, Marcus SM, Bhaumik DK, Erkens JA, et al. Early evidence on the effects of regulators' suicidality warnings on SSRI prescriptions and suicide in children and adolescents. Am J Psychiatry. 2007;164(9):1356–63.
36. Gaynes BN, West SL, Ford CA, Frame P, Klein J, Lohr KN. Screening for suicide risk in adults: a summary of the evidence for the U.S. Preventive Services Task Force. Ann Intern Med. 2004;140(10):822–35.
37. Michel K. Suicide prevention and primary care. In: Hawton K, Heeringen, KV, editors. The international handbook of suicide and attempted suicide. New York: Wiley; 2000.
38. Spicer R, Miller T. Suicide acts in 8 states: incidence and case fatality rates by demographics and method. Am J Public Health. 2000;90(12):1885–91.
39. Kaplan H, Sadock B. Psychiatric emergencies. In: Kaplan H, Sadock B, Grebb J, editors. Synopsis of psychiatry, 7th ed. Baltimore: Williams Wilkins; 1994.

40. Miller M, Azrael D, Hemenway D. The epidemiology of case fatality rates for suicide in the northeast. Ann Emerg Med. 2004;43(6):723–30.
41. Schernhammer ES, Colditz G. Suicide rates among physicians: a quantitative and gender assessment (meta-analysis). Am J Psychiatry. 2004;161(12):2295–302.
42. Heikkinen M, Isometsa E, Marttunen M, Aro H, Lonnqvist J. Social factors in suicide. Br J Psychiatry. 1995;167(6):747–53.
43. Beck A, Steer R, Beck J, Newman C. Hopelessness, depression, suicidal ideation, and clinical diagnosis of depression. Suicide Life Threat Behav. 1993;23(2):139–45.
44. Dannenberg A, McNeil J, Brundage J, Brookmeyer R. Suicide and HIV infection. Mortality follow-up of 4147 HIV-seropositive military service applicants. JAMA. 1996;276(21): 1743–6.
45. Hawton K. Suicide and attempted suicide. In: Pankel E, editor. Handbook of affective disorders, 2nd ed. New York: Guilford; 1992.
46. Agerbo E. Risk of suicide and spouse's psychiatric illness or suicide: nested case-control study. BMJ. 2003;327(7422):1025–6.
47. Moscicki E. Epidemiology of suicide. In: Goldsmith S, editor. Suicide prevention and intervention. Washington: National Academy Press; 2001.
48. Qin P, Mortensen PB. The impact of parental status on the risk of completed suicide. Arch Gen Psychiatry. 2003;60(8):797–802.
49. Trivedi MH, Rush AJ, Ibrahim HM, Carmody TJ, Biggs MM, Suppes T, et al. The Inventory of Depressive Symptomatology, Clinician Rating (IDS-C) and Self-Report (IDS-SR), and the Quick Inventory of Depressive Symptomatology, Clinician Rating (QIDS-C) and Self-Report (QIDS-SR) in public sector patients with mood disorders: a psychometric evaluation. Psychol Med. 2004;34(1):73–82.
50. Hollon SD, Shelton RC, Wisniewski S, Warden D, Biggs MM, Friedman ES, et al. Presenting characteristics of depressed outpatients as a function of recurrence: preliminary findings from the STAR*D clinical trial. J Psychiatr Res. 2006;40(1):59–69.
51. Blom MB, Spinhoven P, Hoffman T, Jonker K, Hoencamp E, Haffmans PM, et al. Severity and duration of depression, not personality factors, predict short term outcome in the treatment of major depression. J Affect Disord. 2007;104(1–3):119–126.
52. Thase ME, Simons AD, Cahalane J, McGeary J, Harden T. Severity of depression and response to cognitive behavior therapy. Am J Psychiatry. 1991;148(6):784–9.
53. Nease DE, Jr., Volk RJ, Cass AR. Does the severity of mood and anxiety symptoms predict health care utilization? J Fam Pract. 1999;48(10):769–77.
54. Von Korff M, Goldberg D. Improving outcomes in depression. BMJ. 2001;323(7319): 948–9.
55. Katzelnick DJ, Simon GE, Pearson SD, Manning WG, Helstad CP, Henk HJ, et al. Randomized trial of a depression management program in high utilizers of medical care. Arch Fam Med. 2000;9(4):345–51.
56. Gensichen J, Beyer M, Muth C, Gerlach FM, Von Korff M, Ormel J. Case management to improve major depression in primary health care: a systematic review. Psychol Med. 2006;36(1):7–14.
57. Lin EH, Simon GE, Katzelnick DJ, Pearson SD. Does physician education on depression management improve treatment in primary care? J Gen Intern Med. 2001;16(9):614–9.
58. Morey E, Thacher JA, Craighead WE. Patient preferences for depression treatment programs and willingness to pay for treatment. J Ment Health Policy Econ. 2007;10(2):73–85.
59. Lin EH, Von Korff M, Katon W, Bush T, Simon GE, Walker E, et al. The role of the primary care physician in patients' adherence to antidepressant therapy. Med Care. 1995;33(1): 67–74.
60. Schulberg HC, Raue PJ, Rollman BL. The effectiveness of psychotherapy in treating depressive disorders in primary care practice: clinical and cost perspectives. Gen Hosp Psychiatry. 2002;24(4):203–12.
61. Keller MB, McCullough JP, Klein DN, Arnow B, Dunner DL, Gelenberg AJ, et al. A comparison of nefazodone, the cognitive behavioral-analysis system of psychotherapy, and their combination for the treatment of chronic depression. N Engl J Med. 2000;342(20):1462–70.

62. Wolf NJ, Hopko DR. Psychosocial and pharmacological interventions for depressed adults in primary care: A critical review. Clin Psychol Rev. 2008;28(1):131–61.
63. Depression Guideline Panel. Depression in Primary Care: Treatment of Major Depression: Clinical Practice Guideline. Rockville, MD: US Dept of Health and Human Services, Public Health Service, Agency for Health Care Policy and Research. AHCPR publication 93-0551; 1993.
64. Hansen RA, Gartlehner G, Lohr KN, Gaynes BN, Carey TS. Efficacy and safety of second-generation antidepressants in the treatment of major depressive disorder. Ann Intern Med. 2005;143(6):415–26.
65. Van der Kooy K, van Hout H, Marwijk H, Marten H, Stehouwer C, Beekman A. Depression and the risk for cardiovascular diseases: systematic review and meta analysis. Int J Geriatr Psychiatry. 2007;22(7):613–26.
66. Serebruany VL, Glassman AH, Malinin AI, Atar D, Sane DC, Oshrine BR, et al. Selective serotonin reuptake inhibitors yield additional antiplatelet protection in patients with congestive heart failure treated with antecedent aspirin. Eur J Heart Fail. 2003;5(4):517–21.
67. Glassman AH, Bigger JT, Gaffney M, Van Zyl LT. Heart rate variability in acute coronary syndrome patients with major depression: influence of sertraline and mood improvement. Arch Gen Psychiatry. 2007;64(9):1025–31.
68. Siepmann T, Ziemssen T, Mueck-Weymann M, Kirch W, Siepmann M. The effects of venlafaxine on autonomic functions in healthy volunteers. J Clin Psychopharmacol. 2007;27(6):687–91.
69. Fava M, Judge R, Hoog SL, Nilsson ME, Koke SC. Fluoxetine versus sertraline and paroxetine in major depressive disorder: changes in weight with long-term treatment. J Clin Psychiatry. 2000;61(11):863–7.
70. Hemeryck A, Belpaire FM. Selective serotonin reuptake inhibitors and cytochrome P-450 mediated drug-drug interactions: an update. Curr Drug Metab. 2002;3(1):13–37.
71. Murphy GM, Jr., Kremer C, Rodrigues HE, Schatzberg AF. Pharmacogenetics of antidepressant medication intolerance. Am J Psychiatry. 2003;160(10):1830–5.
72. Cyranowski JM, Frank E, Cherry C, Houck P, Kupfer DJ. Prospective assessment of sexual function in women treated for recurrent major depression. J Psychiatr Res. 2004;38(3): 267–73.
73. Zisook S, Rush AJ, Haight BR, Clines DC, Rockett CB. Use of bupropion in combination with serotonin reuptake inhibitors. Biol Psychiatry. 2006;59(3):203–10.
74. Rush AJ. STAR*D: what have we learned? Am J Psychiatry. 2007;164(2):201–4.
75. Triezenberg D, Vachon D, Helmen J, Schneider D. Clinical inquiries: how should you manage a depressed patient unresponsive to an SSRI? J Fam Pract. 2006;55(12):1081–2; 7.
76. Nierenberg AA, Fava M, Trivedi MH, Wisniewski SR, Thase ME, McGrath PJ, et al. A comparison of lithium and T(3) augmentation following two failed medication treatments for depression: a STAR*D report. Am J Psychiatry. 2006;163(9):1519–30; quiz 665.
77. Papakostas GI, Shelton RC, Smith J, Fava M. Augmentation of antidepressants with atypical antipsychotic medications for treatment-resistant major depressive disorder: a meta-analysis. J Clin Psychiatry. 2007;68(6):826–31.
78. Dunn AL, Trivedi MH, Kampert JB, Clark CG, Chambliss HO. Exercise treatment for depression: efficacy and dose response. Am J Prev Med. 2005;28(1):1–8.
79. Blumenthal JA, Babyak MA, Doraiswamy PM, Watkins L, Hoffman BM, Barbour KA, et al. Exercise and Pharmacotherapy in the Treatment of Major Depressive Disorder. Psychosom Med. 2007;(69):587–596.
80. Ostacher MJ. Comorbid alcohol and substance abuse dependence in depression: impact on the outcome of antidepressant treatment. Psychiatr Clin North Am. 2007;30(1):69–76.
81. Paykel ES, Ramana R, Cooper Z, Hayhurst H, Kerr J, Barocka A. Residual symptoms after partial remission: an important outcome in depression. Psychol Med. 1995;25(6):1171–80.
82. Judd LL, Akiskal HS, Maser JD, Zeller PJ, Endicott J, Coryell W, et al. Major depressive disorder: a prospective study of residual subthreshold depressive symptoms as predictor of rapid relapse. J Affect Disord. 1998;50(2–3):97–108.

83. Kennedy N, Foy K. The impact of residual symptoms on outcome of major depression. Curr Psychiatry Rep. 2005;7(6):441–6.
84. Ezquiaga E, Garcia A, Pallares T, Bravo MF. Psychosocial predictors of outcome in major depression: a prospective 12-month study. J Affect Disord. 1999;52(1–3):209–16.
85. Paykel ES. Continuation and maintenance therapy in depression. Br Med Bull. 2001;57:145–59.
86. Thase ME. Preventing relapse and recurrence of depression: a brief review of therapeutic options. CNS Spectr. 2006;11(12 suppl 15):12–21.
87. Anon. Practice guideline for the treatment of patients with major depressive disorder (revision). American Psychiatric Association. Am J Psychiatry. 2000;157(4 suppl):1–45.
88. Demyttenaere K, Enzlin P, Dewe W, Boulanger B, De Bie J, De Troyer W, et al. Compliance with antidepressants in a primary care setting, 1: Beyond lack of efficacy and adverse events. J Clin Psychiatry. 2001;62(suppl 22):30–3.
89. Rush AJ, Kraemer HC, Sackeim HA, Fava M, Trivedi MH, Frank E, et al. Report by the ACNP Task Force on response and remission in major depressive disorder. Neuropsychopharmacology. 2006;31(9):1841–53.
90. American Psychiatric Association., American Psychiatric Association. Task Force on DSM-IV. Diagnostic and statistical manual of mental disorders: DSM-IV-TR. 4th ed. Washington: American Psychiatric Association; 2000.
91. Kroenke K, Spitzer R. The PHQ-9: a new depression and diagnostic severity measure. Psychiatr Ann. 2002;32:509–21.

Treatment of Depression in the Medically Ill

Wei Jiang and K. Ranga Rama Krishnan

Introduction

Depression and ischemic heart disease (IHD) are the two most prevalent health problems afflicting patients not only in the United States but worldwide (1). The lifetime prevalence of major depressive disorder in the general population of the United States has been found to be 16.2% (2). The prevalence of depression in medically ill patients is much higher, ranging 20–50%. Depression is a major contributor to work place absenteeism, diminished or lost productivity, and increased use of health services (3). It is also known to increase disability, morbidity, and mortality among the medically ill.

Because of the high prevalence of depression and its risk for the wellbeing and prognosis of the medically ill, treating depression becomes an extremely important issue (1–3). Even though depression with medical comorbidity is the norm, rather than the exception, most studies on treatment methods in depressive patients have included primarily individuals in good physical health and have excluded those with comorbid medical illness.

Recognizing the medical and socioeconomic significance of late-life depression, a multicenter randomized trial (the Improving Mood-Promoting Access to Collaborative Treatment study) began examining the benefits of integrating depression intervention into the primary care for elderly patients (4). In the study, patients were randomly assigned to the Improving Mood-Promoting Access to Collaborative Treatment intervention ($n = 906$) or to usual care ($n = 895$). Improving Mood-Promoting Access to Collaborative Treatment patients had access for up to 12 months to a depression care manager who was supervised by a psychiatrist and a primary care expert. The care manager offered education, care management, and support of antidepressant management by the patient's primary care physician or a brief psychotherapy for depression, Problem Solving Treatment in Primary Care. At 12 months, 45% of

W. Jiang (✉)
Department of Psychiatry and Behavioral Sciences,
Duke University, Durham, NC, USA
e-mail: jiang001@mc.duke.edu

D.A. Ciraulo and R.I. Shader (eds.), *Pharmacotherapy of Depression*,
DOI 10.1007/978-1-60327-435-7_11, © Springer Science+Business Media, LLC 2011

intervention patients had a 50% or greater reduction in depressive symptoms from baseline compared with 19% of usual care participants. This suggests that effective treatment of depression is possible in the context of a primary care setting, i.e., probably those with comorbid medical conditions.

Kurzthaler et al. have suggested that selective serotonin reuptake inhibitors (SSRIs) are effective and reasonably safe in elderly depressive patients with comorbid physical illness, based on a small open-label study using multiple SSRIs (5). He noted, however, that adverse effects were more common than what has been observed in younger and physically healthy patients.

We evaluated the effect of the SSRI sertraline with respect to treatment response in patients with major depression and comorbid vascular disease (6). Patients were retrospectively categorized into 1 of 3 clinical groups: (1) individuals with a current diagnosis of hypertension but no cardiovascular illness (HTN), (2) individuals with a current or past history of cardiovascular illness other than hypertension (VASC), and (3) individuals with no hypertension or comorbid vascular illness (NoVASC). Response was defined as much or very much improved on the Clinical Global Improvement scale. At study end point, sertraline treatment yielded similar levels of response in all three groups on a complete analysis (HTN, 86%; VASC, 89%; NoVASC, 77%), although the level of response at 12 weeks was higher in those VASC patients than in the other two groups. Sertraline treatment was well tolerated, with no between-group differences in rates of adverse events or in discontinuation caused by adverse events.

This study essentially reaffirmed the opinion of Kurzthaler et al., that antidepressants are effective for depression in primary care setting (5). However, it is of critical importance to understand the impact of treating depression in patients who present with specific medical illness. This article briefly reviews depression treatments with reference to diabetes, stroke, cardiovascular disease, and neurological disorders.

Diabetes

The prevalence of depression in diabetic patients varies depending on study criteria and procedures (7). Anderson et al. conducted a meta-analysis of 42 published studies that included 21,351 adults (8). They found that the prevalence of major depression in people who had diabetes was 11% and the prevalence of clinically relevant depression was 31%. There is overwhelming evidence that the coexistence of diabetes and depression is associated with poor diabetes outcomes, including poor glycemic control (9), high rate of diabetes complications (10, 11), decreased function and increased odds of lost productivity(12–14), increased health care costs (15), less compliance to treatment protocol and self-care behaviors (15–21). Furthermore, coexisting depression increased the risk for death in people who have diabetes (11, 22–24). Although studies of depression treatment among patients with diabetes suggest that depression itself is amenable to treatment, there is disagreement on how this affects diabetes.

Both TCA and SSRIs have been studied among diabetic patients with depression in randomized clinical trials. SSRIs treatment improves depression and may be associated with improved diabetes symptoms. Fluoxetine at a dose of up to 60 mg/day is effective in treating depression and produced reductions in weight, fasting glucose, and HbA1c in diabetic patients (25). Similar results have been repeated with sertraline but in an open label study. In contrast, although it was effective in reducing depressive symptoms, the tricyclic nortriptyline led to worsening of glucose control (25).

The effect of SSRI on diabetic neuropathy was examined with citalopram by Sindrup et al. 11 in a double-blind, placebo-controlled, crossover study for two consecutive 3-week periods. Citalopram, at doses of 40 mg/day, significantly reduced the pain of neuropathy compared with placebo. In diabetic neuropathy, antidepressants that inhibit norepinephrine reuptake as well as serotonin reuptake (such as tricyclics, high-dose paroxetine, venlafaxine and especially duloxetine) may be more effective than serotonin-specific agents, but tricyclics appear to increase fasting blood glucose levels (25). Depression was not a study endpoint in those studies.

The Pathways Study (26), a trial in which 329 diabetic patients with major depression were randomized to either standard medical care or to collaborative care integrating antidepressant therapy or problem-solving therapy, reported that patients receiving depression intervention had depression improved but did not exhibit improved glycemic control. Cognitive behavior therapy (CBT) also appears to be effective in the treatment of depression in diabetes. Lustman et al. studied patients who were randomly assigned to a group that received 10 weeks of individual CBT or to a control condition that received usual treatment (27). All patients also participated in a diabetes education program, which was designed to control the effects of attention. Depression was measured using the Beck Depression Inventory scale (BDI); glucose control was measured using glycosylated hemoglobin concentrations. At 6 months, more patients (17 of 20 [85%]) had achieved remission of depression (BDI score ≤9) in the CBT group than in the control group (6 of 22 [27%]). At follow-up, 70% (14 of 20) of patients in the CBT group achieved remission in contrast to a third (7 of 21) of the controls. Of interest, post treatment glycosylated hemoglobin (HgA1C) levels were no different between the two groups. At 6-month follow-up, mean HgA1C levels were significantly better in the CBT group than in the control group. Such a find is probably explained by the nature of the HgA1C which correlates best with mean blood glucose over the previous 8–12 weeks. Nonremission of depression was associated with lower compliance with blood glucose monitoring and higher glycosylated hemoglobin levels (28). In the CBT group, the presence of diabetes complications and lower compliance with blood glucose monitoring were independent predictors of poor response. These findings show that factors related to the medical illness, such as the presence of complications, can negatively affect recovery from depression. Whether the same factors are operating in depression treated with antidepressants is not known.

Ischemic Heart Disease

Major depression is a common problem in patients with IHD and is associated with an increased risk of cardiac morbidity and mortality (29). It is commonly believed that the efficacy of treating depression is comparable across available antidepressants;

their cardiovascular safety varies substantially. Nevertheless, there are few studies which examined the efficacy and safety of depression treatment in patients with IHD. Studies to evaluate whether treating depression will improve medical prognosis are as well scanty.

The cardiovascular effects of TCAs are well characterized, including orthostatic hypotension, slowed cardiac conduction, type 1A antiarrhythmic activity, and increased heart rate (30). Orthostatic hypotension is a particular concern in the elderly, and slowing of cardiac conduction contraindicates the use of TCAs in patients with pre-existing conduction problems. The Cardiac Arrhythmia Suppression Trials (CAST) (31, 32) demonstrated that class 1C antiarrhythmic agents encainide and flecainide and class 1A antiarrhythmic agent morcizine actually led to *increased* excess mortality compared with placebo. Though these results have been available since the early 90s, cardiac patients continue to be prescribed TCAs, which share type 1A antiarrhythmic activity, and thus should be considered unsafe in patients with IHD. The results of the CAST trial initially presented in August 1989. The only head-to-head comparison of a TCA, nortiptyline, and an SSRI, paroxetine, in IHD patients provided clear evidence that therapeutic plasma levels of a TCA led to negative cardiac effects in patients with IHD (33, 34). Patients with major depressive disorder were randomly assigned to double-blind treatment with paroxetine (flexible dose range of 20–30 mg/day) or nortriptyline (adjusted to reach plasma concentration of 50–150 ng/mL) for 6 weeks. Twenty-seven (66%) of 41 patients treated with paroxetine and 29 (75.5%) of 40 patients treated with nortriptyline had >50% improvement in Hamilton Rating Scale for Depression (HRSD) scores. However, more patients on nortriptyline discontinued treatment compared with paroxetine (35 vs. 10%), and more patients on nortriptyline were terminated secondary to significant adverse events than patients on paroxetine (25 vs. 5%). Moreover, patients treated with nortriptyline had increased heart rate and a reduction in heart rate variability, whereas no effects on heart rate rhythm or heart rate variability were observed with paroxetine treatment. Seven (18%) of 40 patients treated with nortriptyline had adverse cardiac events, compared with one patient treated with paroxetine. Thus, TCAs should be avoided in patients with IHD due to their negative cardiac side effect profile.

SSRIs have been proven to be relatively safe in patients with IHD (30, 35–38). The Sertraline Antidepressant Heart Attack Recovery Trial (SADHART), which examined the safety and efficacy of sertraline for major depressive disorder among 369 patients post acute MI or unstable angina in a randomized, double-blind, placebo-controlled trial, demonstrated that 24 weeks of treatment with sertraline led to no significant effects on heart rate, blood pressure, left ventricular ejection fraction, electrocardiographic changes, treatment-emergent increase in ventricular premature complex runs or other cardiac measures (37). The Canadian Cardiac Randomized Evaluation of Antidepressant and Psychotherapy Efficacy (CREATE) trial further supports the safety of another SSRI in its examination of citalopram in patients with IHD, suggesting that such safety is likely a class effect (38).

Despite this, it remains unclear if treating depression in patients with IHD might decrease the negative effects of depression on cardiovascular prognosis and mortality.

In theory, adequate treatment of depression could affect both physiologic and psychosocial factors that are dysregulated, therefore leading to improved cardiac outcomes. There has been physiologic evidence to support beneficial pleiotropic effects of antidepressant medications in IHD, such as the reduction of platelet activity (39–41) and improvement in low heart rate variability with both sertraline and paroxetine (42–44). SADHART revealed that patients receiving sertraline had fewer cardiac events such as death, MI, stroke, worsened angina, and/or onset of CHF as compared with patients taking placebo. The relative risk ratio for having at least one cardiac event was 0.68, however, the reduction of risk was not statistically significant (95% confidence interval, 0.43–1.09) (37). The study was not designed to have enough power to detect such differences (37). A case-control study following patients suffering their first MI examined the prognostic effect of SSRIs (45). Detailed information regarding antidepressant medication was obtained by telephone interview from 653 smokers hospitalized with a first MI and among 2,990 control subjects. Using multivariate logistic regression to adjust for age, sex, race, education, exercise, quantity smoked per day, body mass index, aspirin use, family history of MI, number of physician encounters, and history of coronary disease, diabetes, hypertension, and hypercholesterolemia, the odds ratio for MI among those prescribed an SSRI (fluoxetine, fluvoxamine, paroxetine, or sertraline) compared to those not taking an SSRI was significantly decreased at 0.35 (95% CI 0.18–0.68; $p<0.01$). Non-SSRI antidepressants (amitriptyline, amoxapine, bupropion, clomipramine, desipramine, doxepin, imipramine, maprotiline, mirtazapine, nefazodone, nortriptyline, phenelzine, protriptyline, trazodone, tranylcypromine, or venlafaxine) were associated with a nonsignificant reduction in MI with wide confidence intervals (adjusted OR 0.48, CI 0.17–1.32; $p=0.15$). The Enhancing Recovery in Coronary Heart Disease (ENRICHD) trial enrolled 2,481 patients after myocardial infarction with depression and/or low perceived social support. Subjects were randomized to usual care or cognitive behavioral therapy (CBT), which was then supplemented, in a nonrandomized fashion, by antidepressant therapy, for those with persistent depressive symptoms (46). Although there was no evidence of an impact of CBT on the combined end point of death or nonfatal MI, the 20.6% of the patients in the usual care group and 28% of those in the treatment group receiving antidepressants by the end of the follow-up period, likely attenuated the effect of the CBT intervention. Interestingly, use of antidepressant was associated with a more than 40% lower risk of either death or nonfatal MI, with a crude HR of 0.61 (95% CI, 0.41–0.90) and an adjusted HR of 0.53 (95% CI, 0.38–0.84) (47). Nonetheless, the prescription of an antidepressant was at the discretion of the study physicians and thus, not randomized nor controlled, limiting the interpretation of these results.

Mirtazapine, an antagonizer of α_2-adrenergic and serotonin 5-HT2 receptors, has been recently studied for post-MI depression by the Mycocardial Infarction Depression Intervention Trial (MIND-IT) using a randomized, placebo-controlled design (48). This trial failed to find a significant treatment effect for depression or for cardiac outcomes (49). Such results may have been related to a lack of statistical power as only 209 treated patients were compared to 122 patients receiving usual care. This trial also raises the question as to whether any non-TCA antidepressant would have beneficial effects on cardiovascular outcomes, or if such an effect would be limited to the SSRI class.

Bleeding time, however, increased in 12 patients in the SADHART study, leading to an investigation of the effects of sertraline on platelet function parameters (50). Both sertraline and its metabolite *N*-desmethylsertraline were assayed in vitro for their effects on platelet function. Whole-blood platelet aggregation was also reduced significantly when induced by collagen. Surface expression of CD9, glycoprotein Ib, glycoprotein IIb/IIIa, very late antigen 2, P selectin, and platelet endothelial cell adhesion molecule 1, but not the vitronectin receptor, was reduced after sertraline and *N*-desmethylsertraline pretreatment. Platelet-function assay suggested glycoprotein IIb/IIIa inhibition, secondary to sertraline, and its metabolite *N*-desmethylsertraline. Both exhibited dose-dependent inhibition of human platelet activity. These anti-platelet effects of sertraline and *N*-desmethylsertraline are reported to be akin to that seen with citalopram and paroxetine and may contribute to the added benefits of SSRIs after ischemic events, including MI and stroke.

Surprisingly, the effects of psychotherapeutic interventions in treating depression in patients with IHD are not as well documented as in non-medically ill patients. The Montreal Heart Attack Readjustment Trial (MHART), a randomized controlled trial of 1,376 post-MI patients (903 men, 473 women) was conducted by Frasure-Smith et al. (51). This study, although not specific to major depression, was interesting in that it focused on psychological distress. Patients were assigned to the intervention program ($n=692$) or usual care ($n=684$) for 1 year. Intervention had no overall impact on survival. Higher cardiac (9.4 vs. 5.0%) and all-cause mortality (10.3 vs. 5.4%) among women in the intervention group was of particular concern, whereas there was no evidence of either benefit or harm among men (cardiac mortality, 2.4 vs. 2.5%; all-cause mortality, 3.1 vs. 3.1%) in the study. These findings suggest that psychosocial treatment may not be routinely warranted among cardiac patients; they also raise the issue of sex as an important covariant in treatment outcome. The ENRICHED study demonstrated CBT intervention modestly improved depression in post-MI patients, but it did not affect late cardiac mortality (52). The Canadian Cardiac Randomized Evaluation of Antidepressant and Psychotherapy Efficacy (CREATE) trial, conducted by Lespe´rance et al., using a randomized, controlled, 12-week, parallel-group, 2×2 factorial design, examined the effects of citalopram and/or interpersonal psychotherapy (IPT), in conjunction with weekly routine clinical management among 284 patients with IHD and moderate to severe MDD (53). Citalopram was superior to placebo in reducing depressive symptoms. However, there was no evidence of a benefit of IPT over clinical management alone or in combination of citalopram.

Post-stroke

Post-stroke depression (PSD) occurs in up to 40% of stroke patients in acute care or rehabilitation facilities and has been linked to worse functional outcome, slower recovery, worse quality of life, and increased mortality (54, 55). The North East

Melbourne Stroke Incidence Study determined that along with physical impairment, depression and anxiety significantly contribute to handicap after stroke (56). Williams et al. followed 51,119 hospitalized patients with ischemic stroke and demonstrated that patients with recorded diagnosis of depression post-stroke had higher death over 3-year period (Hazard ratio = 1.13, 95% confidence interval = 1.06–1.21), independent of other chronic conditions. Another study looked at a cohort of 448 patients within a randomized controlled trial of psychological therapy. Depression was measured by the General Health Questionnaire-28 (GHQ) 1 month after stroke. GHQ-D score ≥1 indicated presence of significant depression, which was associated with increased mortality of 12- and 24-month (odds ration 2.4 for both with p value 0.007 and 0.002 respectively) (57). Thus, studies have attempted to search the proper management of post-stroke depression in order to reduce morbidity and mortality.

A meta-analysis of randomized, placebo-controlled trials of antidepressants in patients with PSD examined a total of 1,320 subjects from 16 trials that met the selection criteria of the study (58). Antidepressants in these studies included aniracetam 600 mg/day, citalopram 10–20 mg/day, fluoxetine 10–40 mg/day, nortriptyline 20–100 mg/day, paroxetine 20 mg/day, reboxetine 20 mg/day, sertraline 50–100 mg/day, and trazodone 300 mg/day, with duration of the trials ranging between 4 and 26 weeks. The pooled response rates in the active and placebo groups were 65.18% (234/359) and 44.37% (138/311), respectively. The pooled RD (rate difference) was 0.23 (95% CI = 0.03–0.43), indicating a significantly higher response rate in the active group compared with the placebo group. From baseline to endpoint, patients in the active group had significantly greater improvement in depressive symptoms compared with patients in the placebo group. Longer duration of treatment was positively correlated with the degree of improvement in depressive symptoms (Spearman's correlation, $[\rho] = -0.93$, $p = 0.001$). However, no consistent evidence was found for positive antidepressant effects on the recovery of neurologic impairments and improvements in ADLs. However, whether antidepressant treatment may reduce morbidity and mortality was not assessed.

Dam et al. conducted a unique study to examine the antidepressant effects on neurologic impairment, involving 52 patients in stroke induced hemiplegia (59). The study consisted of three randomly assigned arms: placebo, maprotiline (150 mg/day), or fluoxetine (20 mg/day). Before and at the end of the 3-month treatment period, activities of daily living by the Barthel Index, degree of neurological deficit by a neurological scale, and depressive symptoms by the HRSD were assessed. At the end of the study, the greatest improvement of depression was observed with fluoxetine treatment, whereas the least improvement was seen in the maprotiline-treated group. Fluoxetine yielded a significantly larger number of patients with good functional recovery compared with maprotiline or placebo. Interestingly, these effects were not related to the treatment of depression. This study suggests that fluoxetine may facilitate, whereas maprotiline may hinder, recovery in post-stroke patients undergoing rehabilitation.

Despite the observed benefit of fluoxetine in this study, the effect of fluoxetine in post-stroke depression remains circumspect, as indicated by Robinson et al. (60).

In a comparative study of nortriptyline and fluoxetine, Robinson et al. studied 104 patients with acute stroke and randomized them to 12 weeks of double-blind treatment with nortriptyline (25–100 mg/day), fluoxetine (10–40 mg/day), or placebo (60). Response to treatment was defined as a >50% reduction in HRSD scores and failure to meet diagnostic criteria for major or minor depression. At the end of 12 weeks of treatment, nortriptyline produced a significantly higher response rate than fluoxetine or placebo in treating post-stroke depression.

Different antidepressants may vary in efficacy in patients with specific symptom clusters or depressive symptom types. A comparative study investigating the efficacy and safety of citalopram and reboxetine, in PSD patients demonstrated that both citalopram and reboxetine showed good safety and tolerability. In addition, citalopram exhibited greater efficacy in anxious depressed patients, while reboxetine was more effective in retarded depressed patients (61).

There has been only one study by Robinson et al. so far which examined the effects of antidepressants on post-stroke mortality in patients with and without depression (60). In this study, a total of 104 patients were randomly assigned to receive a 12-week double-blind course of nortriptyline, fluoxetine, or placebo during the first 6 months following the stroke. Mortality data were obtained for all 104 patients 9 years after initiation of the study. Fifty patients (48.1%) had died by the time of the follow-up. More patients in the antidepressants arms were alive (67.9%) compared with 35.7% of placebo-treated patients ($p=0.004$). Logistic regression analysis showed that the beneficial effect of antidepressants remained significant both in patients who were depressed and in those who were non-depressed at enrollment, after the effects of other factors associated with mortality (i.e., age, coexisting diabetes mellitus, and chronic relapsing depression) were controlled. There were no inter-group differences in severity of stroke, impairment in cognitive functioning and activities of daily living impairment, and other medications received.

Whether antidepressants may prevent PSD has been tested as well. One study examined the effects of sertraline 50 mg daily for 24 weeks in comparison to placebo, in randomized, double-blinded controlled fashion, among a total of 111 stroke patients (62). Analysis revealed that there was no significant difference in the incidence of depressive symptoms during the 24 weeks of treatment (16.7% sertraline vs. 21.6% placebo, $p=0.590$). About a half of the participants terminated the study prematurely. Another study gave patients with ischemic stroke either mirtazapine 30 mg daily or no antidepressant medication from day 1 after the stroke in an open, randomized study design for up to a total of 360 days (63). The authors reported a 40% of the non-treated patients and 5.7% of the patients treated with mirtazapine developed PSD. The inconsistent findings are probably contributed by the limited design and number of studies.

In addition, a double-blind placebo-controlled study of nortriptyline to evaluate the effects of treatment on cognitive impairment included patients with both major and minor depression after stroke (55). In this study, depression was measured by HRSD scores, and cognitive impairment was assessed by the Mini-Mental State Examination. At study end, patients whose post-stroke depression remitted experienced greater recovery in cognitive function than patients whose mood disorder did not remit.

Other common problems after stroke are emotional disturbances such as pathological crying and aggression, without presence of mood disorder. In 26 consecutive patients with episodes of involuntary crying after brain damage, the efficacy and tolerability of paroxetine and citalopram were compared in an open-label study in which the first 13 patients received paroxetine, and the next 13 patients received citalopram in single daily doses of 10–40 mg (64). Within one to two doses, a highly significant improvement of pathological crying was observed after treatment with both paroxetine and citalopram. Citalopram 10–20 mg/day also has been shown to be rapidly effective and well tolerated in a double-blind, placebo-controlled crossover study of 16 patients with pathological crying post-stroke (65). One study by Chan et al. examined the effects of nortriptyline, fluoxetine, or placebo, in double-blinded assignment, on post-stroke irritability and aggression after stroke (58). Results of this study suggested that successful treatment of depression may reduce aggressive behavior. Another study by Choi-Kwon et al. tested the effects of fluoxetine vs. placebo among Koreans, demonstrating improvement in emotional incontinence and anger proneness with fluoxetine (66). However, the effect of it on PSD was not definitive.

Dementia (See Also, Chapter "Antidepressant Treatment of Geriatric Depression")

Population-based studies reveal 20–30% of patients with dementia have depression (67). Diagnosis of depression in patients with dementia can be very difficult. Denial and cognitive impairment may compromise self-report of depressive symptoms by people with dementia. As the dementing illness progresses, the presentation of depression may alter, with non-verbal manifestations (e.g., demanding behavior, clinging) being more apparent than cognitive features (68). Moreover, neurovegetative symptoms such as poor concentration and anhedonia are features of depression and dementia. Not surprisingly, there is no consensus on how best to diagnose depression in demented patients. Symptom depression scales may overestimate, whereas structured diagnostic interviews may underestimate the prevalence of depression in people with dementia. Given the complexity of the issues impinging on accurate diagnosis it is not surprising that estimates of the incidence and prevalence rates of depression in dementing patients has varied between 0 and 86%. Larger studies using standardized criteria for major depressive disorder in Alzheimer's disease provide estimates of prevalence at 10–20% (69).

Despite the high prevalence of depression in patients with dementia, few treatment studies of depression in dementia are considered having had adequate design (70). Early studies with tricyclic antidepressants were not encouraging and often showed no difference compared with placebo (71). Randomized double-blind comparisons of fluoxetine and amitriptyline and of paroxetine and imipramine in the treatment of depression in patients with dementia found equivalent improvements in depression, but significantly more adverse events in patients treated with the tricyclics compared with the SSRIs (72, 73). Lyketsos and Lee recommend initiating depression treatment with non-pharmacological interventions and, considering their relative safety, using SSRIs as first-line pharmacotherapy for psychotherapy-resistant depression (74).

As many individual trials of antidepressants have been too small to provide precise estimates of the moderate benefits that might realistically be expected, Bains et al. of the Cochrane Dementia and Cognitive Improvement Group conducted a review in 2005, attempting to combine information from all appropriate trials to provide a better estimate of the likely effects of treatment (70). Of their intensive literature search between 1861 and 2005, only seven studies met the inclusion and exclusion of the review. Those studies used different antidepressants, three used TCAs or related compounds, one used a reversible monoamine oxidase inhibitor, and only three used an SSRI (75–77).

Lyketsos et al. evaluated SSRI sertraline in the Depression in Alzheimer'sDisease Study, a randomized, placebo-controlled, flexible-dose trial (74, 76). Response to treatment was measured with the Cornell Scale for Depression in Dementia, as well as with the HRSD, activities of daily living scale, Mini-Mental State Examination, and Neuropsychiatric Inventory. After 12 weeks, 9 (75%) of 12 patients who received sertraline and 2 (20%) of 10 patients given placebo were classified as partial or full responders with respect to depression. Patients receiving sertraline had greater reduction from baseline in depression symptoms measured by the Cornell Scale for Depression in Dementia, compared with those who received placebo. Antidepressant response occurred by the third week of treatment. Responders also had a higher rating on the activities of daily living scale. However, no improvement in cognition was observed, as there was no difference between treatment groups in the Mini-Mental State Examination or Neuropsychiatric Inventory scores over time.

Nyth et al. conducted a preliminary trial of citalopram in severe dementia – Alzheimer's type and Alzheimer's disease, finding a reduction in depressed mood and other emotional disturbances (78). Subsequently, they evaluated the efficacy of citalopram in 98 patients with both moderate Alzheimer's disease and vascular dementia (75). After 4 weeks of double-blind treatment, patients with Alzheimer's disease treated with citalopram showed significant improvement in symptoms such as irritability, anxiety, fear/panic, depressed mood, and restlessness. These changes were not seen in patients who received placebo. No effect was found in vascular dementia, and no improvements were recorded in motor or cognitive function.

Parkinson's Disease

Although few prospective trials have examined the incidence of depression in Parkinson's disease (PD), the Global Parkinson's Disease Survey, which included 1,000 patients in five countries, demonstrated that approximately 50% had depressive symptoms that significantly affected daily functioning (79). Despite the large number of individuals with PD affected by depression, there have been no well-designed clinical trials evaluating the efficacy of antidepressant agents in this population.

Open label studies with SSRIs have shown benefit but have raised concern regarding a worsening of the motor dysfunction in PD. Dell'Agnello et al. assessed the effects of 4 SSRIs (citalopram, fluoxetine, fluvoxamine, and sertraline) on motor performance and depression in 62 depressed patients with PD (80). Extrapyramidal symptoms were evaluated using the Unified Parkinson's Disease Rating Scale, whereas effect on depression was measured using the Beck Depression Inventory and HRSD. At 1, 3, and 6 months, researchers observed that Unified Parkinson's Disease Rating Scale scores were not significantly affected by SSRIs, although depressive symptoms improved from baseline to the end of the trial with all SSRIs. A recent 8-week open-label trial of citalopram in ten patients with PD and major depression found significant improvement in depression, anxiety, and functional impairment (81). Although 7 (70%) experienced at least one adverse event, only one withdrawal occurred because of worsening depression and one because of persistent nausea and worsening of motor symptoms. Of the eight completing the trial, none exhibited worsening of motor skills as measured by the Unified Parkinson's Disease Rating Scale or decline of cognitive function as measured by the Mini-Mental State Examination. Together, these findings suggest that there may be less need for a warning against the use of SSRIs in PD patients, although larger controlled trials are needed to clarify the safety and efficacy of SSRIs in this area.

Two early studies of the TCA's imipramine and desipramine in PD employed a double-blind, placebo-controlled design and demonstrated improvement in both depression and Parkinsonian motor features (82, 83). However, these included a heterogeneous population of patients (e.g., post-encephalitic and post-thalamotomy patients were included), did not use standardized clinical rating scales for depression and motor function, and the presence of depression was not itself an inclusion requirement. Another placebo-controlled, double-blind, cross-over design in 19 depressed PD patients reported nortriptyline was effective in treating depressive symptoms without effecting PD motor features (84). However, the rating scales employed to assess these outcomes were not specified. TCAs frequently cause side effects that are poorly tolerated by patients with PD. One of the most common side effects of TCAs is orthostatic hypotension, which is particularly problematic for PD patients because of underlying sympathetic nervous system dysfunction combined with the autonomic side effects of anti-Parkinsonian medications. TCAs also have anticholinergic side effects. Although anticholinergic effects may provide some benefit to PD motor function, they may also produce intolerable symptoms such as dry mouth, blurred vision, constipation, urinary retention, tachycardia, memory impairment, and confusion. Buproprion was another antidepressant that was studied in 20 PD patients with 12 of them being depressed (85). Although depression improved in 5 of the 12 depressed patients, this study was not, however, designed to assess the effect of the drug on depression but rather on motor function, and dosages were not specifically adjusted to treat depression. None of these trials in PD specified the type of depressive disorder present in treated subjects.

Conclusions

Not only is depression more prevalent among medically ill patients, but it also contributes significantly in the progression of those medical ills. Although the available evidence is limited, it suggests that depression concomitant with medical illness can be treated. One or more of the SSRIs have demonstrated potential usefulness in modifying depression in patients with IHD, diabetes, dementia, and Parkinson's disease, and in patients after stroke and after MI. Large-scale trials are needed to assess not only the safety and effectiveness of agents for the treatment of depression in comorbid illness, but also the treatment effects of depression on improving the comorbidities and mortalities associated with depression among the medical illness.

References

1. Murray CJ, Lopez AD, eds. The Global Burden of Disease. Cambridge: Harvard University Press; 1996.
2. Kessler RC, Berglund P, Demler O, et al. The epidemiology of major depressive disorder: results from the National Comorbidity Survey Replication (NCS-R). JAMA. 2003;289:3095–105.
3. US Department of Health and Human Services, Mental Health: A Report of the Surgeon General. Rockville: US Department of Health and Human Services, Substance Abuse and Mental Health Services Administration, Center for Mental Health Services, National Institutes of Health, National Institute of Mental Health; 1999.
4. Unutzer J, Katon W, Williams JW Jr, et al. Improving primary care for depression in late life: the design of a multicenter randomized trial. Med Care. 2001;39:785–99.
5. Kurzthaler I, Hotter A, Miller C, et al. Risk profile of SSRIs in elderly depressive patients with co-morbid physical illness. Pharmacopsychiatry. 2001;34:114–8.
6. Krishnan KR, Doraiswamy PM, Clary CM. Clinical and treatment response characteristics of late-life depression associated with vascular disease: a pooled analysis of two multicenter trials with sertraline. Prog Neuropsychopharmacol Biol Psychiatry. 2001;25:347–61.
7. Musselman DL, Betan E, Larsen H, et al. Relationship of depression to diabetes types 1 and 2: epidemiology, biology, and treatment. Biol Psychiatry. 2003;54:317–29.
8. Anderson RJ, Freedland KE, Clouse RE, et al. The prevalence of comorbid depression in adults with diabetes: a meta- analysis. Diabetes Care. 2001;24:1069–78.
9. Lustman PJ, Anderson RJ, Freedland KE, et al. Depression and poor glycemic control: a meta-analytic review of the literature. Diabetes Care. 2000;23:934–42.
10. de Groot M, Anderson R, Freedland KE, et al. Association of depression and diabetes complications: a meta-analysis. Psychosom Med. 2001;63:619–30.
11. Black SA, Markides KS, Ray LA. Depression predicts increased incidence of adverse health outcomes in older Mexican Americans with type 2 diabetes. Diabetes Care. 2003;26:2822–8.
12. Egede LE. Diabetes, major depression, and functional disability among US adults. Diabetes Care. 2004;27:421–8
13. Egede LE. Effects of depression on work loss and disability bed days in individuals with diabetes. Diabetes Care. 2004;27:1751–3.
14. Goldney RD, Phillips PJ, Fisher LJ, et al. Diabetes, depression, and quality of life: a population study. Diabetes Care. 2004;27:1066–70.
15. Ciechanowski PS, Katon WJ, Russo JE. Depression and diabetes: impact of depressive symptoms on adherence, function, and costs. Arch Intern Med. 2000;160:3278–85.
16. Lin EH, Katon W, Von Korff M, et al. Relationship of depression and diabetes self-care, medication adherence, and preventive care. Diabetes Care. 2004;27:2154–60.

17. Egede LE, Zheng D, Simpson K. Comorbid depression is associated with increased health care use and expenditures in individuals with diabetes. Diabetes Care. 2002;25:464–70.
18. Egede LE, Zheng D. Modifiable cardiovascular risk factors in adults with diabetes: prevalence and missed opportunities for physician counseling. Arch Intern Med. 2002;162:427–33.
19. Nelson KM, Reiber G, Boyko EJ. Diet and exercise among adults with type 2 diabetes: findings from the third National Health and Nutrition Examination Survey (NHANES III). Diabetes Care. 2002;25:1722–8.
20. Harris MI. Frequency of blood glucose monitoring in relation to glycemic control in patients with type 2 diabetes. Diabetes Care. 2001;24:979–82.
21. McKellar JD, Humphreys K, Piette JD. Depression increases diabetes symptoms by complicating patients' self-care adherence. Diabetes Educ. 2004;30:485–92.
22. Zhang X, Norris SL, Gregg EW, et al. Depressive symptoms and mortality among persons with and without diabetes. Am J Epidemiol. 2005;161:652–60.
23. Egede LE, Nietert PJ, Zheng D. Depression and all-cause and coronary heart disease mortality among adults with and without diabetes. Diabetes Care. 2005;28:1339–45.
24. Katon WJ, Rutter C, Simon G, et al. The association of comorbid depression with mortality in patients with type 2 diabetes. Diabetes Care. 2005;28:2668–72.
25. Goodnick PJ. Use of antidepressants in treatment of comorbid diabetes mellitus and depression as well as in diabetic neuropathy. Ann Clin Psychiatry. 2001;13:31–41.
26. Katon WJ, Von Korff M, Lin EH, et al. The Pathways Study: a randomized trial of collaborative care in patients with diabetes and depression. Arch Gen Psychiatry. 2004;61:1042–9.
27. Lustman PJ, Griffith LS, Freedland KE, et al. Cognitive behavior therapy for depression in type 2 diabetes mellitus. A randomized, controlled trial. Ann Intern Med. 1998;129:613– 21.
28. Lustman PJ, Freedland KE, Griffith LS, et al. Predicting response to cognitive behavior therapy of depression in type 2 diabetes. Gen Hosp Psychiatry. 1998;20:302–6.
29. Baker RA, Andrew MJ, Schrader G, et al. Preoperative depression and mortality in coronary artery bypass surgery: preliminary findings. ANZ J Surg. 2001;71:139–42.
30. Roose SP, Spatz E. Treating depression in patients with ischaemic heart disease. Which agents are best to use and to avoid? Drug Safety. 1999;20:459–65.
31. Cardiac Arrhythmia Suppression Trial (CAST) Investigators. Preliminary report: effect of encainide and flecainide on mortality in a randomized trial of arrhythmia suppression after myocardial infarction. N Engl J Med. 1989;321:406–12.
32. Cardiac Arrhythmia Suppression Trial (CAST) II Investigators. Effect of the antiarrhythmic agent moricizine on survival after myocardial infarction. N Engl J Med. 1992;327:227–33.
33. Roose SP, Laghrissi-Thode F, Kennedy JS, et al. Comparison of paroxetine and nortriptyline in depressed patients with ischemic heart disease. JAMA. 1998;279:287–91.
34. Nelson JC, Kennedy JS, Pollock BG, et al. Treatment of major depression with nortriptyline and paroxetine in patients with ischemic heart disease. Am J Psychiatry. 1999;156:1024–8.
35. Roose SP, Glassman AH, Attia E, et al. Cardiovascular effects of fluoxetine in depressed patients with heart disease. Am J Psychiatry. 1998;155:660–65.
36. Strik JJ, Honig A, Lousberg R, et al. Efficacy and safety of fluoxetine in the treatment of patients with major depression after first myocardial infarction: findings from a double-blind, placebo-controlled trial. Psychosom Med. 2000;62:783–9.
37. Glassman AH, O'Connor CM, Califf RM, et al. Sertraline Antidepressant Heart Attack Randomized Trial (SADHART) Group. Sertraline treatment of major depression in patients with acute MI or unstable angina. JAMA. 2002;288:701–9.
38. Lesperence F, Frasure-Smith N, Koszycki D, et al. Effects of citalopram and interpersonal psychotherapy on depression in patients with coronary artery disease: The Candaian cardiac randomized evaluation of antidepressant and psychotherapy efficacy (CREATE) trial. JAMA. 2007;297:367–79.
39. Pollock BG, Laghrissi-Thode F, Wagner WR. Evaluation of platelet activation in depressed patients with ischemic heart disease after paroxetine or nortriptyline treatment. J Clin Psychopharmacol. 2000;20:137–40.
40. Musselman DL, Marzec UM, Manatunga A, et al. Platelet reactivity in depressed patients treated with paroxetine – preliminary findings. Arch Gen Psychiatry. 2000;57:875–82.

41. Serebruany VL, Glassman AH, Malinin AI, et al. Sertraline AntiDepressant Heart Attack Randomized Trial Study Group. Platelet/endothelial biomarkers in depressed patients treated with the selective serotonin reuptake inhibitor sertraline after acute coronary events: the Sertraline Antidepressant Heart Attack Randomized Trial (SADHART) Platelet Substudy. Circulation. 2003;108:939–44.
42. Yeragani VK, Pesce V, Jayaraman A, et al. Major depression with ischemic heart disease: effects of paroxetine and nortriptyline on long-term heart rate variability measures. Biol Psychiatry. 2002;52:418–29.
43. Yeragani VK, Roose S, Mallavarapu M, et al. Major depression with ischemic heart disease: effects of paroxetine and nortriptyline on measures of nonlinearity and chaos of heart rate. Neuropsychobiology. 2002;46:125–35.
44. Rechlin T. The effects of psychopharmacological therapy on heart rate variation. Nervenarzt. 1995;66:678–85.
45. Sauer WH, Berlin JA, Kimmel SE. Selective serotonin reuptake inhibitors and myocardial infarction. Circulation. 2001;104:1894–8.
46. Berkman LF, Blumenthal J, Burg M, et al. Enhancing Recovery in Coronary Heart Disease Patients Investigators (ENRICHD). Effects of treating depression and low perceived social support on clinical events after myocardial infarction: the Enhancing Recovery in Coronary Heart Disease Patients (ENRICHD) Randomized Trial. JAMA. 2003;289:3106–16.
47. Taylor CB, Youngblood ME, Catellier D, Veith RC, Carney RM, Burg MM, Kaufmann PG, Shuster J, Mellman T, Blumenthal JA, Krishnan R, Jaffe AS, ENRICHD Investigators. Effects of antidepressant medication on morbidity and mortality in depressed patients after myocardial infarction. Arch Gen Psychiatry. 2005;62:792–8.
48. Van den Brink RHS, Van Melle JP, Honig A, et al. Treatment of depression after myocardial infarction and the effects on cardiac prognosis and quality of life: rationale and outline of the myocardial infarction and depression-intervention trial (MIND-IT). Am Heart J. 2002;144:219–25.
49. De Jonge P, Hong A, Schene AH, et al. Effects of antidepressive therapy for the treatment of depression following myocardial infarction: results from the Myocardial Infarction and Depression Intervention Trial (MIND_IT). Psychosom Med. 2006;68:A-7.
50. Serebruany VL, Gurbel PA, O'Connor CM. Platelet inhibition by sertraline and N-desmethylsertraline: a possible missing link between depression, coronary events, and mortality benefits of selective serotonin reuptake inhibitors. Pharmacol Res. 2001;43:453–62.
51. Frasure-Smith N, Lesperance F, Prince RH, et al. Randomised trial of home-based psychosocial nursing intervention for patients recovering from myocardial infarction. Lancet. 1997;350:473–9.
52. Enrichd Investigators. Enhancing Recovery in Coronary Heart Disease (ENRICHD Investigators) study intervention: rationale and design. Psychosom Med. 2001;63:747–55.
53. Franc¸ois Lespe´rance, Nancy Frasure-Smith, Diana Koszycki, Marc-Andre´ Laliberte´, Louis T. van Zyl, Brian Baker, John Robert Swenson, Kayhan Ghatavi, Beth L. Abramson, Paul Dorian, Marie-Claude Guertin, for the CREATE Investigators. Effects of Citalopram and Interpersonal Psychotherapy on Depression in Patients With Coronary Artery Disease__The Canadian Cardiac Randomized Evaluation of Antidepressant and Psychotherapy Efficacy (CREATE) Trial. JAMA. 2007;297:367–79.
54. Robinson RG. Poststroke depression: prevalence, diagnosis, treatment, and disease progression. Biol Psychiatry. 2003;54:376–87.
55. Kimura M, Robinson RG, Kosier JT. Treatment of cognitive impairment after poststroke depression: a double-blind treatment trial. Stroke. 2000;31:1482–6.
56. Sturm JW, Donnan GA, Dewey HM, et al. Determinants of handicap after stroke: the North East Melbourne Stroke Incidence Study (NEMESIS). Stroke. 2004;35:715–20.
57. House A, Knapp P, Bamford J, Vail A. Mortality at 12 and 24 months after stroke may be associated with depressive symptoms at 1 month. Stroke. 2001;32:696–701.
58. Chan KL, Campayo A, Moser DJ, Arndt S, Robinson RG. Aggressive behavior in patients with stroke: association with psychopathology and results of antidepressant treatment on aggression. Arch Phys Med Rehabil. 2006;87:793–8.

59. Dam M, Tonin P, DeBoni A, et al. Effects of fluoxetine and maprotiline on functional recovery in poststroke hemiplegic patients undergoing rehabilitation therapy. Stroke. 1996;27:1211–4.
60. Robinson RG, Schultz SK, Castillo C, et al. Nortriptyline versus fluoxetine in the treatment of depression and in short-term recovery after stroke: a placebo-controlled, double-blind study. Am J Psychiatry. 2000;157:351–9.
61. Rampello L, Chiechio S, Nicoletti G, Alvano A, Vecchio I, Raffaele R, Malaguarnera M. Prediction of the response to citalopram and reboxetine in post-stroke depressed patients. Psychopharmacology. 2004;173:73–8.
62. Almeida OP, Waterreus A, Hankey GJ. Preventing depression after stroke: results from a randomized placebo-controlled trial. J Clin Psychiatry. 2006;67:1104–9.
63. Niedermaier N, Bohrer E, Schulte K, Schlattmann P, Heuser I. Prevention and treatment of poststroke depression with mirtazapine in patients with acute stroke. J Clin Psychiatry. 2004;65:1619–23.
64. Muller U, Murai T, Bauer-Wittmund T, et al. Paroxetine versus citalopram treatment of pathological crying after brain injury. Brain Inj. 1999;13:805–11.
65. Andersen G, Vestergaard K, Riis JO. Citalopram for post-stroke pathological crying. Lancet. 1993;342:837–9.
66. Choi-Kwon S, Han SW, Kwon SU, Kang DW, Choi JM, Kim JS. Fluoxetine treatment in poststroke depression, emotional incontinence, and anger proneness: a double-blind, placebo-controlled study. Stroke. 2006;37:156–61.
67. Lyketsos CG, Sheppard JM, Steele CD, et al. Randomized, placebo-controlled, double-blind clinical trial of sertraline in the treatment of depression complicating Alzheimer's disease: initial results from the Depression in Alzheimer's Disease study. Am J Psychiatry. 2000;157:1686–89.
68. Vida S, DesRosiers P, Carrier L, et al. Prevalence of depression in Alzheimer's disease and validity or research diagnostic criteria. J Geriatr Psychiatry Neurol 1994;7:238–44.
69. Loreck DJ, Folstein MF. Depression in Alzheimer disease. In: Starkstein SE, Robinson RG editors. Depression in neurologic disease. The John Hopkins series in pyschiatry and neuroscience. Baltimore: John Hopkins University Press; 1993:50–62.
70. Bains J, Birks JS, Dening TD. Cochrane Dementia and Cognitive Improvement Group Antidepressants for treating depression in dementia Date of Most Recent Update: This version first published online: October 21. 2002; and Last assessed as up-to-date: April 27. 2005. http://www2.cochrane.org/reviews/en/ab003944.html
71. Reifler BV, Teri L, Raskind M, et al. Double-blind trial of imipramine in Alzheimer's disease patients with and without depression. Am J Psychiatry. 1989;146:45–9.
72. Taragano FE, Lyketsos CG, Mangone CA, et al. A double-blind, randomized, fixed-dose trial of fluoxetine vs. amitriptyline in the treatment of major depression complicating Alzheimer's disease. Psychosomatics. 1997;38:246–52.
73. Katona CL, Hunter BN, Bray J. A double-blind comparison of the efficacy and safely of paroxetine and imipramine in the treatment of depression with dementia. Int J Geriatr Psychiatry. 1998;13(2):100–8.
74. Lyketsos CG, Lee HB. Diagnosis and treatment of depression in Alzheimer's disease. A practical update for the clinician. Dement Geriatr Cogn Disord. 2004;17:55–64.
75. Nyth AL, Gottfries CG, Lyby K, et al. A controlled multicenter clinical study of citalopram and placebo in elderly depressed patients with and without concomitant dementia. Acta Psychiatr Scand. 1992;86:138–45.
76. Lyketsos CG, DelCampo L, Steinberg M, et al. Treating depression in Alzheimer disease: efficacy and safety of sertraline therapy, and the benefits of depression reduction: the DIADS. Arch Gen Psychiatry. 2003;60:737–46.
77. Petracca GM, Chemerinski E, Starkstein SE. A double-blind, placebo-controlled study of fluoxetine in depressed patients with Alzheimer's disease. Int Psychogeriatr. 2001;13:233–40.
78. Nyth AL, Gottfries CG. The clinical efficacy of citalopram in treatment of emotional disturbances in dementia disorders. A Nordic multicentre study. Br J Psychiatry. 1990;157:894–901.

79. Global Parkinson's Disease Survey Steering Committee. Factors impacting on quality of life in Parkinson's disease: results from an international survey. Mov Disord. 2002;17:60–7.
80. Dell'Agnello G, Ceravolo R, Nuti A, et al. SSRIs do not worsen Parkinson's disease: evidence from an open-label, prospective study. Clin Neuropharmacol. 2001;24:221–7.
81. Menza M, Marin H, Kaufman K, et al. Citalopram treatment of depression in Parkinson's disease: the impact on anxiety, disability, and cognition. J Neuropsychiatry Clin Neurosci. 2004;16:315–9.
82. Strong RR. Imipramine in treatment of parkinsonism: a double blind placebo study. Br Med J. 1965;2:33–4.
83. Laitinen L. Desipramine in treatment of Parkinson's disease. Acta Neurol Scand. 1969;45:109–13.
84. Anderson J, Aabro E, Gulmann N. Anti-depressive treatment in Parkinson's disease. A controlled trial of the effect of nortriptyline in patients with Parkinson's disease treated with l-dopa. Acta Neurol Scan. 1980;62:210–9.
85. Goetz CG, Tanner CM, Klawans HL. Buproprion in Parkinson's disease. Neurology. 1984;34:1092–4.

Index

A
Alzheimer's disease, 132
Amitriptyline
  antipsychotics, 189–190
  geriatric depression, 156–157
Anticholinergic adverse effects, 143–144
Antidepressants, clinical pharmacology
  augmentation strategiesE
    amantadine, 100
    atypical antipsychotic augmentation, 95–96
    buspirone, 96
    estrogen, 98–99
    medications combination, 94
    psychostimulants, 96–97
    testosterone, 98
    thyroid hormone, 97–98
  geriatric depression, non-MDD subtypes
    complicated grief, 160–161
    dementia, 159–160
    dysthymia and subsyndromal depression, 158–159
    insomnia, 159
    post-stroke depression, 161–162
  MAOIs
    adverse effects, 91–93
    clinical use, 90
    history, 86
    overdose, 93
    pharmacology, 87–90
  novel agents
    buproprion, 288
    mirtazapine, 287–288
    MOA-I, 288–289
    nefazadone, 287
    tetracyclic, 289
    trazadone, 287
    tricyclic, 289
  omega-3-fatty acids, 104–105
  pharmacogenetics
    cythochromes, 35
    FKBP5 receptor, 36
    P-glycoprotein, 35–36
    pharmacodynamic genetic studies, 36
    serotonin, 36–37
  pharmacokinetics and pharmacodynamics, 33–34
  S-adenosyl-L-methionine 1,4-butanedisulfonate (SAMe), 103–104
  SNRI
    duloxetine, 287
    venlafaxine, 286
  SSRIs
    adverse effects, 53–60
    atypical antipsychotic augmentation 95–96
    citalopam (*see* escitaloqpram)
    dosages, 49–50
    drug interactions/P450 metabolism, 53
    efficacy, 62–64
    FDA-approved indications, 47
    fluoxetine, 282–283
    fluvoxamine, 285
    history, 46
    mechanism of action, 50–53
    paroxetine, 283–284
    pharmacokinetic, 46–49
    pharmacology, 48
    safety, 60–62
    sertraline, 284–285
  St. John's Wort
    adverse effects, 100–101
    drug–drug interactions, 101
    efficacy, 101–103
    pharmacology, 100
  TCA
    adult doses and formulations, 67
    adverse effects, 69–72

D.A. Ciraulo and R.I. Shader (eds.), *Pharmacotherapy of Depression*,
DOI 10.1007/978-1-60327-435-7, © Springer Science+Business Media, LLC 2011

Antidepressants, clinical pharmacology (*cont.*)
antidepressants, 75–81
clinical use, 73–75
history, 64
mechanism of action, 69
mixed action antidepressants role, 83
non-SSRI antidepressant metabolites, 68
overdose, 72–73, 82–83
pharmacokinetics, 65–69
pharmacology, 64–65
without US FDA approval, 83–86
treatment
continuation therapy, 45
doses trial, 44–45
illness, prominent psychiatric symptoms, 38–42
medical conditions, 43
meta-analysis, 37–44
response and remission, 45
high-risk behaviors, 363
long-term developmental effects, 365
Antipsychotic depression
atypical
clozapine, 216–217
olanzapine, 217–218
quetiapine, 218
risperidone, 217
treatment, 188–189
vs. typical, 219
ziprasidone and aripiprazole, 218–219
efficacy, 189–191
safety, 191–192

B

Beck depression inventory scale (BDI), 401
Beck's scale, for suicide ideation, 134
Biological theories and treatments
depression cascade, 11
effects of, 1
genetic studies
antidepressants action, 2
heritability, 1–2
identical twins, 2–3
neurobiology evaluation, 3–4
neuroendocrine systems
HPA axis, 5–11
HPT axis, growth hormone and prolactin, 11–13
interaction of, 10
neuromodulators, 17–21
neurotransmitters, 13–17
physiological function alterations
appetite, 21
circardian rhythmns, 20
sleep and pain perception, 20–21
unipolar major depressive disorder, 1
Bipolar depression
antidepressant uses, 204–205
atypical antipsychotic agents
clozapine, 216–217
olanzapine, 217–218
quetiapine, 218
risperidone, 217
vs. typical, 219
ziprasidone and aripiprazole, 218–219
detection and intervention, 225–226
ECT, 223–224
implications for, 199–200
lamotrigine monotherapy, 200
long-term prevention, 223
mood stabilizers
carbamazepine, 207–208
gabapentin (pregabalin), 212–213
lamotrigine, 209–212
levetiracetam, 214–215
lithium, 206–207
oxcarbazepine, 214
tiagabine, 215–216
topiramate, 213–214
valproate, 208–209
zonisamide, 215
potential reasons, 199
psychosocial treatment, 225
reasons, 199
rTMS, 224
second generation antidepressants
bupropion, 202
mirtazepine, 2033
pramipexole, 203–204
SNRIs, 203
SSRIs, 202–203
sequential treatment
acute episode, 220–221
inositol, 222–223
omega-3-fatty acids, 222
supraphysiologic thyroid hormone augmentation, 221
VNS, 224–225
Brain-derived neurotrophic factor (BDNF), 9, 198
Breast-feeding
benefits of, 336
blood levels measurement, 337–338
CYP450 enzymes, 338

foremilk or hind milk, 336–337
milk plasma ratio (M/P), 336
neuro-behavioral impact, 338–339
relative infant dose (RID), 337
treatment, 336
Brofaromine, 89
Bupropion, 75–77, 202
Buspirone, 96

C
Calgary depression scale for schizophrenia (CDSS), 186
Carbamazepine, 207–208
Cardiac arrhythmia suppression trials (CAST), 71, 402
Cardiovascular effects, 144–145
CBT. *See* Cognitive-behavioral therapy
CDSS. *See* Calgary depression scale for schizophrenia
Clozapine, 192, 216–217
Cocaine, abuse substance
disorders, 258
dopamine and norepinephrine depletion, 258–259
fluoxetine, 259
mood stabilizing anticonvulsants, 260
selegeline, 260
venlafaxine, 259
Cochrane meta-analysis, 140
Cognitive-behavioral therapy (CBT), 359, 401
Congenital malformations
cardiac malformation, 323
cohort study, 324
first trimester period, 322
MAOIs, 324
paroxetine, 323
SSRIs, 324–325
teratogenic risk, 323
Corticotrophin releasing factor (CRF), 5–6
Corticotropin releasing hormone (CRH), 280

D
Dementia, depression treatment
neurovegetative symptoms, 407
reversible monoamine oxidase inhibitor, 408
Depression-executive dysfunction syndrome, 130
Desipramine, 189–190
Desvenlafaxine, 78
Dextroamphetamine, 97
Diabetes, depression treatment
CBT, 401
TCA, 400
Dialectical behavioral therapy (DBT), 137
Differential diagnosis, primary care management
age, sex, and race, 383
family history, genetics, 384
hopelessness, 383
impulsivity, 383
lifetime rate, 382
marital and work status, 383
past history, 384
PHQ-9 instrument, 383
protective factors, 384
weapons, 384
Dopamine (DA), 16–17

E
Electroconvulsive therapy (ECT)
geriatric depression, 162–163
schizophrenia, 189
somatic treatments, 331–332
Enhancing recovery in coronary heart disease (ENRICHD) trial, 403
Episode, 366
Escitaloqpram, 285

F
False-positive screening, 377
Fetal programming hypothesis, 319
Fluoxetine, pediatric depression
CBT, 359
double-blind placebo-controlled clinical trials, 358
Frailty, 126

G
Gabapentin (pregabalin), 212–213
Gamma-amino butyric acid (GABA), 5–6, 19
Geriatric depression
aging physiology
anticholinergic adverse effects, 143–144
cardiovascular effects, 144–145
orthostatic hypotension, 145–146
pharmacodynamics, 143
pharmacokinetics, 140–143
SIADH, 146–147

Geriatric depression (*cont.*)
antidepressants, non-MDD subtypes
complicated grief, 160–161
dementia, 159–160
dysthymia and subsyndromal depression, 158–159
post-stroke depression, 161–162
diagnosis, 128–129
electroconvulsive therapy, 162–163
epidemiology
frailty, 126
MCI, 127
pharmacological treatment, 138–140
phenomenology, 127–128
psychosocial treatments, 163
SSRIs
citalopram, 148–149
paroxetine, 151–153
sertraline, 149–151
subtypes and comorbidity
Alzheimer's disease, 132
anxiety, 136
cognitive impairment, 133
concurrent substance abuse, 135–136
depression and personality disorders, 136–137
medical illness, 137–138
psychotic depression, 134
suicidality, 134–135
vascular depression, 130–131
TCAs
amitriptyline, 156–157
clinical use, 157
imipramine, 156
nortriptyline, 154–156
Geriatric suicide ideation scale (GSIS), 134
Growth hormone, 11–13
GSIS. *See* Geriatric suicide ideation scale

H
Hamilton rating scale for depression (HRSD), 402
Hypnotics, 290–291
Hypothalamic pituitary adrenal (HPA) axis, neuroendocrine systems
anxiety and stress, 6
CRF and ACTH, 5–6
hippocampus, 8
interaction, 10
limbic-cortical-striatal-pallidal-thalamic (LCSPT) tract
interconnected brain structures, 6–7
role, 8
volume reduction evaluation, 7
neuronal plasticity and brain-derived neurotrophic factor (BDNF), 9
stress, role of, 9–11

I
Inositol, 222–223
Ischemic heart disease (IHD)
interpersonal psychotherapy (IPT), 404
mirtazapine, 403
orthostatic hypotension, 402
platelet activity reduction, 403
whole-blood platelet aggregation, 404

L
Lamotrigine
advantage, 211
monotherapy, 200
prophylactic antidepressant effects, 210
SJS and TEN, 211
Levetiracetam, 214–215
Lifetime prevalence rate, 356

M
MADRAS. *See* Montgomery-Asberg depression rating scale
Major depressive disorder (MDD), 239–240
Manic switching, 368
Medically ill patients, treatment of
antidepressants, 400
dementia
neurovegetative symptoms, 407
reversible monoamine oxidase inhibitor, 408
diabetes
CBT, 401
TCA, 400
IHD, 401–404
Parkinson's disease (PD), 408–409
PSD, 404–407
SSRIs, 400
Melantonergic agents, 86
Methylphenidate, 96–97
MHART. *See* Montreal heart attack readjustment trial
Mifepristone, 85
Mild cognitive impairment (MCI), 127
Mirtazapine, 81, 203
MOA-I. *See* Monoamine oxidase inhibitors

Moclobemide, 89
Monoamine hypothesis
  dopamine, 16–17
  norepinephrine, 15–16
  role, 13–14
  serotonin, 14–15
Monoamine oxidase inhibitors (MAOIs)
  adverse effects
    drug–drug interactions, 93
    hypertensive crises, 91–92
  clinical use, 90
  history, 86
  novel antidepressant, 288–289
  overdose, 93
  pharmacology
    classification, 87
    Emsam™, 89
    location, 87
    mechanism action, 89–90
    moclobemide and brofaromine, 89
    phenelzine, 88, 90
    RIMA, 87–88
    selegiline, 87
    tranylcypromine, 88, 90
Montgomery-Asberg depression rating scale (MADRAS), 361
Montreal heart attack readjustment trial (MHART), 404
Mood disorder questionnaire (MDQ), 382
Mood stabilizers, bipolar depression
  antidepressant trials, 256–258
  carbamazepine, 207–208
  gabapentin (pregabalin), 212–213
  lamotrigine, 209–212
  levetiracetam, 214–215
  lithium, 206–207
  oxcarbazepine, 214
  tiagabine, 215–216
  topiramate, 213–214
  valproate, 208–209
  zonisamide, 215
Mycocardial infarction depression intervention trial (MIND-IT), 403

N
National Comorbidity Survey (NCS), 240–242
National Epidemiologic Survey on Alcohol and Related Conditions (NESARC), 242
Nefazodone, 79–81, 256
Neuroendocrine systems
  HPT axis, growth hormone and prolactin, 11–13
  hypothalamic pituitary adrenal (HPA) axis
    anxiety and stress, 6
    brain-derived neurotrophic factor (BDNF), 9
    corticotrophin releasing factor (CRF), 5–6
    hippocampal neuronal cells, 8
    limbic-cortical-striatal-pallidal-thalamic (LCSPT) tract, 6–8
    stress role, 9–11
  neuromodulators
    cytokines, 17
    GABA, 19
    glutamate, 18–19
    substance P receptors, 18
  neurotransmitters
    dopamine (DA), 16–17
    monoamine hypothesis, 13–17
    norepinephrine (NE), 15–16
    serotonin, 14–15
Neuropsychiatric inventory (NPI), 132
Non-antidepressant somatic therapies
  a_1 adrenoreceptor agonists, 296
  a_2 adrenoreceptor agonists, 296
  agonists, 297
  antipsychotics, 293
  anxiolytics (*see* Hypnotics)
  aripiprazole, 295
  mood stabilizers, 291
  newer agents, 292–293
  olanzapine, 295
  older agents, 291–292
  other antipsychotics, 295–296
  prevention medication, 297–298
  quetiapine, 294
  repetitive transcranial magnetic stimulation, 298
  risperidone, 293–294
Norepinephrine (NE), 15–16
NPI. *See* Neuropsychiatric inventory

O
Obsessive-compulsive disorder (OCD), 363
OCD. *See* Obsessive-compulsive disorder
Olanzapine, 217–218
Omega-3-fatty acids (OFAs), 104–105, 222
Opiate, substance abuse
  addiction treatment, 263–264
  incidence, 261
  patient profiles, 263
  SSRIs, 262
  TCAs, 262
Orthostatic hypotension, 145–146
Oxcarbazepine, 214

P
PANSS. *See* Positive and negative syndrome scale
Parkinson's disease (PD), 408–409
Paroxetine, pediatric depression
clinical global impression-improvement (CGI-I) scale, 361
Hamilton rating scale score, 360
MADRAS, 361
serious adverse events, 360
Pediatric depression
antidepressant treatment
application, 363–365
citalopram, escitalopram, 362
fluoxetine, 358–359
paroxetine, 360–361
second-generation, 362–363
sertraline, 359–360
venlafaxine, 361
diagnosis and course
attention deficit hyperactivity disorder (ADHD), 356
bipolar II disorder, 357
DSM-IV diagnostic criteria, 356–357
dysthymic disorder, 356
epidemiology, 356
recommendations, clinical practice, 369
safety controversy
clinical practice, 368–369
FDA warning effect, 367–368
suicidal ideation and behavior, 366–367
youth suicide, antidepressants, 365–366
Peritraumatic dissociation, 276
Persistent pulmonary hypertension (PPHTN), 327
P-glycoprotein, 49
Pharmacokinetics, aging physiology
absorption, 141
bupropion, 143
distribution and excretion, 141
fluoxetine and paroxetine, 142
Phenelzine, 88
Positive and negative syndrome scale (PANSS), 294
Postpartum depression
prevalence and risk factors
challenges, 333
hormonal changes, 334
public health problem, 334
risk posed, mother and infant, 335
treatment, 335–336
Post-stroke depression (PSD)
antidepressant effects, 405
logistic regression analysis, 406
pathological crying and aggression, 407
rehabilitation, 405
Posttraumatic stress disorder (PTSD)
acute stress disorder (ASD), 275–276
disorders of extreme stress (DES), 276
epidemiology
co-morbid/co-occurring disorders, 277–279
traumatic events, 276–277
neurobiology, 279–281
non-antidepressant somatic therapies
a_1 adrenoreceptor agonists, 296
a_2 adrenoreceptor agonists, 296
agonists, 297
antipsychotics, 293
anxiolytics (*see* Hypnotics)
aripiprazole, 295
mood stabilizers, 291
newer agents, 292–293
olanzapine, 295
older agents, 291–292
other antipsychotics, 295–296
prevention medication, 297–298
quetiapine, 294
repetitive transcranial magnetic stimulation, 298
risperidone, 293–294
novel antidepressants
buproprion, 288
mirtazapine, 287–288
MOA-I, 288–289
nefazadone, 287
trazadone, 287
tricyclic, tetracyclic, 289
pharmacotherapy, 282
psychosocial treatments, 38–39
SNRI antidepressants
duloxetine, 287
venlafaxine, 286
SSRI antidepressants
citalopam (*see* escitaloqpram)
fluoxetine, 282–283
fluvoxamine, 285
paroxetine, 283–284
sertraline, 284–285
Pramipexole, 203–204
Pregnancy and lactation
adverse effects, on fetus and pregnancy outcome
cortisol stress and fetal programming, 320
course of labor, 316
fetal programming hypothesis, 319
impact, on fetal development, 317
infant, 318–319

neonate, impact on, 318
prenatal stress, 319
preterm labor/delivery, 315–316
stress and anxiety impact, 317–318
antidepressants impact, on neonate
neonatal adaptation, 326–327
non-SSRIs, 328
persistent pulmonary hypertension (PPHTN), 327
developmental risk, 329–330
electroconvulsive therapy (ECT), 331–332
factors
biopsychosocial nature, 312
environmental, 312
hormonal factors, 312
social relationships, 313
subsyndromal symptoms, 312
managing mood disorders, postpartum period
breast-feeding, 336–339
drug selection, 339–340
medication continuation guidelines, 340–341
postpartum blues and depression, 333–336
pharmacologic treatment
co-morbid disorders, 321
history of, 322
malformations risk, 322–325
medication choice, 322
preterm birth and fetal growth restriction, 325–326
spontaneous abortion risk, 325
prescribing antidepressants
dosing considerations, 331
metabolism, 330–331
risk
co-morbidity, 310
prevalence of, 310–312
transcranial magnetic stimulation (TCMS), 332–333
treatment consideration, 320–321
umbilical cord levels, 328–329
untreated depression risk
attention, 313
reduced health quality, 314
Premenstrual dysphoria, 379
Primary care, depression management
adherence and treatment outcomes, 388–389
diagnostic screening
conditions, 376
dysthymia, 377
PHQ-9(7) instruments, 378
risk factors, 378–379
somatic symptoms, 376
task force, 376
two-step process, 377
differential diagnosis
anxiety disorders, 380
bereavement, 381
bipolar disorder, 382
confirmation, 379
GAD-7, 381
hypothyroidism, 381
risk assessment, 382–385
substance abuse, 381
symptom severity assessment, 385–387
epidemiology, 375
goals, of treatment
antidepressant therapy, 392
remission attainment, 391
office nurse, 387
treatment approaches
antiplatelet aggregation effect, 390
cytochrome P450 2D6 enzyme, 390
exercise prescription, 391
psychotherapy/medication, 389
selective serotonin reuptake inhibitors (SSRIs), 390
STAR-D, 390
Prolactin, 11–13
Psychotherapeutic strategies, 387

R

Reboxetine
adverse effects, 84
efficacy, 84–85
pharmacokinetics, 83–84
Risperidone, 217

S

S-Adenosyl-L-methionine 1,4-butanedisulfonate (SAMe), 103–104
SADHART. *See* Sertraline antidepressant heart attack recovery trial
Schizophrenia
antipsychotics
atypical, 188–189
efficacy, 189–191
safety, 191–192
differential diagnosis, 187–188
electroconvulsive therapy, 189
functional consequences, 187
prevalence, 185–186

Screening risk factors
bereavement, 378
chronic illness, 379
trauma, 378
Selective serotonin reuptake inhibitors (SSRIs), 400
adverse effects
CNS, 55–56
discontinuation/withdrawal syndrome, 60
endocrine system, 57–58
gastrointestinal, 55
hematologic, 58
overview, 53–54
serotonin syndrome, 57
sexual, 58–60
suicidality, 56–57
atypical antipsychotic augmentation 95–96
bipolar depression, 202–203
citalopram, 254
dosages, 49–50
drug interactions/P450 metabolism, 53
efficacy, 62–64, 255
escitalopram, 254
FDA-approved indications, 47
fluoxetine, 253
geriatric depression
citalopram, 148–149
paroxetine, 151–153
sertraline, 149–151
history, 46
mechanism of action
clinical studies, 52
degree of selectivity, 50–51
5-HT reuptake pump, 51–52
paroxetine, 52–53
presynaptic 5-HT_{1A} role, 52
pharmacokinetics
clinical importance, 46–47
membrane transport proteins, 47–49
stereochemistry, 47
pharmacology, 48
safety
overdose, 60–61
pregnancy and lactation, 61–62
sertraline, 254
tianeptine, 253
trazodone, 255
trials of, 254–255
Selegiline (eldepryl), 87–89
Serotonin, 14–15
Serotonin norepinephrine reuptake inhibitors (SNRIs), 203
Sertraline antidepressant heart attack recovery trial (SADHART), 402
Sertraline treatment, 400
SIADH. *See* Syndrome of inappropriate antidiuretic hormone secretion
Sigma agonists, 86
SJS. *See* Stevens Johnson syndrome
SNRIs. *See* Serotonin norepinephrine reuptake inhibitors
SSRIs. *See* Selective serotonin reuptake inhibitors
Stevens Johnson syndrome (SJS), 211
St John's Wort
adverse effects, 100–101
drug–drug interactions, 101
efficacy, 101–103
pharmacology, 100
Substance abuse
clinical presentations
alcohol dependence and depression, 247–248
alcoholic hypophoria, 248
depression and acute intoxication, 247
cocaine
disorders, 258
dopamine and norepinephrine depletion, 258–259
fluoxetine, 259
mood stabilizing anticonvulsants, 260
selegeline, 260
studies, 260–261
venlafaxine, 259
co-morbid depression functional consequences, 244–24
diagnosis and clinical evaluation
adequate history, 245
dysthymia, 246
MDD *vs*. substance-induced mood disorder, 245–246
prolonged sobriety, 246–247
suicide risk evaluation, 246
major depressive disorder (MDD), 239–240
opiate
addiction treatment, 263–264
incidence, 261
patient profiles, 263
SSRIs, 262
TCAs, 262
pharmacotherapy, alcoholic
antidepressants clinical pharmacology, 248–250
mood stabilizing antidepressants, 256–258
nefazodone, 256
SSRIs, 253–255
TCAs, 250–252
prevalence and co-morbidity

depression and substance related disorders, cooccurrence of, 243–244
epidemiological catchment area (ECA) study, 240
major depressive episodes, 242–243
National Comorbidity Survey (NCS), 240–242
National Epidemiologic Survey on Alcohol and Related Conditions (NESARC), 242
psychopathology relation, 239
treatment failures, 264
Substance P (SP)-neurokinin-1 (NK1) receptor, 18, 85
Subsyndromal depression, 128
Supraphysiologic thyroid hormone augmentation, 221
Syndrome of inappropriate antidiuretic hormone secretion (SIADH), 146–147

T
TCAs. *See* Tricyclic antidepressants
TEN. *See* Toxic epidermal necrolysis
Tiagabine, 215–216
Topiramate, 213–214
Total sleep deprivation (TSD), 225
Toxic epidermal necrolysis (TEN), 211
Transcranial magnetic stimulation (TCMS), 332–333
Tranylcypromine, 88
Trazodone, 79–81
Tricyclic antidepressants (TCAs)
adult doses and formulations, 67
adverse effects
anticholinergic activity, 69–70
conduction effects, cardiovascular, 70–71
orthostatic hypotension, cardiovascular, 70
sexual dysfunction, 71–72
antidepressants
bupropion, 75–77
mirtazapine, 81
nefazodone and trazodone, 79–81
venlafaxine, 77–78
clinical use
efficacy, 73–74
gender differences, 74–75
desipramine, 252
efficacy, 250
geriatric depression
amitriptyline, 156–157
clinical use, 157
imipramine, 156
nortriptyline, 154–156
history, 64
imipramine, 252
mechanism of action, 69
mixed action antidepressants role, 83
non-SSRI antidepressant metabolites, 68
overdose, 72–73, 82–83
pharmacokinetics, 65–69
pharmacology, 64–65
studies, 252–253
without US FDA approval
melantonergic agents, 86
mifepristone, 85
reboxetine, 83–85
sigma agonists, 86
substance P, 85
TSD. *See* Total sleep deprivation

U
Unified Parkinson's disease rating scale, 409

V
Vagal nerve stimulation (VNS), 221
Valproate, 208–209
Venlafaxine, 77–78
VNS. *See* Vagal nerve stimulation

Z
Zonisamide, 215

CPSIA information can be obtained at www.ICGtesting.com
Printed in the USA
LVOW01*1101150614

390115LV00010B/350/P

9 781603 274340